For Reference

Not to be taken from this room

The GALE
ENCYCLOPEDIA *of*
NEUROLOGICAL
DISORDERS

The GALE
ENCYCLOPEDIA *of*
NEUROLOGICAL
DISORDERS

VOLUME

1

A - L

STACEY L. CHAMBERLIN, BRIGHAM NARINS, EDITORS

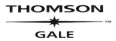

THOMSON

GALE

Detroit • New York • San Francisco • San Diego • New Haven, Conn. • Waterville, Maine • London • Munich

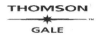

The Gale Encyclopedia of Neurological Disorders

Project Editors
Stacey L. Chamberlin, Brigham Narins

Editorial
Erin Watts

Editorial Support Services
Andrea Lopeman

Indexing Services
Synapse

Rights Acquisitions Management
Margaret Chamberlain, Jackie Jones, Shalice Shah-Caldwell

Imaging and Multimedia
Randy Basset, Lezlie Light, Dan Newell, Robyn V. Young

Product Design
Michelle DiMercurio, Tracey Rowens, Kate Scheible

Composition and Electronic Prepress
Evi Seoud, Mary Beth Trimper

Manufacturing
Wendy Blurton, Dorothy Maki

LIBRARY OF CONGRESS CATALOGING-IN-PUBLICATION DATA

The Gale encyclopedia of neurological disorders / Stacey L. Chamberlin, Brigham Narins, editors.
        p.   ; cm.
   Includes bibliographical references and index.
   ISBN 0-7876-9150-X (set hardcover : alk. paper) — ISBN
0-7876-9151-8 (v. 1) — ISBN
0-7876-9152-6 (v. 2)
   1. Neurology—Encyclopedias.
   [DNLM: 1. Nervous System Diseases—Encyclopedias—English. 2. Nervous System Diseases—Popular Works. WL 13 G151 2005] I. Title: Encyclopedia of neurological disorders. II. Chamberlin, Stacey L. III. Narins, Brigham, 1962– IV. Gale Group.

RC334.G34 2005
616.8'003—dc22   2004021644

This title is also available as an e-book.
ISBN 0-7876-9160-7 (set)
Contact your Gale sales representative for ordering information.

Printed in Canada
10 9 8 7 6 5 4 3 2 1

CONTENTS

List of Entries vii

Introduction xiii

Advisory Board...xv

Contributors xvii

Entries

    Volume 1: A–L..1

    Volume 2: M–Z...**511**

Glossary 941

General Index..973

LIST OF ENTRIES

A

Abulia
Acetazolamide
Acupuncture
Acute disseminated encephalomyelitis
Adrenoleukodystrophy
Affective disorders
Agenesis of the corpus callosum
Agnosia
AIDS
Alcohol-related neurological disease
Alexander disease
Alpers' disease
Alternating hemiplegia
Alzheimer disease
Amantadine
Amnestic disorders
Amyotrophic lateral sclerosis
Anatomical nomenclature
Anencephaly
Aneurysms
Angelman syndrome
Angiography
Anosmia
Anticholinergics
Anticonvulsants
Antiepileptic drugs
Antimigraine medications
Antiparkinson drugs
Antiviral drugs
Anxiolytics
Aphasia
Apraxia
Arachnoid cysts
Arachnoiditis
Arnold-Chiari malformation
Arteriovenous malformations
Aspartame
Asperger's disorder
Assistive mobile devices
Ataxia-telangiectasia
Ataxia
Atomoxetine
Attention deficit hyperactivity
    disorder
Autism
Autonomic dysfunction

B

Back pain
Bassen-Kornzweig syndrome
Batten disease
Behçet disease
Bell's palsy
Benign positional vertigo
Benzodiazepines
Beriberi
Binswanger disease
Biopsy
Blepharospasm
Bodywork therapies
Botulinum toxin
Botulism
Brachial plexus injuries
Brain anatomy
Brain and spinal tumors
Brown-Séquard syndrome

C

Canavan disease
Carbamazepine
Carotid endarterectomy
Carotid stenosis
Carpal tunnel syndrome
Catechol-O-methyltransferase
    inhibitors
Central cord syndrome
Central nervous system
Central nervous system stimulants
Central pain syndrome
Cerebellum
Cerebral angiitis
Cerebral cavernous malformation
Cerebral circulation
Cerebral dominance
Cerebral hematoma
Cerebral palsy
Channelopathies
Charcot-Marie-Tooth disorder
Cholinergic stimulants
Cholinesterase inhibitors
Chorea

Chronic inflammatory demyelinating
    polyneuropathy
Clinical trials
Congenital myasthenia
Congenital myopathies
Corpus callosotomy
Corticobasal degeneration
Craniosynostosis
Craniotomy
Creutzfeldt-Jakob disease
CT scan
Cushing syndrome
Cytomegalic inclusion body disease

D

Dandy-Walker syndrome
Deep brain stimulation
Delirium
Dementia
Depression
Dermatomyositis
Devic syndrome
Diabetic neuropathy disease
Diadochokinetic rate
Diazepam
Dichloralphenazone
Dichloralphenazone, Isometheptene,
    and Acetaminophen
Diencephalon
Diet and nutrition
Disc herniation
Dizziness
Dopamine receptor agonists
Dysarthria
Dysesthesias
Dysgeusia
Dyskinesia
Dyslexia
Dyspraxia
Dystonia

E

Electric personal assistive mobility
    devices

List of Entries

Electroencephalography
Electromyography
Empty sella syndrome
Encephalitis and Meningitis
Encephalitis lethargica
Encephaloceles
Encephalopathy
Endovascular embolization
Epidural hematoma
Epilepsy
Exercise

F

Fabry disease
Facial synkinesis
Fainting
Fatigue
Febrile seizures
Felbamate
Fisher syndrome
Foot drop
Fourth nerve palsy
Friedreich ataxia

G

Gabapentin
Gaucher disease
Gene therapy
Gerstmann-Straussler-Scheinker disease
Gerstmann syndrome
Glossopharyngeal neuralgia
Glucocorticoids
Guillain-Barré syndrome

H

Hallucination
Headache
Hearing disorders
Hemianopsia
Hemifacial spasm
Hereditary spastic paraplegia
Holoprosencephaly
HTLV-1 Associated Myelopathy
Huntington disease
Hydantoins
Hydranencephaly
Hydrocephalus
Hydromyelia
Hypersomnia
Hypotonia
Hypoxia

I

Idiopathic neuropathy

Inclusion body myositis
Incontinentia pigmenti
Infantile spasms
Inflammatory myopathy
Interferons

J

Joubert syndrome

K

Kennedy's disease
Klippel Feil syndrome
Krabbe disease
Kuru

L

Lambert-Eaton myasthenic syndrome
Laminectomy
Lamotrigine
Learning disorders
Lee Silverman voice treatment
Leigh disease
Lennox-Gastaut syndrome
Lesch-Nyhan syndrome
Leukodystrophy
Levetiracetam
Lewy body dementia
Lidocaine patch
Lissencephaly
Locked-in syndrome
Lupus
Lyme disease

M

Machado-Joseph disease
Magnetic resonance imaging (MRI)
Megalencephaly
Melodic intonation therapy
Ménière's disease
Meninges
Mental retardation
Meralgia paresthetica
Metachromatic leukodystrophy
Microcephaly
Mitochondrial myopathies
Modafinil
Moebius syndrome
Monomelic amyotrophy
Motor neuron diseases
Movement disorders
Moyamoya disease
Mucopolysaccharidoses
Multi-infarct dementia
Multifocal motor neuropathy

Multiple sclerosis
Multiple system atrophy
Muscular dystrophy
Myasthenia, congenital
Myasthenia gravis
Myoclonus
Myofibrillar myopathy
Myopathy
Myotonic dystrophy

N

Narcolepsy
Nerve compression
Nerve conduction study
Neurofibromatosis
Neuroleptic malignant syndrome
Neurologist
Neuromuscular blockers
Neuronal migration disorders
Neuropathologist
Neuropsychological testing
Neuropsychologist
Neurosarcoidosis
Neurotransmitters
Niemann-Pick Disease

O

Occipital neuralgia
Olivopontocerebellar atrophy
Opsoclonus myoclonus
Organic voice tremor
Orthostatic hypotension
Oxazolindinediones

P

Pain
Pallidotomy
Pantothenate kinase-associated
    neurodegeneration
Paramyotonia congenita
Paraneoplastic syndromes
Parkinson's disease
Paroxysmal hemicrania
Parsonage-Turner syndrome
Perineural cysts
Periodic paralysis
Peripheral nervous system
Peripheral neuropathy
Periventricular leukomalacia
Phantom limb
Pharmacotherapy
Phenobarbital
Pick disease
Pinched nerve
Piriformis syndrome
Plexopathies
Poliomyelitis

Polymyositis
Pompe disease
Porencephaly
Positron emission tomography (PET)
Post-polio Syndrome
Primary lateral sclerosis
Primidone
Prion diseases
Progressive multifocal
    leukoencephalopathy
Progressive supranuclear palsy
Pseudobulbar palsy
Pseudotumor cerebri

R

Radiation
Radiculopathy
Ramsay-Hunt syndrome type II
Rasmussen's encephalitis
Reflex sympathetic dystrophy
Refsum disease
Repetitive motion disorders
Respite
Restless legs syndrome
Rett syndrome
Reye syndrome

S

Sandhoff disease
Schilder's disease
Schizencephaly
Schizophrenia
Sciatic neuropathy
Sciatica
Seizures
Septo-optic dysplasia
Shaken baby syndrome
Shingles
Single Proton Emission Computed
    Tomography

Sixth nerve palsy
Sjogren-Larsson Syndrome
Sleep apnea
Social workers
Sodium oxybate
Sotos syndrome
Spasticity
Speech synthesizer
Spina bifida
Spinal cord infarction
Spinal cord injury
Spinal muscular atrophy
Spinocerebellar ataxia
Status epilepticus
Stiff person syndrome
Striatonigral degeneration
Stroke
Sturge-Weber syndrome
Stuttering
Subacute sclerosing panencephalitis
Subdural hematoma
Succinamides
Swallowing disorders
Sydenham's chorea
Syringomyelia

T

Tabes dorsalis
Tay-Sachs disease
Temporal arteritis
Temporal lobe epilepsy
Tethered spinal cord syndrome
Third nerve palsy
Thoracic outlet syndrome
Thyrotoxic myopathy
Tiagabine
Todd's paralysis
Topiramate
Tourette syndrome
Transient global amnesia
Transient ischemic attack
Transverse myelitis
Traumatic brain injury

Tremors
Trigeminal neuralgia
Tropical spastic paraparesis
Tuberous sclerosis

U

Ulnar neuropathy
Ultrasonography

V

Valproic acid and divalproex
    sodium
Vasculitic neuropathy
Vasculitis
Ventilatory assistance devices
Ventricular shunt
Ventricular system
Vertebrobasilar disease
Vestibular schwannoma
Visual disturbances
Vitamin/nutritional deficiency
Von Hippel-Lindau disease

W

Wallenberg syndrome
West Nile virus infection
Whiplash
Whipple's Disease
Williams syndrome
Wilson disease

Z

Zellweger syndrome
Zonisamide

PLEASE READ—IMPORTANT INFORMATION

The Gale Encyclopedia of Neurological Disorders is a medical reference product designed to inform and educate readers about a wide variety of diseases, syndromes, drugs, treatments, therapies, and diagnostic equipment. Thomson Gale believes the product to be comprehensive, but not necessarily definitive. It is intended to supplement, not replace, consultation with a physician or other healthcare practitioner. While Thomson Gale has made substantial efforts to provide information that is accurate, comprehensive, and up-to-date, Thomson Gale makes no representations or warranties of any kind, including without limitation, warranties of merchantability or fitness for a particular purpose, nor does it guarantee the accuracy, comprehensiveness, or timeliness of the information contained in this product. Readers are advised to seek professional diagnosis and treatment for any medical condition, and to discuss information obtained from this book with their healthcare providers.

INTRODUCTION

The Gale Encyclopedia of Neurological Disorders (GEND) is a one-stop source for medical information that covers diseases, syndromes, drugs, treatments, therapies, and diagnostic equipment. It keeps medical jargon to a minimum, making it easier for the layperson to use. The Gale Encyclopedia of Neurological Disorders presents authoritative and balanced information and is more comprehensive than single-volume family medical guides.

SCOPE

Almost 400 full-length articles are included in The Gale Encyclopedia of Neurological Disorders. Articles follow a standardized format that provides information at a glance. Rubrics include:

Diseases

- Definition
- Description
- Demographics
- Causes and symptoms
- Diagnosis
- Treatment team
- Treatment
- Recovery and rehabilitation
- Clinical trials
- Prognosis
- Special concerns
- Resources
- Key terms

Drugs

- Definition
- Purpose
- Description
- Recommended dosage
- Precautions
- Side effects
- Interactions
- Resources
- Key terms

Treatments

- Definition
- Purpose
- Precautions
- Description
- Preparation
- Aftercare
- Risks
- Normal results
- Resources
- Key terms

INCLUSION CRITERIA

A preliminary topic list was compiled from a wide variety of sources, including professional medical guides, consumer guides, and textbooks and encyclopedias. The advisory board, made up of seven medical and healthcare experts, evaluated the topics and made suggestions for inclusion. Final selection of topics to include was made by the medical advisors in conjunction with Gale editors.

ABOUT THE CONTRIBUTORS

The essays were compiled by experienced medical writers, physicians, nurses, and pharmacists. GEND medical advisors reviewed most of the completed essays to insure that they are appropriate, up-to-date, and medically accurate.

HOW TO USE THIS BOOK

The *Gale Encyclopedia of Neurological Disorders* has been designed with ready reference in mind:

• Straight **alphabetical arrangement** allows users to locate information quickly.

• Bold faced terms function as print hyperlinks that point the reader to full-length entries in the encyclopedia.

• A list of **key terms** is provided where appropriate to define unfamiliar words or concepts used within the context of the essay.

• **Cross-references** placed throughout the encyclopedia direct readers to where information on subjects without their own entries can be found. Cross-references are also used to assist readers looking for information on diseases that are now known by other names; for example, there is a cross-reference for the rare childhood disease commonly known as Hallervorden-Spatz disease that points to the entry entitled Pantothenate kinase-associated neurodegeneration.

• A **Resources** section directs users to sources of further information, which include books, periodicals, websites, and organizations.

• A **glossary** is included to help readers understand unfamiliar terms.

• A comprehensive **general index** allows users to easily target detailed aspects of any topic.

GRAPHICS

The Gale Encyclopedia of Neurological Disorders is enhanced with over 100 images, including photos, tables, and customized line drawings.

ADVISORY BOARD

An advisory board made up of prominent individuals from the medical and healthcare communities provided invaluable assistance in the formulation of this encyclopedia. They defined the scope of coverage and reviewed individual entries for accuracy and accessibility; in some cases they contributed entries themselves. We would therefore like to express our great appreciation to them:

CONTRIBUTORS

Lisa Maria Andres, MS, CGC
Certified Genetic Counselor and Medical Writer
San Jose, CA

Paul Arthur
Science writer
London, England

Bruno Verbeno Azevedo
Espirito Santo University
Vitória, Brazil

Deepti Babu, MS, CGC
Genetic Counselor
Marshfield Clinic
Marshfield, WI

Laurie Barclay, MD
Neurologist and writer
Tampa, FL

Julia Barrett
Science Writer
Madison, WI

Danielle Barry, MS
Graduate Assisstant
Center of Alcohol Studies
Rutgers University
Piscataway, NJ

Maria Basile, PhD
Medical Writer
Roselle, NJ

Tanja Bekhuis, PhD
Science Writer and Psychologist
TCB Research
Boalsburg, PA

Juli M. Berwald, PhD
Geologist (Ocean Sciences)
Chicago, Illinois

Robert G. Best, PhD
Director
Division of Genetics
University of South Carolina School of Medicine
Columbia, SC

Michelle Lee Brandt
Medical Writer
San Francisco, CA

Dawn J. Cardeiro, MS, CGC
Genetic Counselor
Fairfield, PA

Francisco de Paula Careta
Espirito Santo University
Vitória, Brazil

Rosalyn Carson-DeWitt, MD
Physician and Medical Writer
Durham, NC

Stacey L. Chamberlin
Science Writer and Editor
Fairfax, VA

Bryan Richard Cobb, PhD
Institute for Molecular and Human Genetics
Georgetown University
Washington, D.C.

Adam J. Cohen, MD
Craniofacial Surgery, Eyelid and Facial Plastic Surgery, Neuro-Ophthalmology
Downers Grove, IL

Tish Davidson, AM
Medical Writer
Fremont, CA

James Paul Dworkin, PhD
Professor
Department of Otolaryngology, Voice/Speech Pathology Program and Laboratory
Wayne State University
Detroit, MI

L. Fleming Fallon, Jr., MD, DrPH
Professor
Department of Public Health
Bowling Green State University
Bowling Green, OH

Antonio Farina, MD, PhD
Department of Embryology, Obstetrics, and Gynecology
University of Bologna
Bologna, Italy

Kevin Fitzgerald
Science Writer and Journalist
South Windsor, CT

Paula Anne Ford-Martin
Medical Writer
Warwick, RI

Lisa A. Fratt
Medical Writer
Ashland, WI

Rebecca J. Frey, PhD
Freelance Medical Writer
New Haven, CT

Sandra L. Friedrich, MA
Science Writer
Clinical Psychology
Chicago, IL

Sandra Galeotti, MS
Science Writer
Sao Paulo, Brazil

Larry Gilman, PhD
*Electrical Engineer and Science
    Writer*
Sharon, VT

Laith Farid Gulli, MD
Consulting Psychotherapist
Lathrup Village, MI

**Stephen John Hage, AAAS,
    RT(R), FAHRA**
Medical Writer
Chatsworth, CA

Brook Ellen Hall, PhD
Science Writer
Loomis, CA

Dan Harvey
Medical Writer
Wilmington, DE

Hannah M. Hoag, MSc
Science and Medical Writer
Montreal, Canada

Brian Douglas Hoyle, PhD
Microbiologist
Nova Scotia, Canada

Cindy L. Hunter, CGC
Genetic Counselor
Medical Genetics Department
Indiana University School of
    Medicine
Indianapolis, IN

Alexander I. Ioffe, PhD
Senior Scientist
Geological Institute of the Russian
    Academy of Sciences
Moscow, Russia

Holly Ann Ishmael, MS, CGC
Genetic Counselor
The Children's Mercy Hospital
Kansas City, MO

Joel C. Kahane, PhD
*Professor, Director of the
    Anatomical Sciences
    Laboratory*
The School of Audiology and
    Speech-Language Pathology
The University of Memphis
Memphis, TN

Kelly Karpa, PhD, RPh
Assistant Professor
Department of Pharmacology
Pennsylvania State University
    College of Medicine
Hershey, PA

Karen M. Krajewski, MS, CGC
*Genetic Counselor, Assistant
    Professor of Neurology*
Wayne State University
Detroit, MI

Judy Leaver, MA
*Behavioral Health Writer and
    Consultant*
Washington, D.C.

Adrienne Wilmoth Lerner
University of Tennessee College of
    Law
Knoxville, TN

Brenda Wilmoth Lerner, RN
Nurse, Writer, and Editor
London, UK

K. Lee Lerner
Fellow (rt)
Science Policy Institute
London, UK

**Agnieszka Maria Lichanska,
    PhD**
Department of Microbiology and
    Parasitology
University of Queensland
Brisbane, Australia

Peter T. Lin, MD
Research Assistant
Member: American Academy of
    Neurology, American
    Association of Electrodiagnostic
    Medicine
Department of Biomagnetic
    Imaging
University of California, San
    Francisco
Foster City, CA

**Iuri Drumond Louro, MD,
    PhD**
Adjunct Professor
Human and Molecular Genetics
Espirito Santo University
Vitória, Brazil

Nicole Mallory, MS, PA-C
Medical Student
Wayne State University
Detroit, MI

Igor Medica, MD, PhD
Assistant Professor
School of Medicine
University of Rijeka
Pula, Croatia

Michael Mooney, MA, CAC
Consultant Psychotherapist
Warren, MI

**Alfredo Mori, MD, FACEM,
    FFAEM**
Emergency Physician
The Alfred Hospital
Victoria, Australia
Oxford's Program in Evidence-
    Based Health Care
University of Oxford
Oxford, England

Marcos do Carmo Oyama
Espirito Santo University
Vitória, Brazil

Greiciane Gaburro Paneto
Espirito Santo University
Vitória, Brazil

Borut Peterlin, MD, PhD
*Neurologist; Consultant Clinical
    Geneticist; Director*
Division of Medical Genetics
University Medical Center
Lubiana, Slovenia

Toni I. Pollin, MS, CGC
Research Analyst
Division of Endocrinology,
    Diabetes, and Nutrition
University of Maryland School of
    Medicine
Baltimore, MD

J. Ricker Polsdorfer, MD
Medical Writer
Phoenix, AZ

Scott J. Polzin, MS, CGC
Medical Writer
Buffalo Grove, IL

Jack Raber, PharmD
Principal
Clinipharm Services
Seal Beach, CA

Robert Ramirez, DO
Medical Student
University of Medicine and
    Dentistry of New Jersey
Stratford, NJ

Richard Robinson
Medical Writer
Tucson, AZ

Jennifer Ann Roggenbuck, MS, CGC
Genetic Counselor
Hennepin County Medical Center
Minneapolis, MN

Nancy Ross-Flanigan
Science Writer
Belleville, MI

Stephanie Dionne Sherk
Freelance Medical Writer
University of Michigan
Ann Arbor, MI

Lee Alan Shratter, MD
Consulting Radiologist
Kentfield, CA

Genevieve T. Slomski, PhD
Medical Writer
New Britain, CT

Amie Stanley, MS
Genetic Counselor
Medical Genetics
The Cleveland Clinic
Cleveland, OH

Constance K. Stein, PhD
*Director of Cytogenetics, Assistant
    Director of Molecular
    Diagnostics*
SUNY Upstate Medical University
Syracuse, NY

Roger E. Stevenson, MD
*Senior Clinical Geneticist, Senior
    Clinical Laboratory Geneticist*
Greenwood Genetic Center
Greenwood, SC

Roy Sucholeiki, MD
*Professor, Director of the
    Comprehensive Epilepsy
    Program*
Department of Neurology
Loyola University Health System
Chicago, IL

Kevin M. Sweet, MS, CGC
Cancer Genetic Counselor
James Cancer Hospital, Ohio State
    University
Columbus, OH

David Tulloch
Science Writer
Wellington, New Zealand

Carol A. Turkington
Medical Writer
Lancaster, PA

Samuel D. Uretsky, PharmD
Medical Writer
Wantagh, NY

**Chitra Venkatasubramanian,
    MBBS, MD (internal
    medicine)**
Resident in Neurology
Department of Neurology and
    Neurosciences
Stanford University
Stanford, CA.

Bruno Marcos Verbeno
Espirito Santo University
Vitória, Brazil

Beatriz Alves Vianna
Espirito Santo University
Vitória, Brazil

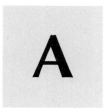

A

Abetalipoproteinemia *see* **Bassen-Kornzweig syndrome**

▌Abulia

Definition

Abulia is a state in which an individual seems to have lost will or motivation.

Description

Abulia is not a separate condition; rather, it is a symptom associated with various forms of brain injury. It may occur in association with a variety of conditions, including **stroke**, brain tumor, traumatic brain damage, bleeding into the brain, and exposure to toxic substances.

Causes and symptoms

Some research suggests that abulia occurs due to malfunction of the brain's dopamine-dependent circuitry. Injuries to the frontal lobe (the area of the brain responsible for higher thinking) and/or the basal ganglia (the area of the brain responsible for movement) can interfere with an individual's ability to initiate speech, movement, and social interaction. Abulia has been noted in patients who have suffered brain injuries due to stroke, bleeding into the brain from a ruptured aneurysm, trauma, brain tumor, neurological disease (such as **Parkinson's disease**), psychiatric condition (such as severe **depression** or **schizophrenia**), and exposure to toxic substances (such as cyclosporin-A).

An individual with abulia may not appear to have much will or motivation to pursue activities or initiate conversation. Such an individual may appear apathetic, disinterested, asocial, quiet or mute, physically slowed or still (hypokinetic), and emotionally remote.

Diagnosis

Abulia is not an individual diagnosis; it is a symptom that usually occurs as part of a constellation of symptoms accompanying a specific disorder. Diagnosis of the underlying disorder depends on the kinds of symptoms that co-exist with abulia. Psychiatric interview, **magnetic resonance imaging (MRI)**, ultrasound, or computed tomography (**CT**) imaging of the brain, EEG, blood tests, and neurological testing may all be used to diagnose an underlying condition.

Treatment team

Treatment of abulia is usually part of a program of general rehabilitation for the symptoms accompanying the underlying condition. A **neurologist** or psychiatrist may lead a treatment team. Other professionals that may be involved include physical therapists, occupational therapists, recreational therapists, and speech and language therapists.

Treatment

There are no specific treatments for abulia. The underlying condition should be treated such as administering antidepressants or electroconvulsive therapy to depressed patients or antipsychotic medications to schizophrenic patients. Patients who have suffered brain injury due to stroke, bleeding, or trauma will benefit from rehabilitation programs that provide stimulation and attempt to re-teach skills.

Research has looked at the possibility of treating abulia with medications that boost the activity of dopamine throughout the brain, but this is far from becoming a standard treatment.

Prognosis

The prognosis of abulia depends on the prognosis of the underlying condition.

Resources

BOOKS

Friedman, Joseph H. "Mood, Emotion, and Thought." In *Textbook of Clinical Neurology*, edited by Christopher G. Goetz. Philadelphia: W. B. Saunders Company, 2003.

PERIODICALS

Al-Adawi, Samir. "Abulia: The Pathology of 'Will' and Dopaminergic Dysfunction in Brain-Injured Patients." *Medical Sciences* 1 (1999): 27–40.

Nishie, M. "Posterior Encephalopathy Subsequent to Cyclosporin A Presenting as Irreversible Abulia." *Internal Medicine* 42, no. 8 (1 August 2003): 750–755.

Pantoni, L. "Abulia and Cognitive Impairment in Two Patients with Capsular Genu Infarct." *Acta Neurologica Scandinavia* 104, no. 3 (1 September 2001): 185–190.

Vijayaraghavan. "Abulia: A Delphi Survey of British Neurologists and Psychiatrists." *Movement Disorders* 17, no. 5 (September 2002): 1052–1057.

Rosalyn Carson-DeWitt, MD

Acanthocytosis *see* **Bassen-Kornzweig syndrome**

Acetazolamide

Definition

Acetazolamide (a-set-a-ZOLE-a-mide) is a carbonic anhydrase inhibitor. Carbonic anhydrase is an enzyme that shifts the rate of reaction to favor the conversion of carbon dioxide and water into carbonic acid, bicarbonate ions, and free protons. Carbonic anhydrase activity is key to the regulation of pH and fluid balance in many different reactions throughout the body.

Fluid buildup can alter the shape of the eye and cause pressure on the optic nerve. Clinically, this condition is described as glaucoma. Inhibition of the enzymatic work of carbonic anhydrase activity (e.g., through the action of a carbonic anhydrase inhibitor) can lower fluid pressure in the eye.

Purpose

Acetazolamide is used to treat a number of disorders, including the control of epileptic **seizures** in those individuals who suffer **epilepsy**.

Acetazolamide is also used to treat non-neurological disorders such as glaucoma (acetazolamide decreases pressure in the eye), and to reduce the symptoms of edema (an excess storage of water by the body that leads to localized swelling or puffiness) and altitude sickness.

Description

Acetazolamide is prescription medication and is available only with a licensed physician's prescription. Acetazolamide is available in oral form in extended release capsules and tablets. Acetazolamide can also be administered by injection.

Recommended dosage

For both adults and children the recommended dosage for use in epilepsy cases is based upon actual body weight. In all cases, the exact dosage is determined by an experienced physician and/or pharmacist. In the most common cases, the normal recommended dosage is 4.5 mg per pound of body weight (10 mg per kg of body weight) and is administered in multiple (divided) doses delivered in the form of tablets or capsules.

Doses must be taken on a regular schedule but individuals should not double dose to make up for a missed dose.

When used to control anticonvulsive seizures, acetazolamide doses should not be stopped all at once. In most cases, physicians usually curtail (gradually lower) the dose an individual takes over time.

Precautions

As with most prescription medicines, acetazolamide should stored in a safe place—away from the reach of children. Acetazolamide should also be stored in a dry area away from excessive heat or light. Outdated medicine (medicines past their expiration date) should be discarded in a container that is safe from the reach of children.

Women who are pregnant, plan to become pregnant, or who are breast-feeding infants should inform their physician of this fact before taking acetazolamide.

Side effects

Unwanted side effects while taking acetazolamide include drowsiness, **fatigue**, or a dizzy lightheaded feeling. Individuals who experience these side effects should not

Key Terms

Carbonic anhydrase An enzyme that shifts the rate of reaction to favor the conversion of carbon dioxide and water into carbonic acid, bicarbonate ions, and free protons.

Optic nerve The bundle of nerve fibers that carry visual messages from the retina to the brain.

operate machinery or drive while experiencing these symptoms. Other common side effects include shortness of breath.

Acetazolamide can also lead to excessive depletion (loss) of potassium from the body. To counter this potential loss, many physicians recommend that patients eat food or drink beverages such as orange juice to replace lost potassium. The loss of potassium does not occur in every case, however, and high levels of potassium can also be dangerous. Individuals who show signs of potassium loss—including, but not limited to, dryness of mouth, increased thirst, or muscle cramps—should alert their physician. Because diet can impact a number of health factors, individuals should only alter their diet after consulting their physician.

Individuals who are diabetic and who take acetazolamide may experience elevated sugar levels in their urine and blood.

Individuals who experience changes in their vision should also consult their physician.

In some rare cases, individuals may suffer **depression**, pains in the area of the kidneys, and bloody or black tarry stools.

Interactions

Physicians and pharmacists are trained to evaluate the potential for adverse interactions by prescription drugs with other drugs. In the case of acetazolamide physicians evaluate potential adverse reactions with a range of drugs that include—but are not limited to—amphetamines, over-the-counter aspirins, cyclosporine, mood altering drugs (e.g., lithium), drugs used to control mental depression, drugs used to control irregular heartbeats, digoxin, diuretics (also known as water pills), and vitamins.

Resources

PERIODICALS

Varadkar S., J. S. Duncan, and H. Cross. "Acetazolamide and Autosomal Dominant Nocturnal Frontal Lobe Epilepsy." *Epilepsia* 44 (July 2003): 986.

OTHER

Medline Plus. U.S. National Library of Medicine and the National Institutes of Health. <http://www.nlm.nih.gov/medlineplus/druginfo/uspdi/202114.html> (May 9, 2004).

ORGANIZATIONS

National Eye Institute. 2020 Vision Place, Bethesda, MD 20892-3655. (301) 496-5248. <http://www.nei.nih.gov/>.

Paul Arthur

Acupuncture

Definition

Acupuncture, one of the main forms of therapy in traditional Chinese medicine (TCM), has been practiced for at least 2,500 years. In acupuncture, certain points on the body are stimulated by the insertion of fine needles. Unlike the hollow hypodermic needles used in mainstream medicine to give injections or to draw blood, acupuncture needles are solid. The points can be needled between 15° and 90° relative to the skin's surface, depending on treatment.

Acupuncture is thought to restore health by removing energy imbalances and blockages in the body. Practitioners of TCM believe that there is a vital force or energy called *qi* (pronounced "chee") that flows through the body and between the skin surface and the internal organs, along channels or pathways called meridians. There are 12 major and eight minor meridians. *Qi* regulates the spiritual, emotional, mental, and physical harmony of the body by keeping the forces of yin and yang in balance. Yang is a principle of heat, activity, brightness, outwardness, while yin represents coldness, passivity, darkness, interiority, etc. TCM does not try to eliminate either yin or yang, but rather keep them in harmonious balance. Acupuncture may be used to raise or lower the level of yin or yang in a specific part of the body in order to restore the energy balance.

Acupuncture was virtually unknown in the United States prior to President Richard Nixon's trip to China in 1972. A reporter for the *New York Times* named James Reston wrote a story for the newspaper about the doctors in Beijing who used acupuncture to relieve his **pain** following abdominal surgery. By 1993, Americans were making 12 million visits per year to acupuncturists, and spending $500 million annually on acupuncture treatments. By 1995, there were an estimated 10,000 certified acupuncturists practicing in the United States; as of 2000, there were 20,000. About a third of the credentialed acupuncturists in the United States as of 2002 are MDs.

Acupuncture's record of success has stimulated a number of research projects investigating its mechanisms

Key Terms

Cardiac tamponade A condition in which blood leaking into the membrane surrounding the heart puts pressure on the heart muscle, preventing complete filling of the heart's chambers and normal heartbeat.

Electroacupuncture A variation of acupuncture in which the practitioner stimulates the traditional acupuncture points electronically.

Endorphins A group of peptide compounds released by the body in response to stress or traumatic injury. Endorphins react with opiate receptors in the brain to reduce or relieve pain.

Hyperemesis gravidarum Uncontrollable nausea and vomiting associated with pregnancy. Acupuncture appears to be an effective treatment for women with this condition.

Meridians In traditional Chinese medicine, a network of pathways or channels that convey *qi* (also sometimes spelled "ki"), or vital energy, through the body.

Moxibustion A technique in traditional Chinese medicine that involves burning a "Moxa," or cone of dried wormwood leaves, close to the skin to relieve pain. When used with acupuncture, the cone is placed on top of the needle at an acupuncture point and burned.

Neurotransmitter A chemical in the brain that transmits messages between neurons, or nerve cells.

Opioids Substances that reduce pain and may induce sleep. Some opioids are endogenous, which means that they are produced within the human body. Other opioids are produced by plants or formulated synthetically in the laboratory.

Pneumothorax A condition in which air or gas is present in the chest cavity.

Qi The Chinese term for energy, life force, or vital force.

Yin and yang In traditional Chinese medicine and philosophy, a pair of opposing forces whose harmonious balance in the body is necessary to good health.

---

as well as its efficacy. Research has been funded not only by the National Center for Complementary and Alternative Medicine (NCCAM), but also by the National Institute on Alcohol Abuse and Alcoholism (NIAAA), the National Institute of Dental Research, the National Institute of Neurological Disorders and Stroke (NINDS), and the National Institute on Drug Abuse. In 1997, a consensus panel of the National Institutes of Health (NIH) presented a report in which it described acupuncture as a sufficiently promising form of treatment to merit further study. In 2000, the British Medical Association (BMA) recommended that acupuncture should be made more readily available through the National Health Service (NHS), and that family doctors should be trained in some of its techniques.

Purpose

The purpose of acupuncture in TCM is the rebalancing of opposing energy forces in different parts of the body. In Western terms, acupuncture is used most commonly as an adjunctive treatment for the relief of chronic or acute pain. In the United States, acupuncture is most widely used to treat pain associated with musculoskeletal disorders, but it has also been used in the treatment of headaches, other painful disorders, and nausea and vomiting. In addition to these disorders, acupuncture has been used to treat a variety of disorders such as asthma, infertility, **depression**, anxiety, HIV infection, and fibromyalgia, although its efficacy in relieving these disorders is largely unproven. Acupuncture should not be used to treat traumatic injuries and other emergency conditions requiring immediate surgery. Also, while it appears to have benefits in relieving symptoms such as pain under the proper circumstances, it has not been shown to alter the underlying course of a disease.

The exact mechanism by which acupuncture works is not known. Studies have demonstrated a variety of physiologic effects such as release in the brain of various chemicals and hormones, alteration of immune function, blood pressure, and body temperature.

Precautions

The risk of infection in acupuncture is minimal if the acupuncturist uses sterile disposable needles. In the United States, the Food and Drug Administration (FDA) mandates the use of sterilized needles made from nontoxic materials. The needles must be clearly labeled as having their use restricted to qualified practitioners.

Patients should also inquire about the practitioner's credentials. People who would prefer to be treated by an MD or an osteopath can obtain a list of licensed physicians

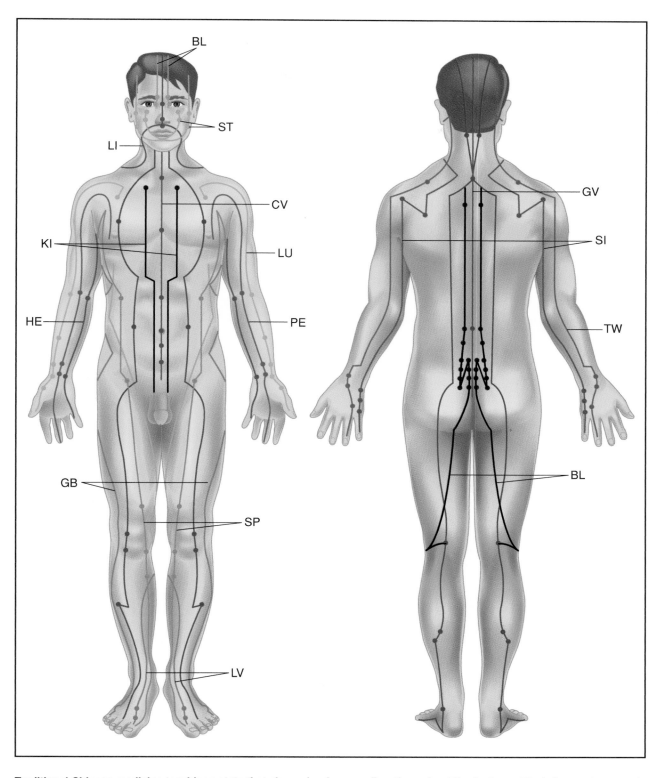

Traditional Chinese medicine teachings state that channels of energy flow throughout the body, and that disease is caused by too much or too little flow of energy along these channels. Points along the channels, called meridians, are manipulated in acupuncture. In the illustration, points are shown on the bladder (BL), conception vessel (CV), gallbladder (GB), governing vessel (GV), heart (HE), kidney (KI), large intestine (LI), liver (LV), lung (LU), pericardium (PE), small intestine (SI), spleen (SP), and stomach (ST), and triple warmer (TW) meridians. *(Illustration by Electronic Illustrators Group.)*

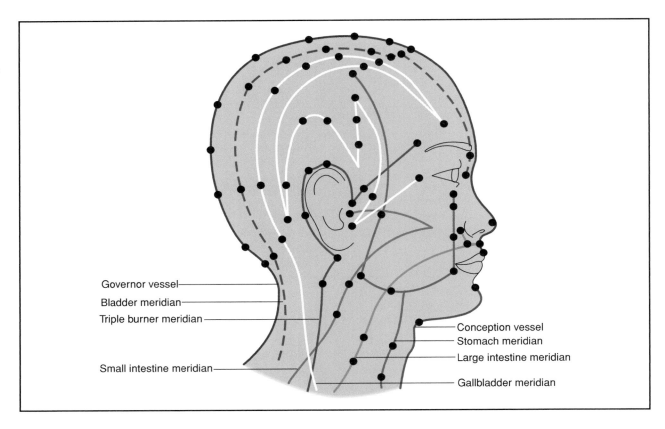

Governor vessel
Bladder meridian
Triple burner meridian

Small intestine meridian

Conception vessel
Stomach meridian
Large intestine meridian
Gallbladder meridian

Acupuncture sites and meridians on the face and neck. *(Illustration by Hans & Cassady, Inc.)*

who practice acupuncture in their area from the American Academy of Medical Acupuncture. With regard to non-physician acupuncturists, 31 states have established training standards that acupuncturists must meet in order to be licensed in those states. In Great Britain, practitioners must qualify by passing a course offered by the British Acupuncture Accreditation Board.

People seeking acupuncture treatment should provide the practitioner with the same information about their health conditions and other forms of treatment that they would give their primary care doctor.

As is true with other forms of medical treatment, a minority of patients do not respond to acupuncture. The reasons for nonresponsiveness are not known at the present stage of research.

Description

In traditional Chinese practice, the needles are twirled or rotated as they are inserted. Many patients feel nothing at all during this procedure, while others experience a prickling or aching sensation, and still others a feeling of warmth or heaviness.

The practitioner may combine acupuncture with moxibustion to increase the effectiveness of the treatment. Moxibustion is a technique in which the acupuncturist lights a small piece of wormwood, called a moxa, above the acupuncture point above the skin. When the patient begins to feel the warmth from the burning herb, it is removed. Cupping is another technique that is a method of stimulation of acupuncture points by applying suction through a metal, wood, or glass jar, and in which a partial vacuum has been created. Cupping produces blood congestion at the site, and the site is thus stimulated.

In addition to the traditional Chinese techniques of acupuncture, the following are also used in the United States:

• Electroacupuncture. In this form of acupuncture, the traditional acupuncture points are stimulated by an electronic device instead of a needle.

• Japanese meridian acupuncture. Japanese acupuncture uses thinner, smaller needles, and focuses on the meridians rather than on specific points along their course.

• Korean hand acupuncture. Traditional Korean medicine regards the hand as a "map" of the entire body, such that any part of the body can be treated by stimulating the corresponding point on the hand.

• Western medical acupuncture. Western physicians trained in this style of acupuncture insert needles into so-called trigger points in sore muscles, as well as into the traditional points used in Chinese medicine.

• Ear acupuncture. This technique regards the ear as having acupuncture points that correspond to other parts of the body. Ear acupuncture is often used to treat substance abuse and chronic pain syndromes.

A standard acupuncture treatment takes between 45 minutes to an hour and costs between $40 and $100, although initial appointments often cost more. Chronic conditions usually require 10 treatment sessions, but acute conditions or minor illnesses may require only one or two visits. Follow-up visits are often scheduled for patients with chronic pain. As of 2000, about 70–80% of health insurers in the United States reimbursed patients for acupuncture treatments.

Preparation

Apart from a medical history and physical examination, no specific preparation is required for an acupuncture treatment. In addition to using sterile needles, licensed acupuncturists will wipe the skin over each acupuncture point with an antiseptic solution before inserting the needle.

Aftercare

No particular aftercare is required, as the needles should not draw blood when properly inserted. Many patients experience a feeling of relaxation or even a pleasant drowsiness after the treatment. Some patients report feeling energized.

Risks

Most complications from acupuncture fall into one of three categories: infections, most often from improperly sterilized needles; bruising or minor soft tissue injury; and injuries to muscle tissue. Rarely, serious side effects from improper application of the needle may result in pneumothorax and cardiac tamponade.

Normal results

Normal results from acupuncture are relief of pain and/or improvement of the condition being treated.

Abnormal results

Abnormal results from acupuncture include infection, a severe side effect, or worsening of the condition being treated.

Resources

BOOKS

Pelletier, Kenneth R., MD. "Acupuncture: From the Yellow Emperor to Magnetic Resonance Imaging (MRI)." Chapter 5 in *The Best Alternative Medicine.* New York: Simon and Schuster, 2002.

Reid, Daniel P. *Chinese Herbal Medicine.* Boston, MA: Shambhala, 1993.

Svoboda, Robert, and Arnie Lade. *Tao and Dharma: Chinese Medicine and Ayurveda.* Twin Lakes, WI: Lotus Press, 1995.

PERIODICALS

Cerrato, Paul L. "New Studies on Acupuncture and Emesis (Acupuncture for Relief of Nausea and Vomiting Caused by Chemotherapy)." *Contemporary OB/GYN* 46 (April 2001): 749.

Kemper, Kathi J., et al. "On Pins and Needles—Pediatric Pain: Patients' Experience with Acupuncture." *Pediatrics* 105 (April 2000): 620–633.

Kirchgatterer, Andreas. "Cardiac Tamponade Following Acupuncture." *Chest* 117 (May 2000): 1510–1511.

Nwabudike, Lawrence C., and Constantin Ionescu-Tirgoviste. "Acupuncture in the Treatment of Diabetic Peripheral Neuropathy." *Diabetes* 49 (May 2000): 628.

Silvert, Mark. "Acupuncture Wins BMA Approval (British Medical Association)." *British Medical Journal* 321 (July 1, 2000): 637–639.

Vickers, Andrew. "Acupuncture (ABC of Complementary Medicine)." *British Medical Journal* 319 (October 9, 1999): 704–708.

ORGANIZATIONS

American Academy of Medical Acupuncture/Medical Acupuncture Research Organization. 5820 Wilshire Boulevard, Suite 500, Los Angeles, CA 90036. (800) 521-2262 or (323) 937-5514; Fax: (323) 937-0959. (May 9, 2004.) <http://www.medical acupuncture.org>.

American Association of Oriental Medicine. 433 Front Street, Catasaqua, PA 18032. (610) 266-1433; Fax: (610) 264-2768. (May 9, 2004.) <http://www.aaom. org>.

National Center for Complementary and Alternative Medicine (NCCAM) Clearinghouse. P.O. Box 7923, Gaithersburg, MD 20898. (888) 644-6226; TTY: (866) 464-3615; Fax: (866) 464-3616. (May 9, 2004.) <http://www.nccam. nih.gov>.

Rebecca Frey, PhD
Rosalyn Carson-DeWitt, MD

Acute disseminated encephalomyelitis

Definition

Acute disseminated encephalomyelitis (ADE) is a neurological disorder involving inflammation of the brain and spinal cord. A hallmark of the disorder is damage to the myelin sheath that surrounds the nerve fibers in the brain, which results in the inflammation.

Description

Acute disseminating encephalomyelitis was first described in the mid-eighteenth century. The English physician who first described the disorder noted its association with people who had recently recovered from smallpox. Symptoms often develop without warning. As well, mental disorientation can occur. The disorder is also known as postinfectious encephalomyelitis and immune-mediated encephalomyelitis. The nerve demyelination that occurs in ADE also occurs in **multiple sclerosis**. However, the two maladies differ in that multiple sclerosis is long lasting and can recur over time, while ADE has a monophasic course, meaning that once it is over, further attacks rarely occur.

Demographics

ADE can occur in both children and adults, although it occurs more commonly in children. ADE is not rare, accounting for approximately 30% of all cases of encephalitis (brain inflammation).

Causes and symptoms

Acute disseminating encephalomyelitis can occur as a consequence of a bacterial or viral infection (including HIV), following recovery from infection with the malarial protozoan, or as a side effect of vaccination or another inoculation. ADE is usually a consequence of a viral illness, and occurs most often after measles, followed by rubella, chicken pox, Epstein-Barr, mumps and pertussis (whooping cough). Typically, symptoms appear two to three weeks after the precipitating infection or immunization. Alternatively, ADE may develop with no known associations.

Despite the different causes, the symptoms that develop are similar. A number of non-specific symptoms, which vary from one person to another, include **headache**, stiff neck, fever, vomiting, and weight loss. These symptoms are quickly followed by lethargic behavior, **seizures**, hallucinations, sight difficulties, and even coma. Paralysis can occur in an arm or leg (monoparesis) or along an entire side of the body (hemiplegia).

These symptoms can last a few weeks to a month. In some people, symptoms can progress from the appearance of symptoms to coma and death in only a few days. Brain damage is largely confined to the white matter. Microscopic examination will typically reveal invasion of white blood cells into small veins. The nerve myelin damage occurs in the regions where the white blood cells accumulate. Examination of the brains of patients who have died of the disorder has not yielded consistent results. Some brains appear normal, while others display the nerve damage and white blood cell congestion.

Diagnosis

Diagnosis is made based on the above symptoms and the patient's medical history (i.e., recent infection or vaccination). In the early stages of the disorder, diagnosis can be confused with diseases including acute meningitis, acute viral encephalitis, and multiple sclerosis. Often, the latter can be ruled out using **magnetic resonance imaging (MRI)** and examination of the cerebrospinal fluid (CSF). Typically, in acute disseminating encephalomyelitis, CSF contains abnormally elevated levels of white blood cells and protein; and magnetic resonance imaging can reveal brain alterations.

Treatment team

The treatment team typically consists of a primary care physician and, when hospitalization is necessary, nurses and specialized medical care personnel.

Treatment

Corticosteroid medication is often prescribed in order to lessen the nerve inflammation. Use of high doses of steroids can often produce a rapid diminishing of the symptoms. Other kinds of treatment depend on the nature of the symptoms that develop. Supportive care includes keeping a patient comfortable and hydrated.

Key Terms

Encephalitis Inflammation of the brain, usually caused by a virus. The inflammation may interfere with normal brain function and cause seizures, sleepiness, confusion, personality changes, weakness in one or more parts of the body, and even coma.

Myelin A fatty sheath surrounding nerves throughout the body that helps them conduct impulses more quickly.

Recovery and rehabilitation

Persons recovering from acute disseminated encephalomyelitis need time to recover their normal consciousness and movements. Problems with memory, especially short-term memory, may be present. The recovering person sometimes has trouble controlling their emotions and is easily frustrated. Frequent periods of rest, alternating with shorter periods of mental and physical **exercise** are prescribed during initial recovery. The maximum possible recovery of brain and motor function may take a period of weeks or months.

Clinical trials

There are no **clinical trials** for the study of ADE recruiting patients or being planned in the United States, as of January 2004. However, organizations such as the National Institute for Neurological Disorders and Stroke undertake and fund studies on disorders that involve damage to the myelin sheath of nerve cells. By understanding the nature of the disorders, it is hoped that detection can be improved and strategies will evolve to prevent or reverse the nerve damage.

Prognosis

Prognosis varies from person to person. Some patients may recover fully, with no residual effects. Others may have some residual damage. Seldomly, ADE is fatal. Early detection and treatment improves a patient's outlook.

Special concerns

Although the incidence of ADE occurring after vaccination is rare, in recent years, public debate has led some parents to choose that their children not receive the recommended childhood vaccinations. The American Academy of Pediatrics asserts that, despite concerns about vaccine safety, vaccination is far safer than accepting the risks for the diseases that the vaccines prevent.

Resources

BOOKS

Icon Health Publications. *The Official Patient's Sourcebook on Acute Disseminated Encephalomyelitis: A Revised and Updated Directory for the Internet Age.* San Diego: Icon Group International, 2002.

PERIODICALS

Anlar, B., C. Basaran, G. Kose, A. Guven, S. Haspolat, A. Yakut, A. Serdaroglu, N. Senbil, H. Tan, E. Karaagaoglu, and K. Oguz. "Acute disseminated encephalomyelitis in children: outcome and prognosis." *Neuropediatrics* (August 2003): 194–199.

Brass, S. D., Z. Caramanos, C. Santos, M. E. Dilenge, Y. Lapierre, and B. Rosenblatt. "Multiple sclerosis vs acute disseminated encephalomyelitis in childhood." *Pediatric Neurology* (September 2003): 227–231.

Koibuchi, T., T. Nakamura, T. Miura, T. Endo, H. Nakamura, T. Takahashi, H. S. Kim, Y. Wataya, K. Washizaki, K. Yoshikawa, and A. Iwamoto. "Acute disseminated encephalomyelitis following Plasmodium vivax malaria." *Journal of Infection and Chemotherapy* (September 2003): 254–256.

Narciso, P., S. Galgani, B. Del Grosso, M. De Marco, A. De Santis, P. Balestra, V. Ciapparoni, and V. Tozzi. "Acute disseminated encephalomyelitis as manifestation of primary HIV infection." *Neurology* (November 2001): 1493–1496.

OTHER

"Acute Disseminated Encephalomyelitis Information Page." National Institute of Neurological Disorders and Stroke. <http://www.ninds.nih.gov/health_and_medical/disorders/acute_encephalomyelitis_doc.htm> (January 26, 2004).

ORGANIZATIONS

National Institute for Neurological Diseases and Stroke (NINDS). 6001 Executive Boulevard, Bethesda, MD 20892. (301) 496-5751 or (800) 352-9424. <http://www.ninds.nih.gov>.

National Organization for Rare Disorders. 55 Kenosia Avenue, Danbury, CT 06813-1968. (203) 744-0100 or (800) 999-6673; Fax: (203) 798-2291. <http://www.rarediseases.org>.

Brian Douglas Hoyle, PhD

ADHD *see* **Attention deficit hyperactivity disorder**

Adrenoleukodystrophy

Definition

Adrenoleukodystrophy (ALD) is a progressive condition that affects both the adrenal glands (located atop the kidneys and responsible for the production of adrenalin) and myelin (the substance that insulates the nerves in the brain, spinal cord, and the limbs).

Description

First described in the early 1900s, adrenoleukodystrophy was originally called Schilder-Addision disease. "Adreno" refers to the adrenal glands, "leuko" is the Greek word for white (myelin is the main component of the white matter in the brain and spinal cord), and "dystrophy" means impaired growth. This disease affects the adrenal glands and the growth of the myelin.

Key Terms

Adrenal insufficiency Problems with the adrenal glands that can be life threatening if not treated. Symptoms include sluggishness, weakness, weight loss, vomiting, darkening of the skin, and mental changes.

Central nervous system (CNS) The CNS is composed of the brain, the cranial nerves, and the spinal cord. It is responsible for the coordination and control of all body activities.

Leukodystrophy A disease that affects the white matter called myelin in the CNS.

Myelin A fatty sheath surrounding nerves in the peripheral nervous system that helps them conduct impulses more quickly.

Peroxisomes Tiny structures in the cells that break down fats so that the body can use them.

Very long chain fatty acid (VLCFA) A type of fat that is normally broken down by the peroxisomes into other fats that can be used by the body.

Types of ALD

There are three types of ALD, each with a different severity of symptoms and age of onset of ALD. All varying degrees of severity have been seen within the same family. Therefore, a family who has many mildly affected members could still have a more severely affected member. Some patients do not fall neatly into one of the three categories, and instead fall somewhere in between. Each type is given a different name, although all have mutations (changes in the genetic code) in the same gene and the same type of inheritance.

The most severe form of ALD is called childhood ALD. About 35% of people with ALD have this type. These children usually have normal development in the first few years of life. Symptoms typically begin between four and eight years of age. Very rarely is the onset before the age of three or after the age of 15. In some boys, the first symptom may be **seizures**. Other children become hyperactive and have behavioral problems that may initially be diagnosed as **attention deficit/hyperactivity disorder** (**ADHD**). Early signs may also include poor school performance due to impaired vision that is not correctable by eyeglasses. Although these symptoms may last for a few months, other more severe problems develop. These include increasing problems with schoolwork and deterioration in handwriting and speech. Affected children usually develop clumsiness, difficulty in reading and comprehension of written material, aggressive or uninhibited

behavior, and various personality and behavioral changes. Most affected boys have problems with their adrenal glands by the time their first symptoms are noticed.

A milder form of ALD, called adrenomyeloneuropathy (AMN), usually has a symptom onset at the age of 20 or later. Approximately 40–45% of people with ALD have AMN. The first symptoms are typically a progressive stiffness and weakness in the legs. Problems with urination and sexual function may also develop. Symptoms slowly progress over many years. Less than 20% of men with AMN will develop significant brain involvement that leads to cognitive and behavioral problems that are severe and may cause a shortened lifespan. About 70% of men with AMN will have problems with their adrenal glands when other symptoms are initially noticed.

A third type of ALD is called Addison disease and affects about 10% of all of those with ALD. In this condition, people do not have the neurologic symptoms associated with ALD and AMN, but they do have problems resulting from adrenal insufficiency. Symptoms typically begin between two years of age and adulthood. The first symptoms are often vomiting, weakness, or coma. People with Addison disease may or may not have darker skin. Many who are initially diagnosed with Addison disease will later develop symptoms of AMN.

In female carriers of ADL, about 20% will develop mild to moderate progressive stiffness and weakness in the legs and sometimes problems with urination. Rarely do they develop adrenal insufficiency. Symptoms in women generally do not begin before middle age.

Demographics

ALD is found in all ethnic groups. About one in every 100,000 people suffers from ALD. Because the most severe form, called classic ALD, is X-linked, many more males than females are affected. Women are carriers of this X-linked form of the disease and may exhibit no or only mild symptoms. Another form of the disease is called neonatal ALD; this form of ALD is not X-linked and therefore both male and female babies exhibit symptoms. An adult-onset type of the disease is commonly called adrenomyeloneuropathy.

Causes and symptoms

ALD causes problems in the peroxisomes, tiny cellular structures that are involved in breaking down large molecules of fats into smaller ones that can be used by the body. In ALD, the peroxisomes cannot break down a type of fat called very long chain fatty acid (VLCFA). As a result, VLCFAs accumulate throughout the body, particularly in the brain and adrenal glands. This accumulation interferes with the adrenal glands' conversion of cholesterol into steroids, and prompts deterioration of the myelin covering nerve cells within the white matter of the brain, thus interfering with nerve function. Additionally, fats that are usually made from the breakdown products of VLCFAs cannot be produced. Because these fats would usually be utilized in the synthesis of myelin, nerve function is further compromised.

The adrenal glands of almost all individuals affected with ALD do not secret a sufficient amount of hormones; this is called adrenal insufficiency. Symptoms include sluggishness, weakness, weight loss, hypoglycemia, nausea, vomiting, darkening of the skin color, and mental changes. Because adrenal insufficiency can cause problems with regulating the balance of sodium and potassium in the body, a person can go into shock and coma, which can be potentially life threatening. As this aspect of ALD is readily treatable, identifying these patients helps prevent these complications.

Diagnosis

When the diagnosis of ALD is suspected, the results of a test called **magnetic resonance imaging (MRI)** are sometimes abnormal. In this test, pictures of the brain are taken. In people with symptoms of ALD, there are usually detectable changes in the white matter. While an MRI can be helpful in making the diagnosis of ALD, a normal MRI does not exclude the diagnosis and an abnormal MRI does not definitively make the diagnosis of ALD.

A more definitive diagnosis of ALD can be made by measuring the level of the VLCFA in the blood. In nearly all males with ALD, the level of the VLCFA in blood is very high.

When ALD is suspected, testing should also be performed to measure the adrenal function. In 90% of boys with symptoms of ALD and 70% of men with AMN, the adrenal glands are affected.

Approximately 85% of female carriers will have higher than normal levels of VLCFA in their blood. However, 15–20% of female carriers will have normal levels of VLCFA in their blood, which gives a "false negative" result. If a woman wants to be certain about her carrier status, genetic testing to look for a specific mutation in the ALD gene can be performed. Before a woman could have testing to determine her carrier status, a mutation in the ALD gene must have already been found in an affected member of the family.

Treatment team

A number of professionals can provide supportive (though not curative) care for patients with adrenoleukodystrophy: neurogeneticists, to help with diagnosis; pediatric or adult neurologists (depending on the type of ALD and age of onset) to monitor and manage the neurological effects; pediatric or adult endocrinologists to manage the adrenal complications; and pediatric or adult urologists to manage bladder complications in both children and adults and sexual problems in adults. In addition, physical therapists, occupational therapists, speech therapists, learning specialists, and behavioral psychologists may be helpful.

Treatment

When the diagnosis of ALD is made, an important first step is to measure the level of adrenal function. If there is adrenal insufficiency, treatment should be given by steroid replacement, which can prove to be lifesaving. Adrenal function should be tested periodically.

Lorenzo's oil

In the early 1990s, a film called *Lorenzo's Oil* presented a fictionalized account of a real ALD patient, a young boy named Lorenzo, and his family's search to find a cure for him. A possible treatment was found and was named Lorenzo's oil. The Lorenzo's oil therapy worked to reduce the level of VLCFA in the blood. The idea was that if the level of VLCFA could be reduced, perhaps it would cure or help the symptoms. After a number of years of use, Lorenzo's oil unfortunately does not seem to be an effective treatment, at least in those with advanced signs and symptoms. Although it does reduce the level of VLCFA in blood, it does not seem to alter a person's symptoms.

Bone marrow transplant

One promising treatment is bone marrow transplant. However, this is a potentially dangerous procedure that has a 10–20% rate of death. As of early 2001, information is available on a limited number of patients. In the very small number of patients who have had a bone marrow transplant, a few had their condition stabilize and a few even made slight improvements. However, all of these people had the bone marrow transplant at an early stage of their disease. This treatment does have drawbacks, including the fact that there are limited numbers of donors who are a suitable match and a significant risk that complications will develop from the transplant. Early data suggests that bone marrow transplant is most effective when it is performed at an early stage of the disease when neurological abnormalities are mild. Additional long-term studies are necessary to determine the overall success of these procedures.

Other treatments

Research is being done with other treatments such as lovastatin and 4-phenylbutyrate, both of which may help lower VLCFA levels in cells, but more work is necessary to determine their effectiveness. **Gene therapy**, a possible method of treatment, works by replacing, changing, or supplementing non-working genes. Although different gene therapy methods are being tested on animals, they are not ready for human trials.

Other types of therapy and supportive care are of benefit to both affected boys and their families. Physical therapy can help reduce stiffness and occupational therapy can help make the home more accessible. Support from psychologists and other families who have been or are in a similar situation can be invaluable. Many men with AMN lead successful personal and professional lives and can benefit from vocational counseling and physical and occupational therapy.

Prenatal diagnosis

Prenatal testing to determine whether an unborn child is affected is possible if a specific ALD mutation has been identified in a family. This testing can be performed at 10–12 weeks gestation by a procedure called chorionic villus sampling (CVS), which involves removing a tiny piece of the placenta and examining the cells. It can also be done by amniocentesis after 14 weeks gestation by removing a small amount of the amniotic fluid surrounding the fetus and analyzing the cells in the fluid. Each of these procedures has a small risk of miscarriage associated with it. Couples interested in these options should have genetic counseling to carefully explore all of the benefits and limitations of these procedures.

An experimental procedure, called preimplantation diagnosis, allows a couple to have a child that is unaffected with the genetic condition. This procedure is only possible for those families in which a mutation in the ALD gene has been identified.

Clinical Trials

A number of **clinical trials** are underway, including testing the efficacy of Lorenzo's oil (combination glyceryl trierucate and glyceryl trioleate), oral bile acid therapy with cholic acid, chenodeoxycholic acid, and ursodeoxycholic acid, and bone marrow or umbilical cord blood transplantation.

Prognosis

The prognosis for people with ALD is highly variable. Those diagnosed with childhood ALD usually have a very rapid course. Symptoms typically progress very fast and these children usually become completely incapacitated and die within three to five years of the onset of symptoms.

The symptoms of AMN progress slowly over decades. Most affected individuals have a normal lifespan.

Resources

PERIODICALS

Laan, L. A. E. M., et al. "Childhood-onset Cerebral X-linked Adrenoleukodystrophy." *The Lancet* 356 (November 4, 2000): 1608–1609.

Moser, H. W., L. Bezman, S. E. Lu, and G. V. Raymond. "Therapy of X-linked Adrenoleukodystrophy: Prognosis Based Upon Age and MRI Abnormality and Plans for Placebo-controlled Trials." *Journal of Inherited Metabolic Disease* 23 (2000): 273–277.

Moser, H. W. "Treatment of X-linked Adrenoleukodystrophy with Lorenzo's Oil." *Journal of Neurology, Neurosurgery and Psychiatry* 67, no. 3 (September 1999): 279–280.

Shapiro, E., et al. "Long-term Effect of Bone Marrow Transplantation for Childhood-onset Cerebral X-linked Adrenoleukodystrophy." *The Lancet* 356, no. 9231 (August 26, 2000): 713–718.

Suzuki, Y., et al. "Bone Marrow Transplantation for the Treatment of X-linked Adrenoleukodystrophy." *Journal of Inherited Metabolic Disease* 23, no. 5 (July 2000): 453–458.

Unterrainer, G., B. Molzer, S. Forss-Petter, and J. Berger. "Co-expression of Mutated and Normal Adrenoleukodystrophy Protein Reduces Protein Function: Implications for Gene Therapy of X-linked Adrenoleukodystrophy." *Human Molecular Genetics* 9, no. 18 (2000): 2609–2616.

Van Geel, B. M., et al, on behalf of the Dutch X-ALD/AMN Study Group. "Progression of Abnormalities in Adrenomyeloneuropathy and Neurologically Asymptomatic X-linked Adrenoleukodystrophy Despite Treatment with 'Lorenzo's Oil.'" *Journal of Neurology, Neurosurgery and Psychiatry* 67, no. 3 (September 1999): 290–299.

Verrips, A., M. A. A. P. Willemsen, E. Rubio-Gozalbo, J. De Jong, and J. A. M. Smeitink. "Simvastatin and Plasma Very Long Chain Fatty Acids in X-linked Adrenoleukodystrophy." *Annals of Neurology* 47, no. 4 (April 2000): 552–553.

ORGANIZATIONS

National Organization for Rare Disorders (NORD). PO Box 8923, New Fairfield, CT 06812-8923. (203) 746-6518 or (800) 999-6673; Fax: (203) 746-6481. (May 9, 2004.) <http://www.rarediseases.org>.

United Leukodystrophy Foundation. 2304 Highland Dr., Sycamore, IL 60178. (815) 895-3211 or (800) 728-5483; Fax: (815) 895-2432. (May 9, 2004.) <http://www.ulf.org>.

WEBSITES

"Entry 300100: Adrenoleukodystrophy, (ALD)." *OMIM— Online Mendelian Inheritance in Man.* (May 9, 2004.) <http://www.ncbi.nlm.nih.gov/htbin-post/Omim/dispmim?300100>.

Moser, Hugo W., Anne B. Moser, and Corinne D. Boehm. "X-linked Adrenoleukodystrophy." March 9, 1999 (May 9, 2004). University of Washington, Seattle. *GeneClinics.*

<http://www.geneclinics.org/profiles/
x-ald/>.

Karen M. Krajewski, MS, CGC
Rosalyn Carson-DeWitt, MD

Affective disorders

Definition

Affective disorders are psychiatric diseases with multiple aspects, including biological, behavioral, social, and psychological factors. Major depressive disorder, bipolar disorders, and anxiety disorders are the most common affective disorders. The effects of these disorders—such as difficulties in interpersonal relationships and an increased susceptibility to substance abuse—are major concerns for parents, teachers, physicians, and the community. Affective disorders can result in symptoms ranging from the mild and inconvenient to the severe and life-threatening; the latter account for more than 15% of deaths due to suicide among those with one of the disorders.

Major depressive disorder (MDD), also known as monopolar **depression** or unipolar affective disorder, is a common, severe, and sometimes life-threatening psychiatric illness. MDD causes prolonged periods of emotional, mental, and physical exhaustion, with a considerable risk of self-destructive behavior and suicide. Major studies have identified MDD as one of the leading causes of work disability and premature death, representing an increasingly worldwide health and economic concern.

Bipolar affective diseases are divided into various types according to the symptoms displayed: Type I (bipolar I, or BPI) and Type II (bipolar II or BPII) disease, cyclothymic disorder, and hypomania disorder. Other names for bipolar affective disease include manic-depressive disorder, cyclothymia, manic-depressive illness (MDI), and bipolar disorder. People with bipolar diseases experience periods of manic (hyper-excitable) episodes alternating with periods of deep depression. Bipolar disorders are chronic and recurrent affective diseases that may have degrees of severity, tending however to worsen with time if not treated. Severe crises can lead to suicidal attempts during depressive episodes or to physical violence against oneself or others during manic episodes. In many patients, however, episodes are mild and infrequent. Mixed states may also occur with elements of mania and depression simultaneously present. Some people with bipolar affective disorders show a rapid cycling between manic and depressive states.

Anxiety disorders are also common psychiatric disorders, and are considered one of the most under-treated

Key Terms

Anxiety disorder A psychiatric disorder involving the presence of anxiety that is so intense or so frequently present that it causes difficulty or distress for the individual.

Bipolar disorder A psychiatric disorder marked by alternating episodes of mania and depression. Also called bipolar illness, manic-depressive illness.

Depressive disorder A psychiatric disorder of varying degrees characterized by feelings of hopelessness, physical responses such as insomnia, and withdrawal from normal activities.

Dysthymia A chronic mood disorder characterized by mild depression.

Manic A period of excess mental activity, often accompanied by elevated mood and disorganized behavior.

Phobia A persistent abnormal fear of an object, experience, or place.

and overlooked health problems. Among its common manifestations are panic syndromes, phobias, chronic generalized anxiety disorder, obsessive-compulsive disorder, and post-traumatic disorder. Anxiety disorders are important contributors to other diseases such as hypertension, digestive and eating disorders, and cardiac arrhythmia. Severe anxiety disorders often lead to tobacco addiction, alcohol abuse, and drug abuse.

Description

People with major depressive disorder (MDD) experience periods of at least two weeks of symptoms that often include sadness, emotional heaviness, feelings of worthlessness, hopelessness, guilt, anguish, fear, loss of interest for normal daily activities, social withdrawal, inability to feel pleasure, physical apathy, difficulty in concentrating, and recurrent thoughts about death. Changes in sleeping pattern, with insomnia during the night and **hypersomnia** (excessive sleep) during the day, chronic **fatigue**, and a feeling of being physically drained and immobile may also occur. Irritability and mood swings may be present, and loss of appetite or overeating are common features. In severe cases, MDD may last for months, with those affected experiencing profound despair and spending most of their time isolated or prostrate in bed, considering or planning suicide. Approximately 50% of MDD patients attempt suicide at least once in their lives.

In bipolar I disease (BPI), the manic episodes are severe, lasting from one week to three months or more if untreated, and often require hospitalization. Manic episodes are characterized by hyperactivity, feelings of grandiosity or omnipotence, euphoria, constant agitation, obsessive work or social activity, increased sexual drive, racing thoughts and surges of creativity, distractibility, compulsive shopping or money spending, and sharp mood swings and aggressive reactions, which may include physical violence against others. Depressive episodes may not occur in some BPI patients, but when present, the signs are similar to those of MDD and tend to last for months if untreated.

In bipolar II disease (BPII), milder and fewer manic episodes occur than for those people suffering from BPI, and at least one major depressive episode is experienced. BPII depression is the most common form of bipolar disease. Depressive episodes are usually more frequent than manic episodes, and can also last for extended periods if untreated.

Cyclothymia disorder is less severe, but tends to be chronic with frequent mood swings and single episodes lasting for at least two years. In some individuals, cyclothymic disorder is the precursor to a progressive bipolar disease. In others, the cyclothymic disorder remains chronic.

Hypomania is a mild degree of mania, manifested as brief and mild episodes of inflated self-esteem and excitability, irritability, impatience, and demanding attitude. Those with hypomania often find it disturbing or impossible to relax or to remain idle. Feelings of urgency to work longer hours and accomplish several tasks simultaneously are common.

Demographics

MDD is a leading cause of suicide, with more than 100,000 attempts per year in the United States alone. Affective disorders account for more than 200,000 suicide attempts in the United States, with an estimated mortality rate of 15%. Affective disorders are, however, a worldwide problem, and there are no racial differences, though Caucasian and Japanese males have been shown to be at higher risk of committing suicide. Suicide due to affective disorders is the second leading cause of mortality in teenagers in the United States and, among young adults, it accounts for 10–30% of deaths.

Causes and symptoms

Cultural influences and social pressures in achievement-oriented societies are important risk factors in affective disorders symptoms. Wars, catastrophic events, severe economic recession, accidents, personal loss, and urban violence are other contributing or triggering factors. Alcohol and drug abuse have a direct impact on brain neurochemistry, as well as some diseases, medical interventions, and medications, constituting a risk factor as well. However, in most cases, alcoholism, tobacco use, and/or drug abuse are the clinical symptoms of an underlying affective disorder that is inherently predisposed to substance abuse. Adaptive neurochemical and structural brain changes occurring in childhood give rise to the symptoms of many affective disorders; the diseases tend to run in families, although specific genetic factors causing the diseases have not yet been identified. Malnutrition and nutritional deficiencies are also important triggering factors in many psychiatric and affective disorders, as well as brain contamination with toxic levels of heavy metals such as methyl-mercury, lead, and bismuth.

The age of onset of bipolar diseases varies from childhood to middle adulthood, with a mean age of 21 years. MDD onset is highly variable, due to the presence of different possible factors such as family history, traumatic childhood, hormonal imbalance or seasonal changes, medical procedures, diseases, stress, menopause, emotional trauma and affective losses, or economical and social factors such as unemployment or social isolation.

Children with one parent affected by MDD or bipolar disease are five to seven times more prone to develop some affective or other psychiatric disorder than the general population. Although an inherited genetic trait is also under suspicion, studies over the past 20 years, as well as ongoing research on brain development during childhood, suggest that many cases of affective disorder may be due to the impact of repetitive and prolonged exposure to stress on the developing brain. Children of bipolar or MDD parents, for instance, may experience neglect or abuse, or be required to cope in early childhood with the emotional outbursts and incoherent mood swings of adults. Many children of those with affective disorders feel guilty or responsible for the dysfunctional adult. Such early exposure to stress generates abnormal levels of toxic metabolites in the brain, which have been shown to be harmful to the neurochemistry of the developing brain during childhood.

The neurochemical effects of stress alter both the quantities and the baseline systems of substances responsible for information processing between neurons such as **neurotransmitters** and hormones. Moreover, the stress metabolites such as **glucocorticoids** cause atrophy and death of neurons, a phenomenon known as neuronal crop, which alters the architecture of a child's brain. Neurotransmitters have specific roles in mood and in behavioral, cognitive, and other physiological functions: serotonin modulates mood, satiety (satisfaction in appetite), and sleeping patterns; dopamine modulates reward-seeking behavior, pleasure, and maternal/paternal and altruistic feelings; norepinephrine determines levels of alertness, danger perception, and fight-or-flight responses; acetylcholine controls memory and cognition processes; gamma amino butyric acid (GABA) modulates levels of reflex/stimuli response and controls or inhibits neuron excitation; and glutamate promotes excitation of neurons. Orchestrated interaction of proper levels of different neurotransmitters is essential for normal brain development and function, greatly influencing affective (mood), cognitive, and behavioral responses to the environment.

Low levels of the neurotransmitters serotonin and norepinephrine were found in people with affective disorders, and even lower levels of serotonin are associated with suicide and compulsive or aggressive behavior. Depressive states with mood swings and surges of irritability also point to serotonin depletion. Lower levels of dopamine are related to both depression and aggressive behavior. Norepinephrine synthesis depends on dopamine, and its depletion leads to loss of motivation and apathy. GABA is an important mood regulator because it controls and inhibits chemical changes in the brain during stress. Depletion of GABA leads to phobias, panic attacks, chronic anxiety pervaded with dark thoughts about the dangers of accidents, hidden menaces, and feelings of imminent death. Acute and prolonged stress, as well as alcohol and drug abuse, leads to GABA depletion. Acetylcholine depletion causes attention and concentration deficits, memory reduction, and **learning disorders**.

Chronic stress or highly traumatic experiences cause adaptive or compensatory changes in brain neurochemistry and physiology, in order to provide the individual with defense and survival mechanisms. However, such adaptive changes come with a high cost, in particular when they are required for an extended period such as in war zones, or other prolonged stressful situations. The adaptive chemicals tend to outlast the situation for which they were required, leading to some form of affective and behavioral disorder.

These adaptive neurochemical changes are especially harmful during early childhood. For instance, neglected or physically, sexually, or emotionally abused children are exposed to harmful levels of glucocorticoids (comparable to those found in war veterans) that lead to neuron atrophy (wasting) and cropping (reduced numbers) in the hippocampus region of the brain. Neuronal atrophy and crop often cause cognitive and memory disorders, anxiety, and poor emotional control. Neuronal crop also occurs in the frontal cortex of the brain's left hemisphere, leading to fewer nerve-cell connections with several other brain areas. These decreased nerve-cell connections favor

epilepsy-like short circuits or microseizures in the brain that occur in association with bursts of aggressiveness, self-destructive behavior, and cognitive or attention disorders. These alterations are also seen in the brains of adults who were abused or neglected during childhood. Time and recurrence of exposure and severity of suffered abuse help determine the extension of brain damage and the severity of psychiatric-related disorders in later stages of life.

Diagnosis

Well-known sets of clinical characteristics associated with MDD, bipolar diseases, or anxiety disorders provide the physician the necessary data for an initial diagnosis of affective disorder. The psychiatrist analyzes the person's pattern of mood, behavioral, and cognitive symptoms, along with the family history and environmental-contributing factors.

Abnormal atrophy, or loss of volume, in the hippocampus and cortex areas of the brain are detectable on **magnetic resonance imaging (MRI)** and computed tomography **(CT) scans**. Postmortem neuropathological (brain tissue) analysis demonstrates reduced cells and/or neuron size reductions in several brain regions of those with affective disorders.

Treatment team

The treatment team for people with affective disorders is primarily the psychiatrist, a medical doctor specializing in mood diseases and chemistry of the brain. Psychologists may also provide counseling and behavioral strategies for coping with the illness. Nurses administer prescribed medicine, along with monitoring behavior and physical condition during acute phases of the illness in the hospital setting. Mental health nurses also support treatment plans for clients in the community and provide a ready link to the psychiatrist. Additional community resources may include school psychologists, counselors, and support groups for affected people, as well as their family.

Treatment

Psychotherapy alone is rarely sufficient for the treatment of affective disorders, as the existing neurochemical imbalance impairs the ability of a person with an affective disorder to respond. However, psychotherapy is important in helping to cope with guilt, low self-esteem, and inadequate behavioral patterns once the neurochemistry is stabilized and more normal levels of neurotransmitters are at work.

Understanding of the devastating effects of stress in the brain of highly stressed or abused children made evident the need of medication as well as psychotherapy in early intervention. Administration of clonidine, a drug that inhibits the fight-or-flight response, and of other medications—or GABA supplementation—that interfere with levels of glucocorticoids in the brain can prevent both harmful neurochemical and architectural changes in the child's **central nervous system**. Family and parental therapy is also crucial in order to reduce the presence of emotional stressors in the child's life.

Teenagers and adults suffering from affective disorders may benefit from prescribed antidepressant medications that reduce symptoms. Recent studies have shown that antidepressants also encourage neuron cells in certain areas of the brain to mature, thus protecting the number of neurons in this area and preventing stress-induced neuronal crop. Lithium is beneficial to some bipolar and MDD patients, and also shows a protective effect against several neural injuries.

Antidepressants that inhibit the fast removal (i.e., re-uptake) of serotonin from the receptors in neurons and that regulate norepinephrine concentrations in the neuronal networks of the brain are very effective in mood stabilization. After a few days of medication, symptoms often recede. Nutrient supplementation, especially with B-complex vitamins, GABA, and essential amino acids, optimizes the synthesis of neurotransmitters and important neuropeptides, which are important for balanced neurochemistry in the central nervous system.

Recovery and rehabilitation

Helping individuals with an affective disorder to recognize their particular symptoms and mood states is essential for recovery and rehabilitation. With recognition, a person may seek additional treatment during recurring episodes early enough to deter the harmful consequences of the disease.

Clinical trials

As of early 2004, the National Institute of Mental Health (NIMH) is offering several **clinical trials** for adults and children with many types of affective disorders. People may participate at the institute's main facility in Bethesda, Maryland, or at several locations throughout the United States. Further information and updates may be found at the NIMH clinical trials web site.

Prognosis

Because affective disorders are usually long-term, cyclic conditions, ongoing treatment should be considered to prevent or modulate episodes of depression, mania, or severe anxiety. With preventative drug therapy, most people with affective disorders can expect to experience stabilization of their moods and anxiety, and can maintain an active role in work and social settings. Without treatment, daily activities and work are usually difficult to maintain within the cycles of mood disturbances, and social isolation, drug abuse, and suicide are often long-term consequences.

Resources

BOOKS

DePaulo, Jr., J. Raymond, and Leslie Alan Horvitz. *Understanding Depression: What We Know and What You Can Do about It.* New York: John Wiley & Sons, Inc., 2002.

Masters, Roger D., and Michael T. McGuire. *The Neurotransmitter Revolution.* Carbondale, IL: Southern Illinois University Press, 1994.

Mondimore, Francis Mark. *Bipolar Disorder: A Guide for Patients and Families.* Baltimore: The Johns Hopkins University Press, 1999.

PERIODICALS

Teicher, Martin H. "Wounds that Won't Heal—The Neurobiology of Child Abuse." *Scientific American* (March 2002): 68–75.

Vogel, G. "Depression Drugs' Powers May Rest on New Neurons." *Science* 301, no. 757 (2003).

OTHER

National Institute of Mental Health. *For the Public.* January 3, 2004 (March 30, 2004). <http://www.nimh.nih.gov/publicat/index.cfm>.

ORGANIZATIONS

National Institute of Mental Health. 6001 Executive Boulevard, Room 8184, MSC 9663, Bethesda, MD 20892-9663. (301) 443-4513 or (866) 615-6464; Fax: (301) 443-4279. nimhinfo@nih.gov. <http://www.nimh.nih.gov>.

Depression and Related Affective Disorders Association (DRADA). 2330 West Joppa Rd., Suite 100, Lutherville, MD 21093. (410) 583-2919. drada@hmi.edu. <http://www.drada.org/Facts/general.html>.

Sandra Galeotti

Agenesis of the corpus callosum

Definition

Agenesis of the corpus callosum (ACC) is an abnormality of brain structure, present at birth, that is characterized by partial or complete absence of the corpus callosum. The corpus callosum is a bundle of nerve fibers that connects the two hemispheres (halves) of the brain and allows information to pass back and forth between both sides.

Description

Agenesis of the corpus callosum is one form of abnormal corpus callosum development. Other corpus callosum disorders include hypoplastic (thin or underdeveloped) corpus callosum and dysgenesis (abnormal formation) of the corpus callosum. In complete ACC, the corpus callosum is entirely missing. In partial ACC, some portion, usually the posterior portion, is absent. Agenesis of the corpus callosum is often found in combination with other brain abnormalities and some degree of mental impairment. Birth defects involving other parts of the body (especially the eyes, face, heart, and skeletal system) may also be present. ACC can occur alone, without other obvious brain abnormalities. In some of these cases, the affected person is healthy and has an IQ (intelligence quotient) in the normal range. Even in these cases however, subtle neuropsychological and cognitive abnormalities may exist.

Demographics

Estimates of the frequency of ACC range between 0.0005% and 0.7% of children. An incidence of 2–3% has been reported in children with developmental disabilities. Between one-half to three-quarters of cases of ACC occur in males. ACC is a feature of Aicardi syndrome, an X-linked (caused by a gene on the X chromosome) condition that occurs almost exclusively in females and is thought to be lethal in males.

Causes and symptoms

The corpus callosum forms during the fifth to sixteenth week of pregnancy. It is thought that ACC occurs when one or more factors interfere with the migration (movement) of cells in the brain that eventually form the corpus callosum. An underlying cause for ACC is found in about one-half of cases. Factors that may affect normal corpus callosum development include:

• prenatal infections, viruses, or toxic exposures such as rubella or fetal alcohol syndrome

• chromosome abnormalities such as trisomy 8, trisomy 13, and trisomy 18

• genetic syndromes such as Aicardi syndrome, acrocallosal syndrome, Andermann syndrome, Shapiro syndrome, and Menkes disease

• blocked growth of the corpus callosum due to cysts or other abnormal structures

• a cerebral dysgenesis syndrome, in which there is abnormal formation of the brain such as **Dandy-Walker syndrome**, **Arnold-Chiari malformation**, **holoprosencephaly**, or **hydrocephalus**

The symptoms of ACC largely depend on the presence or absence of other medical conditions. The majority of children with ACC with other brain abnormalities usually show signs of a neurological disorder by age two. Symptoms in these children can include:

• **seizures**

• developmental delay or mental retardation

• increased or decreased head size

• hydrocephalus (abnormal accumulation of cerebrospinalfluid in the spaces of the brain)

• **cerebral palsy**

• hypotonia (decreased muscle tone)

• failure to thrive

In children with ACC who otherwise have limited neurological problems, there are slight differences in cognition (thought processes) and psychosocial functioning compared with children without ACC. **Neuropsychological testing** has shown that such individuals can have any of the following:

• motor, language, or cognitive delays

• poor motor coordination

• sensitivity to tactile sensations

• high **pain** tolerance

• cognitive and social challenges

Cognitive and social challenges may become more apparent with age. Examples of these challenges include difficulties using language in social settings and with performing tasks that require complex reasoning, creativity, or problem-solving skills. Patients with ACC may display limited insight into one's own behavior, a lack of awareness of others' feelings, misunderstanding of social cues, limited sophistication of humor, and difficulty imagining consequences of behavior.

Diagnosis

A health professional suspicious of ACC may recommend a neurological evaluation that includes imaging studies. The more subtle cognitive and psychosocial problems found in individuals with isolated ACC are less likely to lead to the diagnosis. In some cases, the diagnosis of ACC is incidental, made in the course of an evaluation for other reasons. There may well be many asymptomatic individuals with partial or complete agenesis who never come to medical attention.

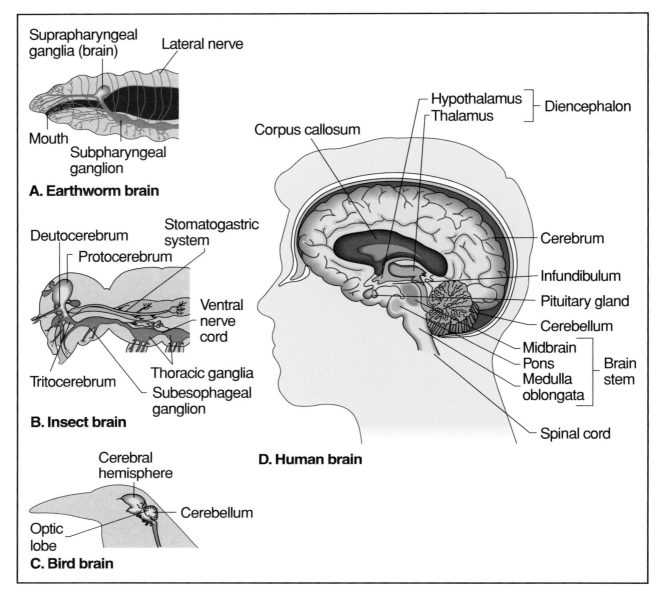

A. Earthworm brain

- Suprapharyngeal ganglia (brain)
- Lateral nerve
- Mouth
- Subpharyngeal ganglion

B. Insect brain

- Deutocerebrum
- Stomatogastric system
- Protocerebrum
- Ventral nerve cord
- Tritocerebrum
- Thoracic ganglia
- Subesophageal ganglion

C. Bird brain

- Cerebral hemisphere
- Cerebellum
- Optic lobe

D. Human brain

- Corpus callosum
- Hypothalamus
- Thalamus
- Diencephalon
- Cerebrum
- Infundibulum
- Pituitary gland
- Cerebellum
- Midbrain
- Pons
- Medulla oblongata
- Brain stem
- Spinal cord

Diagram of the human brain (and others) with the corpus callosum indicated. *(Illustration by Electronic Illustrators Group.)*

Diagnosis of ACC relies on imaging studies such as ultrasound (prenatal or postnatal), **magnetic resonance imaging (MRI),** or computerized axial tomography (**CT** or CAT) scan. Diagnostic findings include:

- absence of the corpus callosum
- widely displaced and parallel lateral ventricles
- selective dilatation of the posterior horns
- widely spaced frontal horns
- upward displacement and enlargement of the third ventricle
- displaced orientation of gyral markings

Fetal ultrasound can detect some but not all cases of ACC, beginning at about 20 weeks of pregnancy. The prenatal or postnatal diagnosis of ACC should be followed by studies aimed to determine the cause for the ACC. Such studies may include chromosome analysis, metabolic screening, and genetic and ophthalmologic consultations.

Treatment team

Treatment for patients with ACC is highly individualized because the severity of symptoms varies from patient to patient. Depending upon the symptoms, many

Key Terms

Arnold-Chiari malformation A condition in which the cerebellum, a structure in the brain, protrudes into the spinal canal.

Cerebral palsy A brain injury that results in inability to use some muscles in the usual way.

Chromosome Thin, rod-like fibers in the nucleus of a cell that contain the genes.

Dandy-Walker syndrome A cyst in the cerebellum that involves the fourth ventricle (a space in the brain) and that may interfere with the body's ability to drain cerebral spinal fluid.

Failure to thrive Failure to grow and gain weight at the expected rate.

Holoprosencephaly Brain, cranial, and facial malformations present at birth that are caused by incomplete cleavage of the brain during embryologic development.

Hydrocephalus Abnormal accumulation of cerebrospinal fluid in the ventricles of the brain.

medical specialists can assist the patient's primary physician or nurse practitioner, including a **neurologist**, ophthalmologist, geneticist, **neuropsychologist**, behavioral psychologist, occupational therapist, physical therapist, speech-language pathologist, and experts in special education and early intervention.

Treatment

There is no cure for ACC. Treatment primarily includes management of associated problems such as seizures, hydrocephalus, and cerebral palsy.

Recovery and rehabilitation

Limited information is available about the optimal remedial strategies for individuals with ACC. Speech therapy, occupational therapy, physical therapy, and early intervention are common services provided to patients with ACC. The goal of these therapies is to maximize the patient's success in school, work, and life in general. Speech therapy can help patients with speech delays, **apraxia** (the inability to make voluntary movements despite normal muscle function), and difficulties with pragmatics or social language use. Occupational therapy can help patients with sensory integration problems. Physical therapy can help address problems such as impaired coordination, motor delays, and **spasticity** (abnormally increased muscle stiffness and restricted movement).

Clinical trials

There are currently no **clinical trials** for patients with agenesis of the corpus callosum. Patients and families may elect to participate in genetic research. Laboratories searching for genes associated with agenesis of the corpus callosum include the laboratory of Elliott H. Sherr M.D., Ph.D, at the University of California, San Francisco, and the Harvard Institutes of Medicine. Both labs accept contact from patients and families.

Prognosis

The prognosis for ACC varies according to the presence and severity of associated problems such as **microcephaly** (small head), seizures, cerebral palsy, and cerebral dysgenesis. In the case of a fetus diagnosed with isolated ACC, prediction of outcome remains imprecise. Estimates of the chance for a normal developmental outcome for a case detected prenatally range from 35–85%. It has also been stated that a so-called "normal" or "asymptomatic" outcome for ACC does not exist. Subtle or cognitive and psychosocial differences have been found in patients with ACC and a normal IQ.

Special concerns

The special educational needs of children with ACC vary. Children with ACC may be eligible for an individual education plan (IEP). An IEP provides a framework from which administrators, teachers, and parents can meet the educational needs of a child with ACC. Depending upon severity of symptoms and the degree of learning difficulties, some children with ACC may be best served by special education classes or a private educational setting.

Resources

BOOKS

Brown, W. S., and M. T. Banich, eds. *Development of the Corpus Callosum and Interhemispheric Interactions: A Special Issue of Developmental Neuropsychology.* Mahwah, NJ: Lawrence Erlbaum Associates, Inc., 2001.

Lassonde, M., and M. Jeeves, ed. *Callosal Agenesis: A Natural Split Brain?* New York: Plenum Press, 1994.

Parker, James N., and Philip M. Parker, eds. *The Official Parent's Sourcebook on Agenesis of the Corpus Callosum: A Revised and Updated Directory for the Internet Age.* San Diego: ICON Health Publications, 2002.

Rourke, B. P., ed. *Syndrome of Nonverbal Learning Disabilities: Neurodevelopmental Manifestations.* New York: Guilford Press, 1995.

PERIODICALS

Brown, W. S., and L. K. Paul. "Cognitive and Psychosocial Deficits in Agenesis of the Corpus Callosum with Normal

Key Terms

Alzheimer's disease A progressive, neurodegenerative disease characterized by loss of function and death of nerve cells in several areas of the brain, leading to loss of mental functions such as memory and learning. Formerly called presenile dementia.

Anoxia Lack of oxygen.

Asperger syndrome A developmental disorder of childhood characterized by autistic behavior but without the same difficulties acquiring language that children with autism have.

Autism A syndrome characterized by a lack of responsiveness to other people or outside stimulus. Often occurs in conjunction with a severe impairment of verbal and non-verbal communication skills.

Huntington's disease A rare hereditary disease that causes progressive chorea (jerky muscle movements) and mental deterioration that ends in dementia. Huntington's symptoms usually appear in patients in their 40s. Also called Huntington's chorea.

Parietal lobe One of two brain hemispheres responsible for associative processes.

Temporal lobes A large lobe of each hemisphere of the brain that is located on the side of the head, nearest the ears. It contains a sensory area associated with hearing.

Intelligence." *Cognitive Neuropsychiatry* 5 (2000): 135–157.

Davila-Gutierrez, G. "Agenesis and Dysgenesis of the Corpus Callosum." *Seminars in Pediatric Neurology* 9 (December 2002): 292–301.

Goodyear, P. W., C. M. Bannister, S. Russell, and S. Rimmer. "Outcome in Prenatally Diagnosed Fetal Agenesis of the Corpus Callosum." *Fetal Diagnosis and Therapy* 16 (May–June 2001): 139–145.

Shevell, M. I. "Clinical and Diagnostic Profile of Agenesis of the Corpus Callosum." *Journal of Child Neurology* 17 (December 2002): 896–900.

Stickles, J. L., G. L. Schilmoeller, and K. J. Schilmoeller. "A 23-Year Review of Communication Development in an Individual with Agenesis of the Corpus Callosum." *International Journal of Disability, Development and Education* 49 (2002): 367–383.

WEBSITES

The National Institute of Neurological Disorders and Stroke (NINDS). *Agenesis of the Corpus Callosum Information Page*. (March 30, 2004.) <http://www.ninds.nih.gov/health_and_medical/disorders/agenesis_doc.htm>.

Corpal Home Page. (March 30, 2004.) <http://www.corpal.org.uk/>.

National Center for Biotechnology Information. *Online Mendelian Inheritance in Man (OMIM) Home Page*. (March 30, 2004.) <http://www.ncbi.nlm.nih.gov/omim/>.

ORGANIZATIONS

Agenesis of the Corpus Callosum (ACC) Network, 5749 Merrill Hall, Room 118, University of Maine, Orono, ME 04469-5749. (207) 581-3119; Fax: (207) 581-3120. UM-ACC@maine.edu.

Aicardi Syndrome Foundation. P.O. Box 3202, St. Charles, IA 60174. (800) 374-8518. aicardi@aol.com. <http://www.aicardisyndrome.org>.

National Organization for Disorders of the Corpus Callosum (NODCC). 18032-C Lemon Drive PMB 363, Yorba Linda, CA 92886. (714) 717-0063. <http://www.corpuscallosum.org>.

Dawn J. Cardeiro, MS, CGC

Agnosia

Definition

Agnosia is a neuropsychological disorder characterized by the inability to recognize common objects, persons, or sounds, in the absence of perceptual disability. There are three major types of agnosia: visual agnosia, auditory agnosia, and tactile agnosia. Agnosia is caused by lesions to the parietal and temporal lobes of the brain, regions involved in storing memories and associations of objects. The condition may arise following head trauma or **stroke**, or following carbon monoxide poisoning or anoxia.

Description

Agnosia, from the Greek "not knowing," describes a collection of disorders where the ability to recognize objects or sounds or retrieve information about them is impaired, in the absence of other perceptual difficulties, including memory, intellectual capabilities, and the capacity for communication. The disorder can affect visual, auditory or tactile object recognition, but visual agnosia is the most common form of the condition, and most often expressed as an inability to recognize people.

Visual Agnosia

In addition to being the most common form of agnosia, visual agnosias are also the best understood. Lissauer was the first scientist to provide a detailed account of agnosia (1888). He hypothesized that disorders in visual object recognition could be classified as either apperceptive agnosia or associative agnosia. This classification continues to be used today although there is some debate as to whether the deficits occur as a dichotomy or as a spectrum.

Apperceptive agnosics can see, but they lack higher-level visual perception, which interferes with object information gathering. Apperceptive agnosics fail shape-recognition and shape-copying tests. In an attempt to copy a drawing of a circle, a patient with apperceptive agnosia my draw a series of concentric scribbles. Conversely, associative agnosics have normal perception, but fail to draw on stored memories or knowledge associated with the object, such as its name, or the way it feels when picked up.

APPERCEPTIVE VISUAL AGNOSIA Carbon monoxide poisoning is a frequent cause of apperceptive visual agnosia. The ensuing brain damage is frequently profuse and located in the posterior region of the brain. Simultanagnosia, a syndrome related to apperceptive visual agnosia, describes a condition where scenes containing multiple objects cannot be interpreted as a whole. Instead patients with simultanagnosia, recognize only portions of the scene at one time, and fail to describe the overall nature of the scene and comprehend its meaning.

Individuals capable of seeing only one object at a time are said to have dorsal simultanagnosia. The condition is associated with lesions in the posterior parietal cortex, which are frequently bilateral. Patients with ventral simultanagnosia retain the ability to recognize whole objects, but the rate of recognition is impaired. The left inferior temporo-occipital cortex is generally implicated in the deficit.

ASSOCIATIVE VISUAL AGNOSIA Even when perception remains intact, some people have difficulty recognizing objects. For these people, who lack language or communication disorders or intellectual impairment, and who are able to create good copies of objects, the deficit lies in retrieving stored information about the object that would permit identification. However, many people can provide semantic information about the object without being able to provide the name. For example, the word "kangaroo" may remain elusive, but descriptors, such as "found in Australia" and "has a pouch" may be offered in its place. Many associative visual agnosics have difficulty recognizing faces (prosopagnosia) or words (pure alexia), others specific types of objects, such as tools, or animals.

Prosopagnosia was first described by Quaglino and Borelli in 1867. Although deficits in face recognition occur in a variety of neurological diseases, including **Alzheimer**'s and **Huntington**'s diseases, Asperger's syndrome and **autism**, the term is best reserved for situations where impaired face recognition appears in absence of other neurological symptoms. Patients are often uncomfortable in social situations, although many learn to recognize people using other visual cues, such as hairstyles, glasses, or scars.

Prosopagnosia can be diagnosed using the Warrington Memory Test for faces, or the Benton Face Recognition test. Although the latter will not indicate prosopagnosia, failing the test does help quantify the degree of impairment. Neuroimaging of the adult with prosopagnosia often reveals lesions in the lingual and fusiform gyri of the medial occipitotemporal cortex, which are frequently bilateral. Children who have acquired the condition *in utero* or genetically, however, may not show these cortical lesions.

Auditory agnosia

Auditory agnosics fail to ascribe values to verbal or non-verbal sounds. Individuals with pure word deafness have intact hearing, but are unable to understand the spoken word, typically the result of bilateral trauma to the temporal cortico-subcortical regions of the brain. Nonverbal auditory agnosics fail to associate sounds with specific objects or events, such as a dog's bark or the slamming of a door. In these patients, the lesions tend to locate to the right hemisphere.

Tactile agnosia

Tactile agnosia, also called astereognosis, is often difficult to recognize as we rarely identify objects solely by feel. Information about the object, including its weight, size, and texture are not given any value. Lesions in the somatosensory cortex are thought to be responsible for the condition.

Resources

BOOKS

"Agnosia," Section 14, Chapter 169. In *The Merck Manual of Diagnosis and Therapy*, Mark H. Beers, and Robert Berkow, eds. Whitehouse Station, NJ: Merck Research Laboratories, 1999.

Farah, M. J. *Disorders of Object Recognition and What They Tell us About Normal Vision*, 2nd edition. Cambridge, MA: The MIT Press, 1995.

Freinberg, T. E. and M. J. Farah. "Cognitive-Motor Disorders, Apraxias, and Agnosias." In *Neurology in Clinical Practice: Principles of Diagnosis and Management*, 3rd edition, W. G. Bradley, R. B. Daroff, G. M. Fenichel, et al., eds. Boston, MA: Butterworth Heinemann, 2000.

PERIODICALS

Barton, J. J. S. "Disorders of face perception and recognition." *Neurologic Clinics of North America* 21 (2003): 521–548.

Hodgson, T. L., and C. Kennard. "Disorders of higher visual function and hemi-spatial neglect." *Current Opinion in Neurology* 13 (2000): 7–12.

Riddoch, M. J. and G. W. Humphreys. "Visual agnosia." *Neurologic Clinics of North America* 21 (May 2003): 501–520.

WEBSITES

National Institute of Neurological Disorders and Stroke (NINDS). *NINDS Agnosia Information Page.* <http://www.ninds.nih.gov/health_and_medical/disorders/agnosia.htm>.

ORGANIZATIONS

National Eye Institute (NEI), National Institutes of Health. Bldg. 31, Rm. 6A32, Bethesda, MD 20892-2510. (301) 496-52482 or (800) 869-2020. 020@b31.nei.nih.gov. <http://www.nei.nih.gov>.

National Institute on Deafness and Other Communication Disorders (NIDCD), National Institutes of Health. Bldg. 31, Rm. 3C35, Bethesda, MD 20892-2320, (301) 496-7243. nidcdinfo@nidcd.nih.gov. <http://www.nidcd.nih.gov>.

National Organization for Rare Disorders (NORD). P.O. Box 1968 (55 Kenosia Avenue), Danbury, CT 06813-1968. (203)744-0100 or (800) 999-NORD (6673); Fax: (203) 798-2291. orphan@rarediseases.org. <http://www.rarediseases.org>.

Hannah M. Hoag, MSc

Aicardi syndrome *see* **Agenesis of the corpus callosum**

AIDS

Definition

Acquired immunodeficiency syndrome (AIDS) is the final and most serious stage of the disease caused by the human immunodeficiency virus. Symptoms begin when an HIV-positive person presents a CD4-cell (also called T cell, a type of immune cell) count below 200. AIDS happens concurrently with numerous opportunistic infections and tumors that are normally associated with the HIV infection.

The most common neurological complications of AIDS involve opportunistic infections of the brain such as progressive multifocal leucoencephalopathy (PML) and meningitis, other opportunistic infections such as herpes zoster (**shingles**), **peripheral neuropathy**, **depression**, and AIDS-related **dementia**.

Key Terms

Hemophiliac A person with the blood disorder hemophilia, an inherited deficiency in blood-clotting ability. Hemophiliacs require regular administration of blood products, and were especially at risk of acquiring AIDS from HIV-contaminated blood during the early years of the evolving AIDS epidemic, before tests were developed to identify the HIV virus in donated blood.

Opportunistic infection An infection in a person with an impaired immune system caused by an organism that does not usually cause disease in people with healthy immune systems.

Pandemic Widespread epidemic.

Western blot A sensitive laboratory blood test for specific antibodies; useful in confirming the diagnosis of AIDS.

Description

AIDS was first recognized in 1981 and has since become a major worldwide pandemic. Abundant evidence indicates that the human immunodeficiency virus (HIV), discovered in 1983, causes AIDS. By leading to the destruction and/or functional impairment of immune cells, notably CD4+ T cells, HIV progressively destroys the body's ability to fight infections and to resist certain cancer formation.

Before the HIV infection became widespread in the human population, AIDS-like syndromes occurred extremely rarely, and almost exclusively in individuals with known causes of immune suppression, such as those receiving chemotherapy or those with underlying cancers. A marked increase in unusual infections and tumors characteristic of severe immune suppression was first recognized in the early 1980s in homosexual men who had been otherwise healthy and had no recognized cause for immune suppression. An infectious cause of AIDS was suggested by geographic clustering of cases, a sexual link among cases, mother-to-infant transmission, and transmission by blood transfusion.

Isolation of the HIV from patients with AIDS strongly suggested that this virus was the cause of AIDS. Since the early 1980s, HIV and AIDS have been repeatedly associated; the appearance of HIV in the blood supply has preceded or coincided with the occurrence of AIDS cases in every country and region where AIDS has been noted. Individuals of all ages from many risk groups, including homosexual men, infants born to HIV-infected mothers, heterosexual women and men, hemophiliacs, recipients of blood and blood products, health care workers and others occupationally exposed to HIV-tainted blood, and injection drug users have all developed AIDS with only one common denominator: HIV.

HIV destroys CD4+ T cells, which are crucial to the normal function of the human immune system. In fact, depletion of CD4+ T cells in HIV-infected individuals is an extremely powerful predictor of the development of AIDS. Studies of thousands of individuals have revealed that most HIV-infected people carry the virus for years before enough damage is done to the immune system for AIDS to develop; however, with time, a near-perfect correlation has been found between infection and the subsequent development of AIDS.

Demographics

In the United States, more than 733,000 people have AIDS, and an estimated one to two million people have HIV infection without the symptoms of AIDS.

Internationally, since the AIDS epidemic began, more than 16 million deaths have been attributed to AIDS. The current estimate of worldwide disease prevalence is more than 33 million HIV infections. Ninety-five percent of these cases are in developing countries, generally in sub-Saharan Africa and Southeast Asia.

Most HIV infections still occur in men; however, the frequency of infection in women is increasing, especially in developing countries. In the United States, fewer than 16% of all HIV cases are in women, whereas worldwide an estimated 46% of all HIV patients are women.

Causes and symptoms

The cause of primary AIDS is infection with the HIV virus, transmitted via infected blood or body fluids. Methods of transmission of the virus include unprotected sex, especially anal intercourse; occupational needle stick or body fluid splash, which has an estimated transmission rate of less than 0.3%; sharing of needles in drug abuse; and receiving contaminated blood products.

Opportunistic infections occur in individuals whose CD4 count is less than 200 cells/mm^3 and those not taking preventative drugs.

Symptoms of AIDS include:

• cough and shortness of breath
• **seizures** and lack of coordination
• difficult or painful swallowing
• confusion and forgetfulness
• severe and persistent diarrhea
• fever
• vision loss
• nausea, abdominal cramps, and vomiting
• weight loss and extreme fatigue
• severe **headaches** with neck stiffness

Neurological complications of AIDS

Almost 30% of people with AIDS develop peripheral neuropathy, causing tingling, numbness, and weakness in the arms and legs due to nerve damage. If severe, peripheral neuropathy can cause difficulty walking. Several drugs used to treat people with AIDS can contribute to the development of peripheral neuropathy.

Several opportunistic infections experienced by people with AIDS involve the nervous system. Progressive multifocal leucoencephalopathy (PML) is a serious viral infection of the brain, most often caused by the JC virus. PML is fatal in more than 90% of cases within six months of diagnosis. Nearly 4% of people with AIDS, especially those with T-cell counts below 100, will develop the disease. Meningitis is an infection of the lining of the spinal cord and brain, and also occurs in some people with AIDS. Cryptococcus, a fungus that normally occurs in the soil and seldom affects persons with intact immune systems, can cause recurring meningitis in people with AIDS whose T-cell count is below 100. The common parasite *Toxoplasma gondii* often present in cat feces, raw meat, raw vegetables, and the soil can also cause encephalitis, or inflammation of the brain, in AIDS patients. Shingles is a painful nerve inflammation caused by a reactivation of the herpes varicella zoster virus, the same virus that causes chicken pox. Although not directly linked to HIV, shingles seems to occur more frequently in people with AIDS.

Other neurological conditions associated with AIDS include depression, occurring at any time during the disease, and dementia, which sometimes occurs in the later stages of AIDS. Depression can stem from living with a chronic and progressive disease. AIDS-related dementia involves problems with thinking, memory, and usually also with controlling the arms and legs, and can stem from direct infection in the brain with the HIV virus. In the initial stages of the pandemic, almost 20% of persons with AIDS developed severe dementia. With the development of combination **antiviral drugs**, the rate of severe dementia in AIDS has been reduced by more than half. The number of persons with HIV and milder dementia has increased, however, as people with HIV live longer.

Diagnosis

In the early stages of infection, HIV often causes no symptoms and the infection can be diagnosed only by testing a person's blood. Two tests are available to diagnose

AIDS

HIV infection, one that looks for the presence of antibodies produced by the body in response to HIV and the other that looks for the virus itself. Antibodies are proteins produced by the body whenever a disease threatens it. When the body is infected with HIV, it produces antibodies specific to HIV. The first test, called ELISA (enzyme-linked immunosorbent assay), looks for such antibodies in the blood.

A positive ELISA has to be confirmed by another test called western blot or immunofluorescent assay (IFA). All positive tests by ELISA are not accurate and hence, western blot and repeated tests are necessary to confirm a person's HIV status. A person infected with HIV is termed HIV positive or seropositive.

Rapid tests that give results in five to 30 minutes are increasingly being used worldwide. The accuracy of rapid tests is stated to be as good as that of ELISA. Though rapid tests are more expensive, researchers have found them to be more cost effective in terms of the number of people covered and the time the tests take.

The HIV antibodies generally do not reach detectable levels in the blood until about three months after infection. This period, from the time of infection until the blood is tested positive for antibodies, is called the window period. Sometimes, the antibodies might take up to six months to be detected. Even if the tests are negative, during the window period the amount of virus is very high in an infected person. If a person is newly infected, therefore, the risk of transmission is higher.

Another test for HIV is called polymerase chain reaction (PCR), which looks for HIV itself in the blood. This test, which recognizes the presence of the virus' genetic material in the blood, can detect the virus within a few days of infection. There are also tests like radio immuno precipitation assay (RIPA), a confirmatory blood test that may be used when antibody levels are difficult to detect or when western blot test results are uncertain.

Treatment team

The treatment team often includes personal caregivers, physical therapists, dietitians, specialists (infectious disease specialists, dermatologists, nephrologists, ophthalmologists, pediatrists, psychiatrists, and neurologists), and **social workers**.

Treatment

Since the early 1990s, several drugs to fight both the HIV infection and its associated infections and cancers have become available, including:

• Reverse transcriptase inhibitors: They interrupt the virus from making copies of itself. These drugs are AZT (zidovudine [Retrovir]), ddC (zalcitabine [Hivid], dideoxyinosine), d4T (stavudine [Zerit]), and 3TC (lamivudine [Epivir]).

• Nonnucleoside reverse transcriptase inhibitors (NNRTIS): These medications are used in combination with other drugs to help keep the virus from multiplying. Examples of NNRTIS are delavirdine (Rescriptor) and nevirapine (Viramune).

• Protease inhibitors: These medications interrupt virus replication at a later step in its lifecycle. These include ritonavir (Norvir), a lopinavir and ritonavir combination (Kaletra), saquinavir (Invirase), indinavir sulphate (Crixivan), amprenavir (Agenerase), and nelfinavir (Viracept). Using both classes of drugs reduces the chances of developing resistance in the virus.

• Fusion inhibitors: This is the newest class of anti-HIV drugs. The first drug of this class (enfuvirtide [Fuzeon]) has recently been approved in the United States. Fusion inhibitors block HIV from entering the human immune cell.

• A combination of several drugs called highly active antiretroviral therapy (HAART): This treatment is not a cure. The virus still persists in various body sites such as in the lymph glands.

The antiretroviral drugs do not cure people of the HIV infection or AIDS. They stop viral replication and delay the development of AIDS. However, they may also have side effects that can be severe. These include decrease of red or white blood cells, inflammation of the pancreas, and painful nerve damage. Other complications are enlarged or fatty liver, which may result in liver failure and death.

Recovery and rehabilitation

As there is no cure for AIDS, the focus is on maintaining optimum health, activity, and quality of life rather than on complete recovery.

Occupational therapy can have a crucial role in assisting people living with HIV/AIDS to reengage with life, particularly through vocational rehabilitation programs. Occupational therapy can provide the patient with a series of learning experiences that will enable the individual to make appropriate vocational choices.

Clinical trials

There are many ongoing **clinical trials** for AIDS. "HIV Vaccine Designed for HIV Infected Adults Taking Anti-HIV Drugs," "When to Start Anti-HIV Drugs in Patients with Opportunistic Infections," and "Outcomes of Anti-HIV Therapy during Early HIV Infection" are some trials that are currently recruiting patients at the National

Institute of Allergy and Infectious Diseases (NIAID). Updated information on these and other trials for the study and treatment of AIDS can be found at the National Institutes of Health website for clinical trials at <http://www.clinicaltrials.gov>.

Prognosis

Presently, there is no cure for HIV infection or AIDS, nor is there a vaccine to prevent the HIV infection. However, there are new medications that help slow the progression of the infection and reduce the seriousness of HIV consequences in many people.

Special concerns

The surest way to avoid AIDS is to abstain from sex, or to limit sex to one partner who also limits his or her sex in the same way (monogamy). Condoms are not 100% safe, but if used properly they will greatly reduce the risk of AIDS transmission. Also, avoiding the use of intravenous drugs (drug abuse, sharing contaminated syringes) is highly recommended.

Resources

BOOKS

Conner, R. F., L. P. Villarreal, and H. Y. Fan. *AIDS: Science and Society.* Sudbury, MA: Jones & Bartlett Publishers, 2004.

Stine, G. J. *AIDS Update 2004.* Essex, England: Pearson Benjamin Cummings, 2003.

PERIODICALS

Grant, A. D, and K. M. De Cock. "ABC of AIDS: HIV Infection and AIDS in the Developing World." *BMJ* 322 (June 2001): 1475–1478.

OTHER

"AIDS Factsheets." *AIDS.ORG.* April 20, 2004 (May 27, 2004). <http://www.aids.org/factSheets/>.

"How HIV Causes AIDS." *National Institute of Allergy and Infectious Disease.* April 20, 2004 (May 27, 2004). <http://www.niaid.nih.gov/factsheets/howhiv.htm>.

UNAIDS. The Joint United Nations Program on HIV/AIDS. April 20, 2004 (May 27, 2004). <http://www.unaids.org/>.

ORGANIZATIONS

Centers for Disease Control (Office of Public Inquiries). Clifton Road, Atlanta, GA 30333. (800) 342-2437. <http://www.cdc.gov>.

National Institute of Allergy and Infectious Disease. 6610 Rockledge Drive MSC 6612, Bethesda, MD 20892-6612. <http://www.niaid.nih.gov/>.

Greiciane Gaburro Paneto
Brenda Wilmoth Lerner, RN
Iuri Drumond Louro, MD, PhD

Alcohol-related neurological disease

Definition

Alcohol-related neurological disease represents a broad spectrum of conditions caused by acute or chronic alcohol intake.

Description

Alcohol, or ethanol, is a poisonous chemical that has direct and toxic effects on nerve and muscle cells. The effects can be profound, and symptoms can include incoordination, weakness, **seizures**, memory loss, and sensory deficits. Alcohol has a profoundly negative effect on both the **central nervous system** (i.e., the brain and spinal cord) and the **peripheral nervous system** (i.e., nerves that send impulses to peripheral structures such as muscles and organs). Alcohol can have negative effects on neurological centers that regulate body temperature, sleep, and coordination.

Alcohol can significantly lower body temperature. It disrupts normal sleep patterns because it decreases rapid eye movement (REM) during the dreaming stage of sleep. It also adversely affects muscle coordination, causing imbalance and staggering—alcohol is a toxic insult to the **cerebellum**, which is responsible for balance.

Additionally, the chronic use of alcohol can cause a broad spectrum of abnormalities in mental functioning. Generally, persons exhibit poor attention, difficulty with abstraction and problem solving, difficulty learning new materials, reduced visuospatial abilities (capacity to discriminate between two-dimensional or three-dimensional space), and often require extra time to integrate visual information. Other related problems include thiamine deficiency (vitamin B-1) and liver disease (liver cirrhosis and possibly liver cancer).

Acute effects of alcohol

When alcohol is ingested, it moves from the bloodstream into every part of the body that contains water, including the brain, lungs, kidneys, and heart. Alcohol distributes itself equally both inside and outside cells. Ninety-five percent of alcohol is eliminated from the body by breakdown in the liver, and 5% is eliminated through urine, sweat, and breath. Alcohol is broken down (metabolized) in the liver by a complex process called zero-order kinetics (broken down at a certain amount at a time). This means that alcohol is metabolized at a rate of 0.3 oz (8.8 ml) of pure ethanol per hour. Within moments after ingestion, alcohol reaches the brain and produces acute effects such as euphoria, sedation (calmness), anesthesia,

Cerebellum Part of the brain that is responsible for muscle control and maintenance of balance.

Cortical atrophy A wasting away and decrease in size of the outer portion of the brain, or cerebral cortex.

Diencephalon The relay station of the brain for impulses concerning sensation and movement.

Euphoria An exaggerated state of psychological and physical well being.

Gray matter Area deep in the brain that functions during thinking and contains nerve cells that have an insulation membrane called a myelin sheath.

Incoordination Loss of voluntary muscle control resulting in irregular movements.

Limbic system Part of the brain that functions in motivational and mood states.

and a sleepy hypnotic state. Further effects include release of inhibitions and judgment, blunting of sexual desire, aggressiveness, and mood changes. Physical effects of intoxication (with continued consumption) include impairment of motor ability, muscle function, eyesight, reaction time, night vision, and depth perception. Continued consumption can be lethal because alcohol can depress heart and lung function, which can slow breathing and circulation. Lethality occurs when levels are high enough to paralyze breathing. However, death due to alcohol consumption is rare because body defenses tend to eliminate the chemical by vomiting or the person becomes comatose. Alcohol "hangovers" usually cause persons to have **headache** (due to dilation of blood vessels in the head), dehydration (alcohol acts as a diuretic increasing urine output), and upset stomach (due to irritation of stomach lining).

Specific neurological damage

The effects of alcohol can include damage or impairment to brain systems and to specific regions in the brain. The limbic system, located deep inside the brain, has several functions, including memory. Long-term users of alcohol often exhibit memory loss due to damage of the limbic system structures called the amygdala and hippocampus, located in the temporal lobes. Damage to other parts of the limbic system can produce symptoms such as abnormalities in emotional functioning and in the ability to use one of the senses (e.g., eyesight or the sense of smell) or in the ability to learn using the senses (e.g., learning through the sense of touch). Damage to the **diencephalon** (major relay station for nerve signals moving within the brain, associated with memory functioning) occurs and is associated with chronic usage and malnutrition (a late-onset condition). The cerebral cortex (folded outer layer of the brain) is composed of nerve cells called gray matter, which functions as the center of intelligent behavior and higher consciousness. Neuroimaging studies reveal that there are definitive signs of morphological change such as cortical atrophy (a decrease in size of the cerebral cortex). Cortical atrophy induced by alcoholism is associated with deficits in spatial memory and visual associations, learning related to or caused by touch, and problem solving. Alcoholic subjects also exhibit a decrease in blood nourishing the frontal lobe (portion of the brain behind the forehead), whose functions include planning, carrying out, and monitoring goal-directed and socially acceptable behaviors.

Neurotransmitter deficits and the progression of alcoholism

Neurotransmitters are brain chemicals that allow nerve cells to communicate. These chemicals are released and picked up by specialized structures (receptors) in a space between nerve cells called a synapse. Alcohol can cause "up"-regulation or "down"-regulation effects on neurotransmitters. Over prolonged periods of alcohol abuse, the levels of receptors change. Genes that produce molecular copies of receptors may by turned off (decreasing activity) or on (increasing activity). Levels of glutamate (an amino acid that is an excitatory neurotransmitter in the brain) are abnormally altered. Glutamate is correlated with long-term potentiation (mechanism vital for learning and memory) in the brain. Even minute amounts of alcohol have profound effects on brain glutamate action. Interference with glutamate chemistry in the brain can cause memory impairment and may account for the short-lived condition called "blackouts." Because alcohol suppresses the excitatory effect of glutamate on nerve cells, this can result in strokes and seizures.

Another neurochemical that is altered due to chronic intake of alcohol is gamma-aminobutyric acid (GABA), a major inhibitory neurotransmitter in the brain. Initially, alcohol increases the effects of GABA, which produces a state of mild sedation. Over time with continued abuse, the GABA system is down regulated and, when alcohol is not present in the system, the inhibitory effects are lost and overexcitation of the brain results.

Alcoholism is a chronic disease, with a natural history that progresses to death if the intake does not completely stop. The progress consists of three stages. During the beginning stage, the alcoholic becomes dependent on the mood-altering effects of alcohol. In the middle stage, drinking starts earlier and there is tolerance (when more alcohol is needed to produce effects); during this stage, alcohol consumption is out of control and alcoholics frequently exhibit denial. Heavy consumption causes symptoms of anxiety, **depression**, **fatigue**, anger, rage, lack of self-esteem, and self-loathing. Symptoms worsen as the disease progresses, and alcoholics develop hand **tremors** and shaking (**delirium** tremens) and morning hangover. The final stages of alcoholism progress to round-the-clock consumption despite extremely negative personal and social consequences. The disease progresses with symptoms of intense guilt and remorse (suppressed by more drinking), fear of crowds and public places, financial debt, legal problems, and ill health (including malnutrition). Late-stage disease typically involves liver degeneration (cirrhosis) and severe, even life-threatening, clinical signs (shakes and convulsions) during withdrawal without treatment. Insanity due to brain damage or death may occur during this stage.

Alcohol can cause thiamine deficiency (vitamin B-1). The Wernicke-Korsakoff syndrome is a late complication due to vitamin B deficiency, resulting from malnutrition. These alcoholics have a condition called hepatic **encephalopathy**, caused by diminished capacity of the liver to metabolize and detoxify chemicals in the body. Symptoms of Wernicke-Korsakoff syndrome include agitation, confusion, and altered personality. There is **peripheral neuropathy** (damage to peripheral nerves), which is symmetrical and affects the lower extremities. If untreated, this syndrome can further cause brain (cerebellum) degeneration, abnormal gait (walking), memory deficits (retrograde amnesia), and difficulty with abstract thinking and the acquisition of new learning (anterograde amnesia). Even if successfully treated with vitamin therapy, patients may still have amnesia (a condition called Korsakoff Syndrome).

Fetal alcohol syndrome is a condition that occurs in infants born to alcoholic mothers. Prenatal exposure to alcohol can impair and retard fetal development and growth. Affected infants have a characteristic appearance that consists of a flat nose, flat mid face, small head size, short stature, and a thin upper lip. Approximately 50% are mentally deficient and most others exhibit intellectual deficits. Affected babies typically suffer from poor coordination, decreased adipose (fat) tissue, cleft palate, **attention deficit hyperactivity disorder** (ADHD), decreased muscle tone, heart defects, eye/ear defects, and smaller jaw.

Alcoholic **myopathy** (disorder affecting muscle tissue) can be either acute (rapid onset of symptoms) or chronic (slower onset to develop symptoms). Acute alcoholic myopathy can involve symptoms such as muscular cramps, weakness, swelling, and tenderness in affected areas of muscle. Chronic alcoholic myopathy can be painless, but is associated with weakness due to nerve atrophy.

Demographics

Alcoholism is a widespread and costly problem. Even though use has declined since 1981, two of three American adults drink alcoholic beverages. Approximately 6.5% to 10% of the total U.S. population are heavy drinkers and they consume 50% of all the alcohol ingested annually. Alcohol is heavily implicated in tragic events and is involved in 50% of all crimes, 50% of all fatal car accidents, 33% of all boat/aviation deaths and drowning, and 50% of all accidental death, suicides, and murder. Approximately 50% of alcoholics are not diagnosed, because alcoholics rarely admit to excessive consumption. In approximately 50% of Chinese, Japanese, and Koreans, an enzyme called aldehyde dehydrogenase is absent. This is the enzyme that breaks down alcohol in the liver. Thus in populations who do not have the enzyme, alcohol-related problems are less likely, because persons with this deficiency will become sick (face flushing, racing heart rate) when they consume alcohol. Persons who develop nerve damage as a result of chronic alcoholism have a greater mortality rate than the general population. Fetal alcohol syndrome is estimated to occur in 5.2 per 10,000 live births in the United States. Women are more likely to develop alcoholic myopathy more than men, because women can develop the complication with 40% less consumption than males.

Causes and symptoms

Studies of adopted twins reveal that children of alcoholics have a greater propensity for alcoholism even though they were adopted away from the alcoholic parents. Additionally, research indicated that children of nonalcoholic parents are less likely to develop alcoholism even when adopted into families with an alcoholic parent(s). Adopted children of alcoholic parents have four times a greater risk of developing alcoholism than those born of nonalcoholic parents. The cause is ultimately a combination of genetic and environmental factors, and poor prevention programs among high-risk target populations.

Diagnosis

Diagnosis of neurologic disease is based on clinical signs and symptoms. Psychometric testing, psychological evaluation, and appropriate medical tests (neuroimaging, blood chemistry, liver profiles, differential cell count) can help establish the diagnosis. Alcoholics can exhibit disorders in multiple organ systems, and careful, comprehensive examination is necessary in order to stage the disease and execute an effective interventional treatment plan. No single test can diagnose alcoholism. The diagnosis can be made once a careful evaluation of all the clinical data is available. Criminal information related to drunk driving can also help establish the diagnosis.

Treatment team

The treatment for medical-related disorders can include a psychiatrist, **neurologist**, and members of an inpatient medical ward in a hospital or psychiatric unit. Professional psychotherapist services are necessary to initiate an interventional treatment program. Monitoring and follow-up care with primary care practitioners and specialists is part of a well-integrated treatment program.

Treatment

Acute management of alcohol intoxication is supportive in nature, and patients are monitored and treated if heart or lung problems develop. Patients may require intravenous fluid replacement (due to fluid loss from sweating and fever). Agitation can be treated with medications called **benzodiazepines**. Wernickes' syndrome can be reversed with IV thiamine replacement, and withdrawal seizures can be treated with antiepileptic medication. Damage to muscles (chronic alcoholic myopathy) can be treated by supplementation of deficient vitamins and special diets. This initial management of detoxification usually requires inpatient treatment ranging from three to 10 days. Patients must undergo intensive inpatient or outpatient psychotherapy, and a long process of recovery and rehabilitation.

Recovery and rehabilitation

Involvement in nonprofessional community-centered support groups such as Alcoholics Anonymous (AA) that utilize the "12-step" recovery approach is helpful for maintaining sobriety. During early recovery, patients still exhibit mood swings and compulsions to drink. Patients should attempt to receive positive support from family and friends, take rest and good nutrition, and seek to share experiences with other alcoholics (e.g., through self-help groups). Patients should also receive professional psychotherapy treatment from a clinician with special certifications in addictions counseling, or from a specialist in forensic psychotherapy. Typical treatment using psychological techniques include cognitive behavioral therapy and motivational enhancement therapy.

Clinical trials

Clinical trials are currently recruiting patients for government-sponsored medical research (National Institute on Alcohol Abuse and Alcoholics). Studies include the role of dopamine in response to alcohol, and the effects of another neurotransmitter, serotonin, in alcoholism.

Prognosis

The prognosis depends on the motivation of the patient to stop drinking alcohol, and the extent of organ damage, which varies with each case. The prognosis can be favorable in some patients (with minimal organ damage) that successfully complete long-term intensive psychotherapy and stop drinking.

Special concerns

Psychotherapy treatment may be long term and complicated. Frequently, there may be psychological problems that occur within families who have an alcoholic. Alcoholics may cause violence to or abuse of family members.

Resources

BOOKS

Goetz, Christopher G., et al., eds. *Textbook of Clinical Neurology*, 1st ed. Philadelphia: W. B. Saunders Company, 1999.

Noble, John., et al., eds. *Textbook of Primary Care Medicine*, 3rd ed. St. Louis: Mosby, Inc., 2001.

Rakel, Robert, A. *Textbook of Family Practice*, 6th ed. Philadelphia: W. B. Saunders Company, 2002.

PERIODICALS

American Academy of Pediatrics. "Fetal Alcohol Syndrome and Alcohol-related Neurodevelopment Disorders (RD9948)." *Pediatrics* 106, no. 2 (August 2000).

Finlayson, R. E., and R. D. Hurt. "Medical Consequences of Heavy Drinking by the Elderly." *Alcohol Problems and Aging* (1998): 193–212.

Fuller, R., and S. Hiller. "Alcoholism Treatment in the United States: An Overview." *Alcohol Research and Health* 23, no. 2 (1999).

Oscar-Berman, M., and C. Epstein. "Impairments of Brain and Behavior: The Neurological Effects of Alcohol." *Alcohol Health and Research World* 21, no. 1 (1997).

Vittadini, G., and G. Biscaldi. "Alcoholic Polyneuropathy: A Clinic and Epidemiological Study." *Alcohol and Alcoholism* 36, no. 5 (2001).

WEBSITES

National Institute on Alcohol Abuse and Alcoholism. <http://www.niaaa.nih.gov/> (May 9, 2004).

ORGANIZATIONS

Alcoholics Anonymous. Grand Central Station, P. O. Box 459, New York, NY 10163. <http://www.aa.org/>.

National Council on Alcoholism and Drug Dependence, Inc., 20 Exchange Place, Suite 2902, New York, NY 10005. (212) 269-7797 or (800) NCA-CALL; Fax: (212) 269-7510. <http://www.ncadd.org/>.

Key Terms

Amniocentesis A procedure performed at 16-18 weeks of pregnancy in which a needle is inserted through a woman's abdomen into her uterus to draw out a small sample of the amniotic fluid from around the baby for analysis. Either the fluid itself or cells from the fluid can be used for a variety of tests to obtain information about genetic disorders and other medical conditions in the fetus.

Astrocytes Types of neuroglial cells in the central nervous system that help support other nerve cells.

Chorionic villus sampling A medical procedure done during weeks 10-12 of a pregnancy. A needle is inserted into the placenta and a small amount of fetal tissue is withdrawn for analysis.

Chromosome A structure in the nucleus of a cell that contains a thread of DNA containing the genetic information (genes). Humans have 46 chromosomes in 23 pairs.

DNA Deoxyribonucleic acid; the genetic material in cells that holds the inherited instructions for growth, development, and cellular functioning.

Histologic Pertaining to histology, the study of cells and tissues at the microscopic level.

Hydrocephalus An abnormal accumulation of cerebrospinal fluid within the brain. This accumulation can be harmful by pressing on and damaging brain structures.

Quadriparesis Partial or incomplete paralysis of all four limbs.

Laith Farid Gulli, MD
Michael Mooney, MA, CAC

Alexander disease

Definition

Alexander disease (ALX) is a rare and often fatal nervous system disorder that primarily occurs in infants and children.

Description

The main features of Alexander disease are progressive mental impairment and loss of motor control. Based on the age of onset and type of symptoms present, ALX has been classified into three forms: infantile, juvenile, and adult. Alexander disease is named for Dr. W. Stewart Alexander, an Australian pathologist who first described an infantile case in 1949. Since that time, 80% of cases described have also been the infantile form. About 14% of patients have the juvenile form, and adult cases are rare. All three forms of ALX are unified by the presence of Rosenthal fibers (RF), microscopic protein aggregates that are found in astrocytes in the brain and spinal cord. Though Rosenthal fibers are associated with other conditions, the numbers and distribution of RF-containing astrocytes are unique to Alexander disease. ALX is one of the leukodystrophies, a group of disorders characterized by imperfect formation or maintenance of white matter, the myelin sheath (insulation) that covers the nerves in the brain and spinal cord. Patients with ALX usually display loss of white matter, most prominently in the frontal lobes of the brain.

Demographics

Alexander disease is thought to be quite rare with approximately 200 cases described. Although there are no known prevalence estimates, the disease has been reported in both males and females and in various ethnic and racial groups.

Causes and symptoms

Most cases of Alexander disease are genetic, caused by a dominant mutation (change) in the glial fibrillary acidic protein (GFAP) gene on chromosome 17. Usually this mutation occurs randomly in an individual without a family history of the disease. There are reports of rare familial cases with affected siblings. Therefore, unaffected parents of a child with ALX are at a low risk to have another affected child. Individuals with ALX who live long enough to reproduce have a 50% chance for an affected child. Since GFAP mutations have not been found in all cases of ALX, there may rarely be other genetic or nongenetic explanations for this disease.

The glial fibrillary acidic protein gene encodes a protein by the same name. GFAP helps to provide structural stability to the astrocytes, which are supporting cells in the brain similar to blood vessels. GFAP is found in Rosenthal fibers. Reports have suggested that GFAP gene mutations result in a toxic gain of function of the protein (GFAP) that leads to a minimal or absent production of myelin. As of 2003, the precise mechanisms by which GFAP mutations cause ALX were unresolved.

In the infantile form of the disease, average age of onset is six months, with a range of birth to two years. Affected children tend to have progressive physical and **mental retardation** with loss of previously attained milestones. Head size becomes increasingly large and the forehead appears prominent as a result of **megalencephaly** (enlarged head and brain). Other disease manifestations include **seizures**, **spasticity** (stiffness of the arms and legs), quadriparesis, feeding problems, and **ataxia** (poor coordination). **Hydrocephalus** may also occur, especially in children with early onset of symptoms.

The juvenile form of ALX usually presents between age four and the early teens. Patients may develop some or all of the following symptoms: speech problems, difficulty swallowing, frequent vomiting, spasticity of the legs, ataxia, gradual intellectual decline, seizures, megalencephaly, or breathing problems. White matter abnormalities in the juvenile form are less prominent than in the infantile form.

The adult form of ALX represents the most variable and least common form of the disorder. Patients with the adult variant may have symptoms that mimic **multiple sclerosis**, or may display symptoms similar to the juvenile form of the disease, except with later onset and slower progression. White matter changes may or may not be present. Some adult cases have been discovered by chance when an autopsy reveals Rosenthal fibers, a characteristic finding of this disease.

Diagnosis

A diagnosis of Alexander disease is usually based on radiologic findings and/or genetic test results in an individual who has symptoms suggestive of this condition. Radiologic studies that may aid in diagnosis include **magnetic resonance imaging (MRI)**, a computerized tomography (**CT**) **scan**, or a head ultrasound. For example, an MRI of an individual with the infantile form typically reveals white matter loss that involves the frontal lobes of the brain, abnormalities of the basal ganglia and thalamus, and possibly, enlargement of the ventricles. Genetic testing is accomplished by looking for known or detectable mutations in the GFAP gene. In up to 94% of cases of ALX, a GFAP mutation is found. Prenatal diagnosis for couples with an affected child can be performed when the mutation responsible for ALX is known. The DNA of a fetus can be tested using cells obtained from chorionic villus sampling (CVS) or amniocentesis.

Prior to the discovery of the gene responsible for the disease, diagnosis of ALX was made by demonstration of Rosenthal fibers in a **biopsy** or autopsy sample from the brain. Though genetic testing has largely replaced these histologic studies, a brain biopsy or autopsy may be indicated in select cases if the diagnosis cannot be made through other means.

Treatment team

Management of ALX usually involves the services of multiple medical specialists. In addition to primary health care professionals, patients may require the care of specialists in neurology, neurosurgery, physical therapy, occupational therapy, social services, orthopedics, and gastroenterology. A genetic specialist, such as a clinical geneticist or a genetic counselor, may be helpful to the patient and family, especially at the time of diagnosis or prior to genetic testing. Families may also benefit from psychological counseling and contact with other families affected by ALX or another **leukodystrophy**.

Treatment

There is no cure for Alexander disease. Treatment, which is symptomatic and supportive, primarily consists of attention to general care and nutritional needs, antibiotic therapy for infections, and management of associated complications such as anti-epileptic drug therapy for seizures. Surgical interventions, including placement of a feeding tube and/or shunting for hydrocephalus, may also be required. Orthopedic surgery for scoliosis has been reported in a case of Alexander disease.

Recovery and rehabilitation

Given the rarity of ALX, the potential for rehabilitation in this disorder is unknown. Depending upon the type, severity, and rate of progression of symptoms in a given individual, interventions such as physical, occupational, and speech therapy may be recommended for management of disease-related complications. In severe cases of ALX, consideration may be given to placement in a residential care facility that can provide 24-hour care and support services.

Clinical trials

As of 2003, there were no **clinical trials** for patients with Alexander disease. As more is learned about how mutations in the GFAP gene cause disease, it is hoped that new therapies may be developed in the future. As of December 2003, two laboratories were conducting research on the GFAP gene; both accept contact from patients and families. They are the Children's National Medical Center—Center for Genetic Medicine (202-884-6065 or <egordon@cnmcresearch.org>) and the University of Alabama at Birmingham, Michael Brenner Research Lab (608-263-9191 or <messing@waisman.wisc.edu>).

Prognosis

The course of Alexander disease is generally one of regression and progressive neurologic degeneration. Prognosis varies according to the form of the disease. Lifespan for patients with the infantile from is significantly reduced; affected individuals live anywhere from one to 10 years of age. For the juvenile form of the disease, survival ranges from several years after onset to the late teens, with rare cases living several decades. Due to the rarity of the adult form, little is known about the prognosis for this ALX variant.

Resources

BOOKS

Johnson, Anne B. "Alexander disease." Chapter 34. In *Handbook of Clinical Neurology*, Vol 22 (66), edited by Hugo Moser. Amsterdam: Elsevier Press, 1996.

PERIODICALS

Johnson, Anne B. "Alexander Disease: A Review and the Gene." *International Journal of Developmental Neuroscience* 20 (June–August 2003): 391–394.

Li, R., A. Messing, J. E. Goldman, and M. Brenner. "GFAP Mutations in Alexander Disease." *International Journal of Developmental Neuroscience* 20 (June–August 2002): 259–268.

Schiffmann, R., and O. Boespflug-Tanguay. "An Update on the Leukodystrophies." *Current Opinion in Neurology* 14 (December 2001): 789–794.

WEBSITES

The National Institute of Neurological Disorders and Stroke (NINDS). *Alexander Disease Information Page.* (February 18, 2004). <http://www.ninds.nih.gov/health_and_medical/disorders/alexand_doc.htm>.

The Waisman Center. *Alexander Disease Project.* (February 18, 2004). <http://www.waisman.wisc.edu/alexander/index.html>.

ORGANIZATIONS

National Organization for Rare Disorders. P.O. Box 1968, 55 Kensonia Avenue, Danbury, CT 06813. (203) 744-0100 or (800) 999-NORD; Fax: (203) 798-2291. orphan@rarediseases.org. <http://www.rarediseases.org>.

United Leukodystrophy Foundation. 2304 Highland Drive, Sycamore, IL 60178. (815) 895-3211 or (800) 728-5483; Fax: (815) 895-2432. ulf@tbcnet.com. <http://www.ulf.org>.

Dawn J. Cardeiro, MS, CGC

▎Alpers' disease

Definition

Alpers' disease is an early-onset, progressive neurological degenerative disease that severely affects the brain and liver. In the familial (inherited) form of the disorder, it is transmitted as a recessive condition, which means that parents are unaffected, but both are carriers. Carrier parents have a 25% risk of having their biological child affected with Alpers' disease.

Description

Alpers' disease was first described by the late **neurologist** Alfons Maria Jakob (1884–1931). The disease was characterized and published by Bernard Jacob Alpers, Erna Christensen, and Knud Haraldsen Krabbe; thus, Alpers' disease is also known as Christensen's disease or Christensen-Krabbe disease. Additionally, the disease is known as progressive sclerosing poliodystrophy. Alpers' disease afflicts children and is eventually fatal. Degeneration in cognitive processes (reasoning ability) and muscular involvement caused by the disease is unrelenting and relatively rapid. Physically, children with Alpers' disease lose control of their muscle movements. The ramifications of this disorder can significantly affect the emotional state of the person with Alpers' disease, along with family members caring for them.

Demographics

Alpers' disease is a rare disorder. Due to complications related to the diagnosis of Alpers' disease, it is difficult to estimate how often it occurs in the population. Both genders are affected with equal frequency.

Causes and symptoms

Children with Alpers' disease usually develop symptoms between the ages of three months and five years old. Initially, the first symptom early in life is **seizures** (convulsions). These children tend to be hypotonic (unable to achieve normal muscle tone) and their limbs seem to be stiff. This is usually followed by the failure to reach cognitive and developmental milestones. **Mental retardation** is progressive in these children.

Among the most devastating features of this disorder is the progressive **dementia**. In children with Alpers' disease, mental deterioration can occur rapidly. The pathological nature of the defect involves an area of the brain called the cerebrum in which a specific part (the gray matter) is affected. Spastic quadriplegia (inability to use and control movements of the arms and legs) can develop in

Key Terms

Hypotonia   Decreased muscle tone.

Mitochondrial DNA   The genetic material found in mitochondria, the organelles that generate energy for the cell. Because reproduction is by cloning, mitochondrial DNA is usually passed along female lines.

Spastic quadriplegia   Inability to use and control movements of the arms and legs.

the later stages of the disorder. Blindness is also observed, and this is usually due to a condition called optic atrophy. In optic atrophy, the optic nerve degenerates, resulting in the inability to process visual information from the eye to the brain.

The liver is also affected. Liver conditions that these children experience are jaundice or complete liver failure in more severe cases. Researchers at the National Institutes of Health (NIH) consider that children with Alpers' disease are often misdiagnosed as having childhood jaundice or liver failure. This is due to the problems associated with making a diagnosis in living patients.

Currently, the specific mechanism, whether genetic, environmental, or both, that causes this disease is unknown. Scientists assume that Alpers' disease is caused by an underlying metabolic defect. Mutations in the DNA of the mitochondria (DNA that is a separate genome from the nucleus) have been associated with this disorder. The mitochondria functions to produce energy to tissues and is particularly important for tissues such as the brain.

Diagnosis

Currently, the only way to arrive at a definitive diagnosis is by autopsy following the death of the child. A postmortem examination of the brain and liver is required.

Treatment team

Because children affected with Alpers' disease usually develop convulsions, they are first directed to a neurologist. An experienced neurologist is always necessary in order to get the appropriate palliative (supportive) care and treatment for these seizures. As the disease progresses, occupational therapists can provide aids for positioning and comfort. Due to the rapid nature of the disorder and the unavailability of treatment to slow the progression, children with Alpers' disease are usually unable to attend school. There are, however, support specialists and organizations that have experience with severe neurological disorders. The National Organization for Rare Disorder can

help affected families find local support organizations. There are also organizations such as the Genetic Alliance that help identify support groups to allow families affected by genetic diseases to find other families with the same or related disorders. These organizations can be a tremendous help in alleviating the many emotional and situational burdens that arise by allowing family members to talk to other families that have experience with diseases such as Alpers' disease. Physical therapy can also be helpful to maintain range of motion in the child's arms and legs for as long as possible.

Treatment

There is no cure for Alpers' disease. Also, there is currently no treatment that will slow the progression of the disease. Therefore, treatment is aimed at symptoms such as the seizures. The neurologist must consider the choice of anticonvulsant carefully to avoid ones that may have an adverse effect on the liver.

Recovery and rehabilitation

As Alpers' disease is progressive and eventually fatal, emphasis is placed not upon recovery, but on maintaining functionality as long as possible. Several lifestyle adaptations must be addressed, as children with Alpers' disease eventually require full-time personal care. Depending on how severely and how rapidly the symptoms develop, families may require structural changes such as wheelchair access or other household modifications.

Clinical trials

As of February 2004, there are no ongoing **clinical trials** designed specifically to treat or study Alpers' diseases.

Prognosis

The prognosis for children with Alpers' disease is poor. Affected individuals typically die within the first decade of life, but in some cases of rapid progression, death can occur in as little as a few months after symptoms become apparent. Seizures can be particularly devastating, as they are often continuous and can lead to death. Other causes of death include complications related to liver disease or cardio-respiratory failure.

Resources

PERIODICALS

Alpers, B. B. "Diffuse Progressive Degeneration of the Grey Matter of the Cerebrum." *Archives of Neurology and Psychiatry* (1931) 25: 469–505.

Blackwood, W., P. H. Buxton, J. N. Cumings, D. J. Robertson, and S. M. Tucker. "Diffuse Cerebral Degeneration in

Infancy (Alpers' Disease)." *Archives of Disease in Childhood* 38, (1963): 193–204.

Boyd, S. G., A. Harden, J. Egger, and G. Pampiglione. "Progressive Neuronal Degeneration of Childhood with Liver Disease ('Alpers' Disease'): Characteristic Neurophysiological Features." *Neuropediatrics* 17, no. 2 (1986 May): 75–80.

Christensen, E., and K. H. Krabbe. "Poliodystrophia Cerebri Progressiva (Infantilis): Report of a Case." *Archives of Neurology* 61 (1949): 28–43.

Fitzgerald, J. F., R. Troncone, and M. A. Del Rosario. "Clinical Quiz. Alpers' Disease." *J Pediatr Gastroenterol Nutr.* 28, no.5 (May 1999): 501, 509.

Narkewicz, M. R., R. J. Sokol, B. Beckwith, J. Sondheimer, and A. Silverman. "Liver Involvement in Alpers' Disease." *J Pediatr.* 119, no.2, (Aug 1991): 260–7.

OTHER

National Institutes of Health (NIH). *NINDS Alpers' Disease Information Page.* February 3, 2004 (March 30, 2004). <http://www.ninds.nih.gov/health_and_medical/disorders/alpersdisease_doc.htm>.

ORGANIZATIONS

Genetic Alliance, Inc. 4301 Connecticut Ave. NW, Suite 404, Washington, DC 20008-2369. (202) 966-5557; Fax: (202) 966-8553. info@geneticalliance.org. <http://www.geneticalliance.org>.

March of Dimes Birth Defects Foundation. 1275 Mamaroneck Avenue, White Plains, NY 10605. (914) 428-7100 or (888) MODIMES; Fax: (914) 428-8203. askus@marchofdimes.com. <http://www.marchofdimes.com>.

National Institute of Diabetes and Digestive and Kidney Diseases (NIDDK). National Institutes of Health, Bldg. 31, Rm. 9A04, Bethesda, MD 20892-2560. (301) 496-3583. <http://www.niddk.nih.gov>.

National Organization for Rare Disorders (NORD). P.O. Box 1968, 55 Kenosia Avenue, Danbury, CT 06813-1968. (203) 744-0100 or (800) 999-NORD; Fax: (203) 798-2291. orphan@rarediseases.org. <http://www.rarediseases.org>.

Bryan Richard Cobb, PhD

Alternating hemiplegia

Definition

Alternating hemiplegia is a very rare condition characterized by recurrent episodes of temporary paralysis.

Description

Alternating hemiplegia usually begins affecting a child before the age of four. Bouts of recurrent, temporary paralysis may involve the arms, legs, facial muscles, and/or eye muscles. The manifestations may range from

> **Key Terms**
>
> **Dystonia** Abnormal muscle movements and stiffening.
>
> **Hemiplegia** Paralysis on one side of the body.
>
> **Migraine** A type of chronic headache caused by a cascade of events in the brain, including initial dilatation or widening of blood vessels, followed by chemical release and then painful spasms of blood vessels in the brain.
>
> **Paralysis** Loss of ability to move a part of the body.

numbness or tingling in the affected body part to complete paralysis. The episodes last between minutes and days, and are usually resolved by sleep. A variety of other neurological problems may also be present in children with alternating hemiplegia.

A less-severe variant of alternating hemiplegia is called "benign nocturnal alternating hemiplegia of childhood." In this variant, a child awakens from sleep to a state of paralysis that resolves completely over 2–15 minutes. Children with this variant do not suffer from other associated neurological problems. This particular condition is thought to be a variant of a migraine **headache**.

Demographics

Alternating hemiplegia is quite rare, with fewer than 100 diagnosed cases in the United States, and fewer than 240 diagnosed patients worldwide.

Causes and symptoms

The underlying cause of alternating hemiplegia is unknown. Benign nocturnal alternating hemiplegia of childhood is thought to be a variant of migraine headache, and therefore may be caused by a similar mechanism (abnormal dilatation of blood vessels in the brain, followed by chemical release and then painful spasms of the blood vessels).

Individual episodes seem to occur spontaneously, although in some individuals they may be precipitated by stress, sleep deprivation, or viral illness.

Symptoms of alternating hemiplegia

Episodes of alternating hemiplegia come on suddenly during wakefulness, and can last between hours and days. Either or both sides of the body may become numb, tingly, or completely paralyzed. Limbs may be limp or stiff (dystonic). Facial and eye muscles are often affected, as well as the limbs. Children with alternating hemiplegia also usually experience progressive difficulty with balance and walking, excess sweating, mental impairment, developmental delay, problems with body temperature, shortness of breath, and **seizures**. Although sleep can ameliorate the symptoms, the symptoms may recur upon awakening.

Symptoms of benign nocturnal alternating hemiplegia of childhood

Symptoms of benign nocturnal alternating hemiplegia of childhood may begin when the child is about two years of age. Boys appear to be more frequently affected than girls. Episodes may be preceded by several days by headache, abnormal irritability, and oppositional behavior. The actual episodes commence when a child is asleep, causing the child to awaken suddenly, screaming or crying and drooling. Although the child may appear to be awake, he or she usually does not respond normally to questions or commands. Usually only one side of the body appears limp and paralyzed. The episodes usually last about fifteen minutes, end with the child falling back into sleep, and are completely resolved when the child awakens again. Some children experience headache and vomiting with each episode, further underscoring the proposed link with migraine headache. Although children with this condition do not seem to exhibit any permanent effects of their hemiplegic episodes, and generally have normal intelligence, there does appear to be an increased risk of hyperactivity, irritability, and oppositional defiant disorder in children who experience episodes of benign nocturnal alternating hemiplegia of childhood.

Diagnosis

There are no available tests to definitively diagnose either form of alternating hemiplegia. These disorders are diagnosed by ruling out other possible reasons for a child's episodes and symptoms.

Treatment team

Children with the more benign form of alternating hemiplegia may not require an extensive treatment team, other than a **neurologist** to help in diagnosis. Children with the more severe form of alternating hemiplegia may require a neurologist, as well as other specialists to help with their progressive problems with walking, such as a physical and occupational therapist. Children with this disorder usually require a specialized educational setting.

Treatment

There is no cure for either form of alternating hemiplegia. A drug called flunarizine has been used to treat the more severe type of alternating hemiplegia, in an effort to decrease the frequency of hemiplegic episodes, as well as

their duration and severity. Some researchers believe that decreasing the number and severity of attacks may improve the child's overall cognitive prognosis, by preventing damage to the brain.

Prognosis

The classic form of alternating hemiplegia has a poor prognosis, with progressively severe impairment of mobility and cognitive functioning, requiring long-term care. About half of all children with benign nocturnal alternating hemiplegia of childhood outgrow their episodes over time.

Resources

PERIODICALS

Chayes-Vischer, V. "Benign alternating hemiplegia of childhood: six patients and long-term follow-up." *Neurology* 57, no. 8 (23 October 2001): 1491–1493.

Grigg-Damberger, M. "Neurologic disorders masquerading as pediatric sleep problems." *Pediatric clinics of North America* 51, no. 1 (1 February 2004): 89–115.

Kavanaugh, M. "Benign alternating hemiplegia of childhood: new features and associations." *Neurology* 62, no. 4 (24 February 2004): 672.

WEBSITES

National Institute of Neurological Disorders and Stroke (NINDS). *NINDS Alternating Hemiplegia Information Page.* January 17, 2002. (June 3, 2004). <http://lwww.ninds.nih.gov/health_and_medical/disorders/alternatinghemiplegia.htm>.

ORGANIZATIONS

Alternating Hemiplegia of Childhood Foundation. Richard George, President. 11700 Merriman Road , Livonia, Michigan 48150. 888-557-5757. richard7@ameritech.net. <http://www.ahckids.org/index.htm>.

Rosalyn Carson-DeWitt, MD

▌Alzheimer disease

Definition

Alzheimer disease is a neurological disorder characterized by slow, progressive memory loss due to a gradual loss of brain cells. Alzheimer disease significantly affects cognitive (thought) capabilities and, eventually, affected individuals become incapacitated. Alzheimer-related issues can cause emotional and financial upheaval for both the individuals with the disease and their families. Alzheimer disease is the most common form of **dementia** (loss of intellectual function) and, according to the National Institutes of Health (NIH), it is the fourth leading cause of death in adults.

Key Terms

Amyloid plaques A waxy protein substance that forms clumps in brain tissues, leading to brain cell death.

Autosomal dominant disorder An inheritance pattern where an affected parent has a 50% chance of passing on a genetic mutation responsible for the disorder to their offspring in each pregnancy.

Dementia Deterioration or loss of intellectual faculties, reasoning power, and memory due to organic brain disease.

Neurofibrillary tangles An accumulation of twisted protein fragments inside nerve cells, and one of the characteristic structural abnormalities found in the brains of patients with Alzheimer disease.

Description

The condition was first described in 1906 by Alois Alzheimer, a German physician. Alzheimer characterized two abnormal structures in the brain of a woman with dementia that are now considered the hallmarks of the disease: amyloid plaques and neurofibrillary tangles. The nature of Alzheimer disease is progressive. Initially, dementia is manifested by barely noticeable memory deficits. Eventually, the memory loss becomes more severe until it is incapacitating. Other symptoms such as confusion, the inability to articulate words correctly, and hallucinations occur with varying degrees. Emotional problems such as easy agitation, poor judgment, and feelings of withdrawal are also common in the early stages. Affected individuals are also likely to develop **seizures**, hypertonicity (increased muscle movements), and incontinence. Without treatment or supervision, death often results from malnutrition or pneumonia. From the initial symptoms, disease progression can last up to 25 years, although typically the duration ranges from eight to 10 years.

Demographics

Dementia is thought to affect between 25–50% of individuals 85 years or older. The risk of developing Alzheimer disease increases with age and is independent of sex or geographical location (although there are environmental toxic agents that can impair various cognitive functions, including memory loss). A genetic association has been found for higher risk of developing Alzheimer disease in individuals with mutations in a particular gene who are also African American or Caribbean Hispanics.

This association is greatest in individuals with a positive family history of dementia.

Approximately 10% of people 65 years or older are at risk for developing significant memory loss. More than half of these individuals (5% of all individuals 65 years or older) have Alzheimer disease. Approximately four in 10,000 individuals between the ages of 40 and 60 are at risk for having Alzheimer disease.

Causes and symptoms

Although there are several known causes of Alzheimer disease, about 75% of cases are sporadic and occur without a clear cause; this percentage represents people without a family history of the disorder. Scientists assume that these cases are due to a combination of unknown genetic predisposing factors and environmental exposures. Although various narcotics, therapeutic drugs, viruses, and toxins have been implicated in the etiology of the disease, there is currently no proof that they can cause Alzheimer disease.

Genetic basis for Alzheimer disease

Of all persons with Alzheimer disease, up to 25% of cases are thought to be part of a familial-based inheritance pattern and therefore are only determined based on family history or genetic test results. In general, these forms of Alzheimer disease are inherited as an autosomal dominant disorder, meaning that affected individuals have a 50% chance of passing on the mutated gene to their offspring in each pregnancy. There is a late-onset familial form (AD2), three early-onset familial forms (AD1, AD3, AD4), and a form of Alzheimer disease associated with Down syndrome.

Down syndrome and Alzheimer disease

Less than 1% of all cases of Alzheimer disease are due to a chromosomal defect called trisomy 21 (also known as Down syndrome). This occurs when there are three copies of genes found on chromosome 21, usually due to a person having an extra chromosome 21. These individuals usually develop Alzheimer disease after the age of 40. The APP gene, which encodes the amyloid precursor protein and is implicated in the pathogenesis of Alzheimer disease, is localized to chromosome 21; it is felt that people with Down syndrome overproduce this protein, resulting in its accumulation in the brain. The excess protein is thought to cause the disease.

Early-onset familial Alzheimer disease

A low percentage (2%) of Alzheimer cases results from a familial form of the disease in which there is an early onset of symptoms (AD1, AD3, and AD4), usually occurring before the age of 60. Age of onset usually occurs around 40–50 years, but can occur as early as 30 years.

The majority of these persons have family members that are also affected. The clinical manifestations are similar to the adult-onset form, with loss of memory and cognitive ability. In this form of Alzheimer disease, there are several chromosomal locations of genes implicated in causing the disease.

AD1 accounts for approximately 10–15% of early-onset Alzheimer disease and involves a protein called presenilin 1 that has a mutation in the gene that encodes it called PSEN1, which is found on chromosome 14. AD3 accounts for 20–70% of the early-onset familial form and is caused by mutations in APP found on chromosome 21, which encodes a protein called amyloid beta A4. AD4 is extremely rare and is caused by mutations in PSEN2, localized to chromosome 1, and encodes a protein called presenilin 2.

Late-onset familial Alzheimer disease

The late-onset familial form of Alzheimer disease (AD2) accounts for approximately 15–25% of all cases. These familial cases are seemingly indistinguishable from sporadic cases when observed clinically, but can be recognized based on molecular genetic testing. However, there is no clear chromosomal location for a gene directly responsible for the disease. Therefore, this complex type may involve many susceptibility genes. These familial cases are most likely due to multiple genes that make these individuals susceptible to developing the disease. For example, the APOE e4 gene on chromosome 19 associated with late-onset Alzheimer disease reduces the age in which symptoms develop by an unknown mechanism. There are many other candidate genes that are thought to modify Alzheimer disease risks and these genes, with various chromosomal locations, have been linked to the disease in different families.

Development (pathogenesis) of Alzheimer disease

Although scientists know how brain cells of persons with Alzheimer disease are affected, and additionally understand some of the genetic explanations of the disease, the precise cause of Alzheimer disease is still unclear. For example, it is known that accumulations of clumps of proteins called amyloid plaques outside brain cells and accumulation of altered proteins inside the cells called neurofibrillary tangles are characteristic of Alzheimer disease; however, it is unclear how these accumulated proteins cause brain cells to die.

According to the Alzheimer's Disease and Related Disorders Association, Inc., there are seven stages that characterize the disease:

- Stage 1: No decline in function is yet noted. This group includes individuals who may carry predictive gene mutations but have no symptoms, or those who will be affected by other unknown mechanisms.

- Stage 2: Normal function in general, although the person is aware of a subtle cognitive decline.

- Stage 3: Early Alzheimer disease. Persons experience difficulty in performing complex tasks that require cognitive skills.

- Stage 4: Mild Alzheimer disease. Persons require assistance with common tasks such as paying bills and balancing a checkbook.

- Stage 5: Moderate Alzheimer disease. Persons require assistance in making personal everyday decisions such as choosing appropriate clothing for the weather or ordering from a menu.

- Stage 6: Moderately severe Alzheimer disease. Persons require assistance dressing, bathing, and using the toilet. Urinary and bowel incontinence may be present.

- Stage 7: Severe Alzheimer disease. The vocabulary shrinks to only a few words; then little or no verbal communication is heard. The ability to walk is lost, followed by an inability to maintain a sitting posture in a chair. Eventually, the person experiences profound lack of purposeful muscle control, is totally dependent for care, and cannot smile or hold up his or her head.

Diagnosis

Alzheimer disease is diagnosed clinically by a physician, postmortem by a histopathologist (a scientist who studies diseased tissues by their various staining patterns), or genetically by identifying mutations in genes associated with the disease.

The gold standard for diagnosis of Alzheimer disease is through autopsy examination by an experienced pathologist. Detection of amyloid plaques in the brain by histopathology is the most conclusive diagnostic tool. This is performed using antibodies that bind to the particular amyloid proteins and can be visualized by microscopic evaluation, as the antibodies are tagged with a fluorescent or colorimetric molecule. A positive result would involve a significantly greater number of plaques compared to age-matched controls. Other brain defects that characterize the disease, such as abnormal nerve cell configurations called intraneuronal neurofibrillary tangles, can also be detected by histopathology by the same methods. A clinical diagnosis by a physician accounts for 80–90% of patients diagnosed with Alzheimer disease.

Clinical diagnosis

A physician can use a number of different tests to assess memory skills, and, combined with any observed changes in the individual's behavior, they can help make a diagnosis of Alzheimer disease. Other tests that are important in diagnosing the disorder can involve laboratory tests that require blood and urine or imaging studies of the

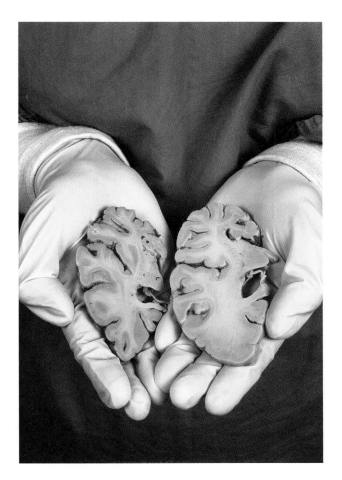

The smaller, darker brain segment on the left is affected by Alzheimer disease; the segment on the right is from a healthy brain. *(Simon Fraser/MRC Unit, Newcastle General Hospital/Science Photo Library. Reproduced by permission.)*

brain. By using neuroimaging studies such as **magnetic resonance imaging (MRI)** scans, physicians have found that patients with Alzheimer disease often have diffuse atrophy (weakening or decrease in size) in a specific area of the brain called the cerebrum.

Genetic diagnosis

It has been shown that there is a significant association of a specific gene called APOE e4 with the development the early-onset form of the disease. There are three different types of Alzheimer disease that have been shown to be caused by mutations in three distinct genes known as APP, PSEN1, and PSEN2. However, determining the genotype (whether a patient carries this associated mutation) is not entirely conclusive. Currently, although APOE e4 mutation analysis can help in diagnosing a patient suspected of having Alzheimer disease, it is not used for predictive testing of these individuals.

Biochemical markers

Although there are no tests to definitively diagnose Alzheimer disease, there are useful biochemical markers that can help distinguish Alzheimer disease from other disorders that involve dementia, including dementia caused by vascular disorders, drugs, or thyroid disease. Fluid that is found in the brain and spinal cord called cerebrospinal fluid can be tested for levels of two proteins, Tau and Aβ42, in patients that develop symptoms of dementia. Aβ42 accumulation in the brain is associated with reduced levels in the cerebrospinal fluid. Accumulation of the Tau protein in the brain is associated with Alzheimer disease. Therefore, increased Tau protein levels and decreased Aβ42 in the cerebrospinal fluid can pinpoint which persons have Alzheimer disease, regardless of the cause or the age of onset.

The score for these tests is numerical and relies heavily on a reference range determined by a patient's age, sex, and the type of equipment used to perform the test. A positive result will only indicate that a patient is at high risk of having Alzheimer disease and requires further analysis for an accurate diagnosis. This test has yet to be widely performed and is, therefore, only available in certain reference laboratories.

Treatment team

Initially, a physician usually recommends counseling by a psychologist or a support group experienced with this disease. After the diagnosis, visits to the physician focus on treating mild behavioral changes such as **depression**. Eventually, treatment requires 24-hour supervision and nursing care. The caretakers are mostly nurses or professionals who are part of various assisted-living programs.

Treatment

Pharmacological treatment

Treatment of Alzheimer disease is mainly palliative (given for comfort) and focuses on mitigating symptoms. Each symptom is treated based on its severity and the other symptoms that are affecting the individual. Most affected individuals will eventually need professional care in assisted living or nursing homes. They require constant supervision as memory loss becomes incapacitating. There are several pharmacological interventions and treatment regimens that are suggested. Patients who have depression are treated with antidepressants. Tacrine is often prescribed to help with some of the behavioral problems and provides modest cognitive benefits in a small percentage of patients. Aricept, Galantamine, and Exelon are more recent drugs used for a similar purpose, and are not believed to cause liver toxicity; the liver must be monitored in those taking Tacrine. Non-steroidal anti-inflammatory drugs

(NSAIDs) are currently being investigated for their use in treating patients with Alzheimer disease.

Coping with the disorder

There are strategies to cope with this disorder and these should be considered in the beginning stages of the disease. Coping mechanisms depend on whether there are family members available for support. If an individual is without family members, relying on community support through neighbors or volunteers of Alzheimer disease organizations will be necessary.

Many precautions can be made early on to avoid difficult or life-threatening situations later, while maintaining everyday activities in the home environment. Dealing with a person with Alzheimer disease with patience is important. Daily tasks should be performed when the person with Alzheimer disease feels best. Informing neighbors of the person's condition is an important first step. Arranging for assistance, depending on the stage of the disorder, will become necessary. As the ability to drive may be compromised fairly early in the disorder, transportation may need to be arranged. There are local chapters of the Alzheimer's Association that offer help with transportation requirements.

In the early period of the disease when memory loss is minimal, it is helpful for family and friends to interact with the affected person, reminding him or her to take medication, eat, keep appointments, and so forth. Family and friends can help sustain the Alzheimer patient's daily living activities. Keeping records is also helpful, particularly if several people are overseeing the patient's care. Additionally, organizing the household so that it is easy to find important items is recommended.

Other helpful coping mechanisms include posting signs to remind patients of important phone numbers, to turn off appliances, and to lock doors. It is important that all electrical cords and appliances are arranged to minimize distraction, and to prevent danger of falling or misuse. Assistance in handling finances is usually necessary. Providing an extra house key for neighbors and setting up a schedule to check on persons with Alzheimer disease is very helpful for both the patient and the family. By utilizing these and other family, neighborhood, and community resources, many people with early Alzheimer disease are able to maintain a successful lifestyle in their home environment for months or years.

Recovery and rehabilitation

For a person with Alzheimer disease, emphasis is placed on maintaining cognitive and physical function for as long as possible. Currently, there is no cure for Alzheimer and, once the symptoms develop, patients do not recover. Instead, they progressively worsen, usually over a period of years. This has many psychosocial and financial ramifications for the patient and the patient's caretakers. Social service workers can help families plan for long-term care, as persons with Alzheimer disease most often eventually require 24-hour assistance with feeding, toileting, bathing, personal safety, and social interaction. Taking care of patients in the later stages can be financially and psychologically draining. Various support systems are available through community mental health centers and national support organizations.

Clinical trials

There are currently many **clinical trials** for the treatment or prevention of Alzheimer disease sponsored by the National Institutes of Health (NIH). Large multi-center clinical trials such as a Phase III clinical trail are aimed at determining whether anti-inflammatory drugs delay age-related cognitive decline. (Contact information: UCLA Neuropsychiatric Institute, Los Angeles, California, 90024. Recruiter: Andrea Kaplan, (310) 825-0545 or her email: akaplan@mednet.ucla.edu.) A Phase III clinical trial is also organized to test the drug Risperidone for the treatment of agitated behavior in Alzheimer's patients. (Contact information: Palo Alto Veterans Administration Health Care System, Menlo Park, California, 94025. Recruiter: Erin L. Cassidy, PhD, (650) 493-5000, ext.27013 or her email: ecassidy@stanford.edu.)

Other trials include:

- A study on Valproate to prevent cognitive and behavioral symptoms in patients. Contact information: Laura Jakimovich, RN, MS, (585) 760-6578 or her email: laura_jakimovich@urmc.rochester.edu.

- The drug Simvastatin, a cholesterol-lowering medication, is being studied to learn if it slows the progression of Alzheimer disease. Contact information: Stanford University, Palo Alto, California, 94304. Recruiter: Lisa M. Kinoshita, PhD, (650) 493-0571 or her email: lisakino@stanford.edu.

- A study of the efficacy and dose of the drug NS 2330 to improve cognition. Contact information: Peter Glassman, MD, PhD, (800) 344-4095, ext. 4776 or his email: pglassma@rdg.boehringer-ingelheim.com.

- A study of investigational medications for the treatment of Alzheimer patients. Contact information: Eli Lilly and Company, (877) 285-4559.

There are also many other studies that are investigating various other pharmacological agents such as vitamin E and other currently available drugs.

Prognosis

There is considerable variability in the rate of Alzheimer disease progression. The Alzheimer Disease Association claims that the time from the onset of clinical symptoms to death can range from three to 20 years, with an average duration of eight years. There are probably many environmental and genetic factors that play a role in the progression of the disease. The accumulation of damage and loss of brain cells eventually results in the failure of many different organ systems in the body. According to the National Institute of Neurological Disorders and Stroke, the most common cause of death is due to infection.

Special concerns

Alzheimer disease should be distinguished from other forms of dementia. In some cases, depression can result in dementia-like symptoms. Other examples include chronic drug use, chronic infections of the **central nervous system**, thyroid disease, and vitamin deficiencies. These causes of dementia can often be treated. It is, therefore, important to obtain an accurate diagnosis to avoid complications associated with the inappropriate treatment and long-term care of these patients. There are also several genetically based syndromes in which dementia plays a role.

Genetic counseling

Genetic counseling is important for family members biologically related to patients with Alzheimer disease because each first-degree relative has as much as a 20% lifetime risk of also being affected. The risk to immediate relatives increases as more family members develop the disease. In the early-onset form of the disease, the inheritance pattern is thought to be autosomal dominant. This means that a carrier (who will eventually be affected) has a 50% chance of passing on the mutated gene to his or her offspring.

The general consensus in the scientific and medical community is to not test children or adolescents in the absence of symptoms for adult-onset disorders. There are many problems associated with predictive testing of asymptomatic individuals who are not yet adults. Children who undergo predictive testing lose the choice later in life (when they are capable of understanding the full ramifications of the disease) to know or not to know this information. It is, therefore, an important consideration that involves ethical and psychological implications.

Resources

BOOKS

Bird, T. D. "Memory Loss and Dementia." In *Harrison's Principles of Internal Medicine*, 15th ed. Edited by A. S.

Franci, E. Daunwald, and K. J. Isrelbacher. New York: McGraw Hill, 2001.

Castleman, Michael, et al. *There's Still a Person in There: The Complete Guide to Treating and Coping with Alzheimer's.* New York: Perigee Books, 2000.

Mace, Nancy L., and Peter V. Rabins. *The 36-Hour Day: A Family Guide to Caring for Persons with Alzheimer Disease, Related Dementing Illnesses, and Memory Loss in Later Life.* New York: Warner Books, 2001.

PERIODICALS

Campion, D., et al. "Early-onset Autosomal Dominant Alzheimer Disease: Prevalence, Genetic Heterogeneity, and Mutation Spectrum." *Am J Hum Genet* 65 (1999): 664–70.

Green, R.C. "Risk Assessment for Alzheimer's Disease with Genetic Susceptibility Testing: Has the Moment Arrived?" *Alzheimer's Care Quarterly* (2002): 3,208–14.

Rogan, S., and C. F. Lippa. "Alzheimer's Disease and Other Dementias: A Review." *Am J Alzheimers Dis Other Demen* (2002) 17: 11–7.

Romas, S. N., et al. "Familial Alzheimer Disease among Caribbean Hispanics: A Reexamination of Its Association with APOE." *Arch Neurol* (2002) 59: 87–91.

Rosenberg, R. N. "The Molecular and Genetic Basis of AD: The End of the Beginning: The 2000 Wartenberg Lecture." *Neurology* 54 (2000): 2045–54.

OTHER

ADEAR Alzheimer Disease Education and Referral Center. *National Institute on Aging about Alzheimer's Disease—General Information.* February 10, 2004 (March 30, 2004). <http://www.alzheimers.org/generalinfo.htm>.

National Institutes of Health. *Alzheimer's Disease.* February 10, 2004 (March 30, 2004). <http://health.nih.gov/result.asp?disease_id=28>.

National Library of Medicine. *Alzheimer's Disease.* MEDLINE plus Health Information. February 10, 2004 (March 30, 2004). <http://www.nlm.nih.gov/medlineplus/alzheimersdisease.html>.

ORGANIZATIONS

Alzheimer's Association. 919 North Michigan Avenue, Suite 1000, Chicago, IL 60611-1676. (312) 335-8700 or (800) 272-3900; Fax: (312) 335-1110. info@alz.org. <http://www.alz.org>.

Alzheimer's Education and Referral Center. PO Box 8250, Silver Springs, MD 20907-8250. (800) 438-4380. adear@alzheimers.org. <http://www.alzheimers.org>.

National Institute on Aging. Building 31, Room 5C27, 31 Center Drive, MSC 2292, Bethesda, MD 20892. (301) 496-1752. <http://www.nia.nih.gov>.

Bryan Richard Cobb, PhD

Amantadine

Definition

Amantadine is a synthetic antiviral agent that also has strong antiparkinsonian properties. It is sold in the United States under the brand name Symmetrel, and is also available under its generic name.

Purpose

Amantadine is used to treat a group of side effects, called parkinsonian side effects, that include **tremors**, difficulty walking, and slack muscle tone. These side effects may occur in patients who are taking antipsychotic medications used to treat mental disorders such as **schizophrenia**. An unrelated use of amantadine is in the treatment of viral infections of some strains of influenza A.

Description

Some medicines, called antipsychotic drugs, that are used to treat schizophrenia and other mental disorders can cause side effects similar to the symptoms of **Parkinson's disease**. The patient does not have Parkinson's disease, but may experience shaking in muscles while at rest, difficulty with voluntary movements, and poor muscle tone. These symptoms are similar to the symptoms of Parkinson's disease.

One way to eliminate these undesirable side effects is to stop taking the antipsychotic medicine. Unfortunately, the symptoms of the original mental disorder usually come back; in most cases, simply stopping the antipsychotic medication is not a reasonable option. Some drugs such as amantadine that control the symptoms of Parkinson's disease also control the parkinsonian side effects of antipsychotic medicines.

Amantadine works by restoring the chemical balance between dopamine and acetylcholine, two neurotransmitter chemicals in the brain. Taking amantadine along with the antipsychotic medicine helps to control symptoms of the mental disorder, while reducing parkinsonian side effects. Amantadine is in the same family of drugs commonly known as anticholinergic drugs, including biperiden and trihexyphenidyl.

Recommended dosage

Amantadine is available in 100 mg tablets and capsules, as well as a syrup containing 50 mg of amantadine in each teaspoonful. For the treatment of drug-induced parkinsonian side effects, amantadine is usually given in a dose of 100 mg orally twice a day. Some patients may need a total daily dose as high as 300 mg. Patients who are

taking other antiparkinsonian drugs at the same time may require lower daily doses of amantadine (e.g., 100 mg daily).

People with kidney disease or who are on hemodialysis must have their doses lowered. In these patients, doses may range from 100 mg daily to as little as 200 mg every seven days.

Precautions

Amantadine increases the amount of the dopamine (a **central nervous system** stimulant) in the brain. Because of this, patients with a history of **epilepsy** or other seizure disorders should be carefully monitored while taking this drug. This is especially true in the elderly and in patients with kidney disease. Amantadine may cause **visual disturbances** and affect mental alertness and coordination. People should not operate dangerous machinery or motor vehicles while taking this drug.

Side effects

Five to 10% of patients taking amantadine may experience nervous system side effects, including:

• dizziness or lightheadedness

• insomnia

- nervousness or anxiety

- impaired concentration

One to 5% of patients taking amantadine may experience other nervous system side effects, including:

- irritability or agitation

- depression

- confusion

- lack of coordination

- sleepiness or nightmares

- fatigue

- headache

In addition, up to 1% of patients may experience hallucinations, euphoria (excitement), extreme forgetfulness, aggressive behavior, personality changes, or **seizures**. Seizures are the most serious of all the side effects associated with amantadine.

Gastrointestinal side effects may also occur in patients taking amantadine. Five to 10% of people taking this drug experience nausea and up to 5% have dry mouth, loss of appetite, constipation, and vomiting. In most situations, amantadine may be continued and these side effects treated symptomatically.

One to 5% of patients taking amantadine have also reported a bluish coloring of their skin (usually on the legs) that is associated with enlargement of the blood vessels (livedo reticularis). This side effect usually appears within one month to one year of starting the drug and subsides within weeks to months after the drug is discontinued. People who think they may be experiencing this or other side effects from any medication should tell their physician.

Interactions

Taking amantadine along with other drugs used to treat parkinsonian side effects may cause increased confusion or even hallucinations. The combination of amantadine and **central nervous system stimulants** (e.g., amphetamines or decongestants) may cause increased central nervous stimulation or increase the likelihood of seizures.

Resources

BOOKS

American Society of Health-System Pharmacists. *AHFS Drug Information 2002*. Bethesda: American Society of Health-System Pharmacists, 2002.

DeVane, C. Lindsay, PharmD. "Drug Therapy for Psychoses." In *Fundamentals of Monitoring Psychoactive Drug Therapy*. Baltimore: Williams and Wilkins, 1990.

Jack Raber, PharmD

Ambenonium *see* **Cholinergic stimulants**

Amnestic disorders

Definition

Amnestic disorders are conditions that cause memory loss.

Description

Memory is the ability to retain and recall new information. Memory can be subdivided into short-term memory, which involves holding onto information for a minute or less, and long-term memory, which involves holding onto information for over a minute. Long-term memory can be further subdivided into recent memory, which involves new learning, and remote memory, which involves old information. In general, amnestic disorders more frequently involve deficits in new learning or recent memory.

There are a number of terms that are crucial to the understanding of amnestic disorders. In order to retain information, an individual must be able to pay close enough attention to the information that is presented; this is referred to as registration. The process whereby memories are established is referred to as encoding or storage. Retaining information in the long-term memory requires passage of time during which memory is consolidated. When an individual's memory is tested, retrieval is the process whereby the individual recalls the information from memory. Working memory is the ability to manipulate information from short-term memory in order to perform some function. Amnestic disorders may affect any or all of these necessary steps.

The time period affecting memory is also described. Anterograde amnesia is more common. Anterograde amnesia begins at a certain point in time and continues to interfere with the establishment of memory from that point forward in time. Retrograde amnesia refers to a loss of memory for information that was learned prior to the onset of amnesia. Retrograde amnesia often occurs in conjunction with head injury, and may result in erasure of memory of events or information from some time period (ranging from seconds to months) prior to the head injury. Over the course of recovery and rehabilitation from a head

Key Terms

Acetylcholine A brain chemical or neurotransmitter that carries information throughout the nervous system.

Anterograde Memory loss for information/events occurring after the onset of the amnestic disorder.

Delirium A condition characterized by waxing-and-waning episodes of confusion and agitation.

Dementia A chronic condition in which thinking and memory are progressively impaired. Other symptoms may also occur, including personality changes and depression.

Retrograde Memory loss for information/events prior to the onset of the amnestic disorder.

Transient ischemic attack (TIA) A stroke-like phenomenon in which a brief blockage of a brain blood vessel causes short-term neurological deficits that are completely resolved within 24 hours of their onset.

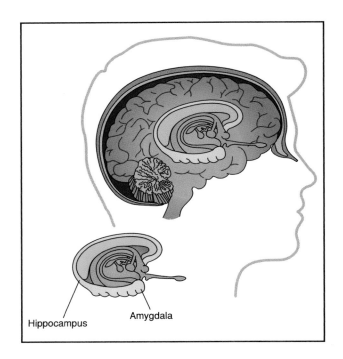

Hippocampus   Amygdala

Memory loss may result from bilateral damage to the limbic system of the brain responsible for memory storage, processing, and recall. *(Illustration by Electronic Illustrators Group.)*

injury, memory may be restored or the period of amnesia may eventually shorten.

Demographics

About 7% of all individuals over the age of 65 have some form of **dementia** that involves some degree of amnesia, as do about 50% of all individuals over the age of 85.

Causes and symptoms

A number of brain disorders can result in amnestic disorders, including various types of dementia (such as **Alzheimer's disease**), **traumatic brain injury** (such as concussion), **stroke**, accidents that involve oxygen deprivation to the brain or interruption of blood flow to the brain (such as ruptured **aneurysms**), encephalitis, tumors in the thalamus and/or hypothalamus, Wernicke-Korsakoff syndrome (a sequelae of thiamine deficiency usually due to severe alcoholism), and **seizures**. Psychological disorders can also cause a type of amnesia called "psychogenic amnesia."

A curious condition called **transient global amnesia** causes **delirium** (a period of waxing and waning confusion and agitation), anterograde amnesia, and retrograde amnesia for events and information from the several hours prior to the onset of the attack. Transient global amnesia usually only lasts for several hours. Ultimately, the individual recovers completely, with no lasting memory deficit. The cause of transient global amnesia is poorly understood; researchers are suspicious that it may be due to either seizure activity in the brain or a brief blockage in a brain blood vessel, which causes a brief stroke-like event that completely resolves without permanent sequelae (similar to a **transient ischemic attack**).

Symptoms of amnestic disorders may include difficulty recalling remote events or information, and/or difficulty learning and then recalling new information. In some cases, the patient is fully aware of the memory impairment, and frustrated by it; in other cases, the patient may seem completely oblivious to the memory impairment or may even attempt to fill in the deficit in memory with confabulation. Depending on the underlying condition responsible for the amnesia, a number of other symptoms may be present as well.

Diagnosis

Diagnosis of amnestic disorders begins by establishing an individual's level of orientation to person, place, and time. Does he or she know who he or she is? Where he or she is? The day/date/time? An individual's ability to recall common current events (who is the president?) may reveal information about the memory deficit. A family member or close friend may be an invaluable part of the examination, in order to provide some background information on the onset and progression of the memory loss, as well as information regarding the individual's original level of functioning.

A variety of memory tests can be utilized to assess an individual's ability to attend to information, utilize short-term memory, and store and retrieve information from long-term memory. Both verbal and visual memory should be tested. Verbal memory can be tested by working with an individual to memorize word lists, then testing recall after a certain amount of time has elapsed. Similarly, visual memory can be tested by asking an individual to locate several objects that were hidden in a room in the individual's presence.

Depending on what types of conditions are being considered, other tests may include blood tests, neuroimaging (**CT**, **MRI**, or **PET** scans of the brain), cerebrospinal fluid testing, and EEG testing.

Treatment team

A **neurologist** and/or psychiatrist may be involved in diagnosing and treating amnestic disorders. Depending on the underlying condition responsible for the memory deficit, other specialists may be involved as well. Occupational and speech and language therapists may be involved in rehabilitation programs for individuals who have amnestic disorders as part of their clinical picture.

Treatment

In some cases, treatment of the underlying disorder may help improve the accompanying amnesia. In mild cases of amnesia, rehabilitation may involve teaching memory techniques and encouraging the use of memory tools, such as association techniques, lists, notes, calendars, timers, etc. Memory exercises may be helpful. Recent treatments for Alzheimer's disease and other dementias have involved medications that interfere with the metabolism of the brain chemical (neurotransmitter) called acetylcholine, thus increasing the available quantity of acetylcholine. These drugs, such as donepezil and tacrine, seem to improve memory in patients with Alzheimer's disease. Research studies are attempting to explore whether these drugs may also help amnestic disorders that stem from other underlying conditions.

Prognosis

The prognosis is very dependent on the underlying condition that has caused the memory deficit, and on whether that condition has a tendency to progress or stabilize. Alzheimer's disease, for example, is relentlessly progressive, and therefore the memory deficits that accompany this condition can be expected to worsen considerably over time. Individuals who have memory deficits due to a brain tumor may have their symptoms improve after surgery to remove the tumor. Individuals with transient global amnesia can be expected to fully recover from their memory impairment within hours or days of its onset. In the case of some traumatic brain injuries, the amnesia may improve with time (as brain swelling decreases, for example), but there may always remain some degree of amnesia for the events just prior to the moment of the injury.

Resources

BOOKS

Cummings, Jeffrey L. "Disorders of Cognition." In *Cecil Textbook of Internal Medicine*, edited by Lee Goldman, et al. Philadelphia: W. B. Saunders Company, 2000.

Gabrieli, John D., et al. "Memory." In *Textbook of Clinical Neurology*, edited by Christopher G. Goetz. Philadelphia: W. B. Saunders Company, 2003.

Mesulam, M.-Marsel. "Aphasias and Other Focal Cerebral Disorders." In *Harrison's Principles of Internal Medicine*, edited by Eugene Braunwald, et al. New York: McGraw-Hill Professional, 2001.

Rosalyn Carson-DeWitt, MD

Amphetamine *see* **Central nervous system stimulants**

Amyotrophic lateral sclerosis

Definition

Amyotrophic lateral sclerosis (ALS) is a disease that breaks down tissues in the nervous system (a neurodegenerative disease) of unknown cause that affects the nerves responsible for movement. It is also known as motor neuron disease and Lou Gehrig's disease, after the baseball player whose career it ended.

Description

ALS is a disease of the motor neurons, those nerve cells reaching from the brain to the spinal cord (upper motor neurons) and the spinal cord to the peripheral nerves (lower motor neurons) that control muscle movement. In ALS, for unknown reasons, these neurons die, leading to a progressive loss of the ability to move virtually any of the muscles in the body. ALS affects "voluntary" muscles, those controlled by conscious thought, such as the arm, leg, and trunk muscles. ALS, in and of itself, does not affect sensation, thought processes, the heart muscle, or the "smooth" muscle of the digestive system, bladder, and other internal organs. Most people with ALS retain function of their eye muscles as well. However, various forms

Key Terms

Aspiration Inhalation of food or liquids into the lungs.

Bulbar muscles Muscles of the mouth and throat responsible for speech and swallowing.

Fasciculations Involuntary twitching of muscles.

Motor neuron A nerve cell that controls a muscle.

Riluzole (Rilutek) The first drug approved in the United States for the treatment of ALS.

Voluntary muscle A muscle under conscious control; contrasted with smooth muscle and heart muscle, which are not under voluntary control.

of ALS may be associated with a loss of intellectual function (**dementia**) or sensory symptoms.

"Amyotrophic" refers to the loss of muscle bulk, a cardinal sign of ALS. "Lateral" indicates one of the regions of the spinal cord affected, and "sclerosis" describes the hardened tissue that develops in place of healthy nerves. ALS affects approximately 30,000 people in the United States, with about 5,000 new cases each year. It usually begins between the ages of 40 and 70, although younger onset is possible. Men are slightly more likely to develop ALS than women.

ALS progresses rapidly in most cases. It is fatal within three years for 50% of all people affected, and within five years for 80%. Ten percent of people with ALS live beyond eight years.

Causes and symptoms

Causes

The symptoms of ALS are caused by the death of motor neurons in the spinal cord and brain. Normally, these neurons convey electrical messages from the brain to the muscles to stimulate movement in the arms, legs, trunk, neck, and head. As motor neurons die, the muscles they enervate cannot be moved as effectively, and weakness results. In addition, lack of stimulation leads to muscle wasting, or loss of bulk. Involvement of the upper motor neurons causes spasms and increased tone in the limbs, and abnormal reflexes. Involvement of the lower motor neurons causes muscle wasting and twitching (fasciculations).

Although many causes of motor neuron degeneration have been suggested for ALS, none has yet been proven responsible. Results of recent research have implicated toxic

molecular fragments known as free radicals. Some evidence suggests that a cascade of events leads to excess free radical production inside motor neurons, leading to their death. Why free radicals should be produced in excess amounts is unclear, as is whether this excess is the cause or the effect of other degenerative processes. Additional agents within this toxic cascade may include excessive levels of a neurotransmitter known as glutamate, which may over-stimulate motor neurons, thereby increasing free-radical production, and a faulty detoxification enzyme known as SOD-1, for superoxide dismutase type 1. The actual pathway of destruction is not known, however, nor is the trigger for the rapid degeneration that marks ALS. Further research may show that other pathways are involved, perhaps ones even more important than this one. Autoimmune factors or premature aging may play some role, as could viral agents or environmental toxins.

Two major forms of ALS are known: familial and sporadic. Familial ALS accounts for about 10% of all ALS cases. As the name suggests, familial ALS is believed to be caused by the inheritance of one or more faulty genes. About 15% of families with this type of ALS have mutations in the gene for SOD-1. SOD-1 gene defects are dominant, meaning only one gene copy is needed to develop the disease. Therefore, a parent with the faulty gene has a 50% chance of passing the gene along to a child.

Sporadic ALS has no known cause. While many environmental toxins have been suggested as causes, to date no research has confirmed any of the candidates investigated, including aluminum and mercury and lead from dental fillings. As research progresses, it is likely that many cases of sporadic ALS will be shown to have a genetic basis as well.

A third type, called Western Pacific ALS, occurs in Guam and other Pacific islands. This form combines symptoms of both ALS and **Parkinson's disease**.

Symptoms

The earliest sign of ALS is most often weakness in the arms or legs, usually more pronounced on one side than the other at first. Loss of function is usually more rapid in the legs among people with familial ALS and in the arms among those with sporadic ALS. Leg weakness may first become apparent by an increased frequency of stumbling on uneven pavement, or an unexplained difficulty climbing stairs. Arm weakness may lead to difficulty grasping and holding a cup, for instance, or loss of dexterity in the fingers.

Less often, the earliest sign of ALS is weakness in the bulbar muscles, those muscles in the mouth and throat that control chewing, swallowing, and speaking. A person with bulbar weakness may become hoarse or tired after speaking at length, or speech may become slurred.

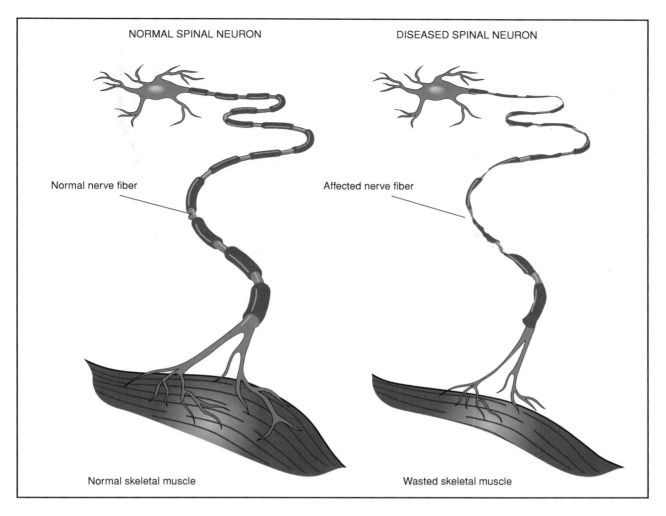

NORMAL SPINAL NEURON

DISEASED SPINAL NEURON

Normal nerve fiber

Affected nerve fiber

Normal skeletal muscle

Wasted skeletal muscle

Amyotrophic lateral sclerosis (ALS) is caused by the degeneration and death of motor neurons in the spinal cord and brain. These neurons convey electrical messages from the brain to the muscles to stimulate movement in the arms, legs, trunk, neck, and head. As motor neurons degenerate, the muscles are weakened and cannot move as effectively, leading to muscle wasting. *(Illustration by Electronic Illustrators Group.)*

In addition to weakness, the other cardinal signs of ALS are muscle wasting and persistent twitching (fasciculation). These are usually seen after weakness becomes obvious. Fasciculation is quite common in people without the disease, and is virtually never the first sign of ALS.

While initial weakness may be limited to one region, ALS almost always progresses rapidly to involve virtually all the voluntary muscle groups in the body. Later symptoms include loss of the ability to walk, to use the arms and hands, to speak clearly or at all, to swallow, and to hold the head up. Weakness of the respiratory muscles makes breathing and coughing difficult, and poor swallowing control increases the likelihood of inhaling food or saliva (aspiration). Aspiration increases the likelihood of lung infection, which is often the cause of death. With a ventilator and scrupulous bronchial hygiene, a person with ALS

may live much longer than the average, although weakness and wasting will continue to erode any remaining functional abilities. Most people with ALS continue to retain function of the extraocular muscles that move their eyes, allowing some communication to take place with simple blinks or through use of a computer-assisted device.

Diagnosis

The diagnosis of ALS begins with a complete medical history and physical exam, plus a neurological examination to determine the distribution and extent of weakness. An electrical test of muscle function, called an electromyogram, or EMG, is an important part of the diagnostic process. Various other tests, including blood and urine tests, x rays, and CT scans, may be done to rule out other possible causes of the symptoms, such as tumors of the skull base or high cervical spinal cord, thyroid disease, spinal arthritis, lead poisoning, or severe vitamin deficiency. ALS is rarely misdiagnosed following a careful review of all these factors.

Treatment

There is no cure for ALS, and no treatment that can significantly alter its course. There are many things which can be done, however, to help maintain quality of life and to retain functional ability even in the face of progressive weakness.

As of early 1998, only one drug had been approved for treatment of ALS. Riluzole (Rilutek) appears to provide on average a three-month increase in life expectancy when taken regularly early in the disease, and shows a significant slowing of the loss of muscle strength. Riluzole acts by decreasing glutamate release from nerve terminals. Experimental trials of nerve growth factor have not demonstrated any benefit. No other drug or vitamin currently available has been shown to have any effect on the course of ALS.

A physical therapist works with an affected person and family to implement **exercise** and stretching programs to maintain strength and range of motion, and to promote general health. Swimming may be a good choice for people with ALS, as it provides a low-impact workout to most muscle groups. One result of chronic inactivity is contracture, or muscle shortening. Contractures limit a person's range of motion, and are often painful. Regular stretching can prevent contracture. Several drugs are available to reduce cramping, a common complaint in ALS.

An occupational therapist can help design solutions to movement and coordination problems, and provide advice on adaptive devices and home modifications.

Speech and swallowing difficulties can be minimized or delayed through training provided by a speech-language pathologist. This specialist can also provide advice on communication aids, including computer-assisted devices and simpler word boards.

Nutritional advice can be provided by a nutritionist. A person with ALS often needs softer foods to prevent jaw exhaustion or choking. Later in the disease, nutrition may be provided by a gastrostomy tube inserted into the stomach.

Mechanical ventilation may be used when breathing becomes too difficult. Modern mechanical ventilators are small and portable, allowing a person with ALS to maintain the maximum level of function and mobility. Ventilation may be administered through a mouth or nose piece, or through a tracheostomy tube. This tube is inserted through a small hole made in the windpipe. In addition to providing direct access to the airway, the tube also decreases the risk aspiration. While many people with rapidly progressing ALS choose not to use ventilators for lengthy periods, they are increasingly being used to prolong life for a short time.

The progressive nature of ALS means that most persons will eventually require full-time nursing care. This care is often provided by a spouse or other family member. While the skills involved are not difficult to learn, the physical and emotional burden of care can be overwhelming. Caregivers need to recognize and provide for their own needs as well as those of people with ALS, to prevent **depression**, burnout, and bitterness.

Throughout the disease, a support group can provide important psychological aid to affected persons and their caregivers as they come to terms with the losses ALS inflicts. Support groups are sponsored by both the ALS Society and the Muscular Dystrophy Association.

Alternative treatment

Given the grave prognosis and absence of traditional medical treatments, it is not surprising that a large number of alternative treatments have been tried for ALS. Two studies published in 1988 suggested that amino-acid therapies may provide some improvement for some people with ALS. While individual reports claim benefits for megavitamin therapy, herbal medicine, and removal of dental fillings, for instance, no evidence suggests that these offer any more than a brief psychological boost, often followed by a more severe letdown when it becomes apparent the disease has continued unabated. However, once the causes of ALS are better understood, alternative therapies may be more intensively studied. For example, if damage by free radicals turns out to be the root of most of the symptoms, antioxidant vitamins and supplements may be used more routinely to slow the progression of ALS. Or, if environmental toxins are implicated, alternative therapies with the goal of detoxifying the body may be of some use.

Prognosis

ALS usually progresses rapidly, and leads to death from respiratory infection within three to five years in most cases. The slowest disease progression is seen in those who are young and have their first symptoms in the limbs. About 10% of people with ALS live longer than eight years.

Prevention

There is no known way to prevent ALS or to alter its course.

Resources

BOOKS

Adams, Raymond D., Maurice Victor, and Allan H. Ropper. *Adams' & Victor's Principles of Neurology,* 6th ed. New York: McGraw Hill, 1997.

Brown, Robert H. "The motor neuron diseases." In *Harrison's Principles of Internal Medicine,* 14th ed., edited by Anthony S. Fauci, et al., pp. 2368-2372. New York: McGraw-Hill, 1998.

Feldman, Eva L. "Motor neuron diseases." In *Cecil Textbook of Medicine,* 21st ed., edited by Lee Goldman and J. Claude Bennett, pp. 2089-2092. Philadelphia: W. B. Saunders, 2000.

Kimura, Jun, and Ryuji Kaji. *Physiology of ALS and Related Diseases.* Amsterdam: Elsevier Science, 1997.

Mitsumoto, Hiroshi, David A. Chad, Erik Pioro, and Sid Gilman. *Amyotrophic Lateral Sclerosis.* New York: Oxford University Press, 1997.

PERIODICALS

Ansevin, C. F. "Treatment of ALS with pleconaril." *Neurology* 56, no. 5 (2001): 691-692.

Eisen, A., and M. Weber. "The motor cortex and amyotrophic lateral sclerosis." *Muscle and Nerve* 24, no. 4 (2001): 564-573.

Gelanis, D. F. "Respiratory Failure or Impairment in Amyotrophic Lateral Sclerosis." *Current treatment options in neurology* 3, no. 2 (2001): 133-138.

Ludolph, A. C. "Treatment of amyotrophic lateral sclerosis— what is the next step?" *Journal of Neurology* 246, Suppl 6 (2000): 13-18.

Pasetti, C., and G. Zanini. "The physician-patient relationship in amyotrophic lateral sclerosis." *Neurological Science* 21, no. 5 (2000): 318-323.

Robberecht, W. "Genetics of amyotrophic lateral sclerosis." *Journal of Neurology* 246, Suppl 6 (2000): 2-6.

Robbins, R. A., Z. Simmons, B. A. Bremer, S. M. Walsh, and S. Fischer. "Quality of life in ALS is maintained as physical function declines." *Neurology* 56, no. 4 (2001): 442-444.

ORGANIZATIONS

ALS Association of America. 27001 Agoura Road, Suite 150, Calabasas Hills, CA 91301-5104. (800) 782-4747 (Information and Referral Service) or (818) 880-9007; Fax: (818) 880-9006. <http://www.alsa.org/als/>

American Academy of Family Physicians. 11400 Tomahawk Creek Parkway, Leawood, KS 66211-2672. (913) 906-6000. fp@aafp.org. <http://www.aafp.org/>.

American Academy of Neurology. 1080 Montreal Avenue, St. Paul, Minnesota 55116. (651) 695-1940; Fax: (651) 695-2791. info@aan.org. <http://www.aan.com/>.

American Medical Association, 515 N. State Street, Chicago, IL 60610. (312) 464-5000. <http://www.ama-assn.org/>.

Centers for Disease Control and Prevention. 1600 Clifton Road, Atlanta, GA 30333. (404) 639-3534 or (800) 311-3435. <http://www.cdc.gov/netinfo.htm>, <http://www.cdc.gov/ncidod/eid/vol7no1/brown.htm>.

Muscular Dystrophy Association. 3300 East Sunrise Drive, Tucson, AZ 85718-3208. (520) 529-2000 or (800) 572-1717; Fax: (520) 529-5300. <www.mdausa.org>.

WEBSITES

ALS Society of Canada. <http://www.als.ca/>.

ALS Survival Guide. <http://www.lougehrigsdisease.net/>.

American Academy of Family Physicians. <http://www.aafp.org/afp/990315ap/1489.html>.

National Organization for Rare Diseases. <http://www.stepstn.com/cgi-win/nord.exe?proc=Redirect&type=rdb_sum&id=57.htm>.

National Institute of Neurological Disorders and Stroke. <http://www.ninds.nih.gov/health_and_medical/disorders/amyotrophiclateralsclerosis_doc.htm>.

National Library of Medicine. <http://www.nlm.nih.gov/medlineplus/amyotrophiclateralsclerosis.html>.

World Federation of Neurology. <http://www.wfnals.org/>.

L. Fleming Fallon, Jr., MD, DrPH

Anatomical nomenclature

Over the centuries, anatomists developed a standard nomenclature, or method of naming anatomical structures. Terms such as "up" or "down" obviously have no meaning unless the orientation of the body is clear. When a body is lying on its back, the thorax and abdomen are at the same level. The upright sense of up and down is lost. Further, because anatomical studies and particularly embryological studies were often carried out in animals, the development of the nomenclature relative to comparative anatomy had an enormous impact on the development of human anatomical nomenclature. There were obvious difficulties in relating terms from quadrupeds (animals that walk on four legs) who have abdominal and thoracic regions at the same level as opposed to human bipeds in whom an upward and downward orientation might seem more obvious.

In order to standardize nomenclature, anatomical terms relate to the *standard anatomical position.* When the human body is in the standard anatomical position it is upright, erect on two legs, facing frontward, with the arms at the sides each rotated so that the palms of the hands turn forward.

In the standard anatomical position, *superior* means toward the head or the *cranial* end of the body.

The term *inferior* means toward the feet or the *caudal* end of the body.

The frontal surface of the body is the *anterior* or *ventral* surface of the body. Accordingly, the terms "anteriorly" and "ventrally" specify a position closer to—or toward—the frontal surface of the body. The back surface of the body is the *posterior* or *dorsal* surface and the terms "posteriorly" and "dorsally" specify a position closer to—or toward—the posterior surface of the body.

The terms *superficial* and *deep* relate to the distance from the exterior surface of the body. Cavities such as the thoracic cavity have internal and external regions that correspond to deep and superficial relationships in the midsagittal plane.

The bones of the skull are fused by sutures that form important anatomical landmarks. Sutures are joints that run jaggedly along the interface between the bones. At birth, the sutures are soft, broad, and cartilaginous. The sutures eventually fuse and become rigid and ossified near the end of puberty or early in adulthood.

The sagittal suture unties the parietal bones of the skull along the midline of the body. The suture is used as an anatomical landmark in anatomical nomenclature to establish what are termed *sagittal planes* of the body. The primary sagittal plane is the sagittal plane that runs through the length of the sagittal suture. Planes that are parallel to the sagittal plane, but that are offset from the midsagittal plane are termed *parasagittal planes*. Sagittal planes run anteriorly and posteriorly, are always at right angles to the coronal planes. The *medial plane* or *midsagittal plane* divides the body vertically into superficially symmetrical *right* and *left* halves.

The medial plane also establishes a centerline axis for the body. The terms *medial* and *lateral* relate positions relative to the medial axis. If a structure is medial to another structure, the medial structure is closer to the medial or center axis. If a structure is lateral to another structure, the lateral structure is farther way from the medial axis. For example, the lungs are lateral to the heart.

The coronal suture unites the frontal bone with the parietal bones. In anatomical nomenclature, the primary *coronal plane* designates the plane that runs through the length of the coronal suture. The primary coronal plane is also termed the *frontal plane* because it divides the body into frontal and back halves.

Planes that divide the body into superior and inferior portions, and that are at right angles to both the sagittal and coronal planes are termed transverse planes. Anatomical planes that are not parallel to sagittal, coronal, or transverse planes are termed oblique planes.

The body is also divided into several regional areas. The most superior area is the *cephalic region* that includes the head. The *thoracic region* is commonly known as the chest region. Although the *celiac region* more specifically refers to the center of the *abdominal region*, celiac is sometimes used to designate a wider area of abdominal structures. At the inferior end of the abdominal region lies the *pelvic region* or *pelvis*. The posterior or dorsal side of the body has its own special regions, named for the underlying vertebrae. From superior to inferior along the midline of the dorsal surface lie the *cervical, thoracic, lumbar*, and *sacral* regions. The buttocks are the most prominent feature of the *gluteal region*.

The term *upper limbs* or *upper extremities* refers to the arms. The term *lower limbs* or *lower extremities* refers to the legs.

The *proximal* end of an extremity is at the junction of the extremity (i.e., arm or leg) with the trunk of the body. The *distal* end of an extremity is the point on the extremity farthest away from the trunk (e.g., fingers and toes). Accordingly, if a structure is proximate to another structure it is closer to the trunk (e.g., the elbow is proximate to the wrist). If a structure is distal to another, it is farther from the trunk (e.g., the fingers are distal to the wrist).

Structures may also be described as being medial or lateral to the midline axis of each extremity. Within the upper limbs, the terms radial and ulnar may be used synonymous with lateral and medial. In the lower extremities, the terms fibular and tibial may be used as synonyms for lateral and medial.

Rotations of the extremities may de described as medial rotations (toward the midline) or lateral rotations (away from the midline).

Many structural relationships are described by combined anatomical terms (e.g., the eyes are anterio-medial to the ears).

There are also terms of movement that are standardized by anatomical nomenclature. Starting from the anatomical position, *abduction* indicates the movement of an arm or leg away from the midline or midsagittal plane. *Adduction* indicates movement of an extremity toward the midline.

The opening of the hands into the anatomical position is *supination* of the hands. Rotation so the dorsal side of the hands face forward is termed *pronation*.

The term *flexion* means movement toward the flexor or anterior surface. In contrast, *extension* may be generally regarded as movement toward the extensor or posterior surface. Flexion occurs when the arm brings the hand from the anatomical position toward the shoulder (a curl) or when the arm is raised over the head from the anatomical position. Extension returns the upper arm and or lower to the anatomical position. Because of the embryological rotation of the lower limbs that rotates the primitive dorsal side to the adult form ventral side, flexion occurs as the thigh is raised anteriorly and superiorly toward the anterior portion of the pelvis. Extension occurs when the thigh is returned to anatomical position. Specifically, due to the embryological rotation, flexion of the lower leg occurs as the foot is raised toward the back of the thigh and extension of the lower leg occurs with the kicking motion that returns the lower leg to anatomical position.

The term *palmar surface* (palm side) is applied to the flexion side of the hand. The term *plantar surface* is applied to the bottom sole of the foot. From the anatomical position, extension occurs when the toes are curled back and the foot arches upward and flexion occurs as the foot is returned to anatomical position.

Rolling motions of the foot are described as *inversion* (rolling with the big toe initially lifting upward) and *eversion* (rolling with the big toe initially moving downward).

K. Lee Lerner

Anencephaly

Definition

Anencephaly is a lethal birth defect characterized by the absence of all or part of the skull and scalp and malformation of the brain.

Description

Anencephaly is one of a group of malformations of the **central nervous system** collectively called neural tube defects. Anencephaly is readily apparent at birth because of the absence of the skull and scalp and exposure of the underlying brain. The condition is also called acrania (absence of the skull) and acephaly (absence of the head). In its most severe form, the entire skull and scalp are missing. In some cases, termed "meroacrania" or "meroanencephaly," a portion of the skull may be present. In most instances, anencephaly occurs as an isolated birth defect with the other organs and tissues of the body forming correctly. In approximately 10% of cases, other malformations coexist with anencephaly.

Demographics

Anencephaly occurs in all races and ethnic groups. The prevalence rates range from less than one in 10,000 births (European countries) to more than 10 per 10,000 births (Mexico, China).

Causes and symptoms

As an isolated defect, anencephaly appears to be caused by a combination of genetic factors and environmental influences that predispose to faulty formation of the nervous system. The specific genes and environmental insults that contribute to this multifactorial causation are not completely understood. It is known that nutritional insufficiency, specifically folic acid insufficiency, is one predisposing environmental factor, and that mutations of genes involved in folic acid metabolism are genetic risk factors. The recurrence risk after the birth of an infant with anencephaly is 3–5%. The recurrence may be anencephaly or another neural tube defect such as **spina bifida**.

Anencephaly is readily apparent at birth because of exposure of all or part of the brain. Not only is the brain malformed, but it is also damaged because of the absence of the overlying protective encasement.

Diagnosis

Anencephaly is diagnosed by observation. Prenatal diagnosis may be made by ultrasound examination after 12–14 weeks' gestation. Prenatal diagnosis of anencephaly can also be detected through maternal serum alpha-fetoprotein screening. The level of alpha-fetoprotein in the maternal blood is elevated because of the leakage of this fetal protein into the amniotic fluid.

There are no treatments for anencephaly. A pregnant woman or couple expecting an anencephalic baby will need a sensitive and supportive health care team, and perhaps some additional psychological support as they face the inevitable death of their infant, usually before or shortly after birth.

Treatment and management

No treatment is indicated for anencephaly. Affected infants are stillborn or die within the first few days of life. The risk for occurrence or recurrence of anencephaly may be reduced by half or more by the intake of folic acid during the months immediately before and after conception. Natural folic acid, a B vitamin, may be found in many foods (green leafy vegetables, legumes, orange juice, liver). Synthetic folic acid may be obtained in vitamin preparations and in certain fortified breakfast cereals. In

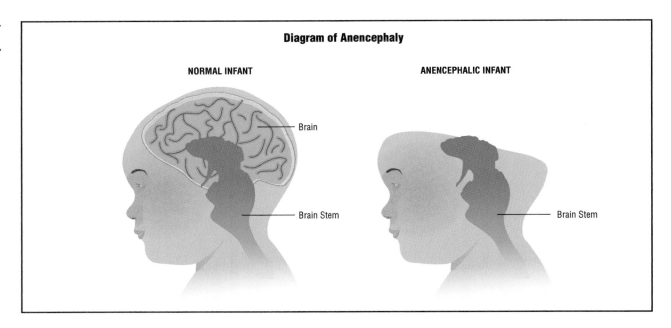

Diagram of Anencephaly

NORMAL INFANT   ANENCEPHALIC INFANT

Brain

Brain Stem   Brain Stem

Infants born with anencephaly have either a severely underdeveloped brain or total brain absence. A portion of the brain-stem usually protrudes through the skull, which also fails to develop properly. *(Gale Group.)*

the United States, all enriched cereal grain flours have been fortified with folic acid.

Clinical Trials

Research is primarily directed at understanding the underlying factors that affect early neurological development in the fetus.

Prognosis

Anencephaly is uniformly fatal at birth or soon thereafter.

Resources

PERIODICALS

Czeizel, A. E., and I. Dudas. "Prevention of the First Occurrence of Neural Tube Defects by Preconceptional Vitamin Supplementation." *New England Journal of Medicine* 327 (1992): 1832–1835.

Medical Research Council Vitamin Study Research Group. "Prevention of Neural Tube Defects: Results of the Medical Research Council Vitamin Study." *Lancet* 338 (1991): 131–137.

Sells, C. J., and J. G. Hall. "Neural Tube Defects." *Mental Retardation and Developmental Disabilities Research Reviews* 4, no. 4, 1998.

ORGANIZATIONS

March of Dimes Birth Defects Foundation. 1275 Mamaroneck Ave., White Plains, NY 10605. (888) 663-4637. resourcecenter@modimes.org. <http://www.modimes.org>.

National Birth Defects Prevention Network. Atlanta, GA. (770) 488-3550. <http://www.nbdpn.org>.

Roger E. Stevenson, MD
Rosalyn Carson-DeWitt, MD

Aneurysms

Definition

Cerebral aneurysm is the enlargement, distention, dilation, bulging, or ballooning of the wall of a cerebral artery or vein. Aneurysms affect arteries throughout the body, including blood vessels in the brain (intracerebral aneurysm). Ruptures of intracerebral aneurysm result in **stroke** (loss of blood supply to tissue) and bleeding into the subarachnoid space). The most common aneurysm is an abdominal aneurysm.

Description

Dilations, or ballooning, of blood vessels to form an aneurysm are particularly dangerous because they increase the chance of arterial rupture and subsequent bleeding into brain tissues (a hemorrhagic stroke). Rupture of an aneurysm can lead to the leakage of blood into the tissues and spaces surrounding the brain. This leaked blood then clots to form an intracranial hematoma. Aneurysms that rupture can result in severe disability or death.

Common complications of cerebral aneurysms that leak include **hydrocephalus** (the excessive accumulation of cerebrospinal fluid) and persistent spasms of blood vessels that adversely affect the maintenance of arterial blood pressure.

Once they rupture or bleed, aneurysms have a tendency toward recurrent bleeding episodes. This tendency to rebleed is particularly high in the first few days following the initial bleed. Intracerebral bleeds are often accompanied by increases in cerebrospinal fluid and an increased intracranial pressure (hydrocephalus).

Once they occur, aneurysms are dynamic and can increase in size over time. The increase in size is not always linear and can advance sporadically until they expand to a critical size. As they grow, aneurysms begin to put pressure on surrounding tissues. In addition, as they grow, aneurysms usually result in progressively more difficult problems.

The larger the size of an aneurysm, regardless of location, the greater the chance it will ultimately bleed. Cerebral aneurysm ruptures usually lead to subarachnoid hemorrhage (SAH).

Demographics

Although more common in adults than children, cerebral aneurysms occur in all age groups. Cerebral aneurysms are more common—and the risk of aneurysm generally increases—with age.

Aneurysm sufferers are rarely young; the incidence of aneurysm is low in those under 20 years of age. In contrast, aneurysms are relatively common in people over 65 years of age. Risk indicators for some groups such as Caucasian males begin to increase at age 55. Some studies indicate that up to 5% of the population over 65 suffer some form of aneurysm.

Incidence of specific aneurysms varies, but in general within the United States they are occur less frequently in Caucasian women, and are relatively uncommon in African Americans.

Of those affected with an aneurysm anywhere in the body, the National Institute of Health (NIH) estimates that approximately 30,000 people in the United States will suffer an aneurysm rupture.

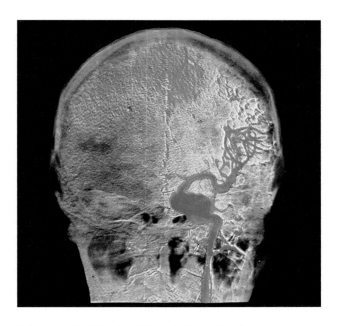

Arteriograph of the head from behind, showing an aneurysm, the balloon-like smooth swelling just below and to the right of center. *(CNRI/National Audubon Society Collection/Photo Researchers, Inc. Reproduced by permission.)*

Cigarette smoking and excess alcohol use substantially increase the risk of aneurysm rupture.

Causes and symptoms

An aneurysm may be a congenital defect in the structure of the muscular wall of affected blood vessels (e.g., the intima of an artery), or arise secondary to trauma, atherosclerosis, or high blood pressure. The defect results in an abnormal thinning of the arterial or venous wall that makes the wall subsequently susceptible to aneurysm.

Research data appears to show that some individuals have a basic genetic susceptibility or predisposition to aneurysms. The genetic inheritance patterns resemble characteristics linked to an autosomal dominant gene. Within some families, rates of aneurysms can run as high as five to 10 times those found in the general population.

Direct causes of intracerebral aneurysms include infection, trauma, or neoplastic disease. If infection is the cause, the infection may be from a remote site. For example, an aneurysm in the brain may result from the loosed embolus such as plaque, fatty deposit, clot, or clump of cells, originating at an infection in another part of the body. The embolus is transported to the site of the future cerebral aneurysm by the bloodstream and **cerebral circulation**. An aneurysm formed in this manner is termed a mycotic aneurysm.

Prior to rupture, the symptoms associated with an aneurysm depend upon its location, size, and rate of expansion. A static aneurysm that does not leak (bleed) or adversely affect cerebral circulation or neighboring tissue may be asymptomatic (without symptoms). In contrast, larger aneurysms or aneurysms with a rapid growth rate may produce pronounced symptoms such as swelling, loss of sensation, blurred vision, etc.

Just prior to an aneurysm rupture, patients typically experience some symptoms commonly associated with stroke. Depending on the size and location of the aneurysm about to rupture, a patient may suffer a severe **headache**, deterioration or disturbances of hearing, and disturbances of vision such as double vision, severe nausea and vomiting, and syncopal episodes (periodic **fainting** or loss of consciousness).

A severe headache that is unresponsive to standard analgesics is the most common sign of a leaking or bleeding aneurysm. Many patients experience a series of sentinel (warning) headaches if the aneurysm begins to leak prior to rupture. A fully ruptured aneurysm presents with a severe headache that is frequently accompanied by fainting or temporary (transient) loss of consciousness, often with severe nausea, vomiting, and rapidly developing stiff neck (nuchal rigidity).

Aneurysms normally rupture while the patient is active and awake.

Diagnosis

The severe headache that accompanies a cerebral aneurysm is often the principle complaint upon which the diagnosis of aneurysm begins to build.

Angiography provides the most definitive diagnosis of an intracerebral aneurysm by determining the specific site of the aneurysm. A computed tomography (**CT**) **scan** can also diagnose a bleeding cerebral aneurysm. Arteriography is an x ray of the carotid artery taken when a special dye is injected into the artery.

The presence of blood in the cerebrospinal fluid withdrawn during a lumbar puncture is also diagnostic evidence for blood leaking into the subarachnoid space.

Magnetic resonance imaging (MRI) studies can also be useful in accessing the extent of damage to surrounding tissues and are often used to study aneurysms prior to leakage or rupture. MRI uses magnetic fields to detect subtle changes in brain tissue content. The benefit of MRI over CT imaging is that MRI is better able to localize the exact anatomical position of an aneurysm. Other types of MRI scans are magnetic resonance angiography (MRA) and functional magnetic resonance imaging (fMRI). Neurosurgeons use MRA to detect stenosis (blockage) of the brain arteries inside the skull by mapping flowing blood. Functional MRI uses a magnet to pick up signals from oxygenated blood and can show brain activity through increases in local blood flow.

Duplex Doppler ultrasound and arteriography are two additional diagnostic imaging techniques used to decide if an individual would benefit from a surgical procedure called **carotid endarterectomy**. This surgery is used to remove fatty deposits from the carotid arteries and can help prevent stroke. Doppler ultrasound is a painless, noninvasive test in which sound waves bounce off the moving blood and the tissue in the artery and can be formed into an image.

Treatment team

Management and treatment of aneurysms require a multi-disciplinary team. Physicians are responsible for caring for general health and providing guidance aimed at preventing a stroke. Neurologists and neurosurgeons usually lead acute-care teams and direct patient care during hospitalization and recovery from surgery. Neuroradiologists help pinpoint the location and extent of aneurysms.

Treatment

Treatment for ruptures of cerebral aneurysms includes measures to stabilize the emergency by assuring cardiopulmonary functions (adequate heart rate and respiration) while simultaneously moving to decrease intracranial pressure and surgically clip (repair and seal) the ruptured cerebral aneurysm.

Surgery is often performed as soon as the patient is stabilized; ideally within 72 hours of the onset of rupture. The goal of surgery is to prevent rebleeding. Surgery is performed to expose the aneurysm and allow the placement of a clip across a strong portion of the vessel to obstruct the flow of blood through the weakened aneurysm. Repeat surgical procedures to seal an aneurysm are not uncommon.

Treatment of unruptured aneurysms is certainly less dramatic, but presents a more deliberate and complex path. Microcoil thrombosis or balloon embolization (the insertion via the arterial catheter of a balloon or other obstruction that blocks blood flow through the region of aneurysm) are alternatives to full surgical intervention.

Other nonsurgical interventions include rest, medications, and hypertensive-hypervolemic therapy to drive blood around obstructed vessels.

Treatment decisions are made between the treatment team and family members with regard to the best course of treatment and the probable outcomes for patients suffering a severe aneurysm rupture with extensive damage to surrounding brain tissue.

Asymptomatic aneurysms allow the treatment team to more fully evaluate surgical and nonsurgical options.

Recovery and rehabilitation

The recovery and rehabilitation of patients suffering a cerebral aneurysm depend on the location and size of the aneurysm. The course of recovery and rehabilitation is also heavily influenced by whether the aneurysm ruptures.

Key to recovery is the prevention of aneurysm re-bleeding, the management of swelling in the **ventricular system** (hydrocephalus), **seizures**, cardiac arrhythmias, and vasospasm. The onset of vasospasm within the first two weeks of the initial bleeding incident is the major cause of death in those who survive the initial rupture of the aneurysm.

Ventricular drains are used to control the buildup of cerebrospinal fluid in the ventricular system.

Clinical trials

As of May 2004, current studies sponsored by the National Institute of Neurological Disorders and Stroke (NINDS) include a study on the effect of the drug ProliNO on brain artery spasms after aneurysm rupture and a study of the role of genetics on the development of intracranial aneurysms (Familial Intracranial Aneurysm Study). Further information is available at <http://www.clinicaltrials.gov>.

Prognosis

The overall prognosis for a patient with a cerebral aneurysm depends on several factors including the size, location, and stability of the aneurysm. Facets of the patient's general health, neurological health, age, and familial history must also be evaluated in forming a prognosis.

Although each patient is different, and each aneurysm must be individually evaluated, in general, the prognosis for patients who have suffered a bleed is guarded at best, with mortality rates up 60% within a year of the initial bleeding incident. Approximately half of the survivors suffer some long-lasting disability. Patients with cerebral aneurysm can, however, fully recover with no long-lasting disorder.

Data regarding the prognosis for unruptured aneurysms is more tentative and not specific for cerebral aneurysms. Some long-term studies give evidence that only 10% of patients might suffer leakage or bleeding from their aneurysm over a period of 10 years and only about a quarter of patients would experience bleeding from the aneurysm over a period of 25 years.

Special concerns

Intracerebral aneurysms are sometimes associated with other diseases such as fibromuscular hyperplasia or other disorders such as high blood pressure (although aneurysms also occur in persons with normal blood pressure.

Other physiological stresses such as pregnancy have not been demonstrated to have a correlation to the rupture of cerebral aneurysm.

Resources

BOOKS

Bear, M., et al. *Neuroscience: Exploring the Brain.* Baltimore: Williams & Wilkins, 1996.

Goetz, C. G., et al. *Textbook of Clinical Neurology.* Philadelphia: W.B. Saunders Co., 1999.

Goldman, Cecil. *Textbook of Medicine*, 21st ed. New York: W.B. Saunders Co., 2000.

Guyton & Hall. *Textbook of Medical Physiology,* 10th ed. New York: W.B.Saunders Co., 2000.

Wiebers, David. *Stroke-Free for Life: The Complete Guide to Stroke Prevention and Treatment.* New York: Harper, 2002.

OTHER

"Stroke Risk Factors." *American Stroke Association.* April 20, 2004 (May 22, 2004). <http://www.strokeassociation.org/presenter.jhtml?identifier=4716>.

ORGANIZATIONS

American Stroke Association: A Division of American Heart Association. 7272 Greenville Avenue, Dallas, TX 75231-4596. (214) 706-5231 or (888) 4STROKE (478-7653). strokeassociation@heart.org. <http://www.strokeassociation.org/>.

Brain Aneurysm Foundation. 12 Clarendon Street, Boston, MA 02116. (617) 723-3870; Fax: (617) 723-8672. information@bafound.org. <http://www.bafound.org>.

National Stroke Association. 9707 East Easter Lane, Englewood, CO 80112-3747. (303) 649-9299 or (800) STROKES (787-6537); Fax: (303) 649-1328. info@stroke.org. <http//www.stroke.org/>.

Paul Arthur

Angelman syndrome

Definition

Angelman syndrome (AS) is a genetic condition that causes severe **mental retardation**, severe speech impairment, and a characteristic happy and excitable demeanor.

Description

Individuals with AS show evidence of delayed development by 6–12 months of age. Eventually, this delay is recognized as severe mental retardation. Unlike some genetic conditions causing severe mental retardation, AS is

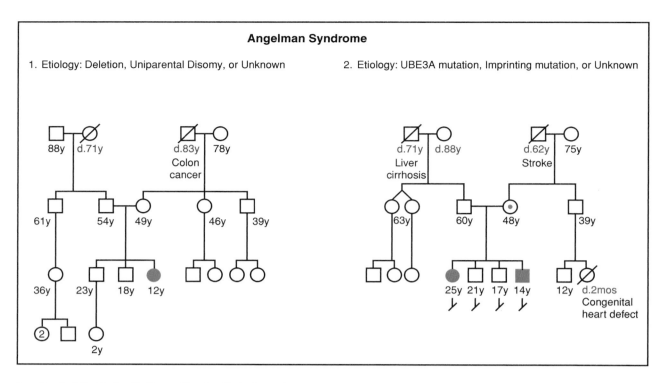

Angelman Syndrome

1. Etiology: Deletion, Uniparental Disomy, or Unknown

2. Etiology: UBE3A mutation, Imprinting mutation, or Unknown

See Symbol Guide for Pedigree Charts. *(Gale Group.)*

not associated with developmental regression (loss of previously attained developmental milestones).

Severe speech impairment is a striking feature of AS. Speech is almost always limited to a few words. However, receptive language skills (listening to and understanding the speech of others) and non-verbal communication are not as severely affected.

Individuals with AS have a balance disorder, causing unstable and jerky movements. This typically includes gait **ataxia** (a slow, unbalanced way of walking) and tremulous movements of the limbs.

AS is also associated with a unique "happy" behavior, which may be the best-known feature of the condition. This may include frequent laughter or smiling, often with no apparent stimulus. Children with AS often appear happy, excited, and active. They may also sometimes flap their hands repeatedly. Generally, they have a short attention span. These characteristic behaviors led to the original name of this condition, the "Happy Puppet" syndrome. However, this name is no longer used as it is considered insensitive to AS individuals and their families.

Demographics

AS has been reported in individuals of diverse ethnic backgrounds. The incidence of the condition is estimated at 1/10,000 to 1/30,000.

Causes and symptoms

Most cases of AS have been traced to specific genetic defects on chromosomes received from the mother. In about 8% of individuals with AS, no genetic cause can be identified. This may reflect misdiagnosis, or the presence of additional, unrecognized mechanisms leading to AS.

The first abnormalities noted in an infant with AS are often delays in motor milestones (those related to physical skills, such as sitting up or walking), muscular **hypotonia** (poor muscle tone), and speech impairment. Some infants seem unaccountably happy and may exhibit fits of laughter. By age 12 months, 50% of infants with AS have **microcephaly** (a small head size). Tremulous movements are often noted during the first year of life.

Seizures occur in 80% of children with AS, usually by three years of age. No major brain lesions are typically seen on cranial imaging studies.

The achievement of walking is delayed, usually occurring between two-and-a-half and six years of age. The child with AS typically exhibits a jerky, stiff gait, often with uplifted and bent arms. About 10% of individuals with AS do not walk. Additionally, children may have drooling, protrusion of the tongue, hyperactivity, and a short attention span.

Many children have a decreased need for sleep and abnormal sleep/wake cycles. This problem may emerge in infancy and persist throughout childhood. Upon awakening at night, children may become very active and destructive to bedroom surroundings.

The language impairment associated with AS is severe. Most children with AS fail to learn appropriate and consistent use of more than a few words. Receptive language skills are less severely affected. Older children and adults are able to communicate by using gestures or communication boards (special devices bearing visual symbols corresponding to commonly used expressions or words).

Some individuals with AS may have a lighter skin complexion than would be expected given their family background.

Diagnosis

The clinical diagnosis of AS is made on the basis of physical examination and medical and developmental history. Confirmation requires specialized laboratory testing.

There is no single laboratory test that can identify all cases of AS. Several different tests may be performed to look for the various genetic causes of AS. When positive, these tests are considered diagnostic for AS. These include DNA methylation studies, UBE3A mutation analysis, and fluorescent in situ hybridization (FISH).

Treatment team

Children with Angelman syndrome will need help from a variety of professionals, including a general pediatrician and pediatric **neurologist**. A child psychiatrist and/or psychologist may be helpful as well, particularly to help design and implement various behavioral plans. Physical, occupational, and speech and language therapists may help support specific deficits. A learning specialist may be consulted for help with an individualized educational plan.

Treatment

There is no specific treatment for AS. A variety of symptomatic management strategies may be offered for hyperactivity, seizures, mental retardation, speech impairment, and other medical problems.

The typical hyperactivity in AS may not respond to traditional behavior modification strategies. Children with AS may have a decreased need for sleep and a tendency to awaken during the night. Drug therapy may be prescribed to counteract hyperactivity or aid sleep. Most families make special accommodations for their child by providing a safe yet confining environment.

Seizures in AS are usually controllable with one or more anti-seizure medications. In some individuals with severe seizures, dietary manipulations may be tried in combination with medication.

Individuals with AS may be more likely to develop particular medical problems which are treated accordingly. Newborn babies may have difficulty feeding and special bottle nipples or other interventions may be necessary. Gastroesophageal reflux (heartburn) may lead to vomiting or poor weight gain and may be treated with drugs or surgery. Constipation is a frequent problem and is treated with laxative medications. Many individuals with AS have strabismus (crossed eyes), which may require surgical correction. Orthopedic problems, such as tightening of tendons or scoliosis, are common. These problems may be treated with physical therapy, bracing, or surgery.

Prognosis

Individuals with AS have significant mental retardation and speech impairment that are considered to occur in all cases. However, they do have capacity to learn and should receive appropriate educational training.

Young people with AS typically have good physical health aside from seizures. Although life span data are not available, the life span of people with AS is expected to be normal.

Special concerns

Educational concerns

Children with AS appear to benefit from targeted educational training. Physical and occupational therapy may improve the disordered, unbalanced movements typical of AS. Children with a severe balance disorder may require special supportive chairs. Speech therapy is often directed towards the development of nonverbal communication strategies, such as picture cards, communication boards, or basic signing gestures.

Legal issues

The most pressing long-term concern for patients with AS is working out a life plan for ongoing care, since many are likely to outlive their parents. The parents of a child diagnosed with AS should consult an estate planner, an attorney, and a certified public accountant (CPA) in order to draft a life plan and letter of intent. A letter of intent is not a legally binding document, but it gives the patient's siblings and other relatives or caregivers necessary information on providing for her in the future. The attorney can help the parents decide about such matters as guardianship as well as guide them through the legal process of appointing a guardian, which varies from state to state.

Resources

PERIODICALS

"Angelman syndrome." *The Exceptional Parent* 30, no. 3 (March 2000): S2.

Lombroso, Paul J. "Genetics of Childhood Disorders: XVI. Angelman Syndrome: A Failure to Process." *Journal of the American Academy of Child and Adolescent Psychiatry* 39, no. 7 (July 2000): 931.

ORGANIZATION

Angelman Syndrome Foundation, Inc. 414 Plaza Drive, Suite 209, Westmont, IL 60559. (800) IF-ANGEL or (630) 734-9267. Fax: (630) 655-0391. Info@angelman.org. <http://www.angelman.org>.

WEBSITES

Williams, Charles A., M.D., Amy C. Lossie, Ph.D., and Daniel J. Driscoll, Ph.D. "Angelman Syndrome." (November 21, 2000). *GeneClinics.* University of Washington, Seattle. <http://www.geneclinics.org/profiles/angelman/details>.

Jennifer Ann Roggenbuck, MS, CGC
Rosalyn Carson-DeWitt, MD

Angiography

Definition

Angiography is the x-ray (radiographic) study of the blood vessels. An angiogram uses a radiopaque substance, or contrast medium, to make the blood vessels visible under x ray. The key ingredient in most radiographic contrast media is iodine.

Purpose

Angiography is used to detect abnormalities, including narrowing (stenosis) or blockages in the blood vessels (called occlusions) throughout the circulatory system and in some organs. The procedure is commonly used to identify atherosclerosis; to diagnose heart disease; to evaluate kidney function and detect kidney cysts or tumors; to map renal anatomy in transplant donors; to detect an aneurysm (an abnormal bulge of an artery that can rupture leading to hemorrhage), tumor, blood clot, or **arteriovenous malformations** (abnormal tangles of arteries and veins) in the brain; and to diagnose problems with the retina of the eye. It is also used to provide surgeons with an accurate vascular map of the heart prior to open-heart surgery, or of the brain prior to neurosurgery. Angiography may be used after penetrating trauma, like a gunshot or knife wound, to detect blood vessel injury. It may also be used to check the position of shunts and stents placed by physicians into blood vessels.

Precautions

Patients with kidney disease or injury may have further kidney damage from the contrast media used for angiography. Patients who have blood-clotting problems, have a known allergy to contrast media, or are allergic to iodine may not be suitable candidates for an angiography procedure. Newer types of contrast media classified as non-ionic are less toxic and cause fewer side effects than traditional ionic agents. Because x rays carry risks of ionizing **radiation** exposure to the fetus, pregnant women are also advised to avoid this procedure.

Description

Angiography requires the injection of a contrast medium that makes the blood vessels visible to x ray. The contrast medium is injected through a procedure known as arterial puncture. The puncture is usually made in the groin area, armpit, inside of the elbow, or neck.

Patients undergoing an angiogram are advised to stop eating and drinking eight hours prior to the procedure. They must remove all jewelry before the procedure and change into a hospital gown. If the arterial puncture is to be made in the armpit or groin area, shaving may be required. A sedative may be administered to relax the patient for the procedure. An intravenous (IV) line is also inserted into a vein in the patient's arm before the procedure begins, in case medication or blood products are required during the angiogram, or if complications arise.

Prior to the angiographic procedure, patients are briefed on the details of the test, the benefits and risks, and the possible complications involved, and asked to sign an informed consent form.

The site is cleaned with an antiseptic agent and injected with a local anesthetic. Then, a small incision is made in the skin to help the needle pass. A needle containing a solid inner core called a stylet is inserted through the incision and into the artery. When the radiologist has punctured the artery with the needle, the stylet is removed and replaced with another long wire called a guide wire. It is normal for blood to spurt out of the needle before the guide wire is inserted.

The guide wire is fed through the outer needle into the artery to the area that requires angiographic study. A fluoroscope displays a view of the patient's vascular system and is used to direct the guide wire to the correct location. Once it is in position, the needle is then removed, and a catheter is threaded over the length of the guide wire until it reaches the area of study. The guide wire is then removed, and the catheter is left in place in preparation for the injection of the contrast medium.

Depending on the type of angiographic procedure being performed, the contrast medium is either injected by hand with a syringe or is mechanically injected with an automatic injector, sometimes called a power injector, connected to the catheter. An automatic injector is used frequently because it is able to deliver a large volume of contrast medium very quickly to the angiographic site. Usually a small test injection is made by hand to confirm

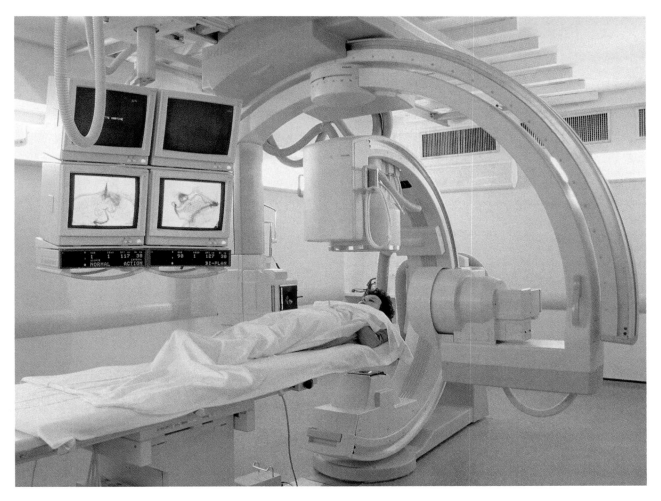

A female patient undergoing a cerebral angiography. The arteries of her brain are seen in the angiograms (arterial x rays) on the monitors at the upper left; a radio-opaque dye has been injected into her arterial system. (© Laurent. Photo Researchers. Reproduced by permission.)

that the catheter is in the correct position. The patient is told that the injection will start, and is instructed to remain very still. The injection causes some mild to moderate discomfort. Possible side effects or reactions include **headache**, **dizziness**, irregular heartbeat, nausea, warmth, burning sensation, and chest **pain**, but they usually last only momentarily. To view the area of study from different angles or perspectives, the patient may be asked to change positions several times, and subsequent contrast medium injections may be administered. During any injection, the patient or the imaging equipment may move.

Throughout the injection procedure, radiographs (x-ray pictures) or fluoroscopic images are obtained. Because of the high pressure of arterial blood flow, the contrast medium dissipates through the patient's system quickly and becomes diluted, so images must be obtained in rapid succession. One or more automatic film changers may be used to capture the required radiographic images. In many

imaging departments, angiographic images are captured digitally, negating the need for film changers. The ability to capture digital images also makes it possible to manipulate the information electronically, allowing for a procedure known as digital subtraction angiography (DSA). Because every image captured is comprised of tiny picture elements called pixels, computers can be used to manipulate the information in ways that enhance diagnostic information. One common approach is to electronically remove or (subtract) bony structures that otherwise would be superimposed over the vessels being studied, hence the name digital subtraction angiography.

Once the x rays are complete, the catheter is slowly and carefully removed from the patient. Manual pressure is applied to the site with a sandbag or other weight for 10–20 minutes to allow for clotting to take place and the arterial puncture to reseal itself. A pressure bandage is then applied, usually for 24 hours.

Key Terms

Arteriosclerosis A chronic condition characterized by thickening and hardening of the arteries and the build-up of plaque on the arterial walls. Arteriosclerosis can slow or impair blood circulation.

Carotid artery An artery located in the neck that supplies blood to the brain.

Catheter A long, thin, flexible tube used in angiography to inject contrast material into the arteries.

Cirrhosis A condition characterized by the destruction of healthy liver tissue. A cirrhotic liver is scarred and cannot function properly (i.e., breaks down the proteins in the bloodstream). Cirrhosis is associated with portal hypertension.

Embolism A blood clot, air bubble, or clot of foreign material that travels and blocks the flow of blood in an artery. When blood supply blocks a tissue or organ with an embolism, infarction (death of the tissue the artery feeds) occurs. Without immediate and appropriate treatment, an embolism can be fatal.

Femoral artery An artery located in the groin area that is the most frequently accessed site for arterial puncture in angiography.

Fluorescein dye An orange dye used to illuminate the blood vessels of the retina in fluorescein angiography.

Fluoroscope An imaging device that displays x rays of the body. Fluoroscopy allows the radiologist to visualize the guide wire and catheter moving through the patient's artery.

Guide wire A wire that is inserted into an artery to guide a catheter to a certain location in the body.

Ischemia A lack of normal blood supply to a organ or body part because of blockages or constriction of the blood vessels.

Necrosis Cellular or tissue death; skin necrosis may be caused by multiple, consecutive doses of radiation from fluoroscopic or x-ray procedures.

Plaque Fatty material that is deposited on the inside of the arterial wall.

Portal hypertension A condition caused by cirrhosis of the liver, characterized by impaired or reversed blood flow from the portal vein to the liver. The resulting pressure can cause an enlarged spleen and dilated, bleeding veins in the esophagus and stomach.

Portal vein thrombosis The development of a blood clot in the vein that brings blood into the liver. Untreated portal vein thrombosis causes portal hypertension.

Most angiograms follow the general procedures outlined above, but vary slightly depending on the area of the vascular system being studied. There is a variety of common angiographic procedures.

Cerebral angiography

Cerebral angiography is used to detect **aneurysms**, stenosis, blood clots, and other vascular irregularities in the brain. The catheter is inserted into the femoral or carotid artery and the injected contrast medium travels through the blood vessels in the brain. Patients frequently experience headache, warmth, or a burning sensation in the head or neck during the injection portion of the procedure. A cerebral angiogram takes two to four hours to complete.

Coronary angiography

Coronary angiography is administered by a cardiologist with training in radiology or, occasionally, by a radiologist. The arterial puncture is typically made in the femoral artery, and the cardiologist uses a guide wire and catheter to perform a contrast injection and x-ray series on

the coronary arteries. The catheter may also be placed in the left ventricle to examine the mitral and aortic valves of the heart. If the cardiologist requires a view of the right ventricle of the heart or of the tricuspid or pulmonic valves, the catheter is inserted through a large vein and guided into the right ventricle. The catheter also serves the purpose of monitoring blood pressures in these different locations inside the heart. The angiographic procedure takes several hours, depending on the complexity of the procedure.

Pulmonary (lung) angiography

Pulmonary, or lung, angiography is performed to evaluate blood circulation to the lungs. It is also considered the most accurate diagnostic test for detecting a pulmonary embolism. The procedure differs from cerebral and coronary angiography in that the guide wire and catheter are inserted into a vein instead of an artery, and are guided up through the chambers of the heart and into the pulmonary artery. Throughout the procedure, the patient's **vital signs** are monitored to ensure that the catheter doesn't cause arrhythmias, or irregular heartbeats. The contrast medium is then injected into the pulmonary artery where it circulates through the lungs' capillaries. The test typically takes up to 90 minutes and carries more risk than other angiography procedures.

Kidney (renal) angiography

Patients with chronic renal disease or injury can suffer further damage to their kidneys from the contrast medium used in a renal angiogram, yet they often require the test to evaluate kidney function. These patients should be well hydrated with an intravenous saline drip before the procedure, and may benefit from available medications (e.g., dopamine) that help to protect the kidney from further injury associated with contrast agents. During a renal angiogram, the guide wire and catheter are inserted into the femoral artery in the groin area and advanced through the abdominal aorta, the main artery in the abdomen, and into the renal arteries. The procedure takes approximately one hour.

Fluorescein angiography

Fluorescein angiography is used to diagnose retinal problems and circulatory disorders. It is typically conducted as an outpatient procedure. The patient's pupils are dilated with eye drops and he or she rests the chin and forehead against a bracing apparatus to keep it still. Sodium fluorescein dye is then injected with a syringe into a vein in the patient's arm. The dye travels through the patient's body and into the blood vessels of the eye. The procedure does not require x rays. Instead, a rapid series of close-up photographs of the patient's eyes are taken, one set immediately after the dye is injected, and a second set approximately 20 minutes later once the dye has moved through the patient's vascular system. The entire procedure takes up to one hour.

Celiac and mesenteric angiography

Celiac and mesenteric angiography involves radiographic exploration of the celiac and mesenteric arteries, arterial branches of the abdominal aorta that supply blood to the abdomen and digestive system. The test is commonly used to detect aneurysm, thrombosis, and signs of ischemia in the celiac and mesenteric arteries, and to locate the source of gastrointestinal bleeding. It is also used in the diagnosis of a number of conditions, including portal hypertension, and cirrhosis. The procedure can take up to three hours, depending on the number of blood vessels studied.

Splenoportography

A splenoportograph is a variation of an angiogram that involves the injection of contrast medium directly into the spleen to view the splenic and portal veins. It is used to diagnose blockages in the splenic vein and portal-vein

thrombosis and to assess the patency and location of the vascular system prior to liver transplantation.

Most angiographic procedures are typically paid for by major medical insurance. Patients should check with their individual insurance plans to determine their coverage.

Computerized tomographic angiography (CTA), a new technique, is used in the evaluation of patients with intracranial aneurysms. CTA is particularly useful in delineating the relationship of vascular lesions with bony anatomy close to the skull base. While such lesions can be demonstrated with standard angiography, it often requires studying several projections of the two-dimensional films rendered with standard angiography. CTA is ideal for more anatomically complex skull-base lesions because it clearly demonstrates the exact relationship of the bony anatomy with the vascular pathology. This is not possible using standard angiographic techniques. Once the information has been captured a workstation is used to process and reconstruct images. The approach yields shaded surface displays of the actual vascular anatomy that are three dimensional and clearly show the relationship of the bony anatomy with the vascular pathology.

Angiography can also be performed using **magnetic resonance imaging** (**MRI**) scanners. The technique is called MRA (magnetic resonance angiography). A contrast medium is not usually used, but may be used in some body applications. The active ingredient in the contrast medium used for MRA is one of the rare earth elements, gadolinium. The contrast agent is injected into an arm vein, and images are acquired with careful attention being paid to the timing of the injection and selection of MRI specific imaging parameters. Once the information has been captured, a workstation is used to process and reconstruct the images. The post-processing capabilities associated with CTA and MRA yield three-dimensional representations of the vascular pathology being studied and can also be used to either enhance or subtract adjacent anatomical structures.

Aftercare

Because life-threatening internal bleeding is a possible complication of an arterial puncture, an overnight stay in the hospital is sometimes recommended following an angiographic procedure, particularly with cerebral and coronary angiography. If the procedure is performed on an outpatient basis, the patient is typically kept under close observation for a period of six to 12 hours before being released. If the arterial puncture was performed in the femoral artery, the patient is instructed to keep his or her leg straight and relatively immobile during the observation period. The patient's blood pressure and vital signs are monitored, and the puncture site observed closely. Pain medication may be prescribed if the patient is experiencing discomfort from the puncture, and a cold pack is often applied to the site to reduce swelling. It is normal for the puncture site to be sore and bruised for several weeks. The patient may also develop a hematoma at the puncture site, a hard mass created by the blood vessels broken during the procedure. Hematomas should be watched carefully, as they may indicate continued bleeding of the arterial puncture site.

Angiography patients are also advised to have two to three days of rest after the procedure in order to avoid placing any undue stress on the arterial puncture site. Patients who experience continued bleeding or abnormal swelling of the puncture site, sudden dizziness, or chest pain in the days following an angiographic procedure should seek medical attention immediately.

Patients undergoing a fluorescein angiography should not drive or expose their eyes to direct sunlight for 12 hours following the procedure.

Risks

Because angiography involves puncturing an artery, internal bleeding or hemorrhage are possible complications of the test. As with any invasive procedure, infection of the puncture site or bloodstream is also a risk, but this is rare.

A **stroke** or heart attack may be triggered by an angiogram if blood clots or plaque on the inside of the arterial wall are dislodged by the catheter and form a blockage in the blood vessels or artery, or if the vessel undergoes temporary narrowing or spasm from irritation by the catheter. The heart may also become irritated by the movement of the catheter through its chambers during pulmonary and coronary angiographic procedures, and arrhythmias may develop.

Patients who develop an allergic reaction to the contrast medium used in angiography may experience a variety of symptoms, including swelling, difficulty breathing, heart failure, or a sudden drop in blood pressure. If the patient is aware of the allergy before the test is administered, certain medications (e.g., steroids) can be administered at that time to counteract the reaction.

Angiography involves minor exposure to radiation through the x rays and fluoroscopic guidance used in the procedure. Unless the patient is pregnant, or multiple radiological or fluoroscopic studies are required, the dose of radiation incurred during a single procedure poses little risk. However, multiple studies requiring fluoroscopic exposure that are conducted in a short time period have been known to cause skin necrosis in some individuals. This risk can be minimized by careful monitoring and documentation of cumulative radiation doses administered to these patients, particularly in those who have therapeutic procedures performed along with the diagnostic angiography.

Results

The results of an angiogram or arteriogram depend on the artery or organ system being examined. Generally, test results should display a normal and unimpeded flow of blood through the vascular system. Fluorescein angiography should result in no leakage of fluorescein dye through the retinal blood vessels.

Abnormal results of an angiogram may display a narrowed blood vessel with decreased arterial blood flow (ischemia) or an irregular arrangement or location of blood vessels. The results of an angiogram vary widely by the type of procedure performed, and should be interpreted by and explained to the patient by a trained radiologist.

Resources

BOOKS

Baum, Stanley, and Michael J. Pentecost, eds. *Abrams' Angiography*, 4th ed. Philadelphia: Lippincott-Raven, 1996.

LaBergem, Jeanne, ed. *Interventional Radiology Essentials*, 1st ed. Philadelphia: Lippincott Williams & Wilkins, 2000.

Ziessman, Harvey, ed. *The Radiologic Clinics of North America, Update on Nuclear Medicine*. Philadelphia: W. B. Saunders Company, 2001.

OTHER

Food and Drug Administration. *Public Health Advisory: Avoidance of Serious X-Ray-Induced Skin Injuries to Patients during Fluoroscopically Guided Procedures. September 30, 1994*. Rockville, MD: Center for Devices and Radiological Health, FDA, 1994.

Radiological Society of North America CMEJ. *Renal MR Angiography*. April 1, 1999 (February 18, 2004). <http://ej.rsna.org/ej3/0091-98.fin/mainright.html>.

Stephen John Hage, AAAS, RT(R), FAHRA
Lee Alan Shratter, MD

Angiomatosis *see* **von Hippel-Lindau disease**

Anosmia

Definition

The term anosmia means lack of the sense of smell. It may also refer to a decreased sense of smell. Ageusia, a companion word, refers to a lack of taste sensation. Patients who actually have anosmia may complain wrongly of ageusia, although they retain the ability to distinguish salt, sweet, sour, and bitter—humans' only taste sensations.

Description

Of the five senses, smell ranks fourth in importance for humans, although it is much more pronounced in other animals. Bloodhounds, for example, can smell an odor that is a thousand times weaker than one perceptible by humans. Taste, considered the fifth sense, is mostly the smell of food in the mouth. The sense of smell originates from the first cranial nerves (the olfactory nerves), which sit at the base of the brain's frontal lobes, right behind the eyes and above the nose. Inhaled airborne chemicals stimulate these nerves.

There are other aberrations of smell beside a decrease. Smells can be distorted, intensified, or hallucinated. These changes usually indicate a malfunction of the brain.

Causes and symptoms

The most common cause of anosmia is nasal occlusion caused by rhinitis (inflammation of the nasal membranes). If no air gets to the olfactory nerves, smell will not happen. In turn, rhinitis and nasal polyps (growths on nasal membranes) are caused by irritants such as allergens, infections, cigarette smoke, and other air pollutants. Tumors such as nasal polyps can also block the nasal passages and the olfactory nerves and cause anosmia. Head injury or, rarely, certain viral infections can damage or destroy the olfactory nerves.

Diagnosis

It is difficult to measure a loss of smell, and no one complains of loss of smell in just one nostril. So a physician usually begins by testing each nostril separately with a common, non-irritating odor such as perfume, lemon, vanilla, or coffee. Polyps and rhinitis are obvious causal agents a physician looks for. Imaging studies of the head may be necessary in order to detect brain injury, sinus infection, or tumor.

Treatment

Cessation of smoking is one step. Many smokers who quit discover new tastes so enthusiastically that they immediately gain weight. Attention to reducing exposure to other nasal irritants and treatment of respiratory allergies or chronic upper respiratory infections will be beneficial. Corticosteroids are particularly helpful.

Alternative treatment

Finding and treating the cause of the loss of smell is the first approach in naturopathic medicine. If rhinitis is the cause, treating acute rhinitis with herbal mast cell stabilizers and herbal decongestants can offer some relief as the body heals. If chronic rhinitis is present, this is often related to an environmental irritant or to food allergies. Removal of the causative factors is the first step to healing. Nasal steams with essential oils offer relief of the blockage and tonification of the membranes. Blockages can sometimes be resolved through naso-specific therapy—a way of realigning the nasal cavities. Polyp blockage can be addressed through botanical medicine treatment as well as hydrotherapy. Olfactory nerve damage may not be regenerable. Some olfactory aberrations, like intensified sense of smell, can be resolved using homeopathic medicine.

Prognosis

If nasal inflammation is the cause of anosmia, the chances of recovery are excellent. However, if nerve damage is the cause of the problem, the recovery of smell is much more difficult.

Resources

BOOKS

Bennett, J. Claude, and Fred Plum, eds. *Cecil Textbook of Medicine.* Philadelphia: W. B. Saunders Co., 1996.

Harrison's Principles of Internal Medicine. Ed. Anthony S. Fauci, et al. New York: McGraw-Hill, 1997.

"Olfactory Dysfunction." In *Current Medical Diagnosis and Treatment, 1996.* 35th ed. Ed. Stephen McPhee, et al. Stamford: Appleton & Lange, 1995.

PERIODICALS

Davidson, T. M., C. Murphy, and A. A. Jalowayski. "Smell Impairment. Can It Be Reversed?" *Postgraduate Medicine* 98 (July 1995): 107-109, 112.

J. Ricker Polsdorfer, MD

Anoxia *see* **Hypoxia**

> **Key Terms**
>
> **Allergen** Any substance that irritates only those who are sensitive (allergic) to it.
>
> **Corticosteroids** Cortisone, prednisone, and related drugs that reduce inflammation.
>
> **Rhinitis** Inflammation and swelling of the nasal membranes.
>
> **Nasal polyps** Drop-shaped overgrowths of the nasal membranes.

Anticholinergics

Definition

Anticholinergics are a class of medications that inhibit parasympathetic nerve impulses by selectively blocking the binding of the neurotransmitter acetylcholine to its receptor in nerve cells. The nerve fibers of the parasympathetic system are responsible for the involuntary movements of smooth muscles present in the gastrointestinal tract, urinary tract, lungs, etc. Anticholinergics are divided into three categories in accordance with their specific targets in the central and/or **peripheral nervous system**: antimuscarinic agents, ganglionic blockers, and **neuromuscular blockers**.

Purpose

Anticholinergic drugs are used to treat a variety of disorders such as gastrointestinal cramps, urinary bladder spasm, asthma, motion sickness, muscular spasms, poisoning with certain toxic compounds, and as an aid to anesthesia.

Description

Antimuscarinic agents are so called because they block muscarine, a poisonous substance found in the *Amanita muscaria*, a nonedible mushroom species. Muscarine is a toxic compound that competes with acetylcholine for the same cholinoreceptors. Antimuscarinic agents are atropine, scopolamine, and ipratropium bromide. Atropine and scopolamine are alkaloids naturally occurring in *Atropa belladonna* and *Datura stramonium* plants, whereas ipratropium bromide is a derivative of atropine used to treat asthma.

Under the form of atropine sulfate, atropine is used in the treatment of gastrointestinal and bladder spasm, cardiac arrhythmias, and poisoning by cholinergic toxins such as organophosphates or muscarine. Atropine is used in ophthalmology as well when the measurement of eye refractive errors (i.e., cyclopegia) is required, due to its papillary dilation properties. Scopolamine shows an effect in the peripheral nervous system similar to those of atropine. However, scopolamine is a **central nervous system** (CNS) depressant and constitutes a highly effective treatment to prevent motion sickness, although at high doses it causes CNS excitement with side effects similar to those caused by high doses of atropine. Its use in ophthalmology is identical in purpose to that of atropine. The main use of ipratropium is for asthma treatment. Ipratropium is also administered to patients with chronic obstructive pulmonary disease.

Benapryzine, benzhexol, orphenadrine, and bornaprine are other examples of anticholinergic drugs used

Key Terms

Acetylcholine   The neurotransmitter, or chemical that works in the brain to transmit nerve signals, involved in regulating muscles, memory, mood, and sleep.

Neuromuscular junction   The junction between a nerve fiber and the muscle it supplies.

Neurotransmitter   Chemicals that allow the movement of information from one neuron across the gap between the adjacent neuron.

Parasympathetic nervous system   A branch of the autonomic nervous system that tends to induce secretion, increase the tone and contraction of smooth muscle, and cause dilation of blood vessels.

alone or in combination with other medications in **Parkinson's disease** to improve motor function. Disturbances in dopaminergic transmissions are associated with the symptoms observed in Parkinson's disease. The beneficial effects of anticholinergics in this disease are due to the resulting imbalance between dopamine and acetylcholine ratio in neurons (e.g., levels of acetylcholine lower than dopamine levels). These anticholinergic agents may interfere with mood and also decrease gastrointestinal movements, causing constipation; and the positive effects on motor functions vary among patients. Other classes of drugs available today that act on the pathways of dopamine and its receptors to treat Parkinson's disease, such as levodopa, tolcapone, and pramipexol, effectively increase the levels of dopamine at dopaminergic receptors in neurons.

Ganglionic blockers are anticholinergic agents that target nicotinic receptors in nerve cells of either sympathetic or parasympathetic systems. The most used ganglionic blockers are trimethaphan and mecamylamine. Trimethaphan is administered by intravenous infusion for the emergency short-term control of extreme high blood pressure caused by pulmonary edema, or in surgeries that require a controlled lower blood pressure, such as the repair of an aortic aneurysm. Mecamylamine is used to treat moderately severe and severe hypertension (high blood pressure), as the drug is easily absorbed when taken orally.

Neuromuscular anticholinergic agents act on motor-nerve cholinoreceptors. They prevent the transmission of signals from motor nerves to neuromuscular structures of the skeletal muscle. Neuromuscular blockers are very useful as muscle relaxants in several surgical procedures, either as an adjuvant to anesthesia or as a pre-anesthetic. Their main therapeutic use is in surgical procedures. Examples of the first group are mivacurium, tubocurarine, metocurine, doxacurium, and atracurium; the second group consists of rocuronium, vecuronium, pipercuronion, and pancuronium.

Precautions

Atropine should be avoided by persons suffering from hepatitis, glaucoma, gastrointestinal obstruction, decreased liver or kidney function, and allergy to anticholinergic agents. Scopolamine is not indicated in cases of glaucoma, asthma, severe colitis, genitourinary or gastrointestinal obstruction, and **myasthenia gravis**, as well as people with hypersensitivity to cholinergic blockers.

The prescription of ganglionic blockers to patients with kidney insufficiency, or coronary or cerebrovascular disorders requires special caution and should only be a choice when other agents cannot be used instead.

Side effects

Atropine may cause severe adverse effects with dose-dependent degrees of severity. Overdoses of atropine, for instance, may induce **delirium**, hallucinations, coma, circulatory and respiratory collapse, and death. Rapid heart rate, dilation of pupils and blurred vision, restlessness, burning **pain** in the throat, marked mouth dryness, and urinary retention are observed with higher doses, while lower dosages may result in decreased salivary, respiratory, and perspiration secretions. Sometimes surgeons administer atropine prior to surgery due to this antisecretory property. Scopolamine's main side effects are similar to those observed with atropine.

The adverse effects of ganglionic blockers include paralysis of gastrointestinal movements, nausea, gastritis, urinary retention, and blurred vision.

Neuromuscular blockers' adverse effects may include apnea (failure in breathing) due to paralysis of the diaphragm, hypotension (low blood pressure), tachycardia, post-surgery muscle pain, increased intraocular pressure, and malignant hyperthermia (uncontrolled high fever).

Resources

BOOKS

Champe, Pamela C., and Richard A. Harvey (eds). *Pharmacology,* 2nd ed. Philadelphia: Lippincott Williams & Wilkins, 2000.

OTHER

"Anticholinergics/Antispasmodics (Systemic)." *Yahoo! Health Drug Index.* May 14, 2004 (May 22, 2004). <http://health.yahoo.com/health/drug/202049/>.

"Anticholinergics/Antispasmodics (Systemic)." *Medline Plus.* National Library of Medicine. May 15, 2004 (May 22, 2004). <http://www.nlm.nih.gov/medlineplus/druginfo/uspdi/202049.html>.

Sandra Galeotti, MS

Anticonvulsants

Definition

Anticonvulsants are a class of drugs indicated for the treatment of various types of **seizures** associated with seizure disorders such as **epilepsy**, a neurological dysfunction in which excessive surges of electrical energy are emitted in the brain, and other disorders.

Some anticonvulsants are indicated for other medical uses. Some **hydantoins**, such as phenytoin, are also used as skeletal muscle relaxants and antineuralgics in the treatment of neurogenic **pain**. Some anticonvulsants and **antiepileptic drugs** (AEDs) are used in psychiatry for the treatment of bipolar disorders (manic-depression).

Purpose

Although there is no cure for the disorder, anticonvulsants are often effective in controlling the seizures associated with epilepsy. The precise mechanisms by which many anticonvulsants work are unknown, and different sub-classes of anticonvulsants are thought to exert their therapeutic effects in diverse ways. Some anticonvulsants are thought to generally depress **central nervous system** (CNS) function. Others, such as GABA inhibitors, are thought to target specific neurochemical processes, suppress excess neuron function, and regulate electrochemical signals in the brain.

Description

There are several sub-classes and types of anticonvulsants. They are marketed in the United States under a variety of brand names.

- Barbiturates, including Mephobarbital (Mebaral), Pentobarbital (Nembutal), and **Phenobarbital** (Luminol, Solfoton).
- Benzodiazepines, including Chlorazepate (Tranxene), Clonazepam (Klonopin), and **Diazepam** (Valium).
- GABA Analogues, including **Gabapentin** (Neurontin) and **Tiagabine** (Gabitril).
- Hydantoins, including Ethotoin (Peganone), Fosphentyoin (Mesantoin), and Phenytoin (Dilantin).
- Oxazolidinediones, including Trimethadione (Tridione).
- Phenyltriazines, including **Lamotrigine** (Lamictal).

Key Terms

Bipolar disorder   A psychiatric disorder marked by alternating episodes of mania and depression. Also called bipolar illness, manic-depressive illness.

Epilepsy   A disorder associated with disturbed electrical discharges in the central nervous system that cause seizures.

Neurogenic pain   Pain originating in the nerves or nervous tissue and following the pathway of a nerve.

Seizure   A convulsion, or uncontrolled discharge of nerve cells that may spread to other cells throughout the brain, resulting in abnormal body movements or behaviors.

- Succinamides, including Ethosuximide (Zarontin), Methsuximide (Celontin), and Phensuximide (Milontin).
- Other anticonvulsants, including **Acetazolamide** (Diamox), **Carbamazepine** (Carbatrol, Tegretol), **Felbamate** (Felbatol), **Levetiracetam** (Keppra), Oxcarbazepine (Trileptal), **Primidone** (Mysoline), **Topiramate** (Topamax), Valproic acid (Depakene, Depakote), and **Zonisamide** (Zonegran).

A physician prescribes anticonvulsant medication, or a combination of anticonvulsant medications, according to seizure type and pattern in individual patients. Some anticonvulsant medications are not appropriate for pediatric patients under 16 years of age.

Recommended dosage

Anticonvulsants are available in oral suspension (syrup), injectable, capsule, tablet, and sprinkle forms, depending on the type of medication. Not all anticonvulsants will be available in all forms. Anticonvulsants are prescribed by physicians in varying daily dosages, depending on the age, weight, and other health concerns of the individual patient, as well as the severity and frequency of their seizures.

It is important to follow the prescribing physicians directions carefully as each individual anticonvulsant medication has its own recommended daily dosages and dose schedule. Some anticonvulsants are taken in a single daily dose; others are taken in divided, multiple daily doses. A double dose of any anticonvulsant medication should not be taken. If a dose is missed, it should be taken as soon as possible. However, if it is within four hours of the next scheduled dose, the missed dose should be skipped. Taking an anticonvulsant at regular intervals and at the same time each day enables consistent levels of the medication to be maintained in the bloodstream, and results in more effective seizure control.

In general, initiating any course of treatment which includes anticonvulsants requires a gradual dose-increasing regimen. Adults and children typically take a smaller daily dose for the first two weeks. Daily dosages of anticonvulsant medication may then be slowly titrated, or increased over time until adequate seizure control is achieved using the lowest dose possible.

When ending a course of treatment of anticonvulsant, physicians typically taper the patient's daily dose over a period of several weeks. Suddenly stopping treatment including anticonvulsants may cause seizures to return or occur with greater frequency. Patients taking anticonvulsants drugs for the treatment of pain or bipolar disorders may experience also have seizures, even if they have never had them before, if they suddenly stop taking the medication.

Precautions

Each anticonvulsant medication may have its own precautions, counter-indications, and side-effects. However, many are common to all anticonvulsant medications.

Consult the prescribing physician before taking any anticonvulsant with non-perscription medications. Patients should avoid alcohol and CNS depressants (medications that make one drowsy or tired, such as antihistimines, sleep medications, and some pain medications) while taking anticonvulsants. Anticonvulsants can exacerbate the side effects of alcohol and other medications. Alcohol may also increase the risk or frequency of seizures.

Anticonvulsants may not be suitable for persons with a history of **stroke**, anemia, thyroid, liver, depressed kidney function, diabetes mellitus, severe gastro-intestinal disorders, porphyria, **lupus**, some forms of mental illness, high blood presure, angina (chest pain), irregular heartbeats, and other heart problems.

Before beginning treatment with anticonvulsants, patients should notify their physician if they consume a large amount of alcohol, have a history of drug use, are nursing, pregnant, or plan to become pregnant.

Physicians generally advise the use of effective birth control while taking many anticonvulsant medications. Patients taking anticonvulsants should be aware that many anticonvulsants may increase the risk of birth defects. Furthermore, many anticonvulsant medications are secreted in breast milk. Patients who become pregnant while taking any anticonvulsant should contact their physician immediately to discuss the risks and benefits of continuing treatment during pregnancy and while nursing.

Some anticonvulsants may be prescribed for children. However, children may experience increased side effects. Research indicates that some children who take high doses of some anticonvulsants (such as hydantoins) for an extended period of time may experience mild learning difficulties or not perform as well in school.

Side effects

In some patients, anticonvulsants may produce usually mild side effects. **Headache**, nausea, and unusual tiredness and weakness are the most frequently reported side effects of anticonvulsants. Other general side effects of anticonvulsants that do not usually require medical attention include:

• mild coordination problems

• mild dizziness

• abdominal pain or cramping

• sinus pain

• sleeplessness or nightmares

• change in appetite

• mild feelings of anxiety

• feeling of warmth

• tingling or prickly feeing on the skin, or in the toes and fingers

• mild tremors

• diarrhea or constipation

• heartburn or indigestion

• aching joints and muscles or chills

• unpleasant taste in mouth or dry mouth

Many of these side effects disappear or occur less frequently during treatment as the body adjusts to the medication. However, if any symptoms persist or become too uncomfortable, the perscribing physician should be consulted.

Other, uncommon side effects of anticonvulsants can be serious or may indicate an allergic reaction. A patient taking any anticonvulsant who experiencs one or more of the following symptoms should contact the prescribing physician immediately:

• rash or bluish, purplish, or white patches on the skin

• jaundice (yellowing of the skin and eyes)

• bloody nose or unusual bleeding

• hallucinations (seeing visions or hearing voices that are not present)

• sores in the mouth or around the eyes

• ringing or vibrations in the ears

• **depression** or suicidal thoughts

• mood or mental changes, including excessive fear, anxiety, hostility

• severe tremors

• prolonged numbness in the extremeties

• general loss of motor skills

• persistent lack of appetite

• altered vision

• frequent or burning urination

• difficulty breathing

• chest pain or irregular heartbeat

• faintness or loss of consciousness

• persistant, severe headaches

• persistant fever or pain.

Interactions

Anticonvulsants may have negative interactions with some antacids, anticoagulants, antihistimines, antidepressants, antibiotics, pain killers (including lidocaine) and monoamine oxidase inhibitors (MAOIs). Other medications such as amiodarone, diazoxide, phenybutazone, sulfonamides (sulfa drugs), corticosteroids, sucralfate, rifampin, and warfarin may also adversely react with anticonvulsants.

Some anticonvulsants should not be used in combination with other anticonvulsants. (For example, phenytoin (a hydantoin) when used with valproic acid, another anticonvulsant, may increase the seizure frequency). However, several anticonvulsant medications are indicated to be used in conjunction with or suppliment other anticonvulsants. If advised and carefully monitored by a physician, a course of treatment including multiple seizure prevention medications can be effective and safe.

Most anticonvulsants decrease the effectiveness of contraceptives that contain estrogens or progestins, including oral contraceptives (birth control pills), progesterone implants (Norplant), and progesterone injections (Depo-Provera).

Resources

BOOKS

Masters, Roger D., Michael T. McGuire. *The Neurotransmitter Revolution.* Southern Illinois University Press, 1994.

Mondimore, Francis Mark. *Bipolar Disorder: A Guide for Patients and Families.* Baltimore: The Johns Hopkins University Press, 1999.

Weaver, Donald F. *Epilepsy and Seizures: Everything You Need to Know.* Firefly Books, 2001.

Key Terms

Absence seizures Also called a petit mal seizure, characterized by abrupt, short-term lack of conscious activity or other abnormal change in behavior.

Atonic seizure A seizure characterized by a sudden loss of muscle tone, causing the individual to fall to the floor.

Epilepsy A disorder associated with disturbed electrical discharges in the central nervous system that cause seizures.

Febrile convulsion Seizures occurring mainly in children between three months and five years of age that are triggered by fever.

Partial seizure An episode of abnormal activity in a localized, specific part of the brain that causes changes in attention, movement, and/or behavior.

Status epilepticus A serious condition involving continuous seizures with no conscious intervals.

Tonic-clonic seizure A seizure involving the entire body characterized by unconsciousness, muscle contraction, and rigidity. Also called grand mal or generalized seizures.

Trigeminal neuralgia A disorder of the trigeminal nerve that causes severe facial pain.

Wyllie, Elaine. *The Treatment of Epilepsy: Principles and Practice.* New York: Lippincott, Williams & Wilkins, 2001.

PERIODICALS

Feely, Morgan. "Drug treatment of epilepsy." *BMJ* 318 (9 January 1999): 106–109.

"Risk of birth defects with anticonvulsants evaluated." *Psychopharmacology Update* 12, no. 5 (May 2001): 3.

OTHER

"Seizure Medicines." *Epilepsy.com.* <http://www.epilepsy.com/epilepsy/seizure_medicines.html> (May 1, 2004).

ORGANIZATIONS

Epilepsy Foundation. 4351 Garden City Drive, Landover, MD 20785-7223. (800) 332-1000. <http://www.epilepsyfoundation.org>.

American Epilepsy Society. 342 North Main Street, West Hartford, CT 06117-2507. <http://www.aesnet.org>.

Adrienne Wilmoth Lerner

Antiepileptic drugs

Definition

Antiepileptic drugs are all drugs used to treat or prevent convulsions, as in **epilepsy**.

Purpose

Antiepileptic drugs (AEDs) are designed to modify the structures and processes involved in the development of a seizure, including neurons, ion channels, receptors, glia, and inhibitory or excitatory synapses. These processes are modified to favor inhibition over excitation in order to stop or prevent seizure activity.

Description

The ideal AED would suppress all **seizures** without causing any unwanted side effects. Unfortunately, the drugs currently used not only fail to control seizure activity in some patients, but frequently cause side effects that range in severity from minimal impairment of the **central nervous system** (CNS) to death from aplastic anemia or liver (hepatic) failure.

Prior to 1993, the choice of an antiepileptic medication was limited to traditional drugs, as **phenobarbital**, **primidone**, phenytoin, **carbamazepine** and valproate. Although these drugs have the advantage of proven efficacy (effectiveness), many patients are left with refractory (break-through) seizures. Since 1993, many new medications have been approved by the United States Food and Drug Administration (FDA), expanding treatment options. The newer AEDs offer the potential advantages of fewer drug interactions, unique mechanisms of action, and a broader spectrum of activity.

The AEDs can be grouped according to their main mechanism of action, although many have several different actions and others work through unknown mechanisms. The main groups include sodium channel blockers, calcium current inhibitors, gamma-aminobutyric acid (GABA) enhancers, glutamate blockers, and drugs with unknown mechanisms of action.

Sodium Channel Blockade

Blocking the sodium channel in the cell membrane is the most common and the most well-characterized mechanism of currently available AEDs. AEDs that target these sodium channels prevent the return of the channels to the active state by stabilizing the inactive form. In doing so, repetitive firing of nerve impulses from the axon of the nerve is prevented. The blockade of sodium channels of nerve axons causes stabilization of the neuronal membranes and limits the development of seizure activity. Sodium channel blocker drugs include: carbamazepine, phenytoin, fosphenytoin, oxcarbazepine, lamotrignine, and zonizamide.

Calcium Current Inhibitors

Calcium channels are small channels in the nerve cell that function as the "pacemakers" of normal rhythmic brain cell activity. Calcium current inhibitors are particularly useful for controlling absence seizures. The drug ethosuximide is a calcium current inhibitor.

GABA Reuptake Inhibitors

GABA reuptake inhibitors boost the levels of GABA, a neurotransmitter, in the brain. **Neurotransmitters** such as GABA are naturally occurring chemicals that transmit messages from one neuron (nerve cell) to another. When one neuron releases GABA, it normally binds to the next neuron, transmitting information and preventing the transmission of extra electrical activity. When levels of GABA are reduced, there may not be enough GABA to sufficiently bond to the neuron, leading to extra electrical activity in the brain and seizures. **Tiagabine** works to block GABA from being re-absorbed too quickly into the tissues, thereby increasing the amount available to bind to neurons.

GABA Receptor Agonist

GABA receptor agonists bind with certain cell-surface proteins and produce changes that mimic that action of GABA, thereby reducing excess electrical activity and seizures. Clonazepam, phenobarbital, and primidone are examples of GABA receptor agonist drugs. Some drugs such as valproate enhance the synthesis of GABA, in addition to other potential mechanisms of action, and thus prevent seizures.

Glutamate Blockers

Glutamate and aspartate are the two most important excitatory neurotransmitters in the brain. By blocking glutamate action, the excess electrical activity that causes seizures is controlled. **Topiramate** and **felbamate** are examples of glutamate blocker drugs, but their use is limited because they sometimes produce hallucinations and behavior changes.

Recommended dosage

Antiepileptic drugs are usually prescribed in an initial dose, then gradually increased over time until maximum seizure control is achieved with a minimum of side effects. Recommended dosages for specific antiepileptic drugs include:

- Carbamazepine: In generalized tonic-clonic seizures or partial seizures, by mouth, ADULT: initially 100 mg twice daily, increased gradually according to response to usual maintenance dose of 0.8–1.2 g; ELDERLY: reduce initial dose; CHILD: 10–20 mg/kg daily in divided doses. **Trigeminal neuralgia**, by mouth, ADULT: initially 100 mg 1–2 times daily increased gradually according to response; usual dose 200 mg 3–4 times daily with up to 1.6 g daily.

- Clonazepam: Epilepsy, by mouth, ADULT: initially 1 mg at night for 4 nights, increased gradually over 2–4 weeks to a usual maintenance dose of 4–8 mg daily in divided doses; ELDERLY: initial dose 500 micrograms increased as above; CHILD: up to 1 year initially 250 micrograms increased as above to 0.5–1 mg daily in divided doses; 1–5 years: initially 250 micrograms increased to 1–3 mg daily in divided doses; 5–12 years: initially 500 micrograms increased to 3–6 mg daily in divided doses.

- **Diazepam**: Emergency management of recurrent epileptic seizures, by slow intravenous injection (at rate of 5 mg/minute), ADULT: 10–20 mg, repeated if necessary after 30–60 minutes; may be followed by intravenous infusion to maximum 3 mg/kg over 24 hours; CHILD: 200 to 300 micrograms/kg (or 1 mg per year of age); by rectum as solution, ADULT and CHILD over 10 kg: 500 micrograms/kg; ELDERLY: 250 micrograms/kg; repeated if necessary every 12 hours. Febrile convulsions, by rectum as solution; CHILD over 10 kg: 500 micrograms/kg (maximum 10 mg), with dose repeated if necessary. Seizures associated with poisoning, by slow intravenous injection (at rate of 5 mg/minute), ADULT: 10–20 mg.

- Ethosuximide: Absence seizures, by mouth, ADULT and CHILD over 6 years: initially 500 mg daily, increased by 250 mg at intervals of 4–7 days to a usual dose of 1–1.5 g daily (occasionally, up to maximum of 2 g daily); CHILD under 6 years: initially 250 mg daily, increased gradually to usual dose of 20 mg/kg daily.

- Felbamate: By mouth, ADULT: 2400–4600 mg per day; CHILD: 40–60 mg/kg per day. Optimal individual maintenance doses will be determined by clinical response.

- Fosphenytoin: For emergency management of repeated seizures, by intravenous injection, 22.5 to 30 mg per kg. For nonemergent therapy, by intravenous injection, 15 to 30 mg per kg, followed by 6 to 12 mg per kg for maintenance therapy.

- **Lamotrigine**: ADULT: by mouth, if added to valproate monotherapy, 25 mg daily for two weeks, then 50 mg daily for two weeks, then titrate up to 150 mg twice daily. If added to carbamazepine, phenytoin, phenobarbital, or primidone, initial dose 50 mg twice daily, subsequent increases up to 100–200 mg twice daily.

CHILD, by mouth, if added to valproate monotherapy, initial dose 0.5 mg/kg/day, final maintenance dose of 1–5 mg/kg/day. If added to carbamazepine, phenytoin, phenobarbital, or primidone: initial doses 2 mg/kg/day, with subsequent increases to 5–15 mg/kg/day.

- Levetiracetam: ADULT: by mouth, 1000–3000 mg/day. CHILD: dosage range not established.

- Oxcarbazepine: ADULT: by mouth, 600–2400 mg per day; CHILD: by mouth, 10–30 mg/kg per day.

- Phenobarbital: Generalized tonic-clonic seizures, partial seizures, by mouth, ADULT: 60-180 mg at night; CHILD: up to 8 mg/kg daily. Febrile convulsions, by mouth, CHILD: up to 8 mg/kg daily. Neonatal seizures, by intravenous injection (dilute injection 1 in 10 with water for injections), NEWBORN: 5–10 mg/kg every 20–30 minutes up to plasma concentration of 40 mg/liter. By intravenous injection (dilute injection 1 in 10 with water for injections), ADULT: 10 mg/kg at a rate of not more than 100 mg/minute (up to maximum total dose of 1 g); CHILD: 5–10 mg/kg at a rate of not more than 30 mg/minute.

- Phenytoin sodium: Generalized tonic-clonic seizures, partial seizures, by mouth, ADULT: initially 3–4 mg/kg daily (as a single dose or in 2 divided doses), increased gradually by 25 mg at intervals of 2 weeks as necessary (with plasma-phenytoin concentration monitoring); usual dose 200–500 mg daily; CHILD: initially 5 mg/kg daily in 2 divided doses; usual dose range 4–8 mg/kg daily (maximum 300 mg).

- Primidone: ADULT: by mouth, 500–1250 mg per day. CHILD: by mouth, 5–20 mg/kg per day. Optimal individual maintenance doses will be determined by clinical response.

- Sodium valproate: Generalized tonic-clonic seizures, partial seizures, absence seizures, atonic seizures; myoclonic seizures, by mouth, ADULT: initially 600 mg daily in 2 divided doses, preferably after food, increased by 200 mg daily at 3-day intervals to maximum of 2.5 g daily in divided doses; usual maintenance dose 1–2 g daily (20–30 mg/kg daily); CHILD: up to 20 kg, initially 20 mg/kg daily in divided doses, may be increased provided plasma concentrations monitored; CHILD over 20 kg: initially 400 mg daily in divided doses, increased until control (usually in range of 20–30 mg/kg daily); maximum 35 mg/kg daily.

- Tiagabine: By mouth, suggested ADULT maintenance dose 32 to 56 mg/day. Dosage titrations of 4–8 mg/day weekly are suggested by the manufacturer.

- Topiramate: ADULT: by mouth, 400 mg per day. An initiation schedule, where the medication dose is increased

by 50 mg/day each week, is recommended to reduce adverse effects; slower rates of initiation are used by some physicians.

- Zonisamide: ADULT: by mouth, 100–400 mg/day; CHILD dosage range not established.

Precautions

Withdrawal

Treatment is normally continued for a minimum of two years after the last seizure. Withdrawal should be extended over a period of several months, as abrupt withdrawal can lead to complications such as **status epilepticus**, a serious event where seizures occur rapidly and continuously. Many adult patients relapse once treatment is withdrawn and it may be justified to continue treatment indefinitely, particularly when the patient's livelihood or lifestyle can be endangered by recurrence of a seizure.

Pregnancy and Breast-feeding

Untreated epilepsy during pregnancy may cause harm to the fetus; there is, therefore, no justification for abrupt withdrawal of treatment. Withdrawal of therapy with antiepileptic medications may be an option if the patient has been seizure-free for at least two years. Resumption of treatment may be considered after the first trimester. If antiepileptics are continued in pregnancy, a single medication with the lowest effective dose is preferred, and blood levels of the medication should be monitored. There is an increased risk of birth defects with the use of AEDs, particularly carbamazepine, valproate, and phenytoin. However, if there is good seizure control, many physicians see no advantage in changing pregnant patients' AEDs. In view of the risks of neural tube and other defects, patients who may become pregnant should be informed of the risks and referred for advice, and pregnant patients should be offered counseling and screening. To counteract the risk of neural tube defects, adequate folic acid supplements are advised for women before and during pregnancy. In view of the risk of bleeding associated with carbamazepine, phenobarbital, and phenytoin, prophylactic phytomenadione (vitamin K1) is recommended for the mother before delivery and the newborn. Use of AEDs can often be continued during breastfeeding.

Driving

Regulations are in place in many countries that may restrict driving by patients with epilepsy. Further, AEDs may cause central nervous system **depression**, particularly in the early stages of treatment. Patients affected by adverse effects such as drowsiness or **dizziness** should not operate machinery or drive.

Side effects

The most common side effects of therapy with antiepileptic drugs are drowsiness and dizziness. Other drug-specific side effects include:

- Carbamazepine: Dizziness, double vision, nausea, loss of coordination, and blurred vision.
- Clonazepam: Sedation, **ataxia** (loss of coordination), hyperactivity, restlessness, irritability, depression, cardiovascular or respiratory depression. Children and infants may have excess saliva production. Occasionally, tonic seizures may be exacerbated.
- Diazepam: Drowsiness, dizziness, tiredness, weakness, dry mouth, diarrhea, upset stomach, changes in appetite, restlessness or excitement, constipation, difficulty urinating, frequent urination, blurred vision, changes in sex drive or ability.
- Ethosuximide: Drowsiness, upset stomach, vomiting, constipation, diarrhea, stomach **pain**, loss of taste and appetite, weight loss, irritability, mental confusion, depression, insomnia, nervousness, and **headache**.
- Felbamate: Insomnia, weight loss, nausea, decreased appetite, dizziness, **fatigue**, ataxia (loss of coordination), and lethargy.
- Fosphenytoin: Burning/tingling sensations, groin pain, itching, nausea, dizziness or drowsiness may occur. Serious side effects may occur: mental/mood changes, loss of coordination, rash, eye/vision problems.
- Lamotrigine: Rash is the main concern associated with this drug. Other commonly reported adverse reactions are headache, blood dyscrasias, ataxia (loss of coordination), double vision, psychosis, tremor, hypersensitivity reactions, and prolonged sleepiness or insomnia.
- Levetiracetam: Sleepiness, asthenia (loss of strength), dizziness, accidental injury, convulsion, infection, pain, pharyngitis, and a flu-like syndrome.
- Oxcarbazepine: Sleepiness, headache, dizziness, rash, low blood sodium level, weight gain, and hair loss.
- Phenobarbital: Thought and behavior alterations, sedation, psychomotor slowing, poor concentration, depression, irritability, ataxia (loss of coordination), and decreased libido.
- Phenytoin sodium: Ataxia (loss of coordination), abnormal rapid eye movements, drowsiness and lethargy, nausea and vomiting, rash, blood disorders, headaches, vitamin K and folate deficiencies, loss of libido, hormonal dysfunction, and bone marrow suppression.
- Primidone: Intense sedation, dizziness, and nausea at the onset of treatment.
- Sodium valproate: Nausea, vomiting, tremor, sedation, confusion or irritability, and weight gain, elevated blood sugar levels, and hair loss or curling of hair.
- Tiagabine: Dizziness, fatigue, depression, confusion, impaired concentration, speech or language problems, lack of energy, weakness, upset stomach, nervousness, tremor, and stomach pain.
- Topiramate: Dizziness, sleepiness, ataxia (loss of coordination), confusion, fatigue, decreased sensation in lower extremities, speech difficulties, double vision, impaired concentration, and nausea.
- Zonizamide: Dizziness, anorexia, headache, ataxia (loss of coordination), confusion, speech abnormalities, mental slowing, irritability, tremor, weight gain, excessive sleepiness, and fatigue.

Interactions

Antiepilectic drugs may be prescribed alone or in combination with other antiepileptic drugs. In general, drugs that cause central nervous system depression, including alcohol, should be used with caution by those taking antiepileptic medications. Many antiepileptic medications also reduce the effectiveness of oral contraceptives (birth control pills). Specific drug interventions include:

- Carbamazepine: Several drugs, such as macrolide antibiotics (erythromycin and clarithromycin), isoniazid, chloramphenicol, calcium channel blockers, cimetidine, and propoxyphene, inhibit liver enzyme function responsible for the metabolic breakdown of carbamazepine, thereby raising its levels in the blood. Phenobarbital, phenytoin, felbamate, and primidone decrease efficiency of carbamazepine. Toxic symptoms or breakthrough seizures may occur if the dose of carbamazepine is not adjusted. Grapefruit juice and St. John's wort can increase carbamazepine levels. Carbamazepine reduces the effectiveness of tricyclic antidepressants, oral contraceptives, cyclosporin A, and warfarin.
- Clonazepam: Clonazepam blood levels are decreased by coadministration of enzyme-inducing drugs. No significant clinical interactions have been reported.
- Diazepam: Diazepam may increase the effects of other drugs that cause drowsiness, including antidepressants, alcohol, antihistamines, sedatives, pain relievers, anxiety medicines, seizure medicines, and muscle relaxants. Antacids may decrease the effects of diazepam.
- Ethosuximide: Ethosuximide may increase the amount of other antiseizure medications in the blood. Such medications include phenytoin, mephenytoin, and ethotoin. These drugs must be monitored if they are used with ethosuximide to prevent the occurrence of dangerous side effects. Ethosuximide may decrease the level of primidone in the blood, which could lead to a loss of

seizure control. Valproic acid may increase or decrease ethosuximide levels and must be used with caution.

• Felbamate: Felbamate increases blood levels of phenytoin. Adjustments in dosage may be necessary. Its levels are increased by carbamazepine. Felbamate also increases levels of valproic acid in blood.

• Fosphenytoin: Fosphenytoin has no specific known interactions.

• Lamotrigine: Levels increase with concomitant use of valproate.

• Levetiracetam: No significant drug interactions have been identified.

• Oxcarbazepine: Interacts with oral contraceptives, thereby reducing their efficacy.

• Phenobarbital: Metabolism of phenobarbital is inhibited by phenytoin sodium, valproate, felbamate, and dextropropoxyphene. Enzyme inducers, such as rifampicin, decrease phenobarbital levels. Because of the potent induction of liver enzymes, phenobarbital increases the metabolism of estrogen, steroids, warfarin, carbamazepine, diazepam, clonazepam, and valproate.

• Phenytoin sodium: Among all AEDs, phenytoin sodium has one of the most problematic drug interaction profiles. Carbamazepine and phenobarbital have variable and unpredictable effects (i.e., increase or decrease) on phenytoin sodium levels. Valproate raises levels of phenytoin sodium by displacing phenytoin sodium from its protein-binding site and inhibiting its metabolism. Other drugs that significantly increase phenytoin sodium levels are isoniazid, cimetidine, chloramphenicol, dicumarol, and sulfonamides. Drugs that lower phenytoin sodium levels are vigabatrin and amiodarone. Phenytoin sodium itself is a strong inducer of liver enzymes and alters levels of other drugs. It decreases levels of carbamazepine, ethosuximide, felbamate, primidone, tiagabine, and phenobarbital. It inhibits dicumarol, warfarin, and corticosteroids; clotting factors and immunosuppression must be monitored and doses adjusted accordingly. Other drugs whose levels are reduced by phenytoin sodium and require monitoring and adjustment include furosemide, cyclosporin, folate, and praziquantel. Levels of chloramphenicol and quinidine are elevated by phenytoin sodium.

• Primidone: Primidone interacts with most other AEDs. **Acetazolamide**, carbamazepine, ethosuximide, and methsuximide may all decrease the effects of primidone, and larger primidone doses may be necessary. Phenytoin, ethotoin, mephenytoin, and isoniazid may increase blood levels of primidone, and an adjustment of primidone dosage may be necessary. Carbamazepine blood levels may be higher during therapy with primidone, and

an adjustment of the carbamazepine dosage may also be necessary.

• Sodium valproate: Increases plasma levels of free fractions of phenytoin sodium, phenobarbital, carbamazepine epoxide, and lamotrigine. It decreases total phenytoin sodium level. The levels of sodium valproate are decreased by enzyme-inducing drugs and are increased by felbamate and clobazam.

• Tiagabine: Causes a small decrease in valproate levels. Hepatic-inducing drugs increase the clearance of tiagabine by two thirds. Drug plasma concentrations are not affected by valproate, cimetidine, or erythromycin.

• Topiramate: Enzyme-inducing drugs, such as phenytoin sodium or carbamazepine, decrease topiramate concentrations in the blood by approximately 50%. Topiramate generally does not affect the steady-state concentrations of the other drugs given in polytherapy, although phenytoin sodium levels may rise occasionally. Topiramate reduces ethyl estradiol levels by 30% and may inactivate the low-dose contraceptive pill. It may cause a mild reduction in digoxin levels.

• Zonisamide: Phenytoin sodium, carbamazepine, phenobarbital, and valproic acid reduce levels of zonizamide in the blood; however, zonizamide does not affect the levels of these drugs.

Resources

BOOKS

Hardman, Joel Greiffith, Lee E. Limbird, and Alfred G. Gilman. *Goodman & Gilman's The Pharmacological Basis of Therapeutics.* New York: McGraw-Hill Professional, 2001.

PERIODICALS

LaRoche, S., and S. Helmers. "The New Antiepileptic Drugs." *JAMA* 291 (2004): 605–614.

OTHER

"Antiepileptic Drugs: An Overview." *eMedicine.* <http://www.emedicine.com/neuro/topic692.htm> (April 26, 2004).

"Seizure Medicines." *Epilepsy.com.* <http://www.epilepsy.com/epilepsy/seizure_medicines.html> (April 26, 2004).

ORGANIZATIONS

The Epilepsy Foundation. 4351 Garden City Drive, Landover, MD 20785-7223. (800) 332-1000. <http://www.epilepsyfoundation.org/

U.S. Food and Drug Administration. 5600 Fishers Lane, Rockville, MD 20857. (888) 463-6332. <http://www.fda.gov>.

Greiciane Gaburro Paneto,
Iuri Drumond Louro, M.D.,Ph.D.

Antimigraine medications

Definition

Antimigraine medications are drugs that are given to lower the risk of a severe migraine attack or to reduce the severity of the **headache** once an attack begins.

Purpose

Treatment that is given to stop or ease the **pain** of a migraine headache after it has started is known as acute or abortive treatment.

Preventive treatment for migraine headaches is called migraine prophylaxis or prophylactic therapy. Prophylactic medications are taken when the patient is *not* having a headache. They have three purposes:

• lower the frequency and severity of the patient's headaches

• make acute migraines more responsive to abortive treatment

• improve the patient's overall quality of life

Not all patients with migraines need prophylactic treatment. Most doctors, however, recommend prophylactic medications in the following circumstances:

• The patient has two or more migraines per month, with disability lasting three or more days

• Acute treatment is contraindicated or is ineffective

• The patient has been using abortive medications more than twice a week

• The patient has a complex form of migraine such as hemiplegic or basilar migraine

• The patient is at risk of permanent neurologic injury from acute attacks

Description

Abortive medications

Abortive medications for migraine are prescribed according to the severity of the patient's headaches, the presence of nausea or vomiting, the patient's response to the drug, and the presence of such comorbid conditions as **depression** or **epilepsy**. With the exception of mild analgesics, however, these drugs cannot be used as preventive treatment; they are taken only when an acute attack begins. Abortive medications are categorized into four major groups.

SELECTIVE SEROTONIN RECEPTOR (5-HT1) AGONISTS Selective serotonin receptor agonists have been used to treat migraines since 1991. They work by activating serotonin receptors in the brain, which block an inflammatory process that affects the blood vessels in the head and leads

to a leakage of blood plasma through the vessel walls. Some researchers think that the serotonin receptor agonists also reduce the pain of migraine by slowing down the firing of nerve cells in pain-sensitive parts of the head. These drugs, which are also known as triptans or 5-hydroxytryptamine 1B agonists, are effective in treating about 70% of migraine patients. Sumatriptan (Imitrex) is the prototype of this class of medications.

Second-generation triptans include such drugs as eletriptan (Relpax), naratriptan (Amerge), rizatriptan (Maxalt), almotriptan (Axert), frovatriptan (Frova), and zolmitriptan (Zomig). The second-generation triptans were developed to increase the speed of the drug's absorption through the digestive tract and thus relieve the patient's pain more rapidly. All the triptans are prescribed for moderately severe or severe migraines; one, sumatriptan, is available as a nasal spray or injection for patients with severe vomiting. One major drawback of the triptans, however, is that moderate-to-severe headache pain tends to recur within 24 hours of the first dose.

ERGOT ALKALOIDS Ergot alkaloids are an older group of drugs that include such compounds as ergotamine tartrate (Ergostat) and dihydroergotamine (DHE-45, Migranal). These drugs are derived from ergot, a compound produced by a fungus (*Claviceps purpurea*) that grows on rye plants. The medications work by causing the blood vessels in the head to constrict or narrow, which counteracts the dilation of the blood vessels that causes pain. Some medications in this group are combinations of ergotamine tartrate and caffeine (Cafergot, Ercaf); the caffeine intensifies the vasoconstrictive effect of the alkaloid. Like the triptans, the ergot alkaloids are used to treat moderate-to-severe migraines. They are not prescribed as frequently as they once were, however, because of the severity of their side effects and because they cannot be given to patients with coronary artery disease or other vascular disorders.

ANALGESICS Analgesics in general are medications given to relieve pain. These drugs are used to treat patients who have infrequent migraine headaches, or who cannot be treated with triptans. There are two main types of analgesics used as acute treatment for migraines, nonsteroidal anti-inflammatory drugs, or NSAIDs, and combination analgesics. NSAIDs include aspirin, naproxen (Naprosyn), diclofenac (Voltaren, Cataflam), ibuprofen (Advil, Motrin), flurbiprofen (Ansaid), ketorolac (Toradol), and ketoprofen (Orudis). Combination analgesics include butalbital plus acetaminophen (Fioricet), butalbital plus aspirin (Fiorinal), and isometheptene plus acetaminophen and **dichloralphenazone** (Midrin).

As of 2004, doctors disagree about the use of opioid (drugs that are or act like narcotics) analgesics to treat migraine pain. On the one hand, opioids are stronger

Key Terms

Analgesic   A type of drug given to relieve pain.

Aneurysm   A blood-filled sac formed by the dilation of a blood vessel, usually caused by a weakness in the vessel wall.

Anticonvulsant   A type of drug given to prevent or relieve seizures. Anticonvulsants are also known as antiepileptics.

Antiemetic   A type of drug given to stop vomiting.

Aura   A group of visual or other sensations that precedes the onset of a migraine attack.

Basilar migraine   A type of migraine with aura that involves the basilar artery at the base of the brain. It occurs most commonly in young women, and may include vision problems, confusion, and loss of consciousness as well as headache.

Comorbid   A term used to refer to a disease or disorder that is not directly caused by another disorder but occurs at the same time.

Ergot   A compound produced by a fungus that grows on rye plants. It is used in the production of some abortive antimigraine drugs.

Gangrene   The death of tissue caused by loss of blood supply. Gangrene is a serious potential side effect of taking ergot alkaloids.

Hemiplegic migraine   Migraine accompanied by temporary paralysis on one side of the body.

Papilledema   Swelling of the optic disk inside the eye, often caused by increased pressure inside the head.

Primary headache   A headache that is not caused by another disease or medical condition. Migraine headaches are one type of primary headache.

Prophylaxis   A measure taken to prevent disease or an acute attack of a chronic disorder.

Rebound headache   A type of primary headache caused by overuse of migraine medications or pain relievers. It is also known as analgesic abuse headache.

Serotonin syndrome   A potentially fatal drug interaction caused by combining drugs that raise the level of serotonin in the patient's nervous system to dangerously high levels. The symptoms of serotonin syndrome include shivering, overreactive reflexes, nausea, low-grade fever, sweating, delirium, mental confusion, and coma.

Status migrainosus   The medical term for an acute migraine headache that lasts 72 hours or longer.

Vasoconstrictive   Causing a blood vessel to become narrower, thus decreasing blood flow.

---

painkillers than NSAIDs or butalbital. On the other hand, they often make the patient quite drowsy or sedated, and they have a high potential for overuse and dependence. Most doctors, however, consider opioids combined with other analgesics—for example, compounds such as oxycodone plus acetaminophen (Percocet) or aspirin with codeine—to be safe for patients with infrequent migraines who can rest if they feel drowsy. Some doctors will prescribe a synthetic opioid known as butorphanol in the form of a nasal spray (Stadol NS) for use as rescue therapy if the patient's usual abortive drug fails to stop an acute attack; this spray, however, is habit forming and is presently classified as a controlled drug.

ANTIEMETICS Antiemetics are medications given to stop vomiting. These may be beneficial if the patient's headaches are often accompanied by nausea and vomiting. The doctor may also prescribe them to enhance the absorption of other medications taken by mouth, because migraines cause the digestive tract to slow down. The most common antiemetics prescribed for migraine patients are droperidol (Inapsine), metoclopramide (Reglan), and

prochlorperazine (Compazine). Prochlorperazine can be given intravenously, by rectal suppositories, or by intramuscular injection if the patient cannot take the drug by mouth.

Prophylactic medications

There are seven major categories of drugs given for migraine prophylaxis.

ANTICONVULSANTS Anticonvulsants, which are also called **antiepileptic drugs**, are considered first-line preventive treatment for migraine. These drugs work by enhancing the neurotransmission of gamma amino-butyric acid, or GABA. GABA is an amino acid that slows down or inhibits the transmission of nerve impulses in the **central nervous system**. Valproic acid (Depakote, divalproex sodium) is the most commonly used anticonvulsant in migraine treatment, and has been shown to reduce migraine frequency by 50%.

Other anticonvulsants that have been used in migraine prophylaxis are **gabapentin** (Neurontin) and **topiramate**

(Topamax). Both drugs are reported to be effective in 50–55% of migraine patients.

BETA-BLOCKERS Beta-blockers are widely prescribed as migraine prophylaxis; they are reported to help 50–70% of patients. The only beta-blockers that have been approved by the Food and Drug Administration (FDA) for migraine therapy, however, are propranolol (Inderal) and timolol (Blocadren). Other beta-blockers that have been used to treat migraines without FDA approval include nadolol (Corgard), atenolol (Tenormin), and metoprolol (Lopressor, Toprol-XL). It is thought that these drugs reduce the frequency of migraines by preventing the blood vessels in the head from dilating and by increasing the release of oxygen to the surrounding tissues. It takes about two months of treatment, however, for patients to benefit from beta-blockers.

CALCIUM CHANNEL BLOCKERS The most common drug in this category used in preventive treatment is verapamil (Calan, Covera, Verelan). Studies of the effectiveness of verapamil, however, have shown mixed results. It appears to be most useful in treating patients who cannot take beta-blockers or have been diagnosed with coexisting hypertension.

TRICYCLIC ANTIDEPRESSANTS (TCAS) The tricyclic antidepressants are another group of drugs used in migraine prophylaxis. Amitriptyline (Elavil) has been shown in well-conducted studies to benefit migraine patients, although doxepin (Sinequan), nortriptyline (Aventyl), and protriptyline (Vivactil, Triptil) have also been used for preventive treatment. TCAs are often given to patients who are suffering from insomnia or depression as well as migraine. Their chief drawback is their long-term side effects, particularly weight gain.

SELECTIVE SEROTONIN REUPTAKE INHIBITORS (SSRIs) These drugs are not as effective for migraine prophylaxis as the tricyclic antidepressants, but a few small-scale studies have shown that they benefit some patients. The SSRIs include such drugs as fluoxetine (Prozac), sertraline (Zoloft), and paroxetine (Paxil).

NONSTEROIDAL ANTI-INFLAMMATORY DRUGS (NSAIDs) Nonsteroidal anti-inflammatory medications can be used for migraine prophylaxis as well as abortive treatment; however, these drugs have a higher risk of adverse effects—particularly in the digestive tract—when they are used preventively.

SEROTONIN ANTAGONISTS Methysergide (Sansert) is a synthetic ergot alkaloid that has been used as prophylactic treatment; its primary disadvantage is the number and severity of possible side effects. Cyproheptadine (Periactin), an antihistamine, is sometimes used for migraine prophylaxis in children even though there is little evidence of its effectiveness.

Complementary and alternative medications (CAM)

There are two herbal preparations used as migraine preventives as of 2004. Feverfew (*Tanacetum parthenium*) is an herb related to the daisy that is traditionally used in England for migraine prophylaxis. Feverfew contains a compound called parthenolide, which is thought to counteract the inflammatory reaction in the cerebral blood vessels that precedes an acute migraine attack.

The second herb is butterbur root (*Petasites hybridus*), which is the active ingredient in Petadolex, a preparation that has been sold in Germany since the 1970s as a migraine preventive. Petadolex has been available in the United States since December 1998. Butterbur root contains compounds known as petasines, which relieve inflammation as well as counteract the spasmodic contraction of blood vessels that occurs during a migraine attack. Researchers reported in 2003 that Petadolex reduced the frequency of migraine attacks in subjects in a multicenter trial by 60%. The butterbur root preparation has fewer and milder side effects than conventional prophylactic drugs; it also appears to be safe for children and adolescents.

It should be noted that, contrary to the popular notion, herbals are drugs that can and do cause side effects; they are not the medical "free ride" many people seem to think they are. They should thus be used with care and caution and in consultation with a physician.

Recommended dosage

Abortive medications

Abortive medications are taken at the first sign of a migraine attack. About 20% of migraine patients have headaches preceded by an aura, or brief period of warning symptoms that may include seeing flashing or shimmering lights, temporary loss of vision, difficulty speaking, weakness in an arm or leg, or tingling sensations in the face or hands. Most patients with migraines, however, do not have auras but experience the headache pain as building gradually over an hour or two. Abortive medications include triptans, ergot alkaloids, NSAIDs, combination analgesics, and antiemetics.

TRIPTANS Sumatriptan is available as a nasal spray or injection as well as in tablet form; the other triptans are available only as tablets. (Sumatriptan should be injected only into the areas the manufacturer recommends; that is, injections into the arms are not recommended because they are much more painful than injections into thighs, the recommended site.) The patient may take 25–100 mg of sumatriptan by mouth at the beginning of an attack, with a second dose of up to 100 mg after two hours. Additional doses may be taken at two-hour intervals, up to 300 mg daily. With the nasal spray, 5–20 mg may be inhaled into one nostril, with a second dose after two hours if the headache returns. Injections of sumatriptan contain 6 mg per dose and may be given twice, at least one hour apart. With zolmitriptan, the initial dose is 2.5–5 mg by mouth, with a second dose at any time after two hours following the first dose; the maximum daily dose is 10 mg. The initial dose of naratriptan is 2.5 mg, which can be repeated four hours after the first dose. Rizatriptan is taken by mouth in an initial dose of 5–10 mg, which may be repeated every two hours up to a maximum daily dose of 30 mg. Almotriptan is taken in an initial dose of 6.25–12.5 mg, which may be repeated only once. Frovatriptan is taken only once, in a dose of 2.5 mg at the beginning of the headache. Eletriptan is taken in an initial dose of 20–40 mg, which may be repeated once after two hours; the maximum daily dose is 80 mg.

ERGOT ALKALOIDS Ergotamine tartrate is taken by mouth in a 1 mg tablet at the beginning of the attack, with additional doses every 30 minutes as needed; total dosage must not exceed 6 mg per attack. Rectal suppositories containing 1–2 mg of the drug may be used at the onset of the headache and repeated every half hour, not to exceed 4 mg per attack. Dihydroergotamine mesylate (DHE-45) may be given by injection in an initial dose of 0.5–1 mg, to be repeated at hourly intervals up to a maximum dose of 3 mg. The drug may also be given intravenously for more rapid relief.

NSAIDS The patient may take an initial dose of 900–1,000 mg of aspirin, with the dose repeated every 1–2 hours as needed. Ibuprofen may be taken by mouth in an initial dose of 400–1,200 mg, to be repeated with a second dose of 400–800 mg in 1–2 hours. The maximum daily dose of ibuprofen is 3,200 mg. Naproxen may be taken in an initial dose of 825 mg, with additional doses of 550 mg after 1–2 hours as needed. Ketorolac may be taken in 10 mg doses every four hours, not to exceed 40 mg per day. Ketorolac should not be used for longer than five days.

COMBINATION ANALGESICS Fiorinal may be taken in an initial dose of 1–2 tablets by mouth every four hours as needed, up to six tablets per day. Midrin is taken in an initial dose of two capsules, then one capsule every hour until the headache is relieved; not to exceed five capsules in a 12-hour period.

ANTIEMETICS Droperidol is given by injection in a dose of 2.5–10 mg. Metoclopramide is given by mouth or by injection in a dose of 10–20 mg. Prochlorperazine may be taken by mouth in a dose of 5–10 mg every 4–6 hours; by injection in a dose of 5–10 mg every 3–4 hours up to a maximum dose of 40 mg per day; or by rectal suppositories in a dose of 25 mg twice a day.

Prophylactic medications

Dosages for these medications vary somewhat depending on the individual patient's response. The general principle of management is to begin with the lowest effective dose of the particular drug, increasing it gradually until the patient begins to benefit or until the maximal safe dose is reached.

ANTICONVULSANTS Valproic acid is given in an initial dose of 150–250 mg per day, gradually increasing to a maximum dose of 1,500 mg per day. Gabapentin is given in an initial dose of 300 mg per day, gradually increasing up to a maximum dose of 2,400 mg per day.

BETA-BLOCKERS Beta-blocker doses are as follows:

• propranolol: initial dose of 40 mg twice a day, up to a maximum of 320 mg per day

• timolol: 10 mg per day initially, maximum daily dose 30 mg

• nadolol: 20 mg four times per day initially, up to a maximum of 240 mg per day

• metoprolol: 50 mg twice a day initially, not to exceed 200 mg per day

CALCIUM CHANNEL BLOCKERS Verapamil is given in an initial dose of 40 mg three times a day; maximal daily dose is 480 mg.

TCAS Amitriptyline, doxepin, and nortriptyline are given by mouth at bedtime in an initial dose of 10–25 mg, with the dose increased by 10–25 mg every two weeks up to a maximum dose of 150–175 mg. Protriptyline is given in an initial dose of 15 mg, up to a maximum daily dose of 40 mg.

SSRIS Fluoxetine is taken on waking in an initial dose of 10 mg, which may be increased every two weeks up to a maximum daily dose of 60 mg. Sertraline may be given in an initial dose of 50 mg per day, increased at weekly intervals up to a daily dose of 200 mg. Paroxetine may be started at a dose of 10 mg per day and gradually increased up to a daily dose of 50 mg.

NSAIDS Naproxen may be taken in a dose of 275 mg three times daily or a dose of 550 mg twice daily.

SEROTONIN ANTAGONISTS Methysergide is given in a daily dose of 2 mg per day, gradually increasing to a maximum of 8 mg per day. Cyproheptadine is given in an initial dose of 2 mg, increasing every three days to a maintenance dose of 8–32 mg per day.

CAM preparations

The recommended dosage of feverfew as a migraine preventive is 125 mg daily of freeze-dried powdered leaf; patients should start out with a lower dose and work up gradually to 125 mg. The dried leaf is available in capsule form. Petadolex is sold as soft gelatin 50-mg capsules. The recommended dose for migraine prophylaxis is 150 mg daily for adults and 50–100 mg daily for children and adolescents.

Precautions

Diagnosis

Migraine headaches are classified by the International Headache Society (IHS) as primary headaches, which means that they are not caused by other diseases or disorders. Severely painful headaches, however, are not necessarily migraines and may be caused by other conditions, some of them potentially life-threatening. Headaches caused by other disorders are known as secondary headaches. They may be associated with space-occupying brain tumors, meningitis, **stroke**, head trauma, pain referred from the neck or jaw, or a ruptured aneurysm inside the head. Patients with any of the following signs or symptoms should be carefully evaluated, including those who have been previously diagnosed with and treated for migraines:

- The patient is not responding to appropriate treatment for the headaches.

- The headache is severe and is sudden in onset. Although a small percentage of patients with migraines have what are called "crash" or "thunderclap" migraines, most migraine headaches build up slowly over a period of one or two hours.

- The headache differs from the usual pattern of the patient's migraines.

- The patient has described the present headache as "the worst ever."

- The patient has abnormal neurological signs or symptoms such as a swollen optic disk (papilledema), seeing double, loss of sensation, or alteration of consciousness.

Some patients may be suffering from another type of primary headache in addition to migraines. It is possible, for example, for people to have both chronic tension headaches and migraines, and each type may require separate treatment.

A third consideration is whether the patient has been diagnosed with any comorbid disorders. The doctor must take such conditions as hypertension, depression, epilepsy, heart problems, and other disorders into account when selecting antimigraine medications for the patient.

Patient education

Effective use of antimigraine drugs depends on good communication between the patient and the doctor. Migraine headaches vary considerably in their frequency, severity, and associated symptoms; in addition, people vary in their responses to a given medication. It may take some months of trial and error to work out the best treatment regimen for an individual patient with respect to the specific drugs used and their dosage levels. Patients should be advised to give each medication a fair trial (usually about two months) before deciding that the drug does not work for them. In addition, they should be told that some drugs—particularly the beta-blockers—must be taken for several months before the patient can expect to see results. Finally, patients who are taking abortive medications or opioid analgesics should be warned about the risks of dependence or rebound headaches from overuse of these drugs.

Rebound headaches

Rebound headaches are also known as analgesic abuse headaches. They result from overuse of abortive drugs, most commonly the ergot alkaloids. According to one survey of primary care physicians, about 20% of patients treated for migraine experience rebound headaches. These headaches have the following characteristics:

- They occur every day or almost every day.

- They are brought on by a very low level of physical or intellectual activity.

- The patient has been using abortive migraine medications more than two days a week.

- The patient has been using the medications above the recommended dosage level.

- The patient develops withdrawal symptoms if the medications are stopped abruptly.

- The headaches are accompanied by restlessness, depression, irritability, difficulty concentrating, or memory problems.

Status migrainosus

About 40% of all migraine attacks do not respond to treatment with triptans or any other medication. If the headache lasts longer than 72 hours (a condition known as status migrainosus), the patient may be given narcotic medications to bring on sleep and stop the attack. Patients with status migrainosus are often hospitalized because they are likely to be dehydrated from severe nausea and vomiting.

Special populations

CHILDREN Migraines in children are not unusual; a study published in 2003 reported that 10% of children between the ages of six and 20 suffer from migraines, and that they lose, on average, almost two more weeks of school each year than their classmates. Treatment of children's migraines, however, is complicated by the fact that most effective medications—whether abortive or prophylactic—have not been adequately evaluated for use in children or are not recommended for children. As of late 2003, however, there have been few rigorous studies of antimigraine drugs in children; much more research is needed in this area. Cyproheptadine, which is the drug most often prescribed for children's migraines, is not always effective; preventive therapy with propranolol, one of the tricyclics, or an anticonvulsant medication appears to be safe as well as effective in children and adolescents.

PREGNANCY AND LACTATION Pregnancy and lactation complicate migraine treatment in that many antimigraine drugs should not be taken by pregnant or nursing women. These include the ergot alkaloids, anticonvulsants, tricyclic antidepressants, methysergide, and the SSRIs. In addition, NSAIDs should not be used during the last trimester of pregnancy.

OLDER ADULTS Some antimigraine medications are not recommended for patients over the age of 60–65, particularly the triptans and the ergot alkaloids. Older adults may also be more susceptible to the side effects of NSAIDs and TCAs.

Patient dissatisfaction

Antimigraine medications as a group have a high rate of reported patient complaints. One reason is the high cost of some of these drugs; another is dosing difficulties. One survey of migraine patients reported the following reasons for discontent with drug therapy: pain relief took too long (87%); pain was only partly relieved (84%); the medication sometimes failed to work (84%); headache returned within a day (71%); the drug had too many side effects (35%). Because of the limitations of antimigraine medications, many doctors advise their patients to supplement drug therapy with such other measures as adequate sleep and **exercise**, a low-fat diet, quitting smoking, stress management techniques, or cognitive-behavioral psychotherapy.

It is also worth noting that managed care (the health insurance industry) accounts for some patient dissatisfaction. Most health plans strictly limit coverage to an "average" number of doses of triptans per month. Patients who need more doses either must have their doctors try to get the insurance company to authorize them, or the patients must pay the full price of the extra medication themselves.

It is possible that new ways of thinking about migraine will lead to improved antimigraine medications in the future. Migraine headaches are no longer regarded as "just headaches," but as features of a largely inherited chronic disorder that increases the risk of long-term damage to the brain. The use of MRIs and other new imaging techniques may eventually answer some unresolved questions about effective migraine treatment.

Side effects

Abortive medications

In addition to the risk of rebound headaches, possible side effects of abortive medications include:

- Triptans: May cause tingling, numbness, sensations of heat or flushing, **dizziness**, drowsiness, or pain at the injection site.
- Ergot alkaloids: May cause nausea, vomiting, diarrhea, weakness, itching, cold skin, thirst, tingling sensations, and severe muscle cramps; also may cause severe rebound headaches. The most serious potential side effect of ergot alkaloids, however, is gangrene—the death of tissue in the fingers or toes due to constriction of the smaller blood vessels and loss of blood supply to the tissue.
- NSAIDs: May cause heartburn, nausea, and vomiting; may also cause drowsiness, dry mouth, or mild depression.
- Combination analgesics: Midrin has been reported to cause temporary dizziness and skin rashes. The most common side effects of Fioricet and Fiorinal include lightheadedness, nausea, and sleep disturbances. Also, the narcotics and barbiturates (Fiorinal) have the potential for drug abuse and dependence.
- Antiemetics: May cause anxiety, dizziness, low blood pressure, sedation, nausea, dry mouth, and restlessness.

Prophylactic medications

The following side effects have been reported for prophylactic medications:

- Anticonvulsants: Valproic acid may cause indigestion and vomiting, but hair loss, weight gain, tremor, hallucinations, and liver damage have also been reported. Gabapentin and topiramate are associated with drowsiness, dizziness, tingling sensations, diarrhea, altered taste, and **fatigue**.
- Beta-blockers: May cause dizziness, fatigue, nausea, memory problems, sexual dysfunction, bradycardia (slowed heartbeat), and hallucinations.
- Calcium channel blockers: May cause low blood pressure and constipation; in addition, the headaches may grow worse for the first few weeks of treatment.
- TCAs: May cause dry mouth, constipation, difficulty urinating, increased appetite, loss of sexual desire, heavy sweating, agitation, tremor, and **seizures**.
- SSRIs: May cause loss of appetite or sexual desire, anxiety, drowsiness, nausea, or flulike symptoms.
- NSAIDs: More likely to cause digestive problems when used for prophylaxis than when used for acute treatment.
- Serotonin antagonists: Methysergide has been reported to cause insomnia, abdominal pain, diarrhea, nausea,

heartburn, increased sensitivity to cold, and depression. Cyproheptadine may cause dry mouth, increased appetite, and weight gain.

CAM preparations

Feverfew should not be used by pregnant women because it may stimulate uterine contractions. It may also cause mild acid indigestion in some people. Patients who use fresh plant leaves rather than standardized preparations may experience mouth ulcers or temporary loss of taste. Also, patients who use fresh plant leaves cannot regulate their doses: one time they may get too much of the drug and another time not enough.

The side effects reported for preparations made from butterbur root are rare, but include an unpleasant taste in the mouth, belching, and a mild skin rash in some patients.

Interactions

Patients who are taking any antimigraine drug should make sure to give the doctor a list of all other medications that they take on a regular basis, including over-the-counter pain relievers, herbal preparations, and any special herbal or medicinal teas or extracts.

Abortive medications

The following interactions have been reported for abortive medications:

- Triptans: All the triptans narrow coronary arteries by 10–20% and will intensify the effects of other vasoconstrictive drugs, including the ergot alkaloids and drugs given for vascular disorders. With the exception of naratriptan, the triptans cannot be taken together with MAO inhibitor antidepressants because of the risk of a rapid and dangerous rise in blood pressure. Rizatriptan has been reported to interact with the beta-blocker propranolol.

- Ergot alkaloids: Cannot be taken together with the triptans. Ergot alkaloids should not be taken together with methysergide because of an additive effect. Should not be taken together with other vasoconstrictive drugs (including beta-blockers, some acid-reducing drugs, some antibiotics, and some antifungal drugs) because of the increased risk of gangrene.

- NSAIDs: These drugs tend to prolong bleeding time and should be used cautiously by patients taking blood-thinning medications. Alcoholic beverages increase the risk of gastric ulcers or bleeding from the use of NSAIDs. In addition, patients should not take more than one NSAID at a time.

- Combination analgesics: These drugs should not be used together with MAO inhibitors or other drugs that contain acetaminophen. They will intensify the actions of other

drugs that may cause drowsiness, including alcohol, TCAs, antihistamines, sedatives, and muscle relaxants.

- Antiemetics: Should not be taken together with alcohol (intensifies central nervous system depression), tricyclic antidepressants (lowers blood pressure), or **phenobarbital**. Patients taking anticonvulsants may need to have their dosage increased if they are given an antiemetic.

Prophylactic medications

The following interactions have been reported for prophylactic medications:

- Anticonvulsants: Valproic acid will intensify the effects of other anticonvulsants, barbiturates, alcohol, and antidepressants. It interacts with aspirin and heparin to increase the risk of spontaneous bleeding. Gabapentin intensifies the effects of morphine, but is less effective when taken together with antacids.

- Beta-blockers: Antacids decrease the absorption of beta-blockers. Cimetidine is reported to intensify the actions of beta-blockers. Beta-blockers may interact with insulin or other diabetes medications to produce high blood sugar levels. They should not be taken together with MAO inhibitors because of the risks of severe high blood pressure. Cocaine also increases the risks of high blood pressure or other heart problems in patients taking beta-blockers.

- Calcium channel blockers: Verapamil may cause low blood pressure or dizziness if taken together with alcohol. It should not be taken with beta-blockers because of a risk of congestive heart failure or slowed heartbeat. Verapamil also intensifies the effects of cyclosporine and lithium.

- TCAs: Should not be taken together with barbiturates, alcohol, sleeping medicines, or sedatives because they intensify central nervous system depression. They may also intensify the effects of certain antibiotics and antifungal medications. They may interact with bupropion to produce seizures. TCAs should never be taken with MAO inhibitors or SSRIs because of the risk of serotonin syndrome, a potentially fatal condition marked by fever, rapid changes in blood pressure, sweating, hyperreactive reflexes, **delirium**, nausea, vomiting, and coma. Serotonin syndrome takes its name from the overly high levels of serotonin in the patient's nervous system that are produced by these drug combinations.

- SSRIs: Should never be taken together with other antidepressant medications because of the risk of serotonin syndrome. They may increase the patient's drowsiness if taken together with antihistamines, sleep medications, opioid analgesics, and muscle relaxants. Patients taking insulin or other diabetes medications may need to have their dosage adjusted if they are also taking an SSRI.

SSRIs should not be taken together with herbal preparations used as mild tranquilizers, particularly compounds containing valerian or St. John's wort.

• Serotonin antagonists: Methysergide should not be taken together with ergot alkaloids or triptans because it intensifies their vasoconstrictive action. Patients taking this drug should give up smoking for the same reason. In addition, methysergide has been reported to counteract the pain-relieving effectiveness of opioid analgesics.

CAM preparations

Feverfew should not be used with anticoagulants (blood thinners), as it intensifies their effects. It may also interfere with the body's absorption of iron. NSAIDs reduce the effectiveness of feverfew. No interactions with prescription drugs have been reported for butterbur root preparations.

Resources

BOOKS

"Headache." Section 14, Chapter 168 in *The Merck Manual of Diagnosis and Therapy*, edited by Mark H. Beers, MD, and Robert Berkow, MD. Whitehouse Station, NJ: Merck Research Laboratories, 2002.

Pelletier, Kenneth R., MD. *The Best Alternative Medicine*, Part II, "CAM Therapies for Specific Conditions: Headache." New York: Simon & Schuster, 2002.

"Psychogenic Pain Syndromes." Section 14, Chapter 167 in *The Merck Manual of Diagnosis and Therapy*, edited by Mark H. Beers, MD, and Robert Berkow, MD. Whitehouse Station, NJ: Merck Research Laboratories, 2002.

Wilson, Billie Ann, RN, PhD, Carolyn L. Stang, PharmD, and Margaret T. Shannon, RN, PhD. *Nurses Drug Guide 2000*. Stamford, CT: Appleton and Lange, 1999.

PERIODICALS

Corbo, J. "The Role of Anticonvulsants in Preventive Migraine Therapy." *Current Pain and Headache Reports* 7 (February 2003): 63–66.

Freitag, F. G. "Preventative Treatment for Migraine and Tension-Type Headaches: Do Drugs Having Effects on Muscle Spasm and Tone Have a Role?" *CNS Drugs* 17 (2003): 373–381.

Kalin, P. "The Common Butterbur (*Petasites hybridus*)—Portrait of a Medicinal Herb." [in German] *Forschende Komplementarmedizin und klassische Naturheilkunde* 10 (April 2003) (Suppl. 1): 41–44.

Kruit, Mark C., MD, Mark A. van Buchem, MD, PhD, Paul A. M. Hofman, MD, PhD, et al. "Migraine as a Risk Factor for Subcortical Brain Lesions." *Journal of the American Medical Association* 291 (January 28, 2004): 427–434.

Malapira, Amelito, MD, and Jorge Mendizabal, MD. "Migraine Headache." *eMedicine* 22 September 2003 (May 9, 2004). <http://www.emedicine.com/neuro/topic218.htm>.

Punay, Nestor C., MD, and James R. Couch, MD, PhD. "Antidepressants in the Treatment of Migraine Headache." *Current Pain and Headache Reports* 7 (February 2003): 51–54.

Sahai, Soma, MD, Robert Cowan, MD, and David Y. Ko, MD. "Pathophysiology and Treatment of Migraine and Related Headache." *eMedicine* 30 April 2002 (May 9, 2004). <http://www.emedicine.com/neuro/topic517.htm>.

Silberstein, S. D., and P. J. Goadsby. "Migraine: Preventive Treatment." *Cephalalgia* 22 (September 2002): 491–512.

Tepper, S. J., and D. Millson. "Safety Profile of the Triptans." *Expert Opinion on Drug Safety* 2 (March 2003): 123–132.

Victor, S., and S. Ryan. "Drugs for Preventing Migraine Headaches in Children." *Cochrane Database System Review* 4 (2003): CD002761.

Waeber, C. "Emerging Drugs in Migraine Treatment." *Expert Opinion on Emerging Drugs* 8 (November 2003): 437–456.

OTHER

Cleveland Clinic Health System. "Migraines in Children and Adolescents." (May 9, 2004.) <http://www.cchs.net/health/health-info/docs/2500/2555.asp?index=9637>.

NINDS. "Migraine Information Page." NINDS, 2003 (May 9, 2004). <http://www.ninds.nih.gov/health_and_medical/pubs/migraineupdate.htm>.

ORGANIZATIONS

American Council for Headache Education (ACHE). 19 Mantua Road, Mt. Royal, NJ 08061. (856) 423-0258; Fax: (856) 423-0082. achehq@talley.com. <http://www.achenet.org>.

International Headache Society (IHS). Oakwood, 9 Willowmead Drive, Prestbury, Cheshire SK10 4BU, United Kingdom. +44 (0) 1625 828663; Fax: +44 (0) 1625 828494. rosemary@ihs.u-net.com. <http://216.25.100.131>.

National Headache Foundation. 820 North Orleans, Suite 217, Chicago, IL 60610. (773) 525-7357 or (888) NHF-5552. <http://www.headaches.org>.

U. S. Food and Drug Administration (FDA). 5600 Fishers Lane, Rockville, MD 20857-0001. (888) INFO-FDA (463-6332). <http://www.fda.gov>.

Rebecca Frey, PhD

Antiparkinson drugs

Definition

Antiparkinson drugs are medicines used to reduce the symptoms of **Parkinson's disease**.

Purpose

Parkinson's disease (PD) is a neurodegenerative disorder that affects movement. In PD, cells in a part of the brain called the substantia nigra die off. The normal function of these cells is to regulate the action of other cells in other brain regions by releasing a chemical called dopamine. When substantia nigra cells release dopamine, the dopamine attaches to dopamine receptors on the other cells, which influences them in various ways depending on the specific type of cell. The actions of these cells work in concert with other systems that influence movement. When all cells are working properly together, the end result is controlled, fluid movement.

When substantia nigra cells die off, however, as they do in PD, less dopamine is available for release. Consequently, the cells that depend on receiving dopamine are not properly regulated. The result is an imbalance in movement control that causes slowed movements, stiffness, and tremor—the classic signs of PD.

Antiparkinson drugs attempt to restore the balance through one of several mechanisms, depending on drug type. The most effective drugs, called dopaminergic drugs, replace dopamine, or mimic its action in the brain. Another group of drugs delays the breakdown of dopamine, thus increasing the level in the brain. Other drugs act on the other systems that influence movement, preventing them from being too active.

Description

Levodopa

Levodopa, also called L-dopa, is the most widely prescribed antiparkinson medication; almost all PD patients eventually receive levodopa. It is a chemical related to dopamine, and it is converted into dopamine within the brain. Dopamine itself cannot cross the barrier between the bloodstream and the brain, while levodopa can. This chemical form of dopamine works in the place of the natural dopamine that is lost due to the disease process.

Levodopa is chemically similar to amino acids, a type of molecule the body needs and absorbs from foods high in protein. In the digestive system, a carrier picks up the levodopa and transports it into the bloodstream. The same transport process occurs between blood and brain. Meals high in protein may interfere with absorption of levodopa from the digestive tract or from the blood into the brain. Patients may be advised to avoid high-protein meals too close to the time they take levodopa.

Once in the bloodstream, levodopa can be converted to dopamine. This is a problem because, as noted, dopamine cannot be taken into the brain. Additionally, dopamine in the periphery (that is, outside the brain)

Key Terms

Dopamine   A neurotransmitter made in the brain that is involved in many brain activities, including movement and emotion.

Dyskinesia   Impaired ability to make voluntary movements.

Orthostatic hypotension   A drop in blood pressure that causes faintness or dizziness and occurs when an individual rises to a standing position. Also known as postural hypotension.

Substantia nigra   One of the movement control centers of the brain.

---

causes nausea, vomiting, and other adverse effects. To minimize these side effects, levodopa is always given with another drug that inhibits its conversion to dopamine in the periphery. In the United States, this drug is carbidopa. Levodopa and carbidopa are available in a single tablet, with doses adjusted for maximum benefit. However, it should be noted that peripheral dopamine is not always undesirable: it has important metabolic functions, including maintaining blood pressure.

Within the brain, levodopa is taken up by remaining substantia nigra cells, converted to dopamine, and released normally. The extra dopamine provided by the levodopa allows the brain to maintain normal movements, even in the face of dying substantia nigra cells. There are limitations because, as the disease progresses and more cells die, it becomes difficult for the few remaining cells to maintain normal function, even with extra dopamine.

Recommended dosage

Levodopa treatment is usually started when the patient's symptoms begin to interfere with daily living or the ability to work. Initial dosage is typically 200–600 mg of levodopa per day, taken in tablets with carbidopa. This amount of drug is contained in 2–6 tablets, which are taken at regular intervals during the day. The dose is adjusted to the point at which symptoms are well controlled. As the disease progresses, the dose is increased.

Precautions

Levodopa itself is not well tolerated, which is why it is combined with carbidopa. Carbidopa decreases peripheral metabolism of levodopa, which allows for lower doses of levodopa and less-severe side effects. The combination is a safe and well-tolerated medication for patients with

Parkinson's disease. Levodopa may cause **orthostatic hypotension**, or low blood pressure upon standing. Patients with low blood pressure or who are susceptible to orthostatic hypotension should be cautious when starting treatment or increasing the dose.

Levodopa can cause sudden and unexpected extreme drowsiness, which some physicians term "sleep attacks." Currently, no reliable predictive criteria have been developed to determine which patients are susceptible. Patients starting levodopa should be aware of this possibility, and discuss with their physician how best to modify their activities (such as driving) to guard against injury in the event of such an incident.

Patients who have had myocardial infarction (heart attack) or other heart abnormalities should be monitored carefully when beginning levodopa treatment.

Side effects

Early on in the disease, levodopa can cause nausea, vomiting, orthostatic hypotension, and drowsiness. Nausea and vomiting typically stop being problems within several months of treatment.

Long-term use of levodopa in PD often leads to dyskinesias, or unwanted and uncontrolled movements. Dyskinesias appear as writhing, shaking, or twitching movements that may involve a small or large part of the body. Early in the disease, lowering the dose of levopoda can help control dyskinesias, but later on, the lower dose leads to significant loss of movement. Balancing the control of symptoms with the control of dyskinesias is a difficult and frustrating challenge for both patient and physician.

Long-term levodopa use can also lead to psychotic symptoms, including hallucinations, vivid and disturbing dreams, paranoia, and confusion.

Interactions

Patients who are taking drugs called nonselective MAO (monoamine oxidase) inhibitors should discontinue these drugs at least two weeks before beginning levodopa. MAO inhibitors are used to treat **depression**. A selective MAO-B inhibitor, such as selegiline, may be taken, and indeed is often prescribed for use in Parkinson's disease.

Description

Dopamine agonists

Dopamine agonists are drugs that mimic the effect of dopamine by stimulating the same cells as dopamine. They have several theoretical advantages over levodopa in the treatment of PD: dopamine agonists do not require uptake and release by substantia nigra cells; they do not compete with amino acids for transport, and so high-protein

meals are not a problem; and the effect of an individual dose lasts longer.

One of the most significant advantages of the dopamine agonists is their ability to delay the onset of dyskinesias when used instead of levodopa at the start of disease. Patients who take a dopamine agonist instead of levodopa for the first 1–2 years tend to develop dyskinesias many months later than those who begin on levodopa. On the other hand, dopamine agonists are not quite as effective as levodopa at controlling other PD symptoms, and may cause more confusion in elderly patients. For this reason, common advice for elderly patients is to begin on levodopa, with the expectation that dyskinesias are less likely to be a serious problem within the treatment timeframe, while younger patients should begin on a dopamine agonist to delay dyskinesias within a much longer timeframe of treatment.

Dopamine agonists prescribed for PD in the United States include pramipexole, ropinirole, pergolide, and bromocriptine. Approval of another, apomorphine, was expected in early 2004. Unlike the others, apomorphine is injected and has a very short duration of action. It is intended for intermittent (not continuous) use as a treatment for emergent symptoms while waiting for the effect of other medications to begin.

Recommended dosage

There are half a dozen dopamine agonists available in oral forms for treatment of PD. The individual dosage and schedule for each vary. In each case, a low dose is used to begin with, with a gradual adjustment over several weeks to achieve the optimum level of symptomatic benefit.

Precautions

Like levodopa, the dopamine agonists may cause sudden and unpredictable episodes of extreme drowsiness.

Side effects

Long-term use of dopamine agonists can cause nausea, vomiting, orthostatic hypotension, and psychotic symptoms, including hallucinations, vivid and disturbing dreams, paranoia, and confusion. While the risk for developing dyskinesias is lower with dopamine agonists, their long-term use does lead to this complication in many patients.

Description

COMT inhibitors

COMT (**Catechol-O-MethylTransferase**) **inhibitors** restrict the action of an enzyme that converts levodopa to dopamine in the periphery (outside the brain). This allows more of the levodopa to reach the brain. In this way, a

COMT inhibitor increases the effectiveness of a dose of levodopa. A COMT inhibitor cannot be used by itself, but must be administered with levodopa.

Recommended dosage

There are two COMT inhibitors approved for use in PD. Entacapone is dosed at 200 mg with each dose of levodopa. Tolcapone is dosed at either 100 or 200 mg three times per day.

Precautions

Tolcapone has been associated with liver damage in a small number of patients, which has led to death in three patients. Tolcapone is only approved for use by patients for whom other therapies are not providing adequate relief of symptoms.

COMT inhibitors increase the effectiveness of levodopa, as well as levodopa's side effects. Consequently, the same precautions apply for use of COMT inhibitors as for levodopa.

Side effects

COMT inhibitors can cause diarrhea. They also can increase the severity of levodopa's side effects, including orthostatic hypotension, hallucinations, and dyskinesias.

Description

MAO-B inhibitors

MAO-B inhibitors restrict the action of monoamine oxidase B, an enzyme that breaks down levodopa in the brain. Thus, an MAO-B inhibitor prolongs the effectiveness of dopamine, as well as a dose of levodopa. The only MAO-B inhibitor in widespread use for Parkinson's disease is selegiline, also called deprenyl.

Selegiline is often used in the early stages of PD, before other drugs, based on its mild symptomatic benefit. It is also often prescribed based on the possibility it may be neuroprotective—that is, it may help slow the death of neurons (brain cells) in the substantia nigra. While some experiments have suggested this may be true, others have shown no effect, and as of late 2003, there was no widespread consensus that selegiline had any effect in PD other than on symptoms.

Recommended dosage

Selegiline is usually prescribed at 5 mg twice daily.

Precautions

At doses higher than those used in PD, selegiline in combination with certain foods can lead to dangerously high blood pressure. These foods include aged cheeses, fermented beverages such as beer or wine, and smoked or pickled meats. This effect is also seen very rarely in patients taking the recommended dose for PD.

Selegiline should not be used with meperidine. Use with other narcotics should only be with the express approval of the patient's physician.

Side effects

Selegiline can cause side effects similar to levodopa, and when taken with levodopa, may worsen those effects. No reports of sudden drowsiness have been published for PD patients on selegiline alone.

Interactions

Interaction between selegiline and certain kinds of antidepressants is possible, and patients should consult with their physician before combining these two types of medications.

Description

Amantadine

Amantadine is prescribed for two different purposes in PD. It has a mild symptomatic effect in early PD, and is often prescribed before levodopa for that reason. It also reduces dyskinesias, and may be prescribed late in the disease once this symptom develops.

Recommended dosage

Amantadine is dosed at 200–300 mg per day.

Precautions

Patients with kidney disease or reduced kidney function require a much lower dose of amantadine.

Side effects

Amantadine can cause side effects similar to levodopa, including hallucinations, confusion, and orthostatic hypotension. Amantadine can also cause mottled skin and swelling in the peripheral tissues such as the legs.

Description

Anticholinergics

Anticholinergics were the first class of antiparkinson medications developed, but are used much less now than in the past, due to the availability of improved drugs. Anticholinergics suppress activity of the acetylcholine system in the brain, which is relatively overactive in PD. They are

Key Terms

Asthenia   muscle weakness.

Cytomegalovirus (CMV)   A type of virus that attacks and enlarges certain cells in the body. The virus also causes a disease in infants.

Herpes simplex   A virus that causes sores on the lips (cold sores) or on the genitals (genital herpes).

HIV   Acronym for human immunodeficiency virus, the virus that causes AIDS.

Parkinsonism   A group of conditions that all have these typical symptoms in common: tremor, rigidity, slow movement, and poor balance and coordination.

Pregnancy category   A system of classifying drugs according to their established risks for use during pregnancy. Category A: Controlled human studies have demonstrated no fetal risk. Category B: Animal studies indicate no fetal risk, but no human studies, or adverse effects in animals, but not in well-controlled human studies. Category C: No adequate human or animal

studies, or adverse fetal effects in animal studies, but no available human data. Category D: Evidence of fetal risk, but benefits outweigh risks. Category X: Evidence of fetal risk. Risks outweigh any benefits.

Prophylactic   Guarding from or preventing the spread or occurrence of disease or infection.

Retrovirus   A group of viruses that contain RNA and the enzyme reverse transcriptase. Many viruses in this family cause tumors. The virus that causes AIDS is a retrovirus.

Shingles   An disease caused by an infection with the Herpes zoster virus, the same virus that causes chicken pox. Symptoms of shingles include pain and blisters along one nerve, usually on the face, chest, stomach, or back.

Virus   A tiny, disease-causing structure that can reproduce only in living cells and causes a variety of infectious diseases.

---

mainly effective against tremor and rigidity, and less so against slowed movements.

Recommended dosage

Different anticholinergics are dosed at different levels and frequencies. A dose is chosen that maximizes benefits and minimizes side effects. The dose is gradually increased to avoid worsening side effects.

Side effects

Anticholinergics can cause significant confusion, **delirium**, and hallucinations, especially in older patients. For this reason, they are seldom used in this group. They can also cause constipation and urinary retention.

Resources

PERIODICAL

Olanow, C. W., R. L. Watts, and W. C. Koller, eds. "An Algorithm (Decision Tree) for the Management of Parkinson's Disease (2001): Treatment Guidelines." *Neurology* 56, Supplement 5 (June 12, 2001): S1–S88.

WEBSITE

Parkinson's Disease: Etiology, Diagnosis and Management— Version 2.2. November 6, 2003 (March 2, 2004).

<http://www.mdvu.org/multimedia/slides/parv2.2/>.

ORGANIZATIONS

National Parkinson Foundation. 1501 N.W. 9th Avenue, Miami, FL 33136-1494. (800) 327-4545. mailbox@parkinson.org. <http://www.parkinson.org>.

Richard Robinson

Antiviral drugs

Definition

Antiviral drugs are medicines that cure or control virus infections.

Purpose

Antivirals are used to treat infections caused by viruses. Unlike antibacterial drugs, which may cover a wide range of pathogens, antiviral agents tend to be narrow in spectrum, and have limited efficacy.

Description

Exclusive of the antiretroviral agents used in HIV (**AIDS**) therapy, there are currently only 11 antiviral drugs available, covering four types of virus. Acyclovir (Zovirax), famciclovir (Famvir), and valacyclovir (Valtrex) are effective against the herpes virus, including herpes zoster and herpes genitalis. They may also be of value in either conditions caused by herpes, such as chicken pox and **shingles**. These drugs are not curative, but may reduce the **pain** of a herpes outbreak and shorten the period of viral shedding.

Amantadine (Symmetrel), oseltamivir (Tamiflu), rimantidine (Flumadine), and zanamivir (Relenza) are useful in treatment of the influenza virus. Amantadine, rimantadine, and oseltamivir may be administered throughout the flu season as preventatives for patients who cannot take influenza virus vaccine.

Cidofovir (Vistide), foscarnet (Foscavir), and ganciclovir (Cytovene) have been beneficial in treatment of cytomegalovirus in immunosupressed patients, primarily HIV-positive patients and transplant recipients. Ribavirin (Virazole) is used to treat respiratory syncytial virus. In combination with **interferons**, ribavirin has shown some efficacy against hepatitis C, and there have been anecdotal reports of utility against other types of viral infections.

As a class, the antivirals are not curative, and must be used either prophylactically or early in the development of an infection. Their mechanism of action is typically to inactivate the enzymes needed for viral replication. This will reduce the rate of viral growth, but will not inactive the virus already present. Antiviral therapy must normally be initiated within 48 hours of the onset of an infection to provide any benefit. Drugs used for influenza may be used throughout the influenza season in high risk patients, or within 48 hours of exposure to a known carrier. Antiherpetic agents should be used at the first signs of an outbreak. Anti-cytomegaloviral drugs must routinely be used as part of a program of secondary prophylaxis (maintenance therapy following an initial response) in order to prevent reinfection in immunocompromised patients.

Recommended dosage

Dosage varies with the drug, patient age and condition, route of administration, and other factors. See specific references.

Precautions

Ganciclovir is available in intravenous injection, oral capsules, and intraoccular inserts. The capsules should be reserved for prophylactic use in organ transplant patients, or for HIV infected patients who cannot be treated with the intravenous drug. The toxicity profile of this drug when administered systemically includes granulocytopenia, anemia, and thrombocytopenia. The drug is in pregnancy category C, but has caused significant fetal abnormalities in animal studies including cleft palate and organ defects. Breast-feeding is not recommended.

Cidofovir causes renal toxicity in 53% of patients. Patients should be well hydrated, and renal function should be checked regularly. Other common adverse effects are nausea and vomiting in 65% or patients, asthenia in 46% and **headache** and diarrhea, both reported in 27% of cases. The drug is category C in pregnancy, due to fetal abnormalities in animal studies. Breast-feeding is not recommended.

Foscarnet is used in treatment of immunocompromised patients with cytomegalovirus infections and in acyclovir-resistant herpes simples virus. The primary hazard is renal toxicity. Alterations in electrolyte levels may cause **seizures**. Foscarnet is category C during pregnancy. The drug has caused skeletal abnormalities in developing fetuses. It is not known whether foscarnet is excreted in breast milk, however the drug does appear in breast milk in animal studies.

Valaciclovir is metabolized to acyclovir, so that the hazards of the two drugs are very similar. They are generally well tolerated, but nausea and headache are common adverse effects. They are both pregnancy category B. Although there have been no reports of fetal abnormalities attributable to either drug, the small number of reported cases makes it impossible to draw conclusions regarding safety in pregnancy. Acyclovir is found in breast milk, but no adverse effects have been reported in the newborn. Famciclovir is similar in actions and adverse effects.

Ribavirin is used by aerosol for treatment of hospitalized infants and young children with severe lower respiratory tract infections due to respiratory syncytial virus (RSV). When administered orally, the drug has been used in adults to treat other viral diseases including acute and chronic hepatitis, herpes genitalis, measles, and Lassa fever, however there is relatively little information about these uses. In rare cases, initiation of ribavirin therapy has led to deterioration of respiratory function in infants. Careful monitoring is essential for safe use.

The anti-influenza drugs are generally well tolerated. Amantadine, which is also used for treatment of Parkinsonism, may show more frequent CNS effects, including sedation and **dizziness**. Rapid discontinuation of amantidine may cause an increase in Parkinsonian symptoms in patients using the drug for that purpose. All are schedule C for pregnancy. In animal studies, they have caused fetal malformations in doses several times higher than the normal human dose. Use caution in breast-feeding.

Interactions

Consult specific references for information on drug interactions.

Use particular caution in HIV-positive patients, since these patients are commonly on multi-drug regimens with

Key Terms

Amygdala An almond-shaped area of the brain involved with coordinating mood, feeling, instinct, and memory.

Buspirone An anxiolytic drug that does not affect GABA, but instead modifies serotonin neurotransmission. Unlike benzodiazepines, it may take 3–6 weeks for buspirone to reach maximal effectiveness. As a result, the drug is only used to treat generalized anxiety disorder.

Generalized anxiety disorder An anxiety disorder characterized by excessive worry or fear about a number of activities or events.

Neurotransmitter A chemical in the brain that transmits messages between neurons, or nerve cells.

Panic disorder A series of unexpected attacks, involving an intense, terrifying fear similar to that caused by a life-threatening danger.

Phobic disorder Persistent fear of social situations, objects, or specific situations.

Selective serotonin reuptake inhibitors (SSRIs) Prescription drugs used as antidepressants and anti-anxiety agents that enhance the actions of the neurotransmitter serotonin.

a high frequency of interactions. Ganciclovir should not be used with other drugs which cause hematologic toxicity, and cidofovir should not be used with other drugs that may cause kidney damage.

Resources

PERIODICALS

Gray, Mary Ann. "Antiviral Medications." *Orthopaedic Nursing* 15 (November-December 1996): 82.

Samuel D. Uretsky, PharmD

Anxiolytics

Definition

Anxiolytics are prescription drugs used to treat and prevent anxiety disorders. Anxiety is an emotional state in which fear dominates a person's life. Drugs that are often prescribed to manage anxiety episodes are known as **benzodiazepines**. Probably the best-known example of a benzodiazepine is the anxiolytic **diazepam**. In the United States, diazepam is sold under the brand name Valium.

All together, there are six other anxiolytics approved for use in the United States. All of these medications are similar to diazepam in their chemical structures and the way they exert their beneficial anxiolytic effects. However, these drugs differ from one another in several important ways. Some drugs work faster than others, while other drugs continue their anxiolytic effects for longer periods of time. Additionally, some anxiolytics differ from one another in the way that they are eliminated from the body, and others are involved with more drug-to-drug interactions than others. In 2002, the two most commonly prescribed anxiolytics were the drugs lorazepam, sold under

the trade name of Ativan, and alprazolam, sold under the brand name of Xanax.

Purpose

Diazepam and other anxiolytics reduce the frequency, severity, and duration of anxiety symptoms in individuals who have medical or psychiatric disorders associated with anxiety. Illnesses associated with anxiety symptoms include heart disease, gastrointestinal diseases, as well as diseases that affect the lungs and make breathing difficult. Anxiety may also occur in the absence of these diseases and is thought to involve abnormal function of several different **neurotransmitters** in a region of the brain known as the amygdala. The amygdala plays a critical role in assessing fear and responding to danger. Examples of common anxiety disorders include generalized anxiety disorder, panic disorder, and phobic disorders. Nearly 25% of the population will develop an anxiety disorder at some time during their life.

Description

Benzodiazepine anxiolytics like diazepam have similar chemical structures, including a benzene ring fused to a diazepine ring. This structure is important for anxiolytic activity. In the brain, anxiolytics are believed to enhance the actions of gamma-aminobutyric acid (GABA), an inhibitory neurotransmitter. By enhancing GABA's inhibitory actions, brain cells are unable to be stimulated by excitatory neurotransmitters, and this inhibition alleviates symptoms of anxiety.

Although benzodiazepines like diazepam alleviate symptoms of anxiety in a manner similar to older anxiolytics like barbiturates, the distinctive feature that sets benzodiazepines apart from barbiturates is the wide margin of safety associated with benzodiazepines. Unlike barbiturates, benzodiazepine anxiolytics have a wide margin of safety, meaning that the doses of benzodiazepines that cause life-threatening toxicities are considerably larger than the doses that are normally used for alleviating anxiety.

Diazepam and related anxiolytics are safe and effective medications for alleviating anxiety symptoms. Until the 1990s, these drugs were the mainstay of pharmacologic treatment for anxiety-related disorders. However, these anxiolytics do possess some unwanted properties. For example, the Drug Enforcement Administration (DEA) classifies diazepam and related anxiolytics as controlled substances because the drugs are sometimes abused, or used for recreational purposes due to their desirable anxiolytic effects. Additionally, physical dependence develops when these medications are used at high doses or for prolonged periods of time. This means that people experience unpleasant withdrawal symptoms if they abruptly stop taking their medication. Common withdrawal symptoms include anxiety, insomnia, restlessness, agitation, muscle tension, and irritability, although **seizures** and **depression** may sometimes occur. The unpleasant withdrawal effects that are experienced when discontinuing these medications cause people to continue using the drugs to avoid unpleasant effects. Because these drugs are sometimes used for non-medicinal purposes and are associated with unpleasant withdrawal symptoms, benzodiazepine anxiolytics are now typically prescribed only for short-term treatment of anxiety disorders, until other anxiolytics like buspirone or selective serotonin reuptake inhibitors (SSRIs) begin working.

Recommended dosage

The usual adult dosage of diazepam is 2–10 mg taken by mouth two to four times a day. In addition to oral tablets, diazepam is also available as an oral liquid or as an injection that can be given either intramuscularly or intravenously to individuals with severe anxiety symptoms.

Dosages for anxiolytics that are chemically related to diazepam vary. Examples include alprazolam given by mouth in dosages of 0.25–0.5 mg three times a day, or lorazepam taken by mouth in dosages of 0.5–2 mg two or three times a day.

The anxiolytic effects of diazepam occur in as little as 15 minutes, but only last for two or three hours. These features make diazepam an ideal drug for quickly eliminating acute anxiety attacks. On the other hand, lorazepam's anxiolytic effects are a little slower in onset but tend to persist for more than six hours. As a result, lorazepam may be better suited to prevent anxiety in people with generalized anxiety disorder.

Elderly patients may be more sensitive to the side effects of diazepam and related anxiolytics than younger adults. As a result, initial doses are usually reduced and increased slowly in the elderly to avoid excessive sedation and other unwanted side effects.

Precautions

Paradoxically, excitement, rage, anger, or hostility may occur in individuals taking anxiolytics for their calming effects. These reactions may occur secondarily to the relief of anxiety and usually occur within the first two weeks of therapy. If these reactions occur, anxiolytic therapy should be stopped.

Because suicidal tendencies may be present in patients who also have accompanying depressive disorders, only small amounts of anxiolytic agents should be dispensed at any given time to minimize the likelihood of intentional drug overdoses.

Side effects

Diazepam and related anxiolytics are often associated with drowsiness, sedation, confusion, and difficulty maintaining balance. These effects are more pronounced at the beginning of therapy and after dosage increases. People should avoid driving or performing tasks that require alertness until they know how the drugs will affect them.

When using anxiolytics like diazepam, **fainting** or **dizziness** sometimes occurs when a person stands up suddenly. Blurred vision may also occur.

When anxiolytics are used in high doses or taken with other drugs that depress the actions of the brain, such as alcohol or barbiturates, the normal breathing responses of the body may be interrupted and patients may stop breathing. For this reason, alcohol and other CNS depressants should be avoided in people taking diazepam and related anxiolytics. It is also best to avoid anxiolytics in those persons with a prior history of drug abuse or those who are suicidal.

Withdrawal symptoms will occur if patients stop taking anxiolytics suddenly. Patients should only discontinue using diazepam and related anxiolytics at the advice of their physician and the dosage of the drugs should be reduced slowly to avoid withdrawal effects.

Interactions

Diazepam will increase the drowsiness or sedative effects of other **central nervous system** depressants like alcohol or barbiturates. These combinations should be avoided.

Certain drugs, especially those eliminated by the liver, may interfere with the elimination of diazepam from the body. **Anticonvulsants**, antidepressants, numerous antibiotics, and cimetidine inhibit the elimination of most anxiolytics from the body, causing higher blood levels and increased side effects.

Resources

BOOKS

Drug Facts and Comparisons, 6th edition. St. Louis, MO: A Wolter Kluwer Company, 2002.

Kirkwood, Cynthia A. *Anxiety Disorders. Pharmacotherapy: A Pathophysiologic Approach*, edited by Joseph T. Dipiro, et al. Stamford, CT: Appleton and Lange, 1999.

Mosby's Medical Drug Reference. St. Louis, MO: Mosby, 1999.

Kelly Karpa, PhD, RPh

Aphasia

Definition

Aphasia is a communication disorder that occurs after language has been developed, usually in adulthood. Not simply a speech disorder, aphasia can affect the ability to comprehend the speech of others, as well as the ability to read and write. In most instances, intelligence per se is not affected.

Description

Aphasia has been known since the time of the ancient Greeks. However, it has been the focus of scientific study only since the mid-nineteenth century. Although aphasia can be caused by a head injury and neurologic conditions, its most common cause is **stroke**, a disruption of blood flow to the brain, which affects brain metabolism in localized areas of the brain. The onset of aphasia is usually abrupt, and occurs in individuals who have had no previous speech or language problems. Aphasia is at its most severe immediately after the event that causes it. Although its severity commonly diminishes over time through both natural, spontaneous recovery from brain damage and from clinical intervention, individuals who remain aphasic for two or three months after its onset are likely to have some residual aphasia for the rest of their lives. However, positive changes often continue to occur, largely with clinical intervention, for many years. The severity of aphasia is related to a number of factors, including the severity of the condition that brought it about, general overall health, age at onset, and numerous personal characteristics that relate to motivation.

Demographics

The National Aphasia Association estimates that approximately 25–40% of stroke survivors develop aphasia. There are approximately one million persons in the United States with aphasia, and roughly 100,000 new cases occur each year. There are more people with aphasia than with **Parkinson's disease**, **cerebral palsy**, or **muscular dystrophy**.

Causes and symptoms

Although aphasia occasionally results from damage to subcortical structures such as basal ganglia or the thalamus that has rich interconnections to the cerebral cortex, aphasia is most frequently caused by damage to the cerebral cortex of the brain's left hemisphere. This hemisphere plays a significant role in the processing of language skills. However, in about half of left-handed individuals (and a few right-handed persons), this pattern of dominance for language is reversed, making right-hemisphere damage the cause of aphasia in this small minority. Because the left side of the brain controls movement on the right side of the body (and vice versa), paralysis affecting the side of the body opposite the side of brain damage is a frequent co-existing problem. This condition is called hemiplegia and can affect walking, using one's arm, or both. If the arm used for writing is paralyzed, it poses an additional burden on the diminished writing abilities of some aphasic individuals. If paralysis affects the many muscles involved in speaking, such as the muscles of the tongue, this condition is called **dysarthria**. Dysarthria often co-occurs with aphasia.

There are a few more problems that can result from the same brain injury that produces aphasia, and complicate its presentation. Most notable among them are the problems collectively called **apraxia**, which influences one's ability to program movement. Apraxic difficulties make voluntary movements difficult and hard to initiate. Apraxia of speech results in difficulty initiating speech and in making speech sounds consistently. It frequently co-occurs with both dysarthria and aphasia. Finally, sensory problems such as visual field deficits (specifically, **hemianopsia**) and changes in (or absence of) sensation in arms, legs, and tongue commonly occur with aphasia.

There are neurological disorders other than aphasia that also manifest difficulty with language. This makes it important to note what aphasia is not. **Traumatic brain injury** and dementias such as **Alzheimer's disease** are excellent examples. Although brain injury is a cause of aphasia, most head injuries produce widespread brain damage and result in other neuropsychological and cognitive disorders. These disorders often create language that is disturbed in output and form, but are typically the linguistic consequences of cognitive disturbances. In Alzheimer's disease, the situation is much the same. Language spoken by individuals with Alzheimer's reflect their cognitive problems, and, as such, differ from the language retrieval problems typically designated as aphasia. In

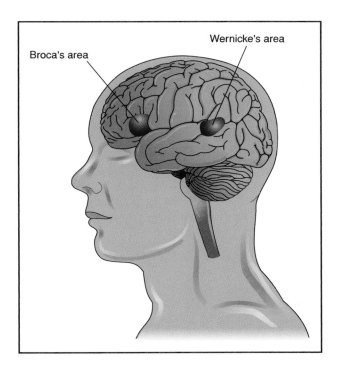
Damage to these areas of the brain can cause types of aphasia. (*Illustration by Electronic Illustrators Group.*)

and fluctuate in a given individual as a result of **fatigue** and other factors. In addition, largely in relationship to lesion size, aphasias differ in overall severity.

Nonfluent aphasia

Frontal cortex is responsible for shaping, initiating, and producing behaviors. Individuals with nonfluent aphasia characteristically have brain damage affecting Broca's area of the cortex and the frontal brain areas surrounding it. These areas are responsible for formulating sound, word, and sentence patterns. Damage to the anterior speech areas results in slow, labored speech with limited output and prosody and difficulty in producing grammatical sentences. Because the motor cortex is closely adjacent, nonfluent Broca's aphasia, by far the most common nonfluent variant, is quite likely to co-occur with motor problems.

Several additional characteristics of nonfluent aphasia can be noted: in nonfluent aphasia verbs and prepositions are disproportionately affected; speech errors occur mostly at the level of speech sounds, producing sound transpositions and inconsistencies; auditory comprehension is only minimally affected; reading abilities parallel comprehension, writing problems parallel speech output, but are sometimes further complicated by hemiplegia; finally, there is an inability to repeat what someone else says.

Fluent aphasia

Fluent aphasias occur when damage occurs in the posterior language areas of the brain, where sensory stimuli from hearing, sight, and bodily sensation converge. In fluent aphasia, the prosody and flow of speech is maintained; one typically must listen closely to recognize that the speech is not normal. Because this posterior damage is located far from the motor areas in the frontal lobes, individuals with fluent aphasia seldom have co-existing difficulty with the mechanics of speech, arm use, or walking. There are three major variants of fluent aphasia, each thought to occur as a function of disruption to different posterior brain regions.

WERNICKE'S APHASIA Wernicke's aphasia results from temporal lobe damage, where auditory input to the brain is received. The essential characteristic is that individuals with this disorder have disproportionate difficulty in understanding spoken and written language. They also have problems comprehending and monitoring their own speech. They are often verbose, and frequently use inappropriate and even jargon words when they speak. Reading and writing are impaired in similar ways to auditory comprehension and speech output. Their comprehension difficulties preclude their being able to repeat others' words.

ANOMIC APHASIA Most people, particularly as they grow older, have trouble with the names of persons and

short, if the damage that results in language problems is general and produces additional intellectual problems, then aphasia is a correct diagnosis. In the absence of other significant intellectual problems, then the language disorder is probably localized to the brain's language processing areas and is properly termed aphasia.

Finally, aphasia is not conventionally used to refer to the developmental language learning problems encountered by some atypically developing children. However, when children who have been previously developing language normally have a stroke or some other type of localized brain damage, then the aphasia diagnosis is appropriate.

Aphasia manifests different language symptoms and syndromes as a result of where in the language-dominant hemisphere the damage has occurred. The advent of neuroimaging has improved the ability to localize the area of brain damage. Nevertheless, the different general patterns of language strengths and weaknesses, as well as unexpected dissociations in language function, can explain how normal language is processed in the brain, as well as provide insights into intervention for aphasia.

Aphasic individuals almost uniformly have some difficulty in using the substantive words of their native language. Most experts in aphasia recognize that aphasia varies along two major dimensions: auditory comprehension ability and fluency of speech output. In reality, aphasic behaviors vary greatly from individual to individual, things; all aphasic persons experience these difficulties. But when brain damage occurs in the area of the posterior brain where information from temporal, parietal, and occipital lobes converge, this problem of naming is much more pervasive than for normal and aphasic speakers alike. Most anomic aphasic individuals have excellent auditory comprehension and read well. But for most of them, writing mirrors speech, and individuals with anomic aphasia can take advantage of words provided by others. Hence, their repetition ability is good. Although anomic aphasia is classified as a fluent syndrome, frequent stops, starts, and word searches typically make speech choppy in between runs of fluency.

CONDUCTION APHASIA Individuals with conduction aphasia are thought to have a discrete brain lesion that disrupts the pathways that underlie the cortex and connect the anterior and posterior speech regions. These individuals have good comprehension, as well as high awareness of the errors that they make. Placement of their brain damage also suggests that there should be little interference with speech production, reading, and writing. However, damage to the neural links between posterior and anterior speech areas makes it quite difficult for these individuals to correct the errors they hear themselves making. Conduction aphasia also affects the ability to repeat the speech of others or to take advantage of the cues others provide. The speech of individuals with this problem includes many inappropriate words, typically involving inappropriate sequences of sounds.

UNUSUAL APHASIA SYNDROMES There are a few other rare aphasic syndromes (called "transcortical aphasias") and unique dissociations in aphasic patterns. The above aphasias represent the most common distinctive syndromes. However, they are estimated to account for only approximately 40% of individuals with aphasia.

MIXED AND GLOBAL APHASIA The remaining majority, about 60% of aphasic individuals, have aphasias that result from brain lesions involving both the anterior and posterior speech areas. Their aphasias, thus, affect both speech production and comprehension. They frequently have reading and writing disorders as well. Individuals with mixed and global aphasia are also very likely to have hemiplegia and dysarthria, as well as a variety of sensation losses. Depending upon the severity of these symptoms, people with mild-to-moderate symptomatology of this type are said to have mixed aphasia; global aphasia describes individuals with extensive difficulties in all language skills.

Diagnosis

As an aid to accurate diagnosis immediately following stroke, it is important to differentiate aphasia from cognitive disorders such as confusion and disorientation. To this end, brief, but general testing of the language functions (naming, comprehension, reading, writing, and repetition) can be incorporated into broader testing that might determine other cognitive functions. Evaluators must remember that language is the medium though which most of these other functions are observed. Therefore, language should be assessed first; if extensive aphasia is present, then only cautious interpretations of other cognitive functions may be given. At present, there are few available objective and standardized measures for testing during the acute phases of disorders such as stroke.

A number of standardized measures are available that provide an inventory of aphasic symptoms. These tests are useful in providing baseline and follow-up assessments to measure progress in treatment, as well as to guide the treatment itself. A fairly general feature of aphasia tests is that individuals without aphasic symptoms should perform with almost no errors on them. Tests are available to measure the extent and severity of language impairments as well as to provide information about functional skills and outcomes. Finally, there are assessments designed specifically to look at quality of life with aphasia.

Treatment team

Because of the various other problems in addition to language that affect most individuals with aphasia, a multidisciplinary team is used in rehabilitation centers for the management of aphasia. Team members, as well as speech-language pathologists, typically include physical and occupational therapists, clinical neuropsychologists, nurses, and **social workers** who are guided by physiatrists and neurologists. Once discharged from rehabilitation centers, aphasic individuals often continue their treatment by speech-language pathologists in settings such as speech and hearing clinics. Self-help groups and support via the Internet are available as well.

Treatment

Most individuals with aphasia are hospitalized for some period of time for treatment of the condition that has resulted in aphasia. Assessment of the extent and type of language disorder is made during that time, as assessment of the ability to swallow (dysphagia). Early medical intervention is important for lessening the long-term effects of stroke.

Recovery and rehabilitation

To date, no pharmacological treatments for aphasia have proven effective, although a number of drugs (dopaminergic, cholinergic, and neurotrophic) continue to be investigated, usually in conjunction with behavioral treatments for aphasia. Various behavioral treatment approaches for aphasia exist. They are usually characterized dichotomously as restorative (restitutive) or compensatory. The goal of restorative treatments is to reestablish disordered language skills. Goals for compensatory approaches are to develop and train alternative approaches to circumvent the language skills that have been affected by aphasia. Most clinicians use both approaches (often simultaneously) to aid in language recovery. Some examples of restorative approaches include practice of carefully selected syntactic structures, naming drills, or practice using self-selected communication needs such as using the telephone.

Compensatory approaches include training conversational partners to modify their own language and communication skills in ways that make it easier for the aphasic individual to communicate, or teaching aphasic individuals to use a relatively intact language skill such as writing or drawing to substitute for talking. Computerized approaches to both restitutive and compensatory aphasia treatment are increasing. Many clinics offer both individual treatment and group treatment, with the latter offering increased psychosocial support. Many clinics also incorporate family support groups.

Clinical trials

Randomized control trials (RCTs) are rare for the behavioral realm of treatments. Aphasia is no exception. To date, only four RCTs have been completed, with three of the four addressing to the efficacy of treatment. A far greater number of phases I and II studies exist, and investigate the value of language intervention, particularly post stroke. The largest testimony comes from single-case designs and qualitative case studies that agree that treatment has a positive influence on outcome. Only one meta-analysis of significant scope has been completed (Robey, 1998).

Prognosis

The traditional view is that most of the language gains made by aphasic individuals will occur in the first six months following injury, except in persons with global aphasia, who may begin the recovery process later, but are shown to make gains through one year. Significantly, it must be noted that most traditional treatment techniques have been validated using aphasic patients whose period of spontaneous recovery has passed. Some people with aphasia may be able to return to work, although the communicative demands of many occupations may affect employment.

As of the late 1990s, research has begun to focus on recovery across the remainder of the lifespan, and it has become apparent that aphasic individuals continue to make progress, often for years after the precipitating event. The factors that explain very late recovery are not clear and will require scientific observation and study.

Special concerns

Despite the prevalence of aphasia, the disorder is neither well recognized nor well understood. Aphasia's psychosocial and vocational consequences are overwhelmingly devastating, but community understanding is at best limited. Similarly, despite substantial evidence concerning the effectiveness of intervention, skepticism about the value of treatment remains. As a consequence of both of these factors, many aphasic individuals and their families are not well informed about either the disorder or what might be done to alleviate it.

Additionally, although a significant and growing number of individuals in the United States is bilingual, there is a surprising lack of research concerning the effects of speaking more than one language on recovery from aphasia. Finally, current funding for only very limited treatment for aphasia is available via third-party reimbursement.

Resources

BOOKS

Davis, G. A. *Aphasology: Disorders and Clinical Practice.* Boston: Allyn and Bacon, 2000.
Goodglass, H. *Understanding Aphasia.* New York: Academic Press, 1993.
Hillis, A. E. *The Handbook of Adult Language Disorders.* New York: Psychology Press, 2002.

PERIODICALS

Robey, R. R. "A Meta-analysis of Clinical Outcomes in the Treatment of Aphasia." *Journal of Speech and Hearing Research* 41 (1998): 172–187.

ORGANIZATIONS

Aphasia Hope Foundation. 2436 West 137th St., Leawood, KS 66224. (913) 402-8306 or (866) 449-5894; Fax: (913) 402-8315. <http://www.aphasiahope.org>.
National Aphasia Association. 29 John Street, New York, NY 10038. (212) 267-2812 or (800) 922-4622. naa@aphasia.org. <http://www.aphasia.org>.

Audrey L. Holland, PhD

Apolipoprotein B deficiency *see* **Bassen-Kornzweig syndrome**

Apraxia

Definition

Apraxia is a neurological disorder. In general, the diagnostic term "apraxia" can be used to classify the inability of a person to perform voluntary and skillful movements of one or more body parts, even though there is no evidence of underlying muscular paralysis, incoordination, or sensory deprivation. Additionally, motor performances in response to commands, imitation tasks, and use of familiar objects may be equally difficult but not attributable to **dementia** or confusion. These types of disturbances usually result from injuries, illnesses, or diseases of different regions of the brain normally responsible for regulating such abilities.

Description

The term apraxia is derived from the Greek word *praxis*, which refers to producing an action or movement. In 1861, Broca described in detail an 84-year-old man who suffered a sudden impairment of speech production, but preservation of oral musculature functions, overall language skills, and intelligence. Broca coined the term "aphemia" to classify the inability to articulate words in the presence of a good language foundation. In 1900, Leipmann reported a 48-year-old patient who was unable to execute various voluntary motor behaviors of the limbs and oral cavity, despite good muscle strength, intactness of certain automatic or previously well-rehearsed speech or bodily movements, and complete understanding of the intended acts. Liepmann popularized the diagnostic term "apraxia" to differentiate individuals with these types of select motor difficulties from those who struggle with movement disturbances because of weakness, paralysis, and incoordination of the muscles involved.

Demographics

There are no undisputed figures regarding the incidence of apraxia in the general population. However, because strokes are common causes, and African-American men are more susceptible to the development of this disease, by default this population may be at the greatest risk for this neurological disorder.

Causes and symptoms

Based on many additional case studies, Liepmann suggested that there are three major types of apraxia, each of which is caused by different sites of brain damage: ideational, ideo-motor, and kinetic.

Autopsy examinations and **magnetic resonance imaging (MRI)** scans have demonstrated that, in general, individuals with ideational, ideo-motor, and kinetic apraxias have pathologies involving either the back (parietal-occipital), middle (parietal), or front (frontal) lobes of the cerebral cortex, respectively. The individual with ideational apraxia cannot consistently produce complex serial actions, particularly with objects, due to disruptions at the conceptual stage of motor planning where the purpose and desire to perform specific movements are formulated. This

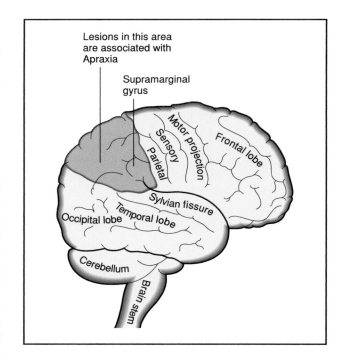

The region of the brain affected by apraxia. (Illustration by Electronic Illustrators Group.)

individual may begin an act with a set purpose and start its performance, but then suddenly cease because the original goal is forgotten. The primary problem is failure to form concepts and/or inability to retain the conceptual plan for a sufficient period of time to allow the desired movements to be effectively programmed and executed. For example, if patients with ideational apraxia are requested to demonstrate proper use of a toothbrush, they might first brush their nails, then hesitate and brush their pants, and finally, with prompting, brush their teeth. Their actions will likely be slow and disorganized, appearing as though they have to think out each movement along the way.

Ideo-motor apraxia is characterized by derailments of bodily movement patterns, due to disturbances in the motor planning stages of a well-conceived behavioral act. Breakdowns most often occur during verbal commands to use objects rather than when the same objects are being used spontaneously. The patient with this disorder fails to translate the idea to perform specific movements into a coordinated and sequential scheme of muscle contractions to achieve the desired motor goal. If asked to demonstrate use of a pair of scissors, unlike ideational apraxics, individuals with ideo-motor apraxia will not make the mistake of using this tool as if it were a screwdriver. Rather, they might grasp the scissors with both hands and repetitively open and close the blades, or pick up the paper in one hand and the scissors in the other and rub them against one another with hesitant motions.

Kinetic apraxia is characterized by coarse, clumsy, groping, and mutilated movement patterns, especially on tasks that require simultaneous, sequential, and smooth contractions of separate muscle groups. These disturbances are usually proportional to the complexity of the task. The disorder does not involve ideation or concept formation, as the desired movement is almost always evident in the struggle. Typing, playing a musical instrument, and handwriting tasks are very difficult for the individual with kinetic apraxia. The problem is not with preliminary motor planning, as in ideo-motor apraxia. Instead, the kinetic apraxic suffers from disturbances in programming the motor plan into subunits of sequential muscle behaviors. Normally, such instructions are then conveyed directly to the primary motor system, which in turn initiates neural commands necessary to execute the intended act.

Apraxia of speech is a subtype of kinetic apraxia. This disorder is often observed following damage to the brain in an area named after Broca. Not infrequently, speech apraxia co-occurs with notable language disturbances, known as **aphasia**. Individuals with speech apraxia struggle with dysfluent articulation problems, as they grope to posture correctly sequential tongue, lip, and jaw movements during speech activities. Numerous, but variable articulatory errors occur, characterized by false starts, re-starts, sound substitutions, sound and word repetitions, and overall slow rate of speech. Multisyllabic words and complex word combinations are most vulnerable to these types of breakdowns.

Diagnosis

Testing for apraxia should employ basic screening tasks to identify individuals who do and do not require deeper testing for the differential diagnosis. Basic limb and orofacial praxis measures include the following commands:

- blow out a match

- protrude the tongue

- whistle

- salute

- wave goodbye

- brush the teeth

- flip a coin

- hammer a nail into wood

- cut paper with scissors

- tap the foot

- stand like a golfer

- jump up and down in place

- thread a needle

- tie a necktie

- recite isolated words, word sequences, and phrases

More detailed testing usually includes many additional tasks of increasing motor complexity.

Treatment team

Because the apraxias are neurological disorders, a clinical **neurologist** is often the team leader. A neurosurgeon may also be on the team, especially if the underlying cause requires surgical attention. Likewise, the primary medical care practitioner plays a very important role in taking care of the individual's overall health-related needs. The responsibilities of the nurse and clinical psychologist should not be underestimated, as many apraxic individuals experience the need for hospitalization, financial aid, social reintegration, and emotional and family counseling. Speech-language and occupational therapists are also key team members in those cases with clinically significant speech and/or limb-girdle movement abnormalities.

Treatment

Occupational therapists may employ exercises to rehabilitate proper use of eating utensils, health care and hygiene products, and self-dressing skills. The speech therapist focuses on retraining fluent and articulate movement patterns to improve overall speech intelligibility. Specific exercises may include tongue, lip, and jaw rate and rhythm activities, as well as combinations of complex sound and word productions.

Clinical trials

As of 2003, the National Institute of Neurological Disorders and Stroke (NINDS) sponsored two **clinical trials** that focused on patients with ideo-motor apraxia. These studies used different techniques to analyze brain activity as patients performed various movements and simple tasks.

The National Institute on Deafness and Other Communication Disorders (NIDCD) is also sponsoring a study. This clinical trial focuses on patients who experience speech and communication complications related to neurological illness.

Further information on these trials can be obtained by contacting the National Institutes of Health Patient Recruitment and Public Liaison Office.

Prognosis

The potential for significant improvements with treatments and self-healing (spontaneous recovery) are most likely in cases of mild apraxia with stable medical courses. For more severe cases, particularly those with progressive or unstable neurological pathologies, the prognoses for notable gains with medical and behavioral interventions remain guarded at the outset. However, many such cases achieve sufficient gains to enable independent lifestyles.

Special concerns

People with apraxia who are elderly and/or who may also have co-morbid medical problems often require ongoing assistance with daily living activities. Nursing home facilities may be necessary for those individuals who do not have the opportunity or resources either to live by themselves or with family members, or to hire a home-based caregiver. Although apraxia most often afflicts adults, school-age children or adolescents with this disorder will require special education considerations and intensive academic and therapeutic programs.

Quality of life

Apraxia may be caused by very serious neurologic diseases or injuries. The quality of life of those afflicted with this disorder is usually influenced by its underlying cause. Many individuals have co-occurring physical, psychological, and intellectual disabilities, which complicate the differential diagnostic process and challenge the potential for meaningful rehabilitation and a fruitful quality of life. Others struggle with less intertwined functional disturbances. These individuals tend to lead more productive lives because they are not as severely impaired.

Resources

BOOKS

Hall, Penelope, Linda Jordan, and Donald Robin. *Developmental Apraxia of Speech: Theory and Clinical Practice.* Austin, TX: Pro Ed, 1993.

Icon Health Publishers. *The Official Patient's Sourcebook on Apraxia: A Revised and Updated Directory for the Internet Age.* San Diego: Icon Group International, 2002.

Vellemen, Shelley L. *Childhood Apraxia of Speech.* San Diego: Singular Publishing, 2002.

PERIODICALS

Geschwind, N. "The Apraxia: Neural Mechanisms of Disorders of Learned Movement." *American Scientist* 63 (1975): 188.

OTHER

Apraxia-Kids. Childhood Apraxia of Speech Association. December 9, 2003 (March 11, 2004). <www.apraxia-kids.org>.

NINDS Apraxia Information Page. National Institute for Neurological Disorders and Stroke. December 17, 2001 (Marhc 11, 2004). <http://www.ninds.nih.gov/health_and_medical/disorders/apraxia.htm>.

ORGANIZATIONS

National Institute of Deafness and Other Communication Disorders. 31 Center Drive, MSC 2320, Bethesda, MD 20892. (800) 411-1222. prpl@mail.cc.nih.gov. <http://www.nidcd.nih.gov/>.

National Institutes of Health Patient Recruitment and Public Liaison Office. 9000 Rockville Pike, Bethesda, MD 20892. (800) 411-1222. prpl@mail.cc.nih.gov. <http://www.nih.gov/>.

National Institute of Neurological Disorders and Stroke. P.O. Box 5801, Bethesda, MD 20824. (301) 496-5751 or (800) 352-9424. <http://www.ninds.nih.gov>.

Wayne State University, Department of Otolaryngology, Head and Neck Surgery. 5E-UHC, 4201 St Antoine, Detroit, MI 48201. (313) 577-0804. <http://www.med.wayne.edu/otohns/index.htm>.

James Paul Dworkin, Ph.D.

Aprosodia *see* **Aphasia, Dysarthria**

Arachnoiditis

Definition

Arachnoiditis literally means "inflammation of the arachnoid," which is the middle of the three membranes (**meninges**) surrounding the brain and spinal cord. The term more generally refers to several rare neurologic disorders caused by inflammation of a portion of the arachnoid and subarachnoid space, affecting the neural tissue that lies beneath. Symptoms of arachnoiditis are quite variable, and may include anything from a skin rash to moderate or severe **pain**, to paralysis. The condition is often progressive, can only rarely be cured, and existing treatments vary in their effectiveness.

Description

Three membranes, including the dura mater, arachnoid, and pia mater, and a layer of cerebrospinal fluid (CSF) surround, protect, and cushion the brain and spinal cord. The pia mater adheres to the brain and spinal cord, and is separated from the arachnoid membrane by the subarachnoid space, which contains the circulating CSF. Arachnoiditis always involves inflammation in one or several restricted areas, but the entire membrane is never affected. Fibrous (scar) tissue growth along the affected section of the membrane usually occurs, projecting down through the subarachnoid space and encompassing neural tissue of the brain (cerebral arachnoiditis) and/or nerve roots of the spinal cord (spinal arachnoiditis). Nerve damage occurs through restricted blood flow (ischemia), compression from accumulated fluids (edema), and secondary effects of the inflammatory process itself.

Key Terms

Arachnoid   One of the three membranes that sheath the spinal cord and brain; the arachnoid is the middle membrane. Also called the arachnoid mater.

Cerebrospinal fluid   The clear, normally colorless fluid that fills the brain cavities (ventricles), the subarachnoid space around the brain, and the spinal cord, and acts as a shock absorber.

Epidural space   The space immediately surrounding the outermost membrane (dura mater) of the spinal cord.

Meningitis   An infection or inflammation of the membranes that cover the brain and spinal cord. It is usually caused by bacteria or a virus.

Subarachnoid space   The space between two membranes surrounding the spinal cord and brain, the arachnoid and pia mater.

Other terms used less frequently for arachnoiditis include arachnitis, chronic adhesive arachnoiditis (CAA), and spinal fibrosis. Other conditions that may be associated with or mimic arachnoiditis include **syringomyelia** (cyst near the spinal cord), cauda equina (lower spinal cord) syndrome, and spinal tumor. Several different types of arachnoiditis have been described, including adhesive (fibrous attachments), ossifying (bony tissue growth), neoplastic (tumor growth), optochiasmatic (optic nerve and chiasm), and rhinosinusogenic (olfactory nerve and area above the sinuses).

Demographics

The true incidence of arachnoiditis is not known, but it is rare. It affects males and females equally, and seems to be less frequent in children than in adults. Rare cases of familial arachnoiditis have been documented, but no particular ethnic groups seem to be at higher risk.

Causes and symptoms

The causes of arachnoiditis are varied, but fall into the following four categories:

- trauma to the membrane due to spinal surgery (often multiple procedures), cranial or spinal injury, or needle insertion to remove CSF for testing
- external agents such as anesthesia, corticosteroids, medications, or medical dyes/chemicals injected near the spinal cord (epidural) or directly into the CSF
- infection of the arachnoid/CSF (meningitis)

- blood in the CSF caused by trauma, spontaneous bleeding, or infection

For reasons that are not entirely clear, different areas of the arachnoid have differing sensitivities to the causative agents. Spinal arachnoiditis due to infection most often occurs in the cervicothoracic (neck and upper back) region, while cases due to external agents most often occur in the lumbosacral (lower back) area. Likewise, spinal arachnoiditis of any type is more common than the cerebral/cranial variety.

Symptoms of cerebral arachnoiditis may include severe headaches, vision disturbances, **dizziness**, and nausea/vomiting. Vision disturbances are especially pronounced in optochiasmatic arachnoiditis. If inflammation and tissue growth in specific areas of the cranial arachnoid membrane divert or obstruct normal flow of the CSF, the result is **hydrocephalus** (increased fluid pressure within the brain).

Typical symptoms of spinal arachnoiditis include **back pain** that increases with activity, pain in one or both legs or feet, and sensory abnormalities of some type, usually involving decreased reflexes. Patients may also exhibit decreased range of motion of the trunk or legs, and urinary sphincter dysfunction (urgency, frequency, or incontinence). In more severe cases, partial or complete paralysis of the lower extremities may occur.

Diagnosis

The most reliable method of establishing the diagnosis of arachnoiditis is a positive computed tomography (CT) or **magnetic resonance imaging (MRI)** scan, combined with one or more of the symptoms. Testing for certain cell types and proteins in the CSF may prove helpful only in the early stages of the inflammation. On the other hand, imaging studies may be negative or equivocal early on, and only later be more definitive as inflammation and tissue growth becomes more pronounced. In some cases, a definitive diagnosis may not be possible.

Treatment team

A **neurologist** is the primary specialist involved in monitoring and treating arachnoiditis. Occupational/physical therapy (OT/PT) might also be suggested to assist with treatment for pain and adaptation to sensory deficits and/or muscular weakness in the back and lower limbs. A neurosurgeon performs any elected surgeries to address the various effects of the inflammation. Many individuals with chronic pain attend pain clinics staffed by physicians (usually anesthesiologists) and nurses who specialize in pain management. Neuropsychiatrists and neuropsychologists specialize in treating the psychological problems specific to individuals who have an underlying neurologic condition.

Treatment

Treatment for arachnoiditis is mostly done with medications, and is geared toward reducing the inflammation and alleviating pain. Medications may include both non-steroidal and steroidal anti-inflammatory drugs, along with non-narcotic and narcotic pain medications. Other possible treatments include epidural steroid injections, transcutaneous electrical nerve stimulation (TENS), topical analgesics, and alternative medical therapies.

Direct spinal cord stimulation is a newer pain management method that involves placement of tiny electrodes under the skin, directly on the affected nerve roots near the spine. Mild current application inhibits pain signals, and is provided by a small, battery-powered unit that is placed under the skin by a surgeon.

Surgery to remove fibrous or ossified tissue at the site of the inflammation is used only if more conservative methods do not provide sufficient relief. Surgical removal of a small portion of one or more vertebrae at the area of the nerve root is called a **laminectomy**. A neurosurgeon treats hydrocephalus by placing a shunt (plastic tube) from the brain to the abdominal cavity to relieve increased pressure. Microsurgical techniques to remove scar tissue from around the nerve roots themselves are a more recent development.

Prognosis

Given the lack of effective treatments for arachnoiditis, the prognosis in most instances is poor, with the neurologic symptoms remaining static or worsening over time. It is not uncommon for people who undergo surgery for the condition to improve at first, but eventually regress within several years.

Resources

BOOKS

Bradley, Walter G., et al., eds. *Neurology in Clinical Practice*, 3rd ed. Boston: Butterworth-Heinemann, 2000.

Victor, Maurice, and Allan H. Ropper. *Adam's and Victor's Principles of Neurology*, 7th ed. New York: The McGraw-Hill Companies, Inc., 2001.

Wiederholt, Wigbert C. *Neurology for Non-Neurologists*, 4th ed. Philadelphia: W.B. Saunders Company, 2000.

PERIODICALS

Chin, Cynthia T. "Spine Imaging." *Seminars in Neurology* 22 (June 2002): 205–220.

Faure, Alexis, et al. "Arachnoiditis Ossificans of the Cauda Equina: Case Report and Review of the Literature." *Journal of Neurosurgery/Spine* 97 (September 2002): 239–243.

Rice, M. Y. K., et al. "Obstetric Epidurals and Chronic Adhesive Arachnoiditis." *British Journal of Anaesthesia* 92 (2004): 109–120.

Wright, Michael H., and Leann C. Denney "A Comprehensive Review of Spinal Arachnoiditis." *Orthopaedic Nursing* 22 (May/June 2003): 215–219.

ORGANIZATIONS

American Paraplegia Society. 75-20 Astoria Boulevard, Jackson Heights, NY 11370-1177. (718) 803-3782. <http://www.apssci.org>.

American Syringomyelia Alliance Project, Inc. P.O. Box 1586, Longview, TX 75606-1586. 800-272-7282. <http://www.asap.org>.

NIH/NINDS Brain Resources and Information Network. PO Box 5801, Bethesda, MD 20824. (800) 352-9424. <http://www.ninds.nih.gov/>.

National Organization for Rare Disorders (NORD). 55 Kenosia Ave, PO Box 1968, Danbury, CT 06813-1968. (800) 999-6673; Fax: (203) 798-2291. <http://www.rarediseases.org>.

National Spinal Cord Injury Association. 6701 Democracy, Bethesda, MD 20817. (800) 962-9629. <http://www.spinalcord.org>.

Spinal Cord Society. 19051 County Hwy 1, Fergus Falls, MN 56537. (218) 739-5252.

Scott J. Polzin, MS, CGC

Arachnoid cysts

Definition

Arachnoid cysts are sacs that are filled with cerebrospinal fluid and form in the surface region of the brain around the cranial base, or on the arachnoid membrane (one of three membranes that covers the brain and spinal cord).

Description

An arachnoid cyst forms when the two lipid (fatty) layers of the arachnoid membrane split apart to form a cavity. Like most membranes, the arachnoid membrane is comprised of two layers (leaflets) of lipid molecules. The hydrophilic (water attracting) region of the lipids is oriented towards an environment rich in water. The hydrophobic (water repelling) portion of the lipids will spontaneously partition away from water, in the interior of the membrane. When an arachnoid cyst forms, the two leaflets of the membrane split apart. Cerebrospinal fluid then fills the cavity.

Arachnoid cysts can be classified according to their location and by the type of tissue making up the cyst wall (arachnoid connective tissue or glioependymal tissue). Cysts that are found in the area of the cerebrum and in the spinal cord tend to be composed of arachnoid tissue, while cysts found in the supracollicular or retrocerebellar regions of the brain tend to be composed of either arachnoid connective tissue or glioependymal tissue.

Key Terms

Arachnoid membrane   A thin layer of tissue that is the middle layer of the three meninges surrounding the brain and spinal cord.

Cerebrospinal fluid   The clear fluid that circulates through the brain and spinal cord.

Intracranial pressure   The overall pressure within the skull.

The expansion of arachnoid cysts may occur when pulses of cerebrospinal fluid become trapped in the cyst cavity. The increasing volume of fluid causes the cyst to grow in size. However, the exact nature of cyst growth is not yet well understood. Arachnoid cysts tend to form on the left side of the brain, where the spinal canal intersects. Typically, a cyst makes up about one percent of the mass of the brain. Arachnoid cysts are also known as intracranial cysts.

Demographics

Infants are most susceptible to developing arachnoid cysts, although cyst formation can occur up through adolescence. Arachnoid cyst development in adults occurs much less frequently. Arachnoid cysts occur predominantly in males. The ratio of affected males to females is 4:1. The true rate of occurrence of arachnoid cysts is unknown, as many people with the disorder do not develop symptoms and the cyst remains undiagnosed.

Causes and symptoms

Arachnoid cysts arise mainly because of an abnormality occurring in development, sometimes as a result of a neonatal (newborn) infection. Other cysts are congenital (present at birth) and presumably result from abnormal formation of the subarachnoid space during embryological development. Cysts can also result from tumors, and complications of surgery or trauma (bleeding).

The symptoms of an arachnoid cyst are related to the size of the cyst and its location. For example, a small cyst may not cause any symptoms at all, and can be discovered accidentally during an unrelated examination. Large cysts can cause the head to change shape or to become enlarged (a phenomenon called macrocephaly). Symptoms associated with a larger cyst include headaches, **seizures**, accumulation of a pronounced amount of cerebrospinal fluid (**hydrocephalus**), increased pressure inside the cranial cavity, delay in mental and physical development, and altered behavior.

Other symptoms can include weakness or complete paralysis along one side of the body (hemiparesis), and the loss of control of muscles (**ataxia**).

Diagnosis

Arachnoid cysts are most commonly diagnosed followed a complaint of headaches, disruption of vision, or delayed development in a child. Even then, the discovery of a cyst is often incidental to another examination. The cysts can also be visualized using computerized tomography (CT) scanning, **magnetic resonance imaging (MRI)**, and cranial **ultrasonography**. Overall, MRI is the preferred diagnostic technique, although cranial ultrasonography is an especially useful technique for newborns.

Arachnoid cysts have also been documented in people who have maladies such as Cockayne syndrome and Menkes disease. However, it is unclear whether this association is typical (and so of diagnostic importance) or merely coincidental.

Treatment team

Treatment can involve medical specialists such as neurosurgeons, imaging technicians, as well as nursing and other care providers. Physical therapists are also often involved.

Treatment

Typically, treatment is for the symptoms caused by the presence of the cyst, rather than for the cyst itself. However, when symptoms warrant, surgery is performed to relieve symptoms of increased intracranial pressure caused by the accumulation of fluid within the arachnoid cyst. Often, a device (shunt) is implanted within the cyst that drains the fluid away from the cyst and into the ventricles of the brain, or into the peritoneum (abdominal space), thus relieving the pressure. An alternative surgery called endoscopic fenestration uses an endoscope (an operative tool with an attached camera) to cut a small hole in the cyst, allowing the fluid to escape into the normal cerebrospinal fluid pathway.

Recovery and rehabilitation

Recovery from either surgical treatment is usually rapid, with symptoms resolving quickly after the excess fluid is redirected, assuming no permanent neurological damage occurred prior to treatment. An active infant or young child often wears a protective helmet during the recovery phase. Physical and mental developmental milestones are usually monitored for infants and children. Follow-up monitoring of the implanted shunt and overall assessment of the cyst are normally required.

Key Terms

Cerebrospinal fluid Fluid that circulates throughout the cerebral ventricles and around the spinal cord within the spinal canal.

Cervico-medullary junction The area where the brain and spine connect.

Hydrocephalus The excess accumulation of cerebrospinal fluid around the brain, often causing enlargement of the head.

Magnetic Resonance Imaging (MRI) A technique that employs magnetic fields and radio waves to create detailed images of internal body structures and organs, including the brain.

Myelomeningocele A sac that protrudes through an abnormal opening in the spinal column.

Posterior fossa Area at the base of the skull attached to the spinal cord.

Spina bifida An opening in the spine.

Syringomyelia Excessive fluid in the spinal cord.

Clinical trials

As of January 2004, the National Institute of Neurological Diseases and Stroke (NINDS) was recruiting patients for a study of **syringomyelia**. The malady arises when cerebrospinal fluid is blocked from its normal circulation, as by an arachnoid cyst. As well, NINDS and other agencies support research that seeks to understand the basis of arachnoid cyst formation.

Prognosis

While many arachnoid cysts cause no symptoms and require no treatment, others, if left untreated, can grow and cause pressure or severe bleeding within the brain (hemorrhage). The result can be permanent neurological damage. However, with treatment, the outlook for most persons with an arachnoid cyst is encouraging and permanent damage can be avoided.

Resources

BOOKS

Parker, J. N., and P. M. Parker. *The Official Patient's Sourcebook on Arachnoid Cysts. A Revised and Updated Directory for the Internet Age.* San Diego. Icon Health Publications, 2002.

OTHER

"Arachnoid Cysts Information Page." *National Institute of Neurological Disorders and Stroke.* <http://www.ninds.nih.gov/health_and_medical/disorders/aracysts_doc.htm> (January 30, 2004).

Khan, A. N. "Arachnoid Cyst." *eMedicine.* <http://www.emedicine.com/radio/topic48.htm> (January 30, 2004).

ORGANIZATIONS

National Institute for Neurological Diseases and Stroke (NINDS). 6001 Executive Boulevard, Bethesda, MD 20892. (301) 496-5751 or (800) 352-9424. <http://www.ninds.nih.gov>.

National Organization for Rare Disorders. 55 Kenosia Avenue, Danbury, CT 06813-1968. (203) 744-0100 or (800) 999-6673; Fax: (203) 798-2291. orphan@rarediseases.org. <http://www.rarediseases.org>.

Brian Douglas Hoyle, Ph.D.

Arnold-Chiari malformation

Definition

Arnold-Chiari malformation is a rare genetic disorder in which parts of the brain are formed abnormally. Malformations may occur in the lower portion of the brain (**cerebellum**) or in the brain stem.

Description

A German pathologist named Arnold-Chiari was the first to describe Arnold-Chiari malformation in 1891. Normally, the brain stem and cerebellum are located in the posterior fossa, an area at the base of the skull attached to the spinal cord. In Arnold-Chiari malformation, the posterior fossa does not form properly. Because the posterior fossa is small, the brain stem, cerebellum, or cerebellar brain tissues (called the cerebellar tonsils) are squeezed downward through an opening at the bottom of the skull. The cerebellum and/or the brain stem may extend beyond the skull or protrude into the spinal column. The displaced tissues may obstruct the flow of cerebrospinal fluid (CSF), the substance that flows around the brain and spinal cord. CSF nourishes the brain and spinal cord.

Although this malformation is present at birth, there may not be any symptoms of a problem until adulthood. For this reason, Arnold-Chiari malformation is often not diagnosed until adulthood. Women have a higher incidence of this disorder than men.

Other names for Arnold-Chiari malformation are Arnold-Chiari syndrome, herniation of the cerebellar tonsils, and cerebellomedullary malformation syndrome. When doctors diagnose Arnold-Chiari malformation, they classify the malformation by its severity. An Arnold-Chiari I malformation is the least severe. In an Arnold-Chiari I malformation, the brain extends into the spinal canal. Doctors measure the length of brain stem located in the spinal canal to further define the malformation.

A type II malformation is more severe than a type I. It is almost always linked with a type of **spina bifida**. A sac protrudes through an abnormal opening in the spinal column. The sac is called a myelomeningocele. It may be filled with part of the spinal cord, spinal membranes, or spinal fluid. Unlike many cases of Arnold-Chiari I malformation, Arnold-Chiari II malformation is diagnosed in childhood. Doctors have identified Arnold-Chiari III and IV malformations, but they are very rare.

Arnold-Chiari malformations may occur with other conditions. There may be excessive fluid in the brain (**hydrocephalus**), opening in the spine (spina bifida), or excessive fluid in the spinal cord (**syringomyelia**), but many people with Arnold-Chiari malformations do not have other medical problems.

Demographics

Arnold-Chiari malformations are rare; no data has been collected to demonstrate the incidence of Arnold-Chiari malformations. However, it is known that Arnold-Chiari malformations are the most common type of malformation of the cervico-medullary junction, the area where the brain and spine connect. About one percent of live newborns have a malformation in the cervico-medullary junction.

Causes and symptoms

Scientists do not know what causes Arnold-Chiari malformations. One hypothesis is that the base of the skull is too small, forcing the cerebellum downward. Another theory focuses on overgrowth in the cerebellar region. The overgrowth pushes the cerebellum downward into the spinal canal.

Some people with Arnold-Chiari I malformations have no symptoms. Typically, with an Arnold-Chiari I malformation symptoms appear as the person reaches the third or fourth decade of life. Symptoms of this disorder vary. Most symptoms arise from the pressure on the cranial nerves or brain stem. The symptoms may be vague or they may resemble symptoms of other medical problems, so diagnosis may be delayed.

One of the most common symptoms of Arnold-Chiari malformations is a **headache**. The headache generally begins in the neck or base of the skull and may radiate through the back of the head. Coughing, sneezing, or bending forward may bring on these headaches. The headaches can last minutes or hours and may be linked with nausea.

There may be **pain** in the neck or upper arm with Arnold-Chiari malformations. Patients often report more pain on one side, rather than equal pain on both sides. There may also be weakness in the arm or hand. Patients may also report tingling, burning, numbness, or pins and needles. Balance can be affected as well. A person may be unsteady on their feet or lean to one side.

Some people with Arnold-Chiari malformation may have difficulty swallowing. They may say that food 'catches' in their throat when they swallow. Another common complaint linked with Arnold-Chiari malformations is hoarseness.

People with Arnold-Chiari malformations may have visual problems, including blurred vision, double vision, or blind spots. There may be bobbing of the eyes.

Diagnosis

An Arnold-Chiari malformation is diagnosed with **magnetic resonance imaging (MRI)**. An MRI uses magnetism and radio waves to produce a picture of the brain and show the crowding of the space between the brain and spinal cord that occurs with Arnold-Chiari malformations. In addition to an MRI, patients will also have a thorough neurologic examination.

Treatment team

Individuals who begin to experience symptoms from an Arnold-Chiari malformation are usually first seen by their primary care physician, who may send them on to a **neurologist** for further evaluation. If the patient is deemed to require surgery, a neurosurgeon will be consulted.

Treatment

The recommended treatment for an Arnold-Chiari I malformation is surgery to relieve the pressure on the cerebellar area. During the surgery, the surgeon removes a small part of the bone at the base of skull. This enlarges and decompresses the posterior fossa. This opening is patched with a piece of natural tissue. In some people with Arnold-Chiari malformation, displaced brain tissue affects the flow of cerebrospinal fluid. Doctors may evaluate the flow of cerebrospinal fluid during surgery for Arnold-Chiari malformation. If they find that brain tissue is blocking the flow of cerebrospinal fluid, they will shrink the brain tissue during surgery.

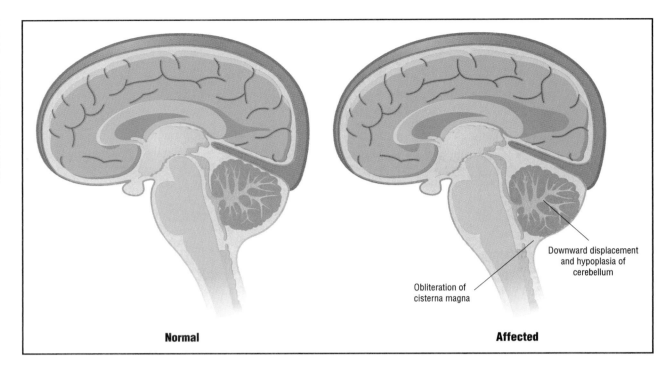

Normal   Affected

Obliteration of cisterna magna

Downward displacement and hypoplasia of cerebellum

A characteristic change that occurs in patients with Arnold-Chiari syndrome, type II, is the downward positioning of the cerebellum. This displacement destroys the area of the cisterna magna. *(Gale Group.)*

Recover and Rehabilitation

Individuals who are recovering from surgery to repair an Arnold-Chiari malformation may require physical and/or occupational therapy as they try to regain strength and fine motor control in their arms and hands. A speech therapist may be helpful in improving both speech and swallowing.

Clinical Trials

The National Institutes of Health are undertaking several research studies exploring aspects of Arnold-Chiari malformations. Efforts are being made to delineate a possible genetic defect leading to such malformations; studies are further exploring the anatomy and physiology of the malformations; and comparisons of the efficacy of various surgical treatments are being made.

Prognosis

Long-term prognosis for persons with Arnold-Chiari I malformations is excellent. Full recovery from surgery may take several months. During that time, patients may continue to experience some of the symptoms associated with Arnold-Chiari malformations.

Prognosis for Arnold-Chiari II malformations depends on the severity of the myelomeningocele and will be equivalent to that of spina bifida.

Resources

ORGANIZATIONS

American Syringomelia Project. PO Box 1586, Longview, Texas 75606-1586. (903) 236-7079.

National Organization for Rare Disorders (NORD). PO Box 8923, New Fairfield, CT 06812-8923. (203) 746-6518 or (800) 999-6673. Fax: (203) 746-6481. <http://www.raredisease.org>.

World Arnold-Chiari Malformation Association. 31 Newton Woods Road, Newton Square, Philadelphia, PA19073. <http://presenter.com?~wacma/milhorat.htm>.

Lisa A. Fratt
Rosalyn Carson-DeWitt, MD

Arteriovenous malformations

Definition

Arteriovenous malformations (AVMs) are blood vessel defects that occur before birth when the fetus is growing in the uterus (prenatal development). The blood vessels appear as a tangled mass of arteries and veins. They do not possess the capillary (very fine blood vessels) bed that normally exists in the common area where the arteries and veins lie in close proximity (artery-vein interface). An arteriovenous malformation may hemorrhage, or bleed, leading to serious complications that can be life-threatening.

Description

AVMs represent an abnormal interface between arteries and veins. Normally, arteries carry oxygenated blood to the body's tissues through progressively smaller blood vessels. The smallest are capillaries, which form a web of blood vessels (the capillary bed) through the body's tissues. The arterial blood moves through tissues by these tiny pathways, exchanging its load of oxygen and nutrients for carbon dioxide and other waste products produced by the body cells (cellular wastes). The blood is carried away by progressively larger blood vessels, the veins. AVMs lack a capillary bed, and arterial blood is moved (shunted) directly from the arteries into the veins.

AVMs can occur anywhere in the body and have been found in the arms, hands, legs, feet, lungs, heart, liver, and kidneys. However, 50% of these malformations are located in the brain, brainstem, and spinal cord. Owing to the possibility of hemorrhaging, such AVMs carry the risk of **stroke**, paralysis, and the loss of speech, memory, or vision. An AVM that hemorrhages can be fatal.

Approximately three of every 100,000 people have a cerebral (brain) AVM and roughly 40–80% of them will experience some bleeding from the abnormal blood vessels at some point. The annual risk of an AVM bleeding is estimated at about 1–4%. After age 55, the risk of bleeding decreases. Pre-existing high blood pressure or intense physical activity do not seem to be associated with AVM hemorrhage, but pregnancy and labor could cause a rupture or breaking open of a blood vessel. An AVM hemorrhage is not as dangerous as an aneurysmal rupture (an aneurysm is a swollen, blood-filled vessel where the pressure of the blood causes the wall to bulge outward). There is about a 10% fatality rate associated with AVM hemorrhage, compared to a 50% fatality rate for ruptured **aneurysms**.

Although AVMs are congenital defects, meaning a person is born with them, they are rarely discovered before age 20. A genetic link has been suggested for some AVMs, but studies have been inconclusive. The majority of AVMs are discovered in people ages 20–40. Medical researchers estimate that the malformations are created during days 45–60 of fetal development. Another theory suggests that AVMs are primitive structures that are left over after fetal blood-circulating systems developed.

However they form, AVMs have blood vessels that are abnormally fragile. The arteries that feed into the malformation are unusually swollen and thin walled. They lack the usual amount of smooth muscle tissue and elastin, a fibrous connective tissue. These blood vessels commonly

Key Terms

Aneurysm A weak point in a blood vessel where the pressure of the blood causes the vessel wall to bulge outwards.

Angiography A mapping of the brain's blood vessels, using x-ray imaging.

Capillary bed A dense network of tiny blood vessels that enables blood to fill a tissue or organ.

Hydrocephalus Swelling of the brain caused by an accumulation of fluid.

Lumbar puncture A diagnostic procedure in which a needle is inserted into the lower spine to withdraw a small amount of cerebrospinal fluid.

Saccular aneurysm A type of aneurysm that resembles a small sack of blood attached to the outer surface of a blood vessel by a thin neck.

accumulate deposits of calcium salts and hyaline. The venous part of the malformation receives blood directly from the artery. Without the intervening capillary bed, the veins receive blood at a higher pressure than they were designed to handle; this part of the malformation is also swollen (dilated) and thin walled. There is a measurable risk of an aneurysm forming near an AVM, increasing the threat of hemorrhage, brain damage, and death. Approximately 10–15% of AVMs are accompanied by saccular aneurysms, a type of aneurysm that looks like a small sac attached to the outer wall of the blood vessel.

Although the malformation itself lacks capillaries, there is often an abnormal proliferation of capillaries next to the defect. These blood vessels feed into the malformation, causing it to grow larger in some cases. As the AVM receives more blood through this "steal," adjacent brain tissue does not receive enough. These areas show abnormal nerve cell growth, cell death, and deposits of calcium (calcification). Nerve cells within the malformation may demonstrate abnormal growth and are believed to be non-functional. This may lead to progressive neurological deficits, or **seizures**, or both.

Causes and symptoms

About half of all patients with AVMs first come to medical attention because of hemorrhage; small AVMs are most likely to hemorrhage. If a hemorrhage occurs, it produces a sudden, severe **headache**. The headache may be focused in one specific area or it may be more general. It can also be mistaken for a migraine in some cases. The headache may be accompanied by other symptoms such as vomiting, stiff neck, sleepiness, lethargy, confusion, irritability, or weakness anywhere in the body. Hemorrhaging from an AVM is generally less dangerous than hemorrhaging from an aneurysm, with a survival rate of 80–90%. Second or subsequent hemorrhages are more dangerous than first hemorrhages.

Almost half of AVM patients first present with seizures. A person may experience decreased, double, or blurred vision. About 25% of patients begin with a progressive neurological deficit such as loss of vision, weakness, or cognitive changes, depending on the exact location of the AVM. Larger AVMs are more likely to cause seizures and progressive deficits than smaller ones. Large AVMs exert pressure against brain tissue, cause abnormal development in the surrounding brain tissue, and slow down or block blood flow. **Hydrocephalus**, a swelling of brain tissue caused by accumulated fluids, may develop.

Additional warning signs of a bleeding AVM are impaired speech or smell, **fainting**, facial paralysis, drooping eyelid, **dizziness**, and ringing or buzzing in the ears.

About 65% of AVM patients have a mild learning disability present long before coming to medical attention for the AVM. There may also be a history of headaches or migraines.

Diagnosis

Based on the clinical symptoms such as severe headache or neurological problems, and after a complete neurologic exam, a computed tomography (CT) scan of the head will be done. In some cases, a whooshing sound from arteries in the neck or over the eye or jaw (called a bruit) can be heard with a stethoscope. The **CT scan** will reveal whether there has been bleeding in the brain and can identify AVMs larger than 1 in (2.5 cm). **Magnetic resonance imaging (MRI)** is also used to identify an AVM. A lumbar puncture, or spinal tap, may follow the **MRI** or CT scan. A lumbar puncture involves removing a small amount of cerebrospinal fluid from the lower part of the spine. Blood cells or blood breakdown products in the cerebrospinal fluid indicate bleeding.

To pinpoint where the blood is coming from, a cerebral **angiography** is done. This procedure uses x rays to map out the blood vessels in the brain, including the vessels that feed into the malformation. The information gained from angiography complements the MRI and helps distinguish the precise location of the AVM. During angiography, an anesthetic may be introduced into the AVM area to determine the precise function of the surrounding region. The patient will be given a variety of tests of language comprehension, speech production, sensation, and other tasks, depending on the precise location of the AVM. These results help determine the risk of treatment.

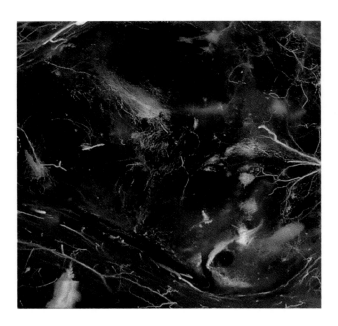

Arteriovenous malformations. *(Photograph by Patricia Barber. Custom Medical Stock Photo. Reproduced by permission.)*

Treatment team

The treatment team consists of a **neurologist**, neuroradiologist, **neuropsychologist**, neurosurgeon, and anesthesiologist.

Treatment

Neurosurgeons consider several factors before deciding on a treatment option. There is some debate over whether or not to treat AVMs that have not ruptured and are not causing any symptoms. The risks and benefits of proceeding with treatment need to be measured on an individual basis, taking into account factors such as the person's age and general health, as well as the AVM's size and location. In older patients at low risk for future hemorrhage, or for those in whom the AVM is located very close to critical brain areas, the doctor and patient may decide that treating symptoms alone is the best course. Antiseizure medications, **pain** relievers for headaches, and migraine medications may provide adequate symptom control for many patients.

To treat the AVM directly, several options are available. These treatment options may be used alone or in combination.

Surgery

Removing the AVM is the surest way of preventing it from causing future problems. Both small and large AVMs can be handled in surgery. Surgery is recommended for superficial AVMs (those close to the surface), but may be too dangerous for deep or very large AVMs. In this procedure, a portion of the skull is opened to expose the AVM. The arteries and veins leading in and out are identified and closed off, and then the AVM itself is removed. Surgery requires general anesthesia and a longer period of recuperation than any other treatment option. It also carries the risk of intracranial bleeding during surgery, and interruption of blood supply to vital brain areas. The blood that no longer flows through the AVM is distributed elsewhere in the brain, and this increase in flow may be dangerous if it is too high for the vessels to handle.

Radiation

Radiation is particularly useful to treat small (under 1 in [2.5 cm]) malformations that are deep within the brain. Ionizing radiation is directed at the malformation, destroying the AVM without damaging the surrounding tissue. Radiation treatment is accomplished in a single session, and it is not necessary to open the skull. However, the radiation takes months to exert its complete effect, and success can only be measured over the course of the following two years. A year after the procedure, 50–75% of treated AVMs are completely blocked; two years after radiation treatment, the percentage increases to 85–95%.

Embolization

Embolization involves plugging up access to the malformation. This technique does not require opening the skull to expose the brain and can be used to treat deep AVMs. Using x-ray images as a guide, a catheter is threaded through the artery in the thigh (femoral artery) to the affected area. The patient remains awake during the procedure and medications can be administered to prevent discomfort. A device is inserted through the catheter into the AVM, and released there to block the blood supply to the malformation. The device may be metal spheres, an adhesive, a hardening polymer, or other such substance.

There may be a mild headache or nausea associated with the procedure, but patients may resume normal activities after leaving the hospital. At least two or three embolization procedures are usually necessary at intervals of 2–6 weeks. At least a three-day hospital stay is associated with each embolization. Embolization rarely provides complete blockage, and may be used prior to one or the other types of treatment.

Recovery and rehabilitation

Recovery and rehabilitation vary with each form of treatment. In general, successful treatment leads to reduction in the risk for cerebral hemorrhage and improvement of symptoms caused by the AVM. Surgical complications, including hemorrhage, infection, and treatment of too large an area, make recovery longer and more difficult, and may leave the patient with permanent neurologic deficits.

Clinical trials

Clinical trials of surgical techniques for treatment of AVMs are conducted in large medical centers.

Prognosis

Approximately 10% of AVM cases are fatal. Seizures and neurological changes may be permanent in another 10–30% cases of AVM rupture. If an AVM bleeds once, it is about 20% likely to bleed again in the next year. As time passes from the initial hemorrhage, the risk for further bleeding drops to about 3–4%. If the AVM has not bled, it is possible, but not guaranteed, that it never will. Untreated AVMs can grow larger over time and rarely go away by themselves. Once an AVM is removed and a person has recovered from the procedure, there should be no further symptoms associated with that malformation.

Resources

BOOKS

The Official Patient's Sourcebook on Arteriovenous Malformations: A Revised and Updated Directory for the Internet Age. San Diego: Icon Health Publications, 2002.

Steig, P., H. H. Batjer, and D. Samson. *Intracranial Arteriovenous Malformations.* New York: Macel Dekker, 2003.

Julia Barrett

Aspartame

Definition

Aspartame, an artificial sweetener that is used as a substitute for sugar in many foods and beverages, is considered by some scientists to be a neurotoxin, a substance that is detrimental to the nervous system. This allegation remains controversial.

Description

Aspartame was introduced as an artificial sweetener by the Monsanto Company in the 1970s. For much of the intervening time, individuals and special interest groups have maintained that aspartame damages the nervous system. Given the number and popularity of the items that are sweetened using aspartame (i.e., yogurts, soft drinks), the special interest groups assert that the general population is at risk for neurological damage caused by the ingestion of aspartame.

Key Terms

Dopamine A neurotransmitter made in the brain that is involved in many brain activities, including movement and emotion.

Fibromyalgia A condition characterized by aching and stiffness, fatigue, and sleep disturbance, as well as pain at various sites on the body.

Neurotoxin A poison that acts directly on the central nervous system.

Alleged harmful effects of aspartame ingestion include **seizures** and a change in the level of dopamine, a brain neurotransmitter. Symptoms associated with **lupus**, **multiple sclerosis**, and **Alzheimer's disease** have been claimed to result from an excess intake of aspartame. As well, aspartame consumption is claimed to increase the difficulty of diet-dependent diabetics in regulating their blood glucose level.

One peer-reviewed scientific study has documented an improvement in fibromyalgia symptoms (**pain** in the muscles, ligaments, and tendons) following the elimination of monosodium glutamate and aspartame from the diet. The influence of aspartame alone, however, was not assessed. Studies conducted prior to the marketing of aspartame and following its introduction have failed to demonstrate these claimed negative effects. The U.S. Food and Drug Administration (FDA) maintains that aspartame is not a health threat to the general population, although individuals who are sensitive to the compound can develop headaches and feel fatigued. Currently, there is no evidence directly linking aspartame with diseases such as lupus, multiple sclerosis, and Alzheimer's.

Demographics

As the association of aspartame with neurological disorders is not proven, statistics relating to how often and how many individuals suffer ill effects from aspartame are unavailable. If the claim of a general population effect is true, and that the effect is cumulative (builds up over time), then aspartame would affect older people more than younger people. There has been no evidence or suggestion of any gender, race, or cultural predilection to negative effects from aspartame.

If, however, only certain people are predisposed to be more sensitive to the presence of aspartame, then the demographics would include this subpopulation. The characteristics of such a group have not been defined.

Causes and symptoms

At elevated temperatures of about 90° Fahrenheit, a component of aspartame can convert to formaldehyde. High concentrations of formaldehyde can kill cells and tissues. Furthermore, formaldehyde can, in turn, be converted to formic acid, which can cause metabolic acidosis. Whether these changes are detrimental to the nervous system is not known.

One research paper published in 2001 reported one patient in whom aspartame exacerbated an ongoing migraine attack. Whether this occurrence is more widespread among the general public is unknown.

Diagnosis

Currently, any symptoms that are directly attributable to aspartame excess have not been conclusively identified. The suspected symptoms such as fibromyalgia and changes in dopamine levels are associated with other maladies including lupus, multiple sclerosis, or Alzheimer's disease. Factors that may trigger migraine **headache** vary among individuals, and physicians may suggest that those suffering from migraine lower their consumption of aspartame.

Treatment

Symptoms may disappear when the use of aspartame is discontinued.

Special concerns

Aspartame poisoning is a contentious issue. Scientific peer-reviewed papers have reported on research performed at companies that have a vested interest in sales of aspartame. While the quality of the scientific data contained in these studies may be sound, other scientists criticize that the evidence presented is difficult to evaluate in light of possible conflicting interests. By the same token, the claims made by special interest groups concerning the dangers of aspartame should be viewed cautiously, as little or no data is presented to support their claims.

Resources

BOOKS

Blaylock, R. L. *Excitotoxins.* Santa Fe, NM: Health Press. 1996.

Roberts, H. J. *Aspartame (Nutrasweet): Is It Safe?* Philadelphia: The Charles Press, 1992.

PERIODICALS

Butchko, H. H., et al. "Aspartame: Review of Safety." *Regulatory Toxicology and Pharmacology* (April 2002): S1–93.

Newman, L. C., and R. B. Lipton. "Migraine MLT-down: An Unusual Presentation of Migraine in Patients with

Key Terms

Autistic psychopathy Hans Asperger's original name for the condition now known as Asperger's disorder. It is still used occasionally as a synonym for the disorder.

DSM Abbreviation for the *Diagnostic and Statistical Manual of Mental Disorders,* a handbook for mental health professionals that includes lists of symptoms that indicate specific diagnoses. The text is periodically revised, and the latest version was published in 2000 and is called *DSM-IV-TR,* for Fourth Edition, Text Revised.

Gillberg's criteria A six-item checklist for AS developed by Christopher Gillberg, a Swedish researcher. It is widely used in Europe as a diagnostic tool.

High-functioning autism (HFA) A subcategory of autistic disorder consisting of children diagnosed with IQs of 70 or higher. Children with AS are often misdiagnosed as having HFA.

Nonverbal learning disability (NLD) A learning disability syndrome identified in 1989 that may overlap with some of the symptoms of AS.

Pervasive developmental disorders (PDDs) A category of childhood disorders that includes Asperger's syndrome and Rett's disorder. The PDDs are sometimes referred to collectively as autistic spectrum disorders.

Semantic-pragmatic disorder A term that refers to the difficulty that children with AS and some forms of autism have with pragmatic language skills. Pragmatic language skills include knowing the proper tone of voice for a given context, using humor appropriately, making eye contact with a conversation partner, maintaining the appropriate volume of one's voice, etc.

Aspartame-triggered Headaches." *Headache* (October 2001): 899–901.

Smith, J. D., C. M. Terpening, S. O. Schmidt, and J. G. Gums. "Relief of Fibromyalgia Symptoms following Discontinuation of Dietary Excitotoxins." *Annals of Pharmacotherapy* (June 2001): 702–706.

OTHER

"Aspartame Information Page." *National Institute of Neurological Disorders and Stroke.* January 21, 2004 (May 17, 2004). <http://www.ninds.nih.gov/ health_and_medical/disorders/aspartame.htm>.

ORGANIZATIONS

Food and Drug Administration. 5600 Fishers Lane, CDER-HFD-210, Rockville, MD 20857. (301) 827-4573 or (888) 463-6332. <http://www.fda.gov>.

Brian Douglas Hoyle, PhD

Asperger's disorder

Definition

Asperger's disorder, which is also called Asperger's syndrome (AS) or autistic psychopathy, belongs to a group of childhood disorders known as pervasive developmental disorders (PDDs) or autistic spectrum disorders. The essential features of Asperger's disorder are severe social interaction impairment and restricted, repetitive patterns of behavior and activities. It is similar to **autism**, but children with Asperger's do not have the same difficulties in acquiring language that children with autism have.

In the mental health professional's diagnostic handbook, the *Diagnostic and Statistical Manual of Mental Disorders* fourth edition text revised, or *DSM-IV-TR,* Asperger's disorder is classified as a developmental disorder of childhood.

Description

AS was first described by Hans Asperger, an Austrian psychiatrist, in 1944. Asperger's work was unavailable in English before the mid-1970s; as a result, AS was often unrecognized in English-speaking countries until the late 1980s. Before *DSM-IV* (published in 1994) there was no officially agreed-upon definition of AS. In the words of ICD-10, the European equivalent of the *DSM-IV,* Asperger's is "a disorder of uncertain nosological validity." (Nosological refers to the classification of diseases.) There are three major reasons for this lack of clarity: differences between the diagnostic criteria used in Europe and those used in the United States; the fact that some of the diagnostic criteria depend on the observer's interpretation rather than objective measurements; and the fact that the clinical picture of Asperger's changes as the child grows older.

Asperger's disorder is one of the milder pervasive developmental disorders. Children with AS learn to talk at the usual age and often have above-average verbal skills. They have normal or above-normal intelligence and the ability to feed or dress themselves and take care of their other daily needs. The distinguishing features of AS are problems with social interaction, particularly reciprocating and empathizing with the feelings of others; difficulties with nonverbal communication (such as facial expressions); peculiar speech habits that include repeated words or phrases and a flat, emotionless vocal tone; an apparent lack of "common sense"; a fascination with obscure or limited subjects (for example, the parts of a clock or small machine, railroad schedules, astronomical data, etc.) often to the exclusion of other interests; clumsy and awkward physical movements; and odd or eccentric behaviors (hand wringing or finger flapping; swaying or other repetitious whole-body movements; watching spinning objects for long periods of time).

Demographics

Although the incidence of AS has been variously estimated between 0.024% and 0.36% of the general population in North America and northern Europe, further research is required to determine its true rate of occurrence—especially because the diagnostic criteria have been defined so recently. In addition, no research regarding the incidence of AS has been done on the populations of developing countries, and nothing is known about the incidence of the disorder in different racial or ethnic groups.

With regard to gender differences, AS appears to be much more common in boys. Dr. Asperger's first patients were all boys, but girls have been diagnosed with AS since the 1980s. One Swedish study found the male/female ratio to be 4:1; however, the World Health Organization's ICD-10 classification gives the male to female ratio as 8 to 1.

Causes and symptoms

There is some indication that AS runs in families, particularly in families with histories of **depression** and bipolar disorder. Asperger noted that his initial group of patients had fathers with AS symptoms. Knowledge of the genetic profile of the disorder continues to be quite limited, however.

In addition, about 50% of AS patients have a history of oxygen deprivation during the birth process, which has led to the hypothesis that the disorder is caused by damage to brain tissue before or during childbirth. Another cause that has been suggested is an organic defect in the functioning of the brain.

Research studies have made no connection between Asperger's disorder and childhood trauma, abuse or neglect.

In young children, the symptoms of AS typically include problems picking up social cues and understanding the basics of interacting with other children. The child may want friendships but find him- or herself unable to make friends.

Most children with Asperger's are diagnosed during the elementary school years because the symptoms of the disorder become more apparent at this point. They include:

- Poor pragmatic language skills. This phrase means that the child does not use the right tone or volume of voice for a specific context, and does not understand that using humorous or slang expressions also depends on social context.
- Problems with hand-eye coordination and other visual skills
- Problems making eye contact with others
- Learning difficulties, which may range from mild to severe
- Tendency to become absorbed in a particular topic and not know when others are bored with conversation about it. At this stage in their education, children with AS are likely to be labeled as "nerds."
- Repetitive behaviors. These include such behaviors as counting a group of coins or marbles over and over; reciting the same song or poem several times; buttoning and unbuttoning a jacket repeatedly; etc.

Adolescence is one of the most painful periods of life for young people with Asperger's, because social interactions are more complex in this age group and require more subtle social skills. Some boys with AS become frustrated trying to relate to their peers and may become aggressive. Both boys and girls with the disorder are often quite naive for their age and easily manipulated by "street-wise" classmates. They are also more vulnerable than most youngsters to peer pressure.

Little research has been done regarding adults with AS. Some have serious difficulties with social and occupational functioning, but others are able to finish their schooling, join the workforce, and marry and have families.

Diagnosis

Currently, there are no blood tests or brain scans that can be used to diagnose AS. Until *DSM-IV* (1994), there was no "official" list of symptoms for the disorder, which made its diagnosis both difficult and inexact. Although most children with AS are diagnosed between five and nine years of age, many are not diagnosed until adulthood. Misdiagnoses are common; AS has been confused with such other neurological disorders as **Tourette's syndrome**, or with **attention-deficit hyperactivity disorder** (ADHD), oppositional defiant disorder (ODD), or obsessive-compulsive disorder (OCD). Some researchers think that AS may overlap with some types of learning disability, such as the nonverbal learning disability (NLD) syndrome identified in 1989.

The inclusion of AS as a separate diagnostic category in *DSM-IV* was justified on the basis of a large international field trial of over a thousand children and adolescents. Nevertheless, the diagnosis of AS is also complicated by confusion with such other diagnostic categories as "high-functioning (IQ higher than 70) autism" or HFA, and "schizoid personality disorder of childhood." Unlike schizoid personality disorder of childhood, AS is not an unchanging set of personality traits—AS has a developmental dimension. AS is distinguished from HFA by the following characteristics:

- Later onset of symptoms (usually around three years of age)
- Early development of grammatical speech; the AS child's verbal IQ (scores on verbal sections of standardized intelligence tests) is usually higher than performance IQ (how well the child performs in school). The reverse is usually true for autistic children
- Less severe deficiencies in social and communication skills
- Presence of intense interest in one or two topics
- Physical clumsiness and lack of coordination
- Family is more likely to have a history of the disorder
- Lower frequency of neurological disorders
- More positive outcome in later life

DSM-IV-TR *criteria for Asperger's disorder*

The *DSM-IV-TR* specifies the following diagnostic criteria for AS:

- The child's social interactions are impaired in at least two of the following ways: markedly limited use of nonverbal communication (facial expressions, for example); lack of age-appropriate peer relationships; failure to share enjoyment, interests, or accomplishment with others; lack of reciprocity (turn-taking) in social interactions.
- The child's behavior, interests, and activities are characterized by repetitive or rigid patterns, such as an abnormal preoccupation with one or two topics, or with parts of objects; repetitive physical movements; or rigid insistence on certain routines and rituals.
- The patient's social, occupational, or educational functioning is significantly impaired.
- The child has normal age-appropriate language skills.
- The child has normal age-appropriate cognitive skills, self-help abilities, and curiosity about the environment.
- The child does not meet criteria for another specific PDD or schizophrenia.

To establish the diagnosis, the child psychiatrist or psychologist would observe the child, and would interview parents, possibly teachers, and the affected child (depending on the child's age), and would gather a comprehensive medical and social history.

Other diagnostic scales and checklists

Other instruments that have been used to identify children with AS include Gillberg's criteria, a six-item list compiled by a Swedish researcher that specifies problems in social interaction, a preoccupying narrow interest, forcing routines and interests on the self or others, speech and language problems, nonverbal communication problems, and physical clumsiness; and the Australian Scale for Asperger's Syndrome, a detailed multi-item questionnaire developed in 1996.

Brain imaging findings

Current research has linked only a few structural abnormalities of the brain to AS. Findings include abnormally large folds in the brain tissue in the left frontal region, abnormally small folds in the operculum (a lid-like structure composed of portions of three adjoining brain lobes), and damage to the left temporal lobe (a part of the brain containing a sensory area associated with hearing). The first single photon emission tomography (SPECT) study of an AS patient found a lower-than-normal supply of blood to the left parietal area of the brain, an area associated with bodily sensations. Brain imaging studies on a larger sample of AS patients is the next stage of research.

Treatment team

The treatment team needed for a child with Asperger's syndrome will vary based on the specifics and the severity of the child's disabilities. Pediatricians, developmental pediatricians, neurologists, and child psychiatrists can all play a part in the diagnosis and the treatment planning for a child with Asperger's syndrome. Physical therapy, occupational therapy, speech and language therapy, individual and group behavioral therapy, and psychoeducational planning are all crucial to helping a child with Asperger's syndrome progress optimally.

Treatments

There is no cure for AS and no prescribed treatment regimen for all AS patients. Specific treatments are based on the individual's symptom pattern.

Medications

Many children with AS do not require any medication. For those who do, the drugs that are recommended most often include psychostimulants (methylphenidate, pemoline), clonidine, or one of the tricyclic antidepressants (TCAs) for hyperactivity or inattention; beta blockers, neuroleptics (antipsychotic medications), or lithium

(lithium carbonate) for anger or aggression; selective serotonin reuptake inhibitors (SSRIs) or TCAs for rituals (repetitive behaviors) and preoccupations; and SSRIs or TCAs for anxiety symptoms. One alternative herbal remedy that has been tried with AS patients is St. John's wort.

Psychotherapy

AS patients often benefit from individual psychotherapy, particularly during adolescence, in order to cope with depression and other painful feelings related to their social difficulties. Many children with AS are also helped by group therapy, which brings them together with others facing the same challenges. There are therapy groups for parents as well.

Therapists who are experienced in treating children with Asperger's disorder have found that the child should be allowed to proceed slowly in forming an emotional bond with the therapist. Too much emotional intensity at the beginning may be more than the child can handle. Behavioral approaches seem to work best with these children. Play therapy can be helpful in teaching the child to recognize social cues as well as lowering the level of emotional tension.

Adults with AS are most likely to benefit from individual therapy using a cognitive-behavioral approach, although many also attend group therapy. Some adults have been helped by working with speech therapists on their pragmatic language skills. A relatively new approach called behavioral coaching has been used to help adults with Asperger's learn to organize and set priorities for their daily activities.

Prognosis

AS is a lifelong but stable condition. The prognosis for children with AS is generally good as far as intellectual development is concerned, although few school districts are equipped to meet the special social needs of this group of children. Adults with AS appear to be at greater risk of depression than the general population. In addition, some researchers believe that people with AS have an increased risk of a psychotic episode (a period of time during which the affected person loses touch with reality) in adolescence or adult life.

Special concerns

Educational considerations

Most AS patients have normal or above-normal intelligence, and are able to complete their education up through the graduate or professional school level. Many are unusually skilled in music or good in subjects requiring rote memorization. On the other hand, the verbal skills of children with AS frequently cause difficulties with teachers, who may not understand why these "bright" children have social and communication problems. Some AS children are dyslexic; others have difficulty with writing or mathematics. In some cases, AS children have been mistakenly put in special programs either for children with much lower levels of functioning, or for children with conduct disorders. AS children do best in structured learning situations in which they learn problem-solving and social skills as well as academic subjects. They frequently need protection from the teasing and bullying of other children, and often become hypersensitive to criticism by their teenage years. One approach that has been found helpful at the high-school level is to pair the adolescent with AS with a slightly older teenager who can serve as a mentor. The mentor can "clue in" the younger adolescent about the slang, dress code, cliques, and other "facts of life" at the local high school.

Employment

Adults with AS are productively employed in a wide variety of fields, including the learned professions. They do best, however, in jobs with regular routines or occupations that allow them to work in isolation. In large companies, employers or supervisors and workplace colleagues may need some information about AS in order to understand the new employee's "eccentricities."

Resources

BOOKS

American Psychiatric Association. *Diagnostic and Statistical Manual of Mental Disorders.* 4th edition, text revised. Washington, DC: American Psychiatric Association, 2000.

"Psychiatric Conditions in Childhood and Adolescence." Section 19, Chapter 274. In *The Merck Manual of Diagnosis and Therapy,* edited by Mark H. Beers, M.D., and Robert Berkow, M.D. Whitehouse Station, NJ: Merck Research Laboratories, 1999.

Thoene, Jess G., ed. *Physicians' Guide to Rare Diseases.* Montvale, NJ: Dowden Publishing Company, 1995.

World Health Organization (WHO). *The ICD-10 Classification of Mental and Behavioural Disorders.* Geneva: WHO, 1992.

PERIODICALS

Bishop, D. V. M. "Autism, Asperger's Syndrome & Semantic-Pragmatic Disorder: Where Are the Boundaries?" *British Journal of Disorders of Communication* 24 (1989): 107–121.

Gillberg, C. "The Neurobiology of Infantile Autism." *Journal of Child Psychology and Psychiatry* 29 (1988): 257–266.

ORGANIZATIONS

Autism Research Institute. 4182 Adams Avenue, San Diego, CA 92116.

Families of Adults Afflicted with Asperger's Syndrome (FAAAS). P.O. Box 514, Centerville, MA 02632. <www.faaas.org>.

National Association of Rare Disorders (NORD). P.O. Box 8923, New Fairfield, CT 06812-8923. (800) 999-NORD or (203) 746-6518.

Yale-LDA Social Learning Disabilities Project. Yale Child Study Center, New Haven, CT. The Project is looking for study subjects with PDDs between the ages of 8 and 24, including AS patients. Contact person: Sanno Zack at (203) 785-3488 or Sanno.Zack@yale.edu. <www.info.med.Yale.edu/chldstdy/autism>.

OTHER

American Academy of Child & Adolescent Psychiatry (AACAP). "Asperger's Disorder." AACAP Facts For Families Pamphlet #69. Washington, DC: American Academy of Child & Adolescent Psychiatry, 1999.

Rebecca Frey, Ph.D.

Assistive mobile devices

Definition

Assistive mobile devices are tools designed to improve the mobility and stability of persons who have difficulty moving independently.

Description

Assistive mobile devices include canes, crutches, walkers, and wheelchairs. The devices are used to allow a person to continue to be mobile; otherwise the person may have difficulty moving about independently. A large variety of medical conditions may lead to the need for a mobility aid. A partial list includes:

- **cerebral palsy**
- **multiple sclerosis**
- **stroke**
- brain or spinal cord injury
- **Parkinson's disease**
- diabetes
- arthritis
- **muscular dystrophies** (progressive muscle-weakening disorders)
- **ataxias** (group of disorders affecting balance and coordination)
- **amyotrophic lateral sclerosis** (ALS), also known as Lou Gehrig's disease, a progressive disease causing muscle weakness

---

Key Terms

Quadriplegia Permanent paralysis of the trunk, lower and upper limbs. It is caused by injury or disease affecting the spinal cord at the neck level.

- trauma of the lower extremities, such as sprain or fracture
- polio
- leg or hip **pain**

The choice of mobility aid will depend less on the patient's disease or disorder and more on the current level of mobility. Factors that affect mobility include leg strength, balance, endurance, **fatigue**, pain, generalized weakness, altered limb sensations, and limb coordination.

Types of Aids

Canes

A cane is appropriate for a person with good strength and endurance, whose balance is impaired either due to slowed movements, loss of isolated muscle control, or ataxia, or who has pain upon full weight bearing on one side. A cane is often used when the impairment is on one side, as from an ankle sprain or localized polio. The cane provides a third point of contact with the ground (along with the two legs), making a tripod that is far more stable than the two legs alone. The cane can support the weight, although prolonged weight bearing is uncomfortable on the wrists. Two canes may be used for extra stability. A cane typically has a rubber tip for traction, and may have a four-pronged base ("quad-cane") for even more stability. The cane and the favored leg move in unison to allow the cane to absorb the weight of the step.

Crutches

Crutches are used in pairs. The patient uses the crutches by gripping them and clasping them between the arm and the side of the chest, or the arms may slip through short tubular "cuffs" to reach the handgrips. The latter style is more commonly used for long-term disabilities such as cerebral palsy, while the former is often used for temporary fractures or sprains. In the case of a fracture or sprain, the goal is to keep weight off the injured limb during healing. Crutches allow the patient to use only a single foot, plus the two crutch tips, for the stable tripod stance. The patient's wrists support the weight, not the armpits. Cuffed crutches may be used when there is limited coordination in the legs, or when (as with polio) the

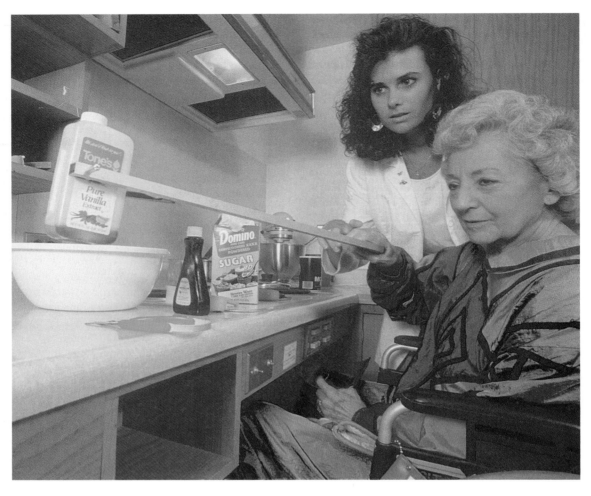

An occupational therapist assists a wheelchair-bound stroke patient. *(© Photo Reasearchers. Reproduced by permission.)*

legs are too weak to support the body's weight in full. The cuff transfers some of the bearing weight to the forearm, relieving the strain on the wrists.

Walkers

Walkers provide the maximum support and stability for a person who walks upright. The walker has four legs, or two legs plus two wheels, or four wheels. The walker's wide base of support provides great stability, important for those patients with balance problems. The frame supports the weight while the patient takes small steps forward. Following that, the patient lifts the walker and moves it forward, or rolls it forward (if it has wheels), and plants it again while taking another set of steps. Walkers move in front of the patient, but can still be useful for a person prone to fall backward. In this case, the height of the walker is lowered to ensure that weight is always tilted forward onto the walker. Wheeled walkers often have hand-operated brakes for greater safety, and may be equipped with a seat to allow the patient to sit down for short periods while ambulating.

Wheelchairs

Wheelchairs are designed for people who cannot support their weight on their legs, or for those whose balance is too impaired to stand. Wheelchairs may be short-term or long-term mobility aids, and may be used intermittently or all the time, depending on the requirements of the patient. There are several major designs for wheelchairs, including folding versus rigid, and manual versus powered. The technological developments in wheelchair design have made them extremely versatile and dependable, but at the same time have increased the cost of the more expensive models into the thousands of dollars. All wheelchairs have adjustable footrests to allow the legs to be held in a variety of positions.

The folding manual wheelchair is perhaps the most widely used style. Older folding chairs, still seen in airport

Key Terms

Alpha-fetoprotein (AFP) A chemical substance produced by the fetus and found in the fetal circulation. AFP is also found in abnormally high concentrations in most patients with primary liver cancer.

Atrophy Wasting away of normal tissue or an organ due to degeneration of the cells.

Cerebellar ataxia Unsteadiness and lack of coordination caused by a progressive degeneration of the part of the brain known as the cerebellum.

Dysarthria Slurred speech.

Dysplasia The abnormal growth or development of a tissue or organ.

Immunoglobulin A protein molecule formed by

mature B cells in response to foreign proteins in the body; the building blocks for antibodies.

Ionizing radiation High-energy radiation such as that produced by x rays.

Leukemia Cancer of the blood-forming organs which results in an overproduction of white blood cells.

Lymphoma A malignant tumor of the lymph nodes.

Recessive gene A type of gene that is not expressed as a trait unless inherited by both parents.

Telangiectasis Very small arteriovenous malformations, or connections between the arteries and veins. The result is small red spots on the skin known as "spider veins."

---

terminals, hospitals, and school nursing offices, have the seat slung between the two sides. This is cheap and durable, but is not designed for maximum comfort or adaptability to the individual patient, and thus is rarely appropriate for long-term use.

More modern folding chairs provide a firm platform for a custom seat, allowing a choice of seating cushion. This is highly important for anyone who will spend long periods in the chair. Lack of proper seating leads to pressure sores, chafing, and skin breakdown. Choice of the right seat is one of the most important decisions in fitting the wheelchair. Seat styles include foam, air cushion, and other materials.

Rigid manual chairs are lighter than folding models, at the expense of some portability. Rigid chairs are also used by wheelchair athletes who compete in marathons and other events, attaining speeds of 30 miles per hour or more. These chairs are custom made for individual athletes, and have little in common with standard manual chairs. All manual chairs do share the same source of power—pushing either by the occupant or by an attendant. Frequent lubrication and maintenance maintains the chair in good shape to make this task as easy as possible.

Power wheelchairs use on-board batteries to drive the wheels, allowing independent mobility to those without enough upper body strength for a long trip in a manual chair. Power chairs are generally controlled by a joystick, although for quadriplegics or others who have lost sufficient arm control, a "sip-and-puff" mechanism is available, in which the patient's inhalations or exhalations into a straw control the direction and speed of the chair.

Resources

BOOKS

Coope, Rory. *Wheelchair Selection and Configuration.* New York: Demos Medical Publishing, 1998.

Short, Ed. *Basic Manual Wheelchair Adjustments: A Handbook.* Fishersville, VA: Woodrow Wilson Rehabilitation Center Foundation, 2000.

WEBSITES

Muscular Dystrophy Association. (April 18, 2004.) <http://www.mdausa.org>.

Richard Robinson

Ataxia-telangiectasia

Definition

Ataxia-telangiectasia (A-T) is a rare, genetic neurological disorder that progressively affects various systems in the body. Children affected with A-T appear normal at birth; however, the first signs of the disease—usually a lack of balance and slurred speech—often appear between one and two years of age.

Description

The onset of cerebellar **ataxia** (unsteadiness and lack of coordination) marks the beginning of progressive degeneration of the **cerebellum**, the part of the brain responsible for motor control (movement). This degeneration gradually leads to a general lack of muscle control, and eventually confines the patient to a wheelchair. Children with A-T become unable to feed or dress themselves without assistance. Because of the worsening ataxia, children with A-T lose their ability to write, and speech also becomes slowed and slurred. Even reading eventually becomes impossible, as eye movements become difficult to control.

Children with A-T usually exhibit another symptom of the disease: telangiectases, or tiny red spider veins (dilated blood vessels). These telangiectases appear in the corners of the eyes—giving the eyes a blood-shot appearance—or on the surfaces of the ears and cheeks exposed to sunlight.

In about 70% of children with A-T, another symptom of the disease is present: an immune system deficiency that usually leads to recurrent respiratory infections. In many patients, these infections can become life threatening. Due to deficient levels of IgA and IgE immunoglobulins—the natural infection-fighting agents in the blood—children with A-T are highly susceptible to lung infections that are resistant to the standard antibiotic treatment. For these patients, the combination of a weakened immune system and progressive ataxia can ultimately lead to pneumonia as a cause of death.

Children with A-T tend to develop malignancies of the blood circulatory system almost 1,000 times more frequently than the general population. Lymphomas (malignant tumors of lymphoid tissues) and leukemias (abnormal overgrowth of white blood cells, causing tumor cells to grow) are particularly common types of cancer, although the risk of developing most types of cancer is high in those with A-T. Another characteristic of the disease is an increased sensitivity to ionizing **radiation** (high-energy radiation such as x rays), which means that patients with A-T frequently cannot tolerate the radiation treatments often given to cancer patients.

Demographics

Both males and females are equally affected by A-T. Epidemiologists estimate the frequency of A-T as between 1/40,000 and 1/100,000 live births. However, it is believed that many children with A-T, particularly those who die at a young age, are never properly diagnosed. Thus, the disease may occur much more often than reported.

It is also estimated that about 1% (2.5 million) of the American population carry a copy of the defective A-T gene. According to some researchers, these gene carriers may also have an increased sensitivity to ionizing radiation and have a significantly higher risk of developing cancer—particularly breast cancer in female carriers.

Causes and symptoms

Ataxia-telangiectasia is called a recessive genetic disorder because parents do not exhibit symptoms; however, each parent carries a recessive (unexpressed) gene that may cause A-T in offspring. The genetic path of A-T is therefore impossible to predict. The recessive gene may lie dormant for generations until two people with the defective gene have children. When two such A-T carriers have a child together, there is a 1-in-4 chance (25% risk) of having a child with A-T. Every healthy sibling of a child with A-T has a 2-in-3 chance (66% risk) of being a carrier, like his or her parents.

Although there is much variability in A-T symptoms among patients, the signs of A-T almost always include the appearance of ataxia between the ages of two and five. Other, less consistent symptoms may include neurological, cutaneous (skin), and a variety of other conditions.

Neurological
Neurological symptoms of A-T include:
- progressive cerebellar ataxia (although ataxia may appear static between the ages of two and five)
- cerebellar **dysarthria** (slurred speech)
- difficulty swallowing, causing choking and drooling
- progressive lack of control of eye movements
- muscle weakness and poor reflexes
- initially normal intelligence, sometimes with later regression to mildly retarded range

Cutaneous
Cutaneous symptoms include:
- progressive telangiectases of the eye and skin develop between two to ten years of age
- atopic dermatitis (itchy skin)
- Café au lait spots (pale brown areas of skin)
- cutaneous atrophy (wasting away)
- hypo- and hyperpigmentation (underpigmented and overpigmented areas of skin)
- loss of skin elasticity
- nummular eczema (coin-shaped inflammatory skin condition)

Other symptoms
Other manifestations of A-T include:
- susceptibility to neoplasms (tumors or growths)
- endocrine abnormalities
- tendency to develop insulin-resistant diabetes in adolescence

- recurrent sinopulmonary infection (involving the sinuses and the airways of the lungs)

- characteristic loss of facial muscle tone

- absence or dysplasia (abnormal development of tissue) of thymus gland

- jerky, involuntary movements

- slowed growth

- prematurely graying hair

Diagnosis

For a doctor who is familiar with A-T, the diagnosis can usually be made on purely clinical grounds and often on inspection. But because most physicians have never seen a case of A-T, misdiagnoses are likely to occur. For example, physicians examining ataxic children frequently rule out A-T if telangiectases are not observed. However, telangiectases often do not appear until the age of six, and sometimes appear at a much older age. In addition, a history of recurrent sinopulmonary infections might increase suspicion of A-T, but about 30% of patients with A-T exhibit no immune system deficiencies.

The most common early misdiagnosis is that of static encephalopathy—a brain dysfunction, or ataxic cerebral palsy—paralysis due to a birth defect. Ataxia involving the trunk and gait is almost always the presenting symptom of A-T. And although this ataxia is slowly and steadily progressive, it may be compensated for—and masked—by the normal development of motor skills between the ages of two and five. Thus, until the progression of the disease becomes apparent, clinical diagnosis may be imprecise or inaccurate unless the patient has an affected sibling.

Once disease progression becomes apparent, **Friedreich ataxia** (a degenerative disease of the spinal cord) becomes the most common misdiagnosis. However, Friedreich ataxia usually has a later onset. In addition, the spinal signs involving posterior and lateral columns along the positive Romberg's sign (inability to maintain balance when the eyes are shut and feet are close together) distinguish this type of spinal ataxia from the cerebellar ataxia of A-T.

Distinguishing A-T from other disorders (differential diagnosis) is ultimately made on the basis of laboratory tests. The most consistent laboratory marker of A-T is an elevated level of serum alpha-fetoprotein (a protein that stimulates the production of antibodies) after the age of two years. Prenatal diagnosis is possible through the measurement of alpha-fetoprotein levels in amniotic fluid and the documentation of increased spontaneous chromosomal breakage of amniotic cell DNA. Diagnostic support may also be offered by a finding of low serum IgA, IgG and/or

IgE. However, these immune system findings vary from patient to patient and are not abnormal in all individuals.

The presence of spontaneous chromosome breaks and rearrangements in lymphocytes in vitro (test tube) and in cultured skin fibroblasts (cells from which connective tissue is made) is also an important laboratory marker of A-T. And finally, reduced survival of lymphocyte (cells present in the blood and lymphatic tissues) and fibroblast cultures, after exposure to ionizing radiation, will confirm a diagnosis of A-T, although this technique is performed in specialized laboratories and is not routinely available to physicians.

When the mutated A-T gene (ATM) has been identified by researchers, it is possible to confirm a diagnosis by screening the patient's DNA for mutations. However, in most cases the large size of the ATM gene and the large number of possible mutations in patients with A-T seriously limit the usefulness of mutation analysis as a diagnostic tool or method of carrier identification.

Treatment team

The child's primary care physician will likely be the first person to begin evaluating the child for the presence of ataxia-telangiectasia. Other consulting physicians may include a **neurologist** (to help manage the neurologic complications), a pulmonologist and/or infectious disease specialist (to help manage the lung infections), and a hematologist/oncologist (to help manage lymphoma or leukemia). Physical therapists, occupational therapists, and speech and language therapists should also be consulted.

Treatment

There is no specific treatment for A-T because **gene therapy** is not yet an available option. Also, the disease is usually not diagnosed until the individual has developed health problems. Treatment is therefore focused on the observed conditions, especially if neoplasms are present. However, radiation therapy must be minimized to avoid inducing further chromosomal damage and tumor growth.

Supportive therapy is available to reduce the symptoms of drooling, twitching, and ataxia, but individual responses to specific medications vary. The use of sunscreens to retard skin changes due to premature aging can be helpful. In addition, early use of pulmonary physiotherapy, physical therapy, and speech therapy is also important to minimize muscle contractures (shortening or tightening of muscles).

Although its use has not been formally tested, some researchers recommend the use of antioxidants (such as vitamin E) in patients with A-T. Antioxidants help to reduce oxidative damage to cells.

Prognosis

A-T is an incurable disease. Most children with A-T depend on wheelchairs by the age of ten because of a lack of muscle control. Children with A-T usually die from respiratory failure or cancer by their teens or early 20s. Although it is extremely rare, some patients with A-T may live into their 40s.

Resources

BOOKS

Vogelstein, Bert, and Kenneth E. Kinzler. *The Genetic Basis of Human Cancer.* New York: McGraw-Hill, 1998.

PERIODICALS

Brownlee, Shanna. "Guilty Gene." *U.S. News and World Report.* (July 3, 1995): 16.

Kum Kum, Khanna. "Cancer Risk and the ATM Gene." *Journal of the American Cancer Institute* 92, no. 6 (May 17, 2000): 795–802.

Stankovic, Tatjana, and Peter Weber, et al. "Inactivation of Ataxia Tlangiectasia Mutated Gene in B-cell Chronic Lymphocytic Leukaemia." *Lancet* 353 (January 2, 1999): 26–29.

Wang, Jean. "New Link in a Web of Human Genes." *Nature* 405, no. 6785 (May 25, 2000): 404–405.

ORGANIZATIONS

A-T Children's Project. 668 South Military Trail, Deerfield Beach, FL 33442. (800) 5-HELP-A-T. <http://www.atcp.org>.

A-T Medical Research Foundation. 5241 Round Meadow Rd., Hidden Hills, CA 91302. <http://pathnet.medsch.ucla.edu/people/faculty/gatti/gat-sign.htm>.

National Ataxia Foundation. 2600 Fernbrook Lane, Suite 119, Minneapolis, MN 55447. (763) 553-0020. Fax: (763) 553-0167. naf@ataxia.org. <http://www.ataxia.org>.

National Organization to Treat A-T. 4316 Ramsey Ave., Austin, TX 78756-3207. (877) TREAT-AT. <http://www.treat-at.org>.

Genevieve T. Slomski, PhD
Rosalyn Carson-DeWitt, MD

Ataxia

Definition

Ataxia, a medical term originated from the Greek language meaning "without order," refers to disturbances in the control of body posture, motor coordination, speech control, and eye movements. Several brain areas, including the **cerebellum** and the spinocerebellar tracts, substantia nigra, pons, and cerebral cortex control these functions. Injuries in one or more of these areas or in the spinal cord may lead to some form of ataxia. Birth trauma, medication toxicity, drug abuse, infections, tumors, degenerative disorders, head injury, **stroke**, or aneurysm, as well as hereditary neurological disorders also may cause ataxia. Many different types of inherited ataxias are presently known. Examples include **Machado-Joseph disease**, **ataxia-telangiectasia**, and **Friedreich ataxia**.

Description

Among children without inherited neurological disorders, important causes of ataxia are medication toxicity and post-infection inflammation of the brain. The later may happen as a complication of other viral diseases, such as measles, chicken pox, or influenza. While most people recover completely, some can have permanent neurological deficits.

Accidental ingestion of some drugs may cause ataxia, **seizures**, sensory neuropathies, or coma and death. The chronic administration of antihistamine medication and anticonvulsive drugs may cause ataxia in children, and should not be administered without instruction of a healthcare provider. Ingestion of seafood contaminated with high levels of methyl-mercury also causes ataxia, as does accidental ingestion of solvents. Some drugs used in treating certain types of tumors, such as those in colorectal cancer, are especially neurotoxic and can induce temporary, but usually reversible ataxia. Alcoholism, metabolic disorders, and vitamin deficiencies may also lead to ataxia.

Demographics

Non-hereditary ataxia is known as sporadic or acquired ataxia. Approximately 150,000 people in the United States alone are presently affected by ataxia, either the acquired or hereditary form. Friedreich ataxia is the most common inherited ataxia, occurring in 1 out of 50,000 population.

Causes and symptoms

Ataxia may be a consequence of brain trauma, stroke, or aneurysm. Chronic and progressive ataxia is generally associated with either brain tumors or with one of the several types of inherited neurodegenerative disorders affecting one or more brain areas involved in movement and coordination control. Other neurodegenerative disorders, such as **Parkinson's disease** and **multiple sclerosis**, may present cerebellar and/or gait ataxia as one of the clinical signs. Another cause of either chronic or progressive

Key Terms

Autosomal Relating to any chromosome besides the X and Y sex chromosomes. Human cells contain 22 pairs of autosomes and one pair of sex chromosomes.

Dystonia Painful involuntary muscle cramps or spasms.

Encephalitis Inflammation of the brain, usually caused by a virus. The inflammation may interfere with normal brain function and may cause seizures, sleepiness, confusion, personality changes, weakness in one or more parts of the body, and even coma.

Hypotonia Having reduced or diminished muscle tone or strength.

Microcephaly An abnormally small head.

Ophthalmoparesis Paralysis of one or more of the muscles of the eye.

ataxia is the congenital (present at birth) malformation of some structures of the **central nervous system**.

Hereditary ataxias are rare diseases, divided into two main categories according to the pattern of inheritance: autosomal dominant ataxias and autosomal recessive ataxias. Hereditary ataxias are additionally classified into types according to the affected structures and gene location of the defective chromosome. Autosomal dominant inheritance requires the presence of the mutation in only one of the two copies of a gene (maternal or paternal) to trigger the onset of the disease at some point in life, whereas autosomal recessive inheritance requires the inheritance of the mutation in both maternal and paternal genes. Other forms of hereditary ataxias are associated with metabolic disorders, such as the Maple Syrup Urine Disease, **Adrenoleukodystrophy**, and **Refsum disease**.

Autosomal Dominant Cerebellar Ataxias (ADCAs) are a group of ataxias divided into Types I, II, and III, according to the symptoms involved. Spinocerebellar ataxias (SCAs) Type 1, 2, 3, 4, 5, 6, 7, 10, and 11 belong to the ADCA group. Dominant Spinocerebellar Ataxias (SCAs) have several overlapping clinical signs, and a common feature to those belonging to the ADCA group is cerebellar ataxia, which manifests in difficulty walking and speaking. SCA1, 2, 3, and 4 may also involve partial paralysis of the eyes, slow eye movements, poor motor coordination, **dementia**, **peripheral neuropathy** (**pain**, numbness, or tingling sensation in the extremities of limbs and

hands), optic neuropathy, and deafness. All of these symptoms are not necessarily present. SCA2 and SCA7 may also result in retinal damage, whereas those with SCA10 exhibit loss of muscle control and generalized seizures without other symptoms.

Inherited ataxias

SCA1 is caused by an abnormal gene expression located on chromosome 6. Genes consist of several different protein sequences, each coding (providing instructions) for one specific amino acid. A sequence error or abnormal repetition of a nucleotide (a building block of DNA and RNA) in a given gene impairs adequate protein synthesis or results in a wrong protein. In SCA1, abnormal amounts of the nucleotide CAG lead to symptoms such as eye-muscle dysfunction and increased tendon reflexes. The onset of symptoms usually occurs around the age of 30, or during the fourth decade of life. Increased amounts of CAG occur in each new generation, resulting in symptoms that usually appear earlier in life. SCA1 is also known as Spinocerebellar Atrophy I, **Olivopontocerebellar atrophy** I, and Menzel Type ataxia.

SCA2 is associated with abnormal gene expression on chromosome 12. Major symptoms include Parkisonism (**tremors** and **spasticity**), **myoclonus** (muscle spasms), Pons atrophy, and slowing of eye movement. SCA2 is subdivided in Episodic Ataxia Type 1 or EA1 (also named Paroxysmal and Myokymia syndrome) and Episodic Ataxia Type 2 or EA2. The onset of EA1 occurs in general around the five to six years of age, with muscles quickly becoming flaccid or rigid, tremors in the head or in the limbs, blurred vision, and/or vertigo. The severity of these episodes varies, and episodes usually last for about ten minutes, although in some cases they may last for as long as six hours. These episodes are generally triggered by stressful situations, anxiety, and abrupt movements, and also occur spontaneously due to a metabolic dysfunction. EA2 symptoms usually begin during school years or adolescence. The crisis starts with vertigo and ataxia, and is often associated with involuntary eye movements. This condition is treatable with daily administration of acetozolamide. When untreated, crisis may occur a few times per month, lasting from 1 to 24 hours. However, most affected individuals will experience a decrease in intensity and number of crises as they mature.

SCA3 ataxia is also known as Machado-Joseph disease and the gene affected is on chromosome 14. **Dystonia** (spasticity or involuntary and repetitive movements) or gait ataxia is usually the initial symptom in children. Gait ataxia is characterized by unstable walk and standing, which slowly progresses with the appearance of some of the other symptoms, such as abnormal hand movements, involuntary eye movements (i.e., nystagmus), muscular wasting of hands, and loss of muscle tone in the face. SCA3 symptoms greatly vary among affected individuals as does the age of onset. Higher numbers of the CAG nucleotide repeats is associated with earlier onset and more severe symptoms. In addition, the number of CAG repeats tends to increase in each new generation, causing earlier onset and increased severity. There is no cure for Machado-Joseph disease.

SCA4 ataxia's genetic defect is located on chromosome 16, and results in major symptoms of cerebellar ataxia and sensory abnormalities. SCA4 may occur in two different forms, type I or type III. Both forms present symptoms 5–7 years earlier per generation. Symptoms usually become evident in type 1 from ages 19 to 59 years; from 45 to 72 years in type III. Difficulty walking, loss of muscle control, loss of fine-movement coordination of hands, and absence of tendon reflexes are the main symptoms observed in this progressive and crippling condition.

SCA5 ataxia is an extremely rare disorder linked to a defect on chromosome 11. Symptoms include mild ataxia and speech disorders. SCA5 ataxia was identified in one family descending from the paternal grandparents of Abraham Lincoln.

SCA6 ataxia is caused by a mutation on at chromosome 19. Clinical signs are varied, with some patients having limb and gait ataxia along with episodic headaches or nausea, and others having gait ataxia, speech difficulty, and abnormal eye movements. Initially, most patients only sense a momentary imbalance and mild vertigo when they make a quick movement or turn. After months or years, balance problems become more pronounced. The disease progresses over 20–30 years and eventually leads to severe disability. The age of onset ranges from 6 to 86 years. Periodic episodes of paralysis occur on one side of the body and last for days. Episodes may be triggered by head injuries and emotional stress. Some persons with SCA6 ataxia experience a more rapid progression and require wheelchair for support and mobility approximately 5 years after onset.

SCA7 ataxia is also known as olivopontocerebellar atrophy III, and results from a defect on chromosome 3. Symptoms of SCA7 ataxia occur earlier with each generation, and earlier onsets are associated with more severe symptoms. The onset of symptoms occurs in younger ages when the mutated copy of the gene is inherited from the paternal side. Ataxia, severe eye problems (retinal and macular degeneration), and early blue-yellow color blindness are typical clinical signs of the disease. Decreased vision occurs in over 80% of individuals with SCA7 ataxia, and almost one third of these persons eventually become blind. Hearing loss is also associated with SCA7 ataxia, and may slowly progress over decades. In more severe cases, usually associated with paternal inheritance of the defective gene, heart failure, liver disorders, muscle loss, and developmental delays can all occur. The degree of severity of SCA7 ataxia, the age of onset, and the rate of progression greatly vary both within and among families.

SCA10 ataxia is caused by an unstable protein repeat on chromosome 22. The main characteristics of SCA10 are generalized motor seizures, irregular eye movements, gait and limb ataxia, and speech difficulties. The age of onset ranges from 10 to 40 years. SCA11 ataxia is a very rare disease, mapped to chromosome 15. SCA11 progresses slowly over decades, with onset between adolescence and young adulthood. All individuals develop gait disorders, increased reflex action, eye disturbances and irregular movements, and speech difficulties.

Some inherited metabolic disorders cause progressive nerve degeneration with ataxia as one of its symptoms, as is the case with the group of diseases known as leukodistrophies. One famous example is Adrenoleukodystrophy (ALD), a rare autosomal dominant disease that causes progressive loss of the myelin sheath that covers the nerve fibers, along with progressive adrenal gland degeneration. ADL has two forms: the X-linked ADL (or X-ADL) and the non X-linked ADL (or ADL). The X-ADL is the more devastating form of the disease, with the onset of symptoms occurring between four and ten years of age. ADL (non X-linked) disease usually begins during adulthood, between 21 and 35 years of age and progresses slowly. In both forms of ADL, the loss of myelin by nerve fibers is due to an abnormal accumulation of saturated long fatty acid chains in the brain, because of a metabolic error involving a protein that transports fatty acids. The gene responsible for X-ADL was identified in 1993. The disorder was presented in the film *Lorenzo's Oil,* based on the story of Lorenzo Odone and his parents' quest to find a cure for the disease. Other X-ADL symptoms are seizures, speech and swallowing difficulties, gait and coordination ataxia, visual loss, progressive dementia, and loss of hearing that ends in deafness. As the mutation is inherited in the X chromosome, ADL is more severe in boys than in girls, because females have two X chromosomes, and the normal copy (or allele) of the affected gene will compensate for the dysfunctional one. Treatment with adrenal hormones can save the child's life and Lorenzo's oil, a mixture of oleic and euric acids, reduces or delays the onset of symptoms in carriers of the mutation without manifested symptoms. Oral intake of DHA (docosahexanoic acid) is prescribed for children and infants with X-ADL. As the neurological degeneration is progressive, prognosis is usually poor with patients dying within 10 years from the onset of symptoms.

Another metabolic disorder causing ataxia is the maple syrup urine disease or MSUD, an inherited disease caused by a metabolic disorder involving the breakdown of certain amino acids by enzymes. MSUD may occur in three different forms: neonatal convulsive crisis (classical form); progressive **mental retardation** (intermediary form); or recurrent ataxia and **encephalopathy** (intermittent form). The disease was first discovered in the Mennonite Community of Lancaster, PA, where MSUD affects 1 out of 176 individuals, although it is rare in other populations. MSUD onset may occur between five months of age and the second year of life. During crisis, the urine presents an odor similar to maple syrup and the blood shows high levels of branched amino acids and ketoacids. Between crises, such concentrations are normal both in urine and blood. Severe crises with high concentrations of ketoacids may be life threatening, requiring dialysis. The standard treatment is protein restriction in the diet; but some patients who respond to the administration of thiamine during crises may benefit from the intake of thiamine on a daily basis.

Refsum disease is caused by a dysfunction in the metabolism of lipids that leads to high concentrations of phytanic acid in tissues and blood plasma. Phytanic acid is a component of chlorophyll, obtained through the diet. The enzyme phytanic acid hydrolase normally helps eliminate phytanic acid from the body. The inheritance is autosomal recessive, and the onset may occur between the first and the third decade of life. One of the first symptoms is night blindness, but the pace of progression varies among affected individuals. Other main symptoms are irregularities in the retina of the eye, bone and skin changes, and the abnormal gait, speech patterns, and muscle movements associated with cerebellar ataxia. Treatment involves dietary restrictions and blood transfusion exchanges aimed at halting the progression of the disease and resolving symptoms.

Friedreich ataxia is the most common form of hereditary ataxia, affecting 1 out of 50,000 individuals. Friedreich ataxia is a progressive disorder affecting the arms and legs, with progressive weakness, loss of deep tendon reflexes, and sensory loss. Diabetes and/or some forms of heart disease may also be present in people with Friedreich ataxia. Onset of symptoms usually occurs before 20 years of age. As symptoms of Friedreich ataxia are similar to those found in other juvenile ataxias, diagnosis requires genetic testing to conform.

Diagnosis

Genetic forms of ataxia must be distinguished from the acquired (non-genetic) ataxias. Diagnosis of inherited ataxias begins with the analysis of the clinical family history, physical examination, and neuro-imaging techniques such as **CT** or **MRI** scans. As similar symptoms are described in many different types of ataxia, genetic screening is the most reliable tool for diagnosis. Genetic tests for

SCA1, SCA2, SCA3, SCA6, SCA7, SCA8, SCA10, SCA12, SCA17, episodic ataxia type 1, episodic ataxia type 2, DRPLA, Friedreich ataxia (FRDA), and Charlevoix-Saguenay ataxia are available.

Treatment team

Neurologists and geneticists are the front line treatment team for people with ataxia, along with specialized nurses and therapists. Both neurologists and geneticists usually participate in the diagnosis of the particular form of ataxia. Neurologists and other physicians provide treatment for the resulting symptoms. Genetic counseling and risk assessment of individuals without symptoms, but with a family history of the disease, is the task of the geneticist.

Treatment

Except for some acquired and reversible forms of ataxia as initially described, there is no cure or preventive treatment for the progressive forms of the disease, or for those ataxias resulting from accidental lesions of motor brain areas and/or the spinal cord. Antispasmodic and/or anticonvulsive medications, and analgesics for some painful neuropathies, may control and relieve the respective symptoms in some ataxia subtypes. Wheelchair, walking devices, and speech aids may be required in different stages of the progressive forms of ataxia.

Recovery and rehabilitation

Whether the ataxia is an acute condition that is likely to improve, or a progressive disease, therapy is aimed at maintaining the highest practical level of muscle function and coordination. Physical therapists provide strengthening exercises where muscle tissue integrity is likely to return or plateau, and range of motion exercises where muscle movement is limited. Gait training is also an important part of rehabilitation for persons with ataxia, as physical therapists help persons adapt to abnormal muscle movements, while safely maintaining posture and walking. As the disease progresses, the goals of therapy adapt to the person's changing abilities. Speech therapists help assess difficulties with speaking and eating, and offer strategies to compensate for them. Occupational therapists also make positional devices available to help maintain posture and comfort.

Clinical trials

Further basic research is needed before **clinical trials** become a possibility for this group of neurodegenerative diseases. Ongoing genetic and molecular research on the mechanisms involved in the disease will eventually yield enough data for the development of further diagnostic

Atomoxetine

markers and, hopefully, allow the design of experimental gene therapies to treat many of the inherited ataxias.

Prognosis

The prognosis for a person with ataxia depends upon the type and nature of the disease. Ataxia as a result of trauma or infection may be a temporary condition, or leave some degree of permanent disability. Hereditary ataxias are usually progressive syndromes, with symptoms becoming more disabling over varying periods of time.

Resources

BOOKS

Fenichel, Gerald M. *Clinical Pediatric Neurology: A Signs and Symptoms Approach,* 4th ed. Philadelphia: W. B. Saunders Company, 2001.

Hamilton, Patricia Birdsong. *A Balancing Act—Living with Spinal Cerebellar Ataxia.* Scripts Publishing, 1996.

Icon Health Publicaitons. *The Official Parent's Sourcebook on Friedreich's Ataxia: A Revised and Updated Directory for the Internet Age.* San Diego: Icon Group Int., 2002.

OTHER

Dystonia Medical Research Foundation. 1 East Wacker Drive, Suite 2430, Chicago, IL, 60601-1905. (312) 755-0198; Fax: (312) 803-0138. Dystonia@dystonia-foundation.org. <http://www.dystonia-foundation.org>.

International Joseph Disease Foundation, Inc. P.O. Box 994268, Redding, CA 96099-4268. (530) 246-4722. MJD@ijdf.net. <http://www.ijdf.net>.

National Ataxia Foundation (NAF). 2600 Fernbrook Lane, Suite 119, Minneapolis, MN 55447-4752. (763) 553-0020; Fax: (763) 553-0167. Naf@ataxia.org. <http://www.ataxia.org>.

National Institute of Neurological Disorders and Stroke. "Friedreich's Ataxia Fact Sheet." <http://www.ninds.nih.gov/health_and_medical/pubs/friedreich_ataxia.htm> (February 11, 2004).

National Institute of Neurological Disorders and Stroke. "Machado-Joseph Disease Fact Sheet." <http://www.ninds.nih.gov/health_and_medical/pubs/machado-joseph.htm> (February 11, 2004).

National Institute of Neurological Disorders and Stroke. "NINDS Ataxias and Cerebellar/Spinocerebellar Degeneration Information Page." <http://www.ninds.nih.gov/health_and_medical/disorders/ataxia.htm> (February 11, 2004).

National Institute of Neurological Disorders and Stroke. "Olivopontocerebellar Atrophy Information Page." <http://www.ninds.nih.gov/health_and_medical/disorders/opca_doc.htm> (February 11, 2004).

National Organization for Rare Disorders (NORD). P.O. Box 1968 (55 Kenosia Avenue), Danbury, CT 06813-1968. (203) 744-0100 or (800) 999-NORD (6673); Fax: (203) 798-2291. Orphan@rarediseases.org. <http://www.rarediseases.org>.

Worldwide Education & Awareness for Movement Disorders (WE MOVE). 204 West 84th Street, New York, NY. (212) 875-8312 or (800) 437-MOV2 (6682). Fax: (212) 875-8389. Wemove@wemove.org. <http://www.wemove.org>.

Sandra Galeotti

Atomoxetine

Definition

Atomoxetine is a prescription drug that is used to treat symptoms of impulsivity, inattentiveness, and hyperactivity, which are hallmark features of **attention deficit hyperactivity disorder** (ADHD). In the United States, atomoxetine is sold under the brand name Strattera.

Purpose

Atomoxetine is the only nonstimulant drug that has proven effective for alleviating all three of the hallmark features of ADHD. The drug is frequently used along with other psychological, educational, or social therapies in ADHD management.

Description

Atomoxetine is a selective norepinephrine inhibitor. By enhancing the activities of norepinephrine in certain areas of the brain, atomoxetine reduces chemical imbalances that are believed to contribute to ADHD symptoms.

Although the exact way that atomoxetine works in the brain is not well understood, the drug is believed to correct chemical imbalances between dopamine and norepinephrine. These two naturally occurring chemicals are commonly referred to as **neurotransmitters**. Their function is to regulate transmission of impulses from one cell to another. Atomoxetine may restore normal attention spans, correct impulsiveness, and calm hyperactivity by counteracting the neurotransmission abnormalities that cause symptoms of ADHD.

Before atomoxetine was approved by the FDA in 2002, all the drugs previously approved for ADHD were stimulants. Stimulants such as amphetamines have the potential to be abused and are sometimes sold illegally. As a result, strict rules are in place to monitor dispensing of prescription stimulants, and patients must obtain new prescriptions from their doctors each month. Because atomoxetine is not a stimulant, it is easy for patients to obtain refills for their medication and fewer physician visits are required. Many patients prefer atomoxetine over stimulants for the convenience the drug offers.

Key Terms

Asthma A condition characterized by spasms of the lung's airways that causes breathing difficulties.

Attention deficit hyperactivity disorder (ADHD) A psychiatric disorder characterized by inattention, hyperactivity, and impulsiveness.

Dopamine A precursor to norepinephrine that is also a neurotransmitter in some regions of the brain.

Neurotransmitter A chemical in the brain that transmits messages between neurons or nerve cells.

Norepinephrine A hormone that controls blood pressure and heart rate. It is also a chemical found in the brain that is thought to play a role in ADHD.

Stimulant Any chemical or drug that has excitatory actions in the central nervous system.

Recommended dosage

In adults or children weighing more than 150 lb (70 kg), the initial dose of atomoxetine is typically 40 mg taken once a day. The dosage can be increased after three days to 80 mg. This can be given either as a single dose in the morning or divided evenly in the morning and late afternoon. If a higher dosage is needed, the dose can be increased after 2–4 weeks to a maximum of 100 mg per day. The dosage must be lowered in individuals that have liver disease, since atomoxetine is broken down by the liver.

Atomoxetine should be initiated at a total daily dose of 1 mg/lb (0.5 mg/kg) in children that weigh less than 150 lb (70 kg). After at least three days, the dose can be increased to 2.4 mg/lb (1.2 mg/kg). Children may either take the entire dose in the morning or may split the dose evenly in the morning and late afternoon.

Improvements in ADHD symptoms may be noticed within 24 hours of first taking atomoxetine, although 3–4 weeks may be required for full benefits to be seen.

Precautions

Atomoxetine may cause changes in heart rate or blood pressure. As a result, this drug may not be appropriate for patients that have high blood pressure, rapid heartbeats, heart disease, or a history of strokes. Patients should have their blood pressure and pulse rate monitored when they start therapy and any time their dosage is increased.

Because of the possibility of severe eye damage, patients with a history of narrow angle glaucoma should not take atomoxetine. Since the liver breaks down the drug, patients with a history of liver disease should only be prescribed a low dose.

Patients who take dietary supplements, herbal remedies, or drugs that are available without a prescription should consult with their doctor prior to taking atomoxetine. It is best to avoid atomoxetine while pregnant and breastfeeding since its effects have not been studied during pregnancy and it is not known whether the drug is excreted in breast milk.

The drug may cause **fatigue**, **dizziness**, and headaches. Patients with a history of low blood pressure may be especially susceptible to these effects. It is best to avoid driving or operating heavy machinery until it is clear whether the drug will alter reaction time or impair judgment.

Side effects

The most common side effects associated with atomoxetine in children and teens are upset stomach, nausea, vomiting, decreased appetite, dizziness, tiredness, and mood swings.

In adults, the effects of constipation, dry mouth, nausea, decreased appetite, dizziness, sleeping difficulties, sexual side effects, difficulty urinating, and menstrual cramps are commonly attributed to atomoxetine.

If patients experience swelling or hives, they should not continue taking atomoxetine since serious allergic reactions may occur.

Interactions

Atomoxetine should not be used with certain types of antidepressants known as monoamine oxidase (MAO) inhibitors since this combination may cause blood pressure and heart rates to increase sharply. Muscle stiffness, muscle spasms, and even death can occur as a result of this drug interaction.

Atomoxetine may also increase heart rate and blood pressure when combined with albuterol, a drug that is commonly used to treat asthma.

Resources

BOOKS

Eli Lilly and Company Staff. *Strattera Package Insert.* Indianapolis, IN: Eli Lilly and Company, 2003.

Eli Lilly and Company Staff. *Strattera Information for Patients or Their Parents or Caregivers Insert.* Indianapolis, IN: Eli Lilly and Company, 2003.

Kelly Karpa, PhD, RPh

Attention deficit hyperactivity disorder

Definition

Attention deficit hyperactivity disorder (ADHD) is not a clinically definable illness or disease. Rather, as of December 2003, ADHD is a diagnosis that is made for children and adults who display certain behaviors over an extended period of time. The most common of these behavioral criteria are inattention, hyperactivity, and marked impulsiveness.

In the American description, there are three types of ADHD, depending on which diagnostic criteria have been met. These are: ADHD that is characterized by inattention, ADHD characterized by impulsive behavior, and ADHD that has both behaviors.

The European description of ADHD places the disorder in a subgroup of what are termed hyperkinetic disorders (hallmarks are inattention and over-activity).

Description

ADHD is also known as attention deficit disorder (ADD), attention deficit disorder with and without hyperactivity, hyperkinesis, hyperkinetic impulse disorder, hyperactive syndrome, hyperkinetic reaction of childhood, minimal brain damage, minimal brain dysfunction, and undifferentiated deficit disorder.

The term attention deficit is inexact, as the disorder is not thought to involve a lack of attention. Rather, there appears to be difficulty in regulating attention, so that attention is simultaneously given to many stimuli. The result is an unfocused reaction to the world. As well, people with ADHD can have difficulty in disregarding stimuli that are not relevant to the present task. They can also pay so much attention to one stimulus that they cannot absorb another stimulus that is more relevant at that particular time.

For many people with ADHD, life is a never-ending shift from one activity to another. Focus cannot be kept on any one topic long enough for a detailed assessment. The constant processing of information can also be distracting, making it difficult for an ADHD individual to direct his or her attention to someone who is talking to him or her. Personally, this struggle for focus can cause great chaos that can be disruptive and diminish self-esteem.

The neurological manifestations of ADHD are disturbances of what are known as executive functions. Specifically, the six executive functions that are affected include:

- the ability to organize thinking
- the ability to shift thought patterns

Key Terms

Dopamine A neurotransmitter made in the brain that is involved in many brain activities, including movement and emotion.

Executive functions A set of cognitive abilities that control and regulate other abilities and behaviors. Necessary for goal-directed behavior, they include the ability to initiate and stop actions, to monitor and change behavior as needed, and to plan future behavior when faced with novel tasks and situations.

Frontal cortex The part of the human brain associated with aggressiveness and impulse control. Abnormalities in the frontal cortex are associated with an increased risk of suicide.

Psychometric The development, administration, and interpretation of tests to measure mental or psychological abilities. Psychometric tests convert an individual's psychological traits and attributes into a numerical estimation or evaluation.

- short-term memory
- the ability to distinguish between emotional and logical responses
- the ability to make a reasoned decision
- the ability to set a goal and plan how to approach that goal

About half or more of those people with ADHD meet criteria set out by the American Psychiatric Association (*Diagnostic and Statistical Manual of Mental Disorders* [DSM-IV]) for at least one of the following other illnesses:

- learning disorder
- restless leg syndrome
- **depression**
- anxiety disorder
- antisocial behavior
- substance abuse
- obsessive-compulsive behavior

Demographics

ADHD is a common childhood disorder. It is estimated to affect 3–7% of all children in the United States, representing up to two million children. The percentage may in fact be even higher, with up to 15% of boys in grades one through five being afflicted. On average, at least one child in each public and private classroom in the United States has ADHD. In countries such as Canada, New Zealand, and Germany, the prevalence rates are estimated to be 5–10% of the population.

The traditional view of ADHD is that boys are affected more often than girls. Community-based samples have found an incidence rate in boys that is double that of girls. In fact, statistics gathered from patient populations have reported male-to-female ratios of up to 4:1. However, as the understanding of ADHD has grown since the early 1990s and as the symptoms have been better recognized, the actual number of females who are affected by ADHD may be more similar to males than previously thought.

Causes and symptoms

The cause of ADHD is unknown. However, evidence is consistent with a biological cause rather than an environmental cause (e.g., home life). Not all children from dysfunctional homes or families have ADHD.

For many years, it was thought that ADHD developed following a physical blow to the head, or from an early childhood infection, leading to the terms "minimum brain damage" and "minimum brain dysfunction." However, these definitions apply to only a very small number of people diagnosed with ADHD, and so have been rejected as the main cause.

Another once-favored theory was that eating refined sugar or chemical additives in food produced hyperactivity and inattention. While sugar can produce changes in behavior, evidence does not support this proposed association. Indeed, in 1982, the results presented at a conference sponsored by the U.S. National Institutes of Health conclusively demonstrated that a sugar- and additive-restricted diet only benefits about 5% of children with ADHD, mostly young children and those with food allergies.

The biological roots of ADHD may involve certain areas of the brain, specifically the frontal cortex and nearby regions. One explanation is that the executive functions are controlled by the frontal lobes of the brain. **Magnetic resonance imaging (MRI)** examination of subjects who are exposed to a sensory cue has identified decreased activity of regions of the brain that are involved in tasks that require attention. Another MRI-based study published in November 2003 also implicates a region of the brain that controls impulsive behavior. Finally, a study conducted by the U.S. National Institute of Mental Health (NIMH) documented that the brains of children and adolescents with ADHD are 3–4% smaller than those of their ADHD-free counterparts. Additionally, the decreased

brain size is not due to the use of drugs in ADHD treatment, the researchers concluded in a paper published in October 2002.

ADHD symptoms can sometimes be relieved by the use of stimulants that increase a chemical called dopamine. This chemical functions in the transmission of impulses from one neuron to another. Too little dopamine can produce decreased motivation and alertness. These observations led to the popular "dopamine hypothesis" for ADHD, which proposed that ADHD results from the inadequate supply of dopamine in the **central nervous system**.

The observations that ADHD runs in families (10–35% of children with ADHD have a direct relative with the disorder) point to an underlying genetic origin. Studies with twins have shown that the occurrence of ADHD in one twin is more likely to be mirrored in an identical twin (who has the same genetic make-up) than in a fraternal twin (whose genetic make-up is similar but not identical).

The genetic studies have implicated the binding, transport, and enzymatic conversion of dopamine. Two genes in particular have been implicated: a dopamine receptor (DRD) gene on chromosome 11 and the dopamine transporter gene (DAT1) on chromosome 5.

There may be environmental factors that influence the development of ADHD. Complications during pregnancy and birth, excessive use of marijuana, cocaine, and/or alcohol (especially by pregnant women), ingestion of lead-based paint, family or marital tension, and poverty have been associated with ADHD in some people. However, many other ADHD sufferers do not display any of these associations.

Heavy use of alcohol by a pregnant woman can lead to malformation of developing nerve cells in the fetus, which can result in a baby of lower than normal birth weight with impaired intelligence. This condition, called fetal alcohol syndrome, can also be evident as ADHD-like hyperactivity, inattention, and impulsive behavior.

Diagnosis

ADHD is sometimes difficult to diagnose. Unlike the flu or a limb fracture, ADHD lacks symptoms that can be detected in a physical examination or via a chemical test. Rather, the diagnosis of ADHD relies on the presence of a number of characteristic behaviors over an extended period of time. Often the specialist will observe the child during high-stimuli periods such as a birthday party and during quieter periods of focused concentration. Diagnosis uses the DSM-IV criteria, originally published in 1994, in combination with an interview and assessment of daily activity by a qualified clinician. (As of December 2003, revised DSM criteria are pending. These revisions will reflect the increased awareness of the greater-than-perceived prevalence of ADHD in girls and women.)

The benchmarks for either inattention or for hyperactivity/impulsive behavior must be met. These benchmarks typically occur by the age of seven and are not exclusive to one particular social setting such as school. These benchmarks must have been present for an extended period of time, at least six months or more. There are nine separate criteria for each category. For diagnosis, six of the nine criteria must be met. Examples of diagnostic signs of inattention include difficulty in maintaining concentration on a task, failure to follow instructions, difficulty in organizing approaches to tasks, repeated misplacement of tools necessary for tasks, and tendency to become easily distracted. Examples of hyperactivity or impulsive behavior include fidgeting with hands or feet, restlessness, difficulty in being able to play quietly, excessive talk, and tendency to verbally or physically interrupt.

Because ADHD can be associated with the use of certain medications or supplements, diagnosis involves screening for the past or present use of medications such as anticonvulsant or antihypertensive agents, and caffeine-containing drugs.

Diagnosis of ADHD can also be complicated by the simultaneous presence of another illness. Diagnosis involves screening for bipolar disorder, depression, eating disorder, learning disability, panic disorder (including agoraphobia), sleep disorder, substance abuse, or Tourette's syndrome. Almost half of all children (mostly boys) with ADHD display what has been termed "oppositional defiant behavior." These children tend to be stubborn, temperamental, belligerent, and can lash out at others over a minor provocation. Without intervention, such children could progress to more serious difficulties such as destruction of property, theft, arson, and unsafe driving.

Other, nonclinical information such as legal infractions (arrests, tickets, vehicle accidents), school reports, and interviews with family members can be valuable, as ADHD can be perceived as antisocial, erratic, or uncommon behavior.

A complete physical examination is recommended as part of the diagnosis. The examination offers the clinician an opportunity to observe the behavior of the person. More specific tests can also be performed. Children can be assessed using the Conner's Parent and Teacher Rating Scale. Adolescent and adult assessment can utilize the Brown Attention Deficit Disorder Scale. Impulsive and inattentive behavior can be assessed using the Conner's Continuous Performance Test (CPT) or the Integrated Visual and Auditory CPT. Girls can be specifically assessed using the Nadeau/Quinn/Littman ADHD Self-Rating Scale.

Treatment team

The treatment team involves behavioral and medical specialists. Concerning behavior, teachers play a very important role. Their daily observation of the child and the use of standard evaluation tests can help in the diagnosis and treatment of ADHD. More specialized consultants within the school system, such as psychometrists, may also be available. Outside of the school setting, psychologists, **social workers**, and family therapists can also be involved in treatment.

The use of medications involves physicians, nurses, and pharmacists.

Treatment

Behavior treatment can consist of the monitoring of school performance and the use of standard evaluation tests. For older children, adolescents, and adults, support groups can be valuable. As well, ADHD patients can learn behavioral techniques that are useful in self-monitoring their behavior and making the appropriate modifications (such as a time out). Behavior treatment is useful in combination with drug therapy or as a stand-alone treatment in those cases in which the use of medication is not tolerated or is not preferred.

Medical treatment can consist of the use of drugs such as Ritalin that are intended to modify over-exuberant behavior, or other drugs that have differing targets of activity. Psychostimulant medications like Ritalin, Cylert, and Dexedrine increase brain activity by increasing the brain concentration of chemicals such as dopamine, which are involved in the transmission of impulses or by stimulating the receptors to which the chemicals bind. Psychostimulant medications can sometimes disrupt sleep, depress appetite, cause stomachaches and **headaches**, and trigger feelings of anger and anxiousness, particularly in people afflicted with psychiatric illnesses such as bipolar disorder or depression. For many people, the side effects are mild and can become even milder with long-term use of the drugs.

Antidepressant medications such as imipramine act by slowing down the absorption of chemicals that function in the transmission of impulses. Central alpha agonists are particularly used in the treatment of hyperactivity. By restricting the presence of neurotransmitter chemicals in the gap between neurons, drugs such as clonidine and guanfacine restrict the flow of information from one neuron to the next. There have been four reported cases of sudden death in people taking clonidine in combination with the drug methylphenidate (Ritalin), and reports of nonfatal heart disturbances in people taking clonidine alone.

Finally, medications known as selective norepinephrine reuptake inhibitors restrict the production of norepinephrine between neurons, which inhibits the sudden and often hyperactive "fight or flight" response.

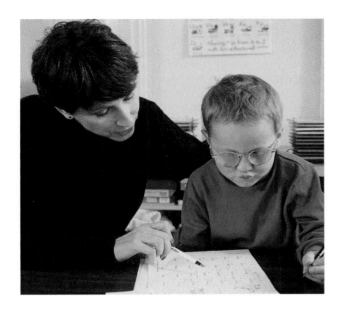

A special education teacher helps a child with ADHD do his math assignment. (© Photo Reasearchers. Reproduced by permission.)

Recovery and rehabilitation

After a patient has been stabilized, typically using medication, follow-up visits to the physician are recommended every few months for the first year. Then, follow-ups every three or four months may be sufficient. The use of medications may continue for months or years.

Recovery and rehabilitation are not terms that apply to ADHD. Rather, a child with ADHD can be assisted to an optimum functionality. Assistance can take the form of special education in the case of those who prove too hyperactive to function in a normal classroom; the child may be seated in a quieter area of the class; or by using a system of rules and rewards for appropriate behavior. Children and adults can also learn strategies to maximize concentration (such as list making) and strategies to monitor and control their behavior.

Clinical trials

Beginning in 1996, the U.S. National Institute of Mental Health (NIMH) and the Department of Education began a clinical trial that included nearly 600 elementary school children ages seven to nine. The study, which compared the effects of medication alone, behavior management alone, or a combination of the two, found the combination to produce the most marked improvement in concentration and attention. Additionally, the involvement of teachers and other school personnel was more beneficial than if the child was examined only a few times a year by their family physician.

As of January 2004, a number of clinical studies were recruiting patients, including:

- Behavioral and functional neuroimaging study of inhibitory motor control. The basis of the inability to control behavior in ADHD was assessed using behavioral tests and the technique of **magnetic resonance imaging (MRI)**.

- Brain imaging in children with ADHD. MRI was used to compare the connections between brain regions in children with and without ADHD.

- Brain imaging of childhood onset psychiatric disorders, endocrine disorders, and healthy children. MRI was used to investigate the structure and activity in the brains of healthy people and those with childhood onset psychiatric disorders, including ADHD.

- Genetic analysis of ADHD. Blood samples from a child with ADHD and his or her immediate family members were collected and analyzed to determine the genetic differences between ADHD and non-ADHD family members.

- Biological markers in ADHD. People with ADHD, their family members, and a control group of healthy people who had previously undergone magnetic resonance examination were assessed using psychiatric interviews, neuropsychological tests, and genetic analysis.

- Study of ADHD using transcranial magnetic stimulation. The technique, in which a magnetic signal is used to stimulate a region of the brain that controls several muscles, was used to investigate whether ADHD patients have a delayed maturation of areas of their nervous system responsible for such activity. Detectable differences could be useful in diagnosing ADHD.

- Clonidine in ADHD Children. The trial evaluated the benefits and side effects of two drugs (clonidine and methylphenidate) used individually or together to treat childhood ADHD.

- Nutrient intake in children with ADHD. The study determined if children with ADHD have a different eating pattern, such as intake of less food or a craving for carbohydrates, than children without ADHD. The information from the study would be used in probing the origins of ADHD and in devising treatment strategies.

- Preventing behavior problems in children with ADHD. The study was designed to gauge the effectiveness of a number of treatment combinations in preventing behavior that is characteristic of ADHD in children.

- Psychosocial treatment for ADHD Type I. The study focused on ADHD that is characterized by inattention. The aim of the study was to develop effective treatment strategies for Type I ADHD.

- Treatment of adolescents with comorbid alcohol use and ADHD. The effectiveness of a drug (bupropion) that is designed to be released at a constant rate over time was evaluated in the treatment of ADHD adolescents (14–18 years) who are also alcohol abusers.

- Behavioral treatment, drug treatment, and combined treatment for ADHD. The effectiveness of the three treatment approaches was compared, and the interactions between different levels of the behavioral and drug treatments were examined.

- Attention deficit disorder and exposure to lead. The effect of past exposure to lead was studied in children with ADHD.

Prognosis

The outlook for a patient with ADHD can be excellent, if the treatment regimen is followed and other existing conditions and disabilities have been identified and are treated. Methylphenidate, the major psychostimulant used in the treatment of ADHD, has been prescribed since the 1960s. The experience gained over this time has established the drug as being one of the safest pharmaceuticals for children. Indeed, intervention can be beneficial. Researchers from the Massachusetts General Hospital reported in 1999 that drug treatment of children diagnosed with ADHD could dramatically reduce the future risk of substance abuse.

Special concerns

The diagnosis of ADHD continues to be controversial. While some children do benefit from the use of medicines, other children who behave differently than is the norm may be needlessly medicated. The inattention, hyperactivity, and impulsive behavior that are the hallmarks of ADHD can be produced by many other conditions. The death of a parent, the discomfort of a chronic ear infection, and living in a dysfunctional household are all situations that can cause a child to become hyperactive, uncooperative, and distracted.

Evidence since the 1960s has led to the consensus that the medications used to treat ADHD, particularly methylphenidate (Ritalin), pose no long-term hazards. However, research published in December 2003 documented that rats exposed to the drug tended to avoid rewarding stimuli and instead became more anxious. More research on the effects of long-term drug treatment in ADHD is scheduled.

Resources

BOOKS

National Institutes of Health. *Attention Deficit Hyperactivity Disorder.* NIH Publication No. 96–3572, 1996.

PERIODICALS

Bolaños, Carlos A., Michel Barrot, Oliver Berton, Deanna Wallace-Black, and Eric J. Nestler. "Methylphenidate Treatment During Pre- and Periadolescence Alters Behavioral Responses to Emotional Stimuli at Adulthood." *Biological Psychiatry* (December 2003).

Castellanos, F. Xavier, Patti P. Lee, Wendy Sharp, et al. "Developmental Trajectories of Brain Volume Abnormalities in Children and Adolescents With Attention-Deficit/Hyperactivity Disorder." *Journal of the American Medical Association* (October 9, 2002) 288: 1740–1748.

Rowland, Andrew S., David M. Umbach, Lil Stallone, A. Jack Naftel, E. Michael Bohlig, and Dale P. Sandler. "Prevalence of Medication Treatment for Attention Deficit-Hyperactivity Disorder among Elementary School Children in Johnston County, North Carolina." *American Journal of Public Health* (February 2002) 92: 231–234.

Sowell, Elizabeth R., Paul M. Thompson, Suzanne E. Welcome, Amy L. Henkenius, Arthur W. Toga, and Bradley S. Peterson. "Cortical Abnormalities in Children and Adolescents with Attention-Deficit Hyperactivity Disorder." *Lancet* (November 2003) 362: 1699–1702.

OTHER

National Institute of Neurological Disorders and Stroke. *NINDS Attention Deficit-Hyperactivity Disorder Information Page.* December 9, 2003 (February 18, 2004). <http://www.ninds.nih.gov/health_and_medical/disorders/adhd.htm>.

ORGANIZATIONS

Attention Deficit Disorder Association (ADDA). PO Box 543, Pottstown, PA 19464. (484) 945-2101; Fax: (610) 970-7520. mail@add.org. <http://www.add.org>.

Children and Adults with Attention-Deficit/Hyperactivity Disorder (CHADD). 8181 Professional Place, Suite 150, Bethesda, MD 20785. (301) 306-7070 or (800) 233-4050; Fax: (301) 306-7090. <http://www.chadd.org>.

National Institute of Mental Health (NIMH). 6001 Executive Boulevard, Bethesda, MD 20892-9663. (301) 443-4513 or (866) 615-6464; Fax: (301) 443-4279. nimhinfor@nih.gov. <http://www.nimh.nih.gov>.

National Institute of Neurological Disorders and Stroke. 6001 Executive Boulevard, Bethesda, MD 20892-9663. (301) 446-5751 or (800) 352-9424. <http://www.ninds.nih.gov>.

Brian Douglas Hoyle

Autism

Definition

Autism is a behavior disorder, characterized by an impairment in social communication, social interaction, and social imagination. Those with autism often have a restricted range of interests and display repetitive behaviors

Key Terms

Cytogenetics The branch of biology that combines the study of genetic inheritance with the study of cell structure.

Fragile X syndrome A genetic condition related to the X chromosome that affects mental, physical, and sensory development. It is the most common form of inherited mental retardation.

Phenylketonuria A rare, inherited, metabolic disorder in which the enzyme necessary to break down and use phenylalanine, an amino acid necessary for normal growth and development, is lacking. As a result, phenylalanine builds up in the body causing mental retardation and other neurological problems.

Schizophrenia A severe mental illness in which a person has difficulty distinguishing what is real from

what is not real. It is often characterized by hallucinations, delusions, and withdrawal from people and social activities.

Thalidomide A mild sedative that is teratogenic, causing limb, neurologic, and other birth defects in infants exposed during pregnancy. Women used thalidomide (early in pregnancy) in Europe and in other countries between 1957 and 1961. It is still available in many places, including the United States, for specific medical uses (leprosy, AIDS, cancer).

Tuberous sclerosis A genetic condition that affects many organ systems including the brain, skin, heart, eyes, and lungs. Benign (non-cancerous) growths or tumors called hamartomas form in various parts of the body, disrupting their normal function.

and mannerisms, along with altered reactions to the everyday environment.

Description

In 1943, the American physician Leo Kanner published his seminal paper, in which he described 11 children who were socially isolated, with "autistic disturbances of affective contact," impaired communication, and behavioral inflexibility. He coined the term "infantile autism" and discussed the causes in terms of biological processes, although at that time, most scientific attention was focused on analytical theories of the disorder. Kanner's paper did not initially receive much scientific credit, and children with autistic symptoms continued to be incorrectly diagnosed with childhood **schizophrenia**. His choice of the term "autism" may have created some confusion, because the word was first used to describe a mental state of fantastical, self-centered thought processes, similar to the symptoms of schizophrenia.

During the development of the disorder, the first year of life is usually marked with no clear discriminating features. Between two and three years of age, children show impairment in language development, especially comprehension; unusual language usage; poor response to name calling; deficient non-verbal communication; minimal recognition or responsiveness to other people's happiness or distress; and limited variety of imaginative play or pretence, and especially social imagination.

During school age, children's abnormalities in language development (including muteness or the use of odd or inappropriate words), their social withdrawal, inability

to join in with the play of other children, or inappropriate attempts at joint play often alert teachers and others to the possibility of an autistic type disorder. The manifestations of autism can also change with time during childhood, depending on other developmental impairments, personality, and the addition of medical or mental health problems.

Demographics

Autism is a disorder that affects predominantly males (four times as many males as females have autism). According to studies, autism is increasing in the pediatric population. In 1966, 4–5 babies per 10,000 births developed autism, while in 2003, two studies showed that between 14–39 babies per 10,000 develop the disorder. Although there is no question that more clinical cases are being detected, the increase in prevalence of autism is in dispute as diagnostic practices have changed over the years and this heightened awareness has changed the evaluation of previously unrecognized cases.

Causes and symptoms

Although autism is behaviorally defined, it is now well recognized to be the endpoint of several organic causes. These include prenatal problems such as rubella (measles) infection, untreated metabolic disorders, and anticonvulsant medication taken during pregnancy, as well as postnatal infections such as encephalitis. A specific medical cause is found in only a minority of people with autism (6–10%, depending on the study). **Epilepsy** occurs more commonly than usual in patients with this disorder

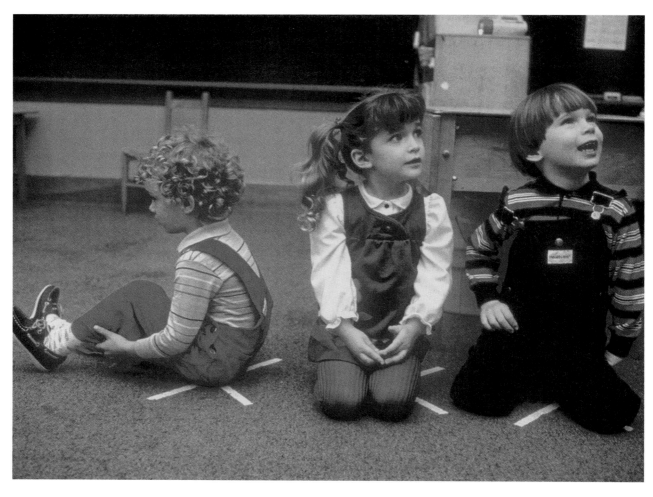

Three autistic children in a classroom. (© Andy Levin/Photo Researchers, Inc. Reproduced by permission.)

and was one of the early indications that this was a neurobiological problem and not one caused by parental behavior or the environment.

In most people with autism, genetic factors play a key role. Multiple genes are likely to be involved, and studies have identified possible candidate genes on chromosomes 2, 7, 16, and 19. Autism has been associated with some genetic abnormalities, especially on chromosome 15, and it is also found associated with the "fragile X syndrome." Despite the fact autism is now agreed to be a neurobiological disorder, results from structural brain scans have not shown consistent features that point to a diagnosis of autism.

Symptoms of autism usually appear during the first three years of childhood and continue throughout life. Some common symptoms are:

• absence or impairment of imaginative and social play

• impaired ability to make friends with peers

• impaired ability to initiate or sustain a conversation with others

• stereotyped, repetitive, or unusual use of language

• restricted patterns of interests that are abnormal in intensity or focus

• apparently inflexible adherence to specific routines or rituals

• preoccupation with parts of objects

Children with some symptoms of autism, but not a sufficient number to be diagnosed with the classical form of the disorder, often receive the diagnosis of pervasive developmental disorder, not otherwise specified (PDD-NOS). People with autistic behavior, but also have well-developed language skills, are often diagnosed with Asperger syndrome. Children who appear normal in their first several years, then lose skills and begin showing autistic behavior, may be diagnosed with childhood disintegrative disorder (CDD). Girls with **Rett syndrome**, a sex-linked genetic disorder characterized by inadequate brain growth, **seizures**, and other neurological problems, may also show autistic behavior. PDD-NOS, Asperger syndrome, CDD, and Rett syndrome are referred to as autism spectrum disorders.

Diagnosis

Currently, there are no objective medical tests for the diagnosis of autism and no reproducible genetic or biological markers for the disorder. The diagnosis is made with a multidisciplinary approach involving a developmental pediatrician, psychologist, speech and language professional, audiologist, and special educator.

Using a standardized rating scale, the specialist closely observes and evaluates the child's language and social behavior. A structured interview is also used to elicit information from parents about the child's behavior and early development. Reviewing family videotapes, photos, and baby albums may help parents recall when each behavior first occurred and when the child reached certain developmental milestones. The specialists may also test for certain genetic and neurological problems.

Treatment team

The treatment of childhood autism traditionally falls within the competence of the psychiatrist and the psychologist and involves the application of various methods of individual therapy. Speech therapists can work with children to help them develop social and language skills because children learn most effectively and rapidly when very young.

Moreover, occupational therapists and physiotherapists are important professionals in the development and life quality improvement for patients and parents. The treatment involves a therapist's work with the child and with the caregivers, who work with the child at home under the therapist's direction. Basic medical assistance is provided by the pediatrician and other physicians.

Treatment

No definitive treatment regimes have thus far been developed for this serious disturbance and therapy is generally merely supportive. Some attempts have been made to support such therapy with psychiatry and psychology, as well as high doses of vitamin B6, vitamin E, and magnesium. Various psychoactive drugs have also been tried, as well as a group of medications called H2 blockers. A "hugging machine" has been built to support therapy by the holding method. This device makes it possible for children with autism to overcome their fear of touch (tactile stimuli).

An alternative treatment approach has been attempted using secretin, which is a hormone secreted by cells in the digestive tract to help control digestion. The history of the application of secretin in the treatment of childhood autism dates back to 1996, when, by coincidence, a significant improvement in mental condition was noticed in a child with autism who had received secretin for diagnostic purposes. When it was administrated, one of the chief symptoms of autism, the avoidance of eye contact, was 75% reduced. Some additional children with autism also showed limited improvement after treatment with secretin. On January 5, 2004, results of a clinical trial revealed that the hormone was of little value in improving the socialization of young children with autism. Nevertheless, many parents and physicians continue to advocate development of the drug and further study.

Recovery and rehabilitation

A wide variety of long-term interventions have been advocated for children with autism. These include applied behavioral analysis, use of pictures for expressive communication (as in the picture exchange communication system), and intensive **exercise** programs. Therapists working in schools now recognize the holistic learning needs of the child, including personal and emotional growth as well as opportunities to broaden their experiences, regardless of whether measurable developmental progress is made.

Clinical trials

As of early 2004, there were numerous open **clinical trials** for autism, including:

- drug treatment for autism at the National Institute of Mental Health (NIMH)
- synthetic human secretin in children with autism, sponsored by Repligen Corporation
- improving attention skills of children with autism at the National Institute of Child Health and Human Development (NICHD) in collaboration with the National Institute of Mental Health (NIMH)
- study of fluoxetine in adults with autistic disorder
- a controlled study of olanzapine in children with autism, sponsored by the FDA Office of Orphan Products Development
- randomized study of fluoxetine in children and adolescents with autism, sponsored by the FDA Office of Orphan Products Development and Mount Sinai Medical Center
- valproate response in aggressive autistic adolescents at the NICHD and the NIMH

• brain imaging of childhood onset psychiatric disorders, endocrine disorders, and healthy children at the NIMH

Prognosis

Among individuals suffering with autism, 75% have a poor outcome and 25% show significant improvement. Acquisition of language before the age of six years old, IQ levels above 50, and having a special skill, such as expertise in computers, predict good outcome. For people with severe autism, independent living and social functioning are unlikely. For those with higher functioning autism, the jobs acquired are often below their education level. The social interactions of most adults with autism are limited or modified.

Special concerns

Most scientists concur that autism has a strong biological basis, with evidence continuing to accumulate for an underlying genetic cause that results in abnormal brain development. Future genetic and brain-imaging studies will undoubtedly contribute to a greater understanding of the disorder's etiology and pathophysiology. The combination of continually evolving methodological and technological advances will, hopefully, bring science closer to the goal of better and earlier intervention in autism.

Resources

BOOKS

Edelson, Stephen M., and Bernard Rimland. *Treating Autism: Parent Stories of Hope and Success.* San Diego, CA: Autism Research Institute, 2003.

Harris, Sandra L., and Beth A. Glasberg. *Siblings of Children With Autism: A Guide for Families (Topics in Autism).* Bethesda, MD: Woodbine House, 2003.

Seroussi, Karyn. *Unraveling the Mystery of Autism and Pervasive Developmental Disorder: A Mother's Story of Research and Recovery.* New York, NY: Broadway, 2002.

PERIODICALS

Baird, G., H. Cass, and V. Slonims. "Diagnosis of Autism." *BMJM* 327 (August 2003): 448–493.

Kamińska, B., et al. "Use of Secretin in the Treatment of Childhood Autism." *Med Sci Monit* 8 (January 2002): RA22–26.

Nicolson, R., and P. Szatmari. "Genetic and Neurodevelopmental Influences in Autistic Disorder." *Canadian Journal of Psychiatry* 8 (September 2003): 526–537.

Tidmarsh, L., and F. Volkmar. "Diagnosis and Epidemiology of Autism Spectrum Disorders." *The Canadian Journal of Psychiatry* 8 (September 2003): 517–525.

Torres, A. "Is Fever Suppression Involved in the Etiology of Autism and Neurodevelopmental Disorders?" *BMC Pediatric* (September 2003): 3–9.

OTHER

Autism Society of America. January 3, 2004 (February 18, 2004). <http://www.autism-society.org>.

National Institute of Mental Health. January 3, 2004 (February 18, 2004). <http://www.nimh.nih.gov>.

ORGANIZATIONS

Autism Society of America. 7910 Woodmont Ave. Suite 300, Bethesda, MD 20814-3067. (301) 657-0881; Fax: (301) 657-0869. info@autism-society.org. <http://www.autism-society.org/>.

Cure Autism Now (CAN) Foundation. 5455 Wilshire Blvd. Suite 715, Los Angeles, CA 90036-4234. (323) 549-0500 or (888) 828-8476; Fax: (323) 549-0547. info@cureautismnow.org. <http://www.cureautismnow.org/>.

National Institute of Child Health and Human Development (NICHD). 9000 Rockville Pike Bldg. 31, Rm. 2A32, Bethesda, MD 20892-2425. (301) 496-5133. NICHDClearinghouse@mail.nih.gov. <http://www.nichd.nih.gov/>.

National Institute of Mental Health (NIMH). 6001 Executive Boulevard, Room 8184, MSC 9663, Bethesda, MD 20892-9663. (301) 443-4513; Fax: (301) 443-4279. nimhinfo@nih.gov. <http://www.nimh.nih.gov/>.

Francisco de Paula Careta
Greiciane Gaburro Paneto
Iuri Drumond Louro

Autonomic dysfunction

Definition

Dysfunction of the autonomic nervous system (ANS) is known as dysautonomia. The autonomic nervous system regulates unconscious body functions, including heart rate, blood pressure, temperature regulation, gastrointestinal secretion, and metabolic and endocrine responses to stress such as the "fight or flight" syndrome. As regulating these functions involves various and multiple organ systems, dysfunctions of the autonomic nervous systems encompass various and multiple disorders.

Description

The autonomic nervous system consists of three subsystems: the sympathetic nervous system, the parasympathetic nervous system and the enteric nervous system. The ANS regulates the activities of cardiac muscle, smooth muscle, endocrine glands, and exocrine glands. The autonomic nervous system functions involuntarily (reflexively) in an automatic manner without conscious control.

In contrast to the somatic nervous system that always acts to excite muscles groups, the autonomic nervous systems can act to excite or inhibit innervated tissue. The ANS achieves this ability to excite or inhibit activity via a dual innervation of target tissues and organs. Most target organs and tissues are innervated by neural fibers from both the parasympathetic and sympathetic systems. The systems can act to stimulate organs and tissues in opposite ways (antagonistic). For example, parasympathetic stimulation acts to decrease heart rate. In contrast, sympathetic stimulation results in increased heart rate. The systems can also act in concert to stimulate activity. The autonomic nervous system achieves this control via two divisions: the sympathetic nervous system and the parasympathetic nervous system. Dysfunctions of the autonomic nervous system are recognized by the symptoms that result from failure of the sympathetic or parasympathetic components of the ANS.

Primary dysautonomias include **multiple system atrophy** (MSA) and familial dysautonomia. The dysfunction can be extensive and manifest as a general autonomic failure or can be confined to a more localized reflex dysfunction.

With multiple system atrophy, a generalized autonomic failure, male patients experience urinary retention or incontinence and impotence (an inability to achieve or maintain a penile erection). Both males and females experience **ataxia** (lack of muscle coordination) and a dramatic decline in blood pressure when they attempt to stand (**orthostatic hypotension**). Symptoms similar to **Parkinson's disease** may develop, such as slow movement, **tremors**, and stiff muscles. **Visual disturbances**, sleep disturbances, and decreased sweating may also occur.

Persons with autonomic dysfunction who do not exhibit the classical symptoms of orthostatic hypotension may exhibit a less dramatic dysfunction termed orthostatic intolerance. These patients experience a milder fall in blood pressure when attempting to stand. However, because the patients have an increased heart rate when standing, they are described as having postural tachycardia syndrome (POTS).

Although not as prevalent in the general population as hypertension, orthostatic intolerance is the second most common disorder of blood pressure regulation and is the most prevalent autonomic dysfunction. Orthostatic hypotension and orthostatic intolerance can result in a wide array of disabilities. Common orthostatic intolerance syndromes include: hyperadrenergic orthostatic hypotension (partial dysautonomia); orthostatic tachycardia syndrome (sympathicotonic orthostatic hypotension); postural orthostatic tachycardia syndrome (mitral valve prolapse syndrome); postural tachycardia syndrome (soldier's heart);

Key Terms

Dysarthria   A group of speech disorders caused by disturbances in the strength or coordination of the muscles of the speech mechanism as a result of damage to the brain or nerves.

Dysautonomia   A disorder or dysfunction of the autonomic nervous system.

Orthostatic hypotension   A sudden fall in blood pressure that occurs when standing.

Parasympathetic nervous system   A branch of the autonomic nervous system that tends to induce secretion, increase the tone and contraction of smooth muscle, and cause dilation of blood vessels.

Stridor   A high-pitched sound made when breathing caused by the narrowing of the airway.

Sympathetic nervous system   A branch of the autonomic nervous system that regulates involuntary reactions to stress such as increased heart and breathing rates, blood vessel contraction, and reduction in digestive secretions.

hyperadrenergic postural hypotension (vasoregulatory asthenia); sympathotonic orthostatic hypotension (neurocirculatory asthenia); hyperdynamic beta-adrenergic state (irritable heart syndrome); and idiopathic hypovolemia (orthostatic anemia).

Demographics

Milder forms of autonomic dysfunction such as orthostatic intolerance affect an estimated 500,000 people in the United States. Orthostatic intolerance more frequently affects women; female-to-male ratio is at least 4:1. It is most common in people less than 35 years of age. More severe forms of dysautonomia such as multiple system atrophy often occur later in life (average age of onset 60 years) and affect men four times as often as women.

Causes and symptoms

Symptoms of the autonomic dysfunction of orthostatic intolerance include lightheadedness, palpitations, weakness, and tremors when attempting to assume an upright posture. Less frequently, patients experience visual disturbances, throbbing headaches, and often complain of **fatigue** and poor concentration. Some patients report **fainting** when attempting to stand.

The cause of lightheadedness, fainting, and similar symptoms is a lack of adequate blood pressure in the cerebral circulatory system.

In addition to orthostatic hypotension and Parkinson-type symptoms, persons with multiple systems atrophy may have difficulty articulating speech, **sleep apnea** and snoring, **pain** in the back of the neck, and fatigue. Eventually, cognitive (mental reasoning) ability declines in about 20% of cases. Multiple systems atrophy occurs sporadically and the cause is unknown.

Diagnosis

Diagnosis of orthostatic intolerance is made when a patient experiences a decrease of blood pressure (not exceeding 20/10 mmHg) when attempting to stand and a heart rate increase of less than 30 beats per minute.

Diagnosis of other types of dysautonomia is difficult, as the disorders are varied and mimic other diseases of the nervous system. As Parkinsonism is the most frequent motor deficit seen in multiple systems atrophy, it is often misdiagnosed as Parkinson's disease. **Magnetic resonance imaging (MRI)** of the brain can sometimes detect abnormalities of striatum, **cerebellum**, and brainstem associated with multiple systems atrophy. But in up to 20% of MSA patients, MRI of the brain is normal. A test with the drug clonidine has also been used to differentiate Parkinson's disease from multiple systems atrophy, as certain hormone levels in the blood will increase in persons with Parkinson's disease after clonidine administration, but not in persons with multiple systems atrophy. Symptoms such as severe **dysarthria** (difficulty articulating speech) and stridor (noisy inspiration) alert the physician to the possibility of multiple systems atrophy, as they occur in the disorder, but are rare in Parkinson's disease.

Treatment team

Caring for a person with a disorder of the autonomic nervous system requires a network of health professionals, community resources, and friends or family members. A **neurologist** usually makes the diagnosis, and the neurologist and primary physician coordinate ongoing treatment and symptom relief. Physical, occupational, speech, and respiratory therapists provide specialized care, as do nurses. Social service and mental health consultants organize support services.

Treatment

At present there is no cure for severe autonomic dysfunction. Treatment is centered on the remediation of symptoms, patient support, and the treatment of underlying diseases and disorders in cases of secondary autonomic dysfunction. In many cases, cure or an improvement in the underlying disease or disorder improves the patient prognosis with regard to remediation of autonomic dysfunction symptoms

With regard to orthostatic hypotension, drug treatment includes fludrocortisone, ephedrine, or midodrine. Medications are accompanied by postural relief such as elevation of the bed at the head and by dietary modifications to provide some relief for the symptoms of **dizziness** and tunnel vision.

In multiple systems atrophy, anti-Parkinson medications such as Sinemet often help with some of the symptoms of muscle rigidity and tremor, and create an overall feeling of well-being. Medications used in the treatment of orthostatic hypotension tend to not perform as well in this group; although they elevate the blood pressure while standing, they decrease the blood pressure while reclining.

Recovery and rehabilitation

Recovery from some dysautonomias can be complicated by secondary conditions such as alcoholism, diabetes, or Parkinson's disease. Some conditions improve with treatment of the underlying disease, while only halting of the progression of symptoms is accomplished in others. Some mild dysautonomias stabilize and, with treatment, cause few limitations to daily activities.

Overall, as there are no cures for most severe or progressive dysautonomias, the emphasis is instead placed upon maintaining mobility and function for as long as possible. Aids for walking and reaching, positioning devices, and strategies for maintaining posture, balance, and blood pressure while rising can be provided by physical and occupational therapists. Speech and nutritional therapists can devise diets and safe strategies for eating, and recommend tube feedings if necessary.

Clinical trials

As of mid-2004, the Mount Sinai Medical Center in New York was recruiting participants for a study related to a new drug for the treatment of multiple systems atrophy. Persons interested in participating in the study (Droxidopa in Treating Patients With Neurogenic Hypotension) should contact the study recruiting coordinator Horacio Kaufmann at telephone: (212) 241-7315. Additional trials for the study and treatment of multiple systems atrophy and other dysautonomias can be found at the National Institutes of Health website for **clinical trials**: <http://www.clinicaltrials.gov>.

Prognosis

The prognosis for persons suffering autonomic dysfunction is variable and depends on specific dysfunction and on the severity of the dysfunction. Autonomic dysfunctions can present as acute and reversible syndromes, or can present in more chronic and progressive forms. Persons with orthostatic intolerance can usually maintain a normal lifespan and active lifestyle with treatment and minimal coping measures, while persons with multiple systems atrophy usually have a lifespan of about 5–7 years after diagnosis.

Resources

BOOKS

Goldstein, David S., and Linda J. Smith. *The NDRF Handbook for Patients with Dysautonomias.* Malden, MA: Blackwell Futura Media, 2002.

OTHER

"Disorders of the Autonomic Nervous System." *National Dysautonomia Research Foundation.* May 16, 2004 (May 22, 2004). <http://www.ndrf.org/autonomic_disorders.htm>.

"NINDS Dysautonomia Information Page." *National Institute of Neurological Disorders and Stroke.* May 16, 2004 (May 22, 2004). <http://www.ninds.nih.gov/health_and_medical/disorders/dysauto_doc.htm>.

ORGANIZATIONS

Dysautonomia Foundation. 633 Third Avenue, 12th Floor, New York, NY 10017-6706. (212) 949-6644; Fax: (212) 682-7625. info@familialdysautonomia.org. <http://www.familialdysautonomia.org>.

Familial Dysautonomia Hope Foundation, Inc. (FD Hope). 1170 Green Knolls Drive, Buffalo Grove, IL 60089. (828) 466-1678. info@fdhope.org. <http://www.fdhope.org>.

National Dysautonomia Research Foundation. 1407 West 4th Street, Red Wing, MN 55066-2108. (651) 267-0525; Fax: (651) 267-0524. ndrf@ndrf.org. <http://www.ndrf.org>.

National Organization for Rare Disorders (NORD). P.O. Box 1968 (55 Kenosia Avenue), Danbury, CT 06813-1968. (203) 744-0100 or (800) 999-NORD; Fax: (203) 798-2291. orphan@rarediseases.org. <http://www.rarediseases.org>.

Shy-Drager/Multiple System Atrophy Support Group, Inc. 2004 Howard Lane, Austin, TX 78728. (866) 737-4999 or (800) 999-NORD; Fax: (512) 251-3315. Don.Summers@shy-drager.com. <http://www.shy-drager.com>.

Paul Arthur

Autonomic dysfunction

B

Back pain

Definition

Back **pain** may occur in the upper, middle, or lower back; it is most often experienced in the lower back. It may originate from the bones and ligaments forming the spine, the muscles and tendons supporting the back, the nerves that exit the spinal column, or even the internal organs.

Description

Back pain can range from mild, annoying discomfort to excruciating agony. Depending on how long it lasts, it can be described as acute or chronic. Acute back pain comes on suddenly but lasts only briefly, and is often intense. While chronic back pain is typically not as severe as acute back pain, it persists for a longer period and may recur frequently. The duration of acute back pain is a few days to a few weeks, with improvement during that time, whereas chronic back pain lasts for more than three months and often gets progressively worse.

The back is composed of bones, muscles, ligaments, tendons, and other tissues that make up the posterior, or back half, of the trunk extending from the neck to the pelvis. Running through and supporting the back is the spinal column, which forms a cage-like structure enclosing the spinal cord. Nerve signals directing movement travel from the brain to the limbs, while nerve signals transmitting pain and other sensations travel from the limbs to the brain. All nerve signals pass through the spinal cord. If the individual vertebrae stacked together to form the spinal column slide out of place, which is referred to as spondylolisthesis, pain may result as the bones rub against each other or as nerves entering the spinal cord are compressed.

Demographics

Lower back pain affects approximately four out of five adults at least once during their lifetime, often interfering with work, recreation, or household chores and

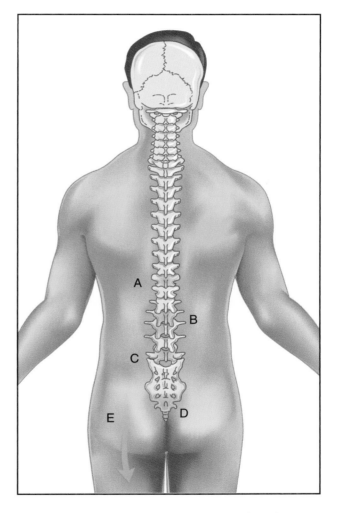

Sites of low back pain. Pain anywhere along the spine (A) can be caused by osteoarthritis. Pain along one or the other side of the spine may be (B) a kidney infection. Trauma to back muscles, joints, or disks (C) causes low back pain. Damage to the coccyx (D) can occur during a fall. Sciatica (E) can cause pain to run from the back and buttocks area down a leg. *(Illustration by Electronic Illustrators Group.)*

other routine activities. It is one of the most common conditions for which Americans seek medical attention, and it is second only to **headache** as the most common neurological condition in the United States. According to the National Institute for Occupational Safety and Health, back pain related to work is one of the most-often diagnosed occupational disorders.

Health care dollars spent on the diagnosis and treatment of low back pain are estimated to be at least $50 billion annually, with additional costs related to disability and delay in return to work.

Back pain strikes equal numbers of men and women, and it typically begins between the fourth and sixth decades. The likelihood of disc disease and spinal degeneration, both prominent causes of back pain, increases with age. A sedentary lifestyle increases vulnerability to back pain, especially when coupled with obesity or sporadic bursts of overexertion.

Because of their greater flexibility and lack of age-related degeneration, children and teenagers are much less prone than adults to develop medically significant back pain.

Causes and symptoms

The spinal column is composed of 24–25 movable bones, or vertebrae, held together by ligaments and separated by intervertebral discs that act as shock absorbers. Although this structure allows great flexibility and range of movement, it also affords many opportunities for injury. Compounding the potential for injury is that the human spine bears weight in the upright position and must therefore counteract gravity. Stresses on the muscles and ligaments that support the spine can cause acute pain or chronic injury.

With normal aging, the fluid cushioning the intervertebral discs tends to dry up, making them more brittle and less protective of the vertebrae. The normal wear and tear of daily activities can eventually erode the vertebral edges, undermining stability and putting pressure on nerves that enter and exit the spinal column to control movement and sensation of the arms and legs.

Heavy physical labor accelerates these processes, but lack of physical activity allows the muscles to lose tone, offering less protection to the spine as it twists and turns. Consequently, regardless of activity levels, back pain becomes more common with increasing age. Bone density and muscle flexibility and strength also tend to decrease with age, further increasing the chance of painful injury.

Obesity increases both the weight that the spine must support and the pressure on the discs, thereby elevating the risk of back pain and injury. Physically demanding sports can also damage the back, especially in the case of "weekend warriors" who overexert themselves on occasion while generally maintaining a low level of physical fitness. Even simple movements like bending over may trigger muscle spasms in individuals with chronic pain.

Injuries unrelated to activity may include motor vehicle accidents or falls that subject the spine and its supporting structures to direct impact or unusual torque. These injuries and those related to overexertion may result in painful sprain, strain, or spasm in the back muscles or ligaments.

Excessive strain or compression of the spine may cause **disc herniation**, in which the disc bulges or even ruptures. The bulging disc or its fragments may be displaced outward, putting pressure on nerve roots entering or exiting the spine and thereby causing pain. Most disc herniations occur in the lumbar or lower part of the spinal column, especially between the fourth and fifth lumbar vertebrae (L4 and L5, respectively) and between the fifth lumbar and first sacral vertebrae (L5 and S1, respectively).

Activities involving hyperextension of the back, such as gymnastics, may result in spondylosis, or disruption of the joint between adjacent vertebrae. A more extreme form of spondylosis is spondylolisthesis, or slippage of one vertebra relative to its neighbor. Impact or excessive mechanical force to the spine may cause spinal fracture. After repeated back injuries, buildup of scar tissue eventually weakens the back and can increase the risk of more serious injury.

Diseases of the bone, such as endocrine conditions or metastatic cancer spreading from the lung, breast, prostate, or other primary site, may cause fractures or other painful conditions in the spinal column. Fractures occurring without apparent traumatic injury, especially in a debilitated or chronically ill person, may be a warning of cancer or other underlying bone disease such as osteoporosis. Osteoporosis is a metabolic bone disease in which progressive decreases in bone strength and density makes the bones brittle, porous, and easily broken.

Other diseases causing back pain include arthritis, which erodes the joints, myopathies and inflammatory conditions, which involve the muscles, and neuropathy, which affects the nerves. Back pain is common in diabetes because this disease may be complicated by **myopathy** (though this is rare) or neuropathy, both of which create gait disturbances that, in turn, cause back pain. In women, fibromyalgia is a fairly common chronic condition associated with musculoskeletal pain, **fatigue**, morning stiffness, and other nonspecific symptoms.

Conditions affecting the spine include spinal degeneration from disc wear and tear, which can narrow the spinal canal and cause back stiffness and pain, especially

Key Terms

Cordotomy Surgery to relieve pain by destroying bundles of nerve fibers on one or both sides of the spinal cord.

Discectomy Surgery to relieve pressure on a nerve root caused by a bulging disc or bone spur.

Discography A test in which dye is injected into a disc space thought to be causing back pain, allowing the surgeon to confirm that an operation on that disc will be likely to relieve pain.

Dorsal root entry zone operation (DREZ) Surgery to relieve pain by severing spinal neurons.

Endorphins Naturally occurring pain relievers produced by the brain.

Fibromyalgia A fairly common chronic condition associated with musculoskeletal pain, fatigue, morning stiffness, and other nonspecific symptoms.

Foraminotomy Surgery to enlarge the bony hole, or foramen, where a nerve root enters or exits the spinal canal.

Intervertebral discs Gelatinous structures separating the spinal vertebrae and acting as shock absorbers.

Kyphosis (dowager's hump) A pronounced rounding of the normal forward curve of the upper back.

Lordosis (swayback) An exaggeration of the normal backward arch in the lower back.

Myelography A test in which dye is injected into the spinal canal and the patient is then tilted in different directions on a special table, allowing dye to outline the spinal cord and nerve roots and to show areas of compression.

Rhizotomy Surgery to relieve pain by cutting the nerve root near its point of entry to the spinal cord.

Sciatica A common form of nerve pain related to compression of fibers from one or more of the lower spinal nerve roots, characterized by burning low back pain radiating to the buttock and back of the leg to below the knee or even to the foot.

Scoliosis An asymmetric curvature of the spine to one side.

Spinal degeneration Wear and tear on the intervertebral discs, which can narrow the spinal canal and cause back stiffness and pain.

Spinal fusion A surgical procedure that stabilizes the spine and prevents painful movements, but with resulting loss of flexibility.

Spinal laminectomy (spinal decompression) Surgical removal of a piece of the bony roof of the spinal canal known as the lamina to increase the size of the spinal canal and reduce pressure on the spinal cord and nerve roots.

Spinal stenosis A narrowing of the spinal canal which is present from birth.

Spondylitis Inflammation of the spinal joints, characterized by chronic back pain and stiffness.

Spondylolisthesis A more extreme form of spondylosis, with slippage of one vertebra relative to its neighbor.

Spondylosis Disruption of the joint between adjacent vertebrae.

Thermography A test using infrared sensing devices to measure differences in temperature in body regions thought to be the source of pain.

Transcutaneous electrical nerve stimulation (TENS) A battery-powered device generating weak electrical impulses applied along the course of nerves to block pain signals traveling to the brain.

Traction Spinal stretching using weights applied to the spine, once thought to decrease pressure on the nerve roots but now seldom used.

upon awakening or after prolonged walking or standing. Spinal stenosis is a narrowing of the spinal canal, a condition that is present from birth. Both conditions increase the likelihood of back pain from disc disease. Spondylitis, or inflammation of the spinal joints, is characterized by chronic back pain and stiffness.

Anatomical abnormalities of the skeleton subject the vertebrae and supporting structures to increased strain, and often manifest as back pain. Scoliosis is an asymmetric curvature of the spine to one side. Kyphosis, or dowager's hump, refers to a pronounced rounding of the normal forward curve of the upper back, whereas lordosis (swayback) is an exaggeration of the normal backward arch in the lower back.

Lifestyle and general medical factors contributing to back pain include smoking, pregnancy, inherited disorders affecting the spine or limbs, poor posture, inappropriate posture for the activity being performed, and poor sleeping position. Psychological stress is a common but often unrecognized source of back pain. Injuries, arthritis, or other conditions affecting the feet, ankles, knees, or hips may result in abnormal walking patterns that exacerbate or cause back pain.

Apart from all the musculoskeletal structures and nerves, the internal organs can also be a source of pain felt in the back. Kidney stones, urinary tract infections, blood clots, stomach ulcers, and diseases of the pancreas can all be experienced as back pain. Fever or other bodily symptoms suggesting infection or involvement of internal organs should prompt a medical evaluation.

The discomfort of back pain may range from the dull ache of muscle soreness, to shooting or stabbing pain if a muscle acutely goes into spasm, to a toothache-like sensation along the course of a spinal nerve. Surprisingly, the severity of the pain may not be correlated with the severity of injury. In uncomplicated back strain, acute muscle spasm can cause agonizing back pain that prevents the person from standing up straight. On the other hand, a massive disc herniation may not produce pain or any other symptoms.

Depending on its source, back pain is usually aggravated by certain movements, although prolonged sitting or standing may also make it worse. Associated symptoms may include limited flexibility and range of motion, difficulty straightening up, or weakness in the arms or legs.

When back pain is caused by **nerve compression**, pain may travel, or radiate, from the back to peripheral areas, usually following the course of the nerve as it supplies the arm or leg. There may be numbness, sensitivity to touch, or "pins and needles" (tingling sensations) along the same distribution. Pain originating from an internal organ may also radiate to an area of the back supplied by the same nerve root as that organ.

Sciatica is a common form of nerve pain related to compression of fibers from one or more of the lower spinal nerve roots, characterized by burning low back pain radiating to the buttock and back of the leg to below the knee or even to the foot. In more severe cases, there may be numbness or tingling in the same regions, as well as weakness. Typically, sciatic pain is caused by a herniated or ruptured disc, but it may also rarely be caused by a tumor or cyst.

Worrisome symptoms associated with back pain that warrant immediate medical attention include loss of control of bowel or bladder, change in bowel and bladder habits, or profound or progressive weakness or sensory loss. Any of these may signal compression of one or more nerve roots, or even of the spinal cord itself, which may result in irreversible paralysis if not treated promptly.

Low back pain is unusual in children, unless caused by motor vehicle accidents and other traumatic injuries. One notable exception is back strain and muscle fatigue caused by carrying an overloaded backpack. According to the U.S. Consumer Product Safety Commission, more than 13,260 injuries caused by backpacks were treated at medical offices, clinics, and emergency rooms in 2000.

Persistent back pain in a young child should raise suspicions of a serious problem such as a tumor or infection of the spine, meriting further evaluation and treatment. Teenagers indulging in extreme sports may subject themselves to compression fractures, stress injuries, spondylosis, and rarely, disc herniation.

Diagnosis

According to the *Clinical Practice Guideline for Understanding Acute Low Back Problems*, published in 1994 by the Department of Health and Human Services Agency for Health Care Policy and Research, the precise cause of back pain is seldom determined, despite the advent of sophisticated diagnostic techniques. Although x rays and other imaging tests typically fail to disclose the reason for back pain, they may be important in ruling out serious conditions demanding specific treatment.

As with most other neurologic conditions, the cornerstone of diagnosis is the history, or analysis, of the patient's complaints, and the physical and neurologic examination. Additional diagnostic testing is needed in only about 1% of individuals with acute back pain. If symptoms do not improve in four to six weeks, further testing may be indicated.

The history focuses on a description of the pain and other symptoms, the circumstances in which the pain first occurred, and conditions that tend to make it better or worse, as well as any injuries and a general medical history. The physical examination should begin with a general medical examination and should include finding areas of back tenderness, testing spinal range of motion and flexibility, and measuring strength, sensation, and reflexes in the legs.

Specialized maneuvers include the straight leg-raising test. While the patient is lying flat on the back, pain in the low back or leg caused by raising a straight leg off the examining table suggests sciatica.

If there is suspicion of a serious cause for back pain, imaging or other tests may be done right away. Reasons for immediate testing include sudden back pain after a fall, suggesting fracture; back pain at night, suggesting a tumor, fever, or other signs of back infection; or loss of bowel or bladder control or progressive leg weakness, suggesting compression of the spinal cord or nerve roots.

Cancer patients who develop back pain should have testing to determine if cancer has spread to the spine, which can lead to spinal cord compression and permanent paralysis if not treated promptly. Children with back pain unrelated to backpacks or sports injuries should also be tested sooner rather than later.

X rays are typically performed first as they are readily available and do a good job of visualizing bony structures, fractures, and deformities. However, they do not usually detect injuries of the muscles or other soft tissues. If x rays are negative and the doctor suspects a tumor, infection, or fracture not easily seen on x ray, bone scans may be helpful. In this test, injecting a low-dose radioactive medication into a vein allows the doctor to study bone structure and function using a special scanning camera.

Because **magnetic resonance imaging (MRI)** provides sharp, clear images of bones, discs, nerves, and soft tissues, it is the best test to show disc herniation and nerve compression. This test uses magnetic signals in water rather than x rays, and therefore poses no risk to the patient other than that associated with a contrast dye, which is not needed in most cases. Although the MRI may show disc bulging, this does not necessarily mean that the disc bulge is causing the back pain or that it needs to be treated. In about half of people without back pain, the MRI shows disc bulges. On the other hand, a bulging disc directly compressing a spinal nerve is more significant and may be causing pain and associated symptoms.

Computed tomography (CT) scan of the spine uses a computer to reconstruct cross-sectional x-ray images. A **CT scan** is good at visualizing bone problems like spinal stenosis, but it is not as sensitive as the MRI in diagnosing soft tissue injuries, and it has the added disadvantage of considerable x-ray exposure.

Because they are painful and carry a small risk of injury to the patient, certain tests are only done in patients who are about to have surgery so that the surgeon can plan the operation better. In myelography, dye is injected into the spinal canal and the patient is then tilted in different directions on a special table, allowing dye to outline the spinal cord and nerve roots and to show areas of compression. In discography, dye is injected into a disc space thought to be causing the pain, allowing the surgeon to confirm that an operation on that disc will likely relieve pain.

If there is evidence of nerve root compression on CT, MRI, history, or physical examination, **electromyography** (EMG), nerve conduction velocity (NCV), and evoked potential (EP) studies help determine the motor and sensory function of the involved nerve(s). These tests are also useful in diagnosing myopathy or neuropathy. During the EMG, fine needles inserted into the muscle determine how rapidly and forcefully the muscle contracts when stimulated. By applying a series of weak electrical shocks over areas supplied by a particular nerve, the NCV helps determine sensory function. Both tests are helpful in pinpointing specific patterns of nerve involvement.

In special cases, thermography and ultrasound imaging may provide additional information. Thermography uses infrared sensing devices to measure differences in temperature in body regions thought to be the source of pain. Ultrasound uses high-frequency sound waves to show tears in ligaments, muscles, tendons, and other soft tissues.

Treatment team

Internists and general practitioners are often the first to see patients with back pain. Depending on the cause and severity of pain, neurologists, orthopedists, physical medicine specialists, pain management specialists, psychologists, psychiatrists, and other medical specialists may offer evaluation and treatment. Physical therapists, chiropractors, acupuncturists, vocational rehabilitation counselors, and radiology technicians may all become involved in management.

Treatment

Most cases of acute musculoskeletal back pain respond in a few days or weeks to limited rest, combined with appropriate **exercise** and education on correct movement patterns to avoid further injury. However, many cases resolve on their own without any treatment during a similar time period.

Although acute back pain was previously treated with complete, prolonged bed rest, this is no longer recommended because it leads to muscular deconditioning and loss of bone calcium, which can make the situation worse. Other complications of bed rest may include **depression** and blood clots in the legs. In 1996, a Finnish study showed that an exercise program to improve back mobility, coupled with resumption of normal activities and avoidance of rest during the day, allowed better back range of motion by the seventh day than did a program of strict bed rest.

Current wisdom is to limit bed rest for low back pain to one day, beginning immediately after injury or acute onset of pain, followed by resuming activities as soon as possible. While resting or sleeping, the best positions are on one side with a pillow between the knees, or on the back with a pillow under the knees.

Exercise speeds up recovery, reduces the risk of future back injuries, and releases the body's natural pain relievers known as endorphins. Doctors may suggest specific back exercises; aerobic exercises that improve conditioning without undue stress on the back include walking, stationary bicycle, and swimming or water aerobics. Any exercise program should be started slowly and built up gradually. Discomfort during exercise is not unusual, especially when starting out. However, patients experiencing pain of moderate or greater severity or lasting more than 15 minutes during exercise should stop exercising and inform their physician.

Local application of an ice pack or heat to the painful area, or use of muscle balms containing menthol, eucalyptus, or camphor may reduce inflammation, feel soothing, and facilitate exercise. Cold packs are recommended within the first 48 hours after back pain begins, with use of hot packs subsequently.

For back pain following an injury, physical therapy may offer strengthening programs and education in posture, movement patterns, and lifting techniques that protect the back to avoid further injury. Exercises designed to increase flexibility, tone, and strength help to replace fluid into dehydrated discs. Ultrasound, moist heat application, hydrotherapy involving pools or spas, or massage of painful areas may relieve pain and spasm, increase local circulation, and improve mobility.

Transcutaneous electrical nerve stimulation (TENS) uses a battery-powered device generating weak electrical impulses applied along the course of affected nerves to block pain signals traveling to the brain. This technique may also stimulate production of endorphins, or naturally occurring pain relievers, by the brain.

Although traction, or spinal stretching using weights applied to the spine, was once thought to decrease pressure on the nerve roots, this treatment has not been proven to be effective and is now seldom used.

Nonsteroidal anti-inflammatory drugs (NSAIDs) may relieve pain by reducing inflammation. These include naproxen (Aleve) and ibuprofen (Nuprin, Motrin IB, and Advil). Because these drugs may cause gastrointestinal bleeding, patients with ulcers, bleeding disorders, or other gastrointestinal conditions should avoid them. Other side effects may include kidney damage, and salt and fluid retention leading to high blood pressure.

COX-2 inhibitors are a more recently developed class of prescription drugs that reduce pain and inflammation with fewer gastrointestinal effects than the NSAIDs. These include celecoxib (Celebrex) and rofecoxib (Vioxx).

For severe back pain caused by inflammation of nerve roots or other structures, steroids may be injected directly into the inflamed area, often combined with local anesthetic. These can be epidural injections targeting the nerve roots, or trigger point injections into tender areas of muscle.

Other medications that may be indicated include analgesics or pain relievers such as aspirin or acetaminophen (Tylenol), muscle relaxants, antidepressants, or **antiepileptic drugs**. Muscle relaxants such as cyclobenzaprine (Flexeril), carisoprodol (Soma), and methocarbamol (Robaxin) may relieve painful spasms, but may also cause drowsiness and should not be used when working, driving, or operating heavy equipment.

Some antidepressants, especially when given in low doses, act as pain relievers in addition to reducing symptoms of depression and insomnia. Among these medications are tricyclic antidepressants such as amitriptyline and desipramine; and newer antidepressants such as the selective serotonin reuptake inhibitors (SSRI)s are being tested for their ability to relieve pain. However, a review of studies published in November 2003 suggests that the tricyclic antidepressants, but not the SSRIs, reduce pain symptoms. Although antiepileptic drugs are primarily used to treat **seizures**, they have a stabilizing effect on nerve cells that makes them effective for certain types of nerve pain.

For severe pain, opioids and narcotics such as oxycodone-release (Oxycontin), acetaminophen with codeine (Tylenol with codeine), and meperidine (Demerol) may be prescribed. However, they may be addicting and associated with troublesome side effects including constipation, impaired judgment and reaction time, and sleepiness. Therefore, these drugs should only be used under a doctor's supervision, only when other medications are ineffective, and only for limited periods. Some pain management specialists believe that habitual use of these drugs may worsen depression and even increase pain.

In some patients, spinal manipulation, also known as osteopathic manipulative therapy or chiropractic, may correct patterns of spinal imbalance that impedes recovery. It may be helpful during the first month of low back pain, but it should be avoided in patients with previous back surgery, back injury related to underlying disease, and back malformations. Before proceeding with chiropractic, it may be wise to get clearance from a medical doctor.

Acupuncture is an alternative medicine technique in which trained practitioners place very-fine needles at precisely specified body locations to relieve pain. Insertion of these needles is thought to unblock the body's normal flow of energy and to release peptides, which are naturally occurring pain relievers. Clinical studies are underway to compare how effective acupuncture is relative to standard treatments for low back pain.

Biofeedback is a treatment recommended by some pain specialists, in conjunction with other treatments. By placing electrodes on the skin and connecting them to a biofeedback machine, the patient learns to modify the response to pain by controlling muscle tension, heart rate, and skin temperature. Meditation or other relaxation techniques may enhance the response to biofeedback training.

Patients who do not respond to the above treatments may be candidates for back surgery if there is a clear abnormality in structure that could be corrected surgically. Although surgery is typically a last resort, it may be done on an urgent basis if the spinal cord or nerve roots are being compromised.

Discectomy is a surgical procedure to relieve pressure on a nerve root caused by a bulging disc or bone spur, whereas foraminotomy enlarges the bony hole, or foramen, where a nerve root enters or exits the spinal canal. In spinal **laminectomy**, or spinal decompression, a piece of the bony roof of the spinal canal known as the lamina is removed on one or both sides to increase the size of the spinal canal and reduce pressure on the spinal cord and nerve roots.

Spinal fusion stabilizes the spine and prevents painful movements, but with resulting loss of flexibility. The spinal discs between two or more vertebrae are removed, and the neighboring vertebrae are joined together with bone grafts and/or metal devices attached by screws. To allow the bone grafts to grow and fuse the vertebrae together, a long recovery period is needed. The Food and Drug Administration (FDA) has approved the intervertebral body fusion device, the anterior spinal implant, and the posterior spinal implant for use in this type of procedure.

To relieve severe chronic pain, spinal cord stimulation devices may be surgically implanted. These devices discharge electrical impulses to stimulate the spinal cord and to block the perception of pain. Other procedures used as a last resort cut nerve fibers to relieve pain, but patients may find the resultant altered sensations more troubling than the pain itself. Rhizotomy involves cutting the nerve root near its point of entry to the spinal cord. Cordotomy destroys bundles of nerve fibers on one or both sides of the spinal cord, and dorsal root entry zone (DREZ) operation severs spinal neurons.

Clinical trials

The National Institute of Neurological Disorders and Stroke (NINDS) and other institutes at the National Institutes of Health (NIH) fund, support, and conduct general pain research, as well as studies of new treatments for pain and nerve damage associated with back pain and other conditions.

Ongoing studies are comparing the effects of different drugs; different treatment approaches such as standard care, chiropractic, or acupuncture; and surgery versus non-surgical treatments. Treatments under investigation include acupuncture and yoga in chronic low back pain, low-dose **radiation** to decrease postsurgical scarring around the spinal cord, and artificial spinal disc replacement surgery.

Studies that are currently recruiting patients include magnets in the treatment of sciatica and a comparison of nortriptyline and MS Contin in sciatica. Contact information for both trials is (800) 411-1222, or prpl@mail.cc.nih.gov.

Prognosis

In about 90% of people, back pain resolves within one month without treatment. Although most people with acute low back pain improve within a few days, others take much longer to recover or develop more serious conditions, especially if left untreated. Fractures, tumors, severe disc herniations, or other spinal conditions compromising nerve roots, spinal cord, or spinal stability may lead to progressive neurologic deterioration if not treated promptly.

Special concerns

Although back pain is usually not a cause for serious concern, it can interfere with work and activities and may even be disabling. Adopting lifestyle habits to prevent back pain and injury are therefore worthwhile, beginning at an early age. These include weight control and nutritionally sound diet, regular exercise, stretching before strenuous exercise, stopping smoking, good posture, and reducing emotional stress contributing to muscle tension.

In the workplace, at home, and while driving, supportive seats can reduce stress and fatigue. Other ergonomically designed furniture, tools, workstations, and living space help protect the body from injury.

Sleeping on the side with knees bent and cradling a pillow, or on the back with a pillow under bent knees, reduces back strain. Proper lifting techniques include bending at the knees rather than the waist, holding the weight close to the body rather than at arm's length, exhaling while lifting a heavy load, not twisting while lifting, and not attempting to lift a load that is too heavy. Frequent stretch breaks while sitting, standing, or working in one position for long periods will reduce muscle fatigue and back discomfort. Wearing comfortable, supportive, low-heeled shoes helps prevent falls and cushions the weight load on the spine during standing and walking.

Children using backpacks should be taught proper lifting techniques, should reduce the amount of books or supplies carried, or should switch to a wheeled carrier.

Resources

PERIODICALS

Birbara, C. A., et al. "Treatment of Chronic Low Back Pain with Etoricoxib, A New Cyclo-Oxygenase-2 Selective Inhibitor: Improvement in Pain and Disability—A Randomized, Placebo-Controlled, 3-Month Trial." *Journal of Pain* 2003 Aug 4(6): 307–15.

Breckenridge, J., and J. D. Clark. "Patient Characteristics Associated with Opioid Versus Nonsteroidal Anti-Inflammatory Drug Management of Chronic Low Back Pain." *Journal of Pain* 2003 Aug 4(6): 344–50.

Lewis, Carol. "What to Do When Your Back Is in Pain." U.S. Food And Drug Administration. *FDA Consumer Magazine* (March-April 1998).

Ohnmeiss, D. D., and R. F. Rashbaum. "Patient Satisfaction with Spinal Cord Stimulation for Predominant Complaints of Chronic, Intractable Low Back Pain." *Spine Journal* 2001 Sep-Oct 1(5): 358–63.

Staiger, T. O., B. Gaster, M. D. Sullivan, and R. A. Deyo. "Systematic Review of Antidepressants in the Treatment of Chronic Low Back Pain." *Spine* 2003 Nov 15 28(22): 2540–5C.

WEBSITES

Clinical Trials. (March 18, 2004.) <http://www.clinicaltrials.gov/ct/action/GetStudy>.

National Institute Of Neurological Disorders and Stroke. NIH Neurological Institute. PO Box 5801, Bethesda, MD 20824. (800) 352-9424. (March 18, 2004.) <http://www.ninds.nih.gov/health_and_medical/disorders/backpain_doc.htm>.

Spine-health.com. 1840 Oak Avenue, Suite 112, Evanston, IL 60201. (March 18, 2004.) <http://www.spine-health.com/topics/cd/kids/kids1.html>.

Spine-health.com. 1840 Oak Avenue, Suite 112, Evanston, IL 60201. (March 18, 2004.) <http://www.spine-health.com/topics/cd/tlbp/type01.html>.

U.S. Food And Drug Administration. 5600 Fishers Lane, Rockville, MD 20857-0001. (888) 463-6332. (March 18, 2004.) <http://www.fda.gov/fdac/features/1998/298_back.html>.

Your Medical Source. (March 18, 2004.) <http://www.yourmedicalsource.com/library/backpain/BAK_types.html>.

Laurie Barclay

Bassen-Kornzweig syndrome

Definition

Bassen-Kornzweig syndrome is a rare genetic disorder that is characterized by an inability to properly absorb dietary fats, resulting in neurological abnormalities, degeneration of the retina of the eye, a typical red blood cell abnormality ("burr-cell" malformation), and failure to thrive (grow and gain weight) during infancy.

Description

Bassen-Kornzweig syndrome is inherited as an autosomal recessive disorder, which means that parents of affected individuals are themselves unaffected carriers, and that they have a 25% risk of having an affected child in each pregnancy. Alternate names for this disorder include abetalipoproteinemia, acanthocytosis, and apolipoprotein

B deficiency. Affected individuals can have severe, irreversible neurological impairments, especially if untreated. Psychological counseling for parents and family members is often helpful. There are support groups that are useful in learning more about other families with affected individuals and how they manage in terms of coping mechanisms, responses to treatment, as well as practical considerations such as lifestyle changes. As the recurrence risk for this disorder is high, genetic counseling is recommended. In some families, prenatal diagnosis is possible.

Demographics

For unclear reasons, males are affected with Bassen-Kornzweig syndrome with greater frequency (70%) than girls, which is uncharacteristic in most autosomal recessive conditions. A majority of the originally described patients (including the first case of an 18-year old girl in 1950) were of Jewish descent. Bassen-Kornzweig syndrome is a rare disorder; estimations of how often it occurs are limited because the responsible genetic mutations were only recently identified and there is more than one gene that contributes to the disorder.

Causes and symptoms

Mutations in two genes have been shown to cause Bassen-Kornzweig syndrome: apolipoprotein B (APOB) and microsomal triglyceride transfer protein (MTP). These proteins are an important part of fat-containing molecules called lipoproteins in the blood. Several of these lipoproteins, such as low-density lipoproteins (LDL) and very-low-density lipoproteins (VLDL), are found in either very low concentrations or are completely absent in the blood. These lipoproteins function to transport fat and are important in fat metabolism. Not having these important lipoproteins can result in malabsorption (poor absorption) of fats, and excessive and wasteful fat excretion in the bile called steatorrhea.

MTP is a gene that encodes a protein responsible for transporting triglycerides, cholesteryl esters, and components of the cell's surface called phospholipids. Biochemical studies revealed that in biopsies from patients that lack lipoproteins (abetalipoproteinemia) and controls, MTP enzyme activity was only detected in control samples. MTP is expressed in the lumen of the liver and intestine and is not only important for transport of lipoproteins, but also for their assembly.

The body requires fats for healthy nerves and muscles. The symptoms that develop in Bassen-Kornzweig syndrome affect a person's sensory perception, coordinating muscle movements, blood chemistry, and vision. People with Bassen-Kornzweig can develop problems related to sensing temperature and touch, particularly on the

Key Terms

Autosomal recessive disorder A genetic disorder that is inherited from parents that are both carriers, but do not have the disorder. Parents with an affected recessive gene have a 25% chance of passing on the disorder to their offspring with each pregnancy.

Lipoproteins Compounds of protein that carry fats and fat-like substances such as cholesterol in the blood.

Malabsorption The inability to adequately or efficiently absorb nutrients from the intestinal tract.

Retinitis pigmentosa A family of genetically linked retinal diseases that causes progressive deterioration of peripheral vision and eventually blindness.

hands and feet, a condition called hypesthesia. The inability to produce lipoproteins leads to several symptoms that can adversely affect infants, who show signs of failure to grow and gain weight, and have fatty, foul-smelling stools that appear to be pale and frothy. A protruding abdomen can often be observed. Brain involvement can be significant, leading to developmental motor delay. Muscle coordination becomes compromised, usually after the child reaches 10 years old. Children with Bassen-Kornzweig syndrome also can have slurred speech that is likely to be secondary to the neurological impairment. Abnormal curvature of the spine, progressively diminished visual abilities, and balance difficulties can also be symptoms experienced by these patients. Finally, affected individuals can develop poor eyesight due to retinitis pigmentosa, along with cataracts and difficulty maintaining eye control.

In Bassen-Kornzweig syndrome, lacking the appropriate concentration of lipoproteins due to defective intestinal absorption of lipids can result in low serum cholesterol levels. Low levels of LDL have also been observed in patients with **AIDS**, certain types of leukemia, and disorders that involve enlargement of the spleen (Gaucher's disease) and should, therefore, not be confused with Bassen-Kornzweig syndrome.

Diagnosis

The initial observations that leads a physician to suspect a fat digestion problem is that affected babies have severe stomach problems with a high level of fats detected in the stool; the stool is often pale and foul smelling. One of the first medical tests usually performed on infants with failure to thrive is a complete blood count (CBC), which shows abnormal, thorny-shaped red blood cells (acanthocytes) that can be visualized using a microscope. A lipid profile demonstrates low levels of total cholesterol and low concentrations of VLDL and LDL in the blood. Apolipoprotein B can be completely absent or detected in reduced amounts in the blood. Due to the inability to digest fats, loss of fat-soluble vitamins such as vitamin A, D, E, or K occurs and can result in a deficiency. An examination by an ophthalmologist might show retinal degeneration leading to visual loss. A **neurologist** might find nerve demyelination (degeneration of the protective layer of the nerve) by performing nerve conduction studies or an EMG. Loss of peripheral nerves can be associated with **ataxia** (abnormal muscle coordination).

Treatment team

In addition to consistent evaluation by an experienced neurologist, it is important to consult with a nutritionist regarding the appropriate dietary restriction, as this can influence the development and well being of an affected individual. There is also a requirement for large doses of fat-soluble vitamin supplements because there is an inability to digest fat from the diet; the body does not retain these vitamins. Because the child with Bassen-Kornzweig syndrome often suffers from **hypotonia** and ataxia, an experienced physical therapist can often help develop strategies to treat the associated symptoms.

Treatment

Persons with Bassen-Kornzweig syndrome are treated primarily to lessen symptoms. The most formidable approach to treatment is dietary restriction and supplementation with the appropriate vitamins (D, E, A, and K) as well as with fats that can be broken down more easily. Supplementation with fat-soluble vitamins may slow the progression of the retinal degeneration. As these patients can develop **movement disorders** such as **tremors**, **chorea** (uncontrollable shaking), difficulty talking (**dysarthria**), and difficulty with tasks that require coordination, speech and occupational therapy is recommended and can be helpful.

Recovery and rehabilitation

Due to the nature of Bassen-Kornzweig syndrome and the biochemical defects, treatment is based solely on monitoring the diet and treating symptoms as well as any biochemical abnormalities that might develop. Currently, there is no cure.

Clinical trials

The National Heart, Lung, and Blood Institute (NHLBI) and the National Institutes of Health (NIH) are sponsoring a clinical trial to investigate circulating lipoproteins in the blood in order to better understand fat metabolism and the role it plays in heart disease. As part of the ongoing studies, healthy patients will receive injections of controlled doses of isolated and purified lipoproteins, along with a specially formulated diet. Patients will have blood drawn and a urinalysis and be monitored during the study. Contact information: National Heart, Lung and Blood Institute (NHLBI), 9000 Rockville Pike, Bethesda, Maryland, 20892; Patient Recruitment and Public Liaison Office (800) 411-1222; e-mail: prpl@mail.cc.nih.gov.

Prognosis

The prognosis depends on the severity of the neurological impairments, which can vary from patient to patient. There have been cases of severe, progressive neurological damage occurring before the person reaches age 30. Neurological damage is irreversible. The visual problems can also be progressive and the extent of retinal degeneration and visual loss can be variable. Mental deterioration can also sometimes occur.

Special concerns

An important consideration for these patients is dietary restriction. Due to the inability to digest dietary fats, the diet of persons with Bassen-Kornzweig syndrome should contain no more than five ounces of lean meat, fish, or chicken per day. This will help mitigate unpleasant intestinal symptoms. Certain high fat foods should be avoided, or foods that contain long-chain triglycerides (fat-containing molecules that are more difficult to breakdown). However, because the body needs some fats, as fat is important for many components of cells and tissues including cell membranes, medium chain triglycerides can be taken to supplement the diet.

All dietary restrictions should be carefully considered by a nutritionist and a physician, and the patient should be monitored for symptoms and responses to such treatments. Failure to supplement with vitamins such as vitamin E can lead to a vitamin deficiency. Vitamin E deficiency is associated with poor transmission of nerve impulses, hypotonia (weak muscles), and retinal degeneration leading to blindness. For these reasons, it is important to supplement with the appropriate vitamins at a dose recommended by a physician.

Resources

PERIODICALS

Rader, D. J., et al. "Abetalipoproteinemia: New Insights into Lipoprotein Assembly and Vitamin E Metabolism from a Rare Genetic Disease." *JAMA*, vol. 270, no. 7 (1993): 865–869.

OTHER

"A-Beta-Lipoproteinemia." *Genetic Information and Patient Services, Inc (GAPS)*. March 10, 2004 (April 27, 2004). <http://www.icomm.ca/geneinfo/abl.htm>.

National Institutes of Health. "Bassen-Kornzweig Syndrome." *Medline Plus*. March 10, 2004 (April 27, 2004). <http://www.nlm.nih.gov/medlineplus/ency/article/001666.htm>.

ORGANIZATIONS

Abetalipoproteinemia Support Group. 14252 Culver drive #543, Irvine, CA 92604. abetalipoproteinemia@yahoogroups.com. <http://groups.yahoo.com/group/Abetalipoproteinemia>.

CLIMB (Children Living with Inherited Metabolic Diseases). The Quadrangle, Crewe Hall, Weston Road, Crewe, Cheshire, CW1-6UR, United Kingdom. (127) 0 2-50221. Lesley@climb.org.uk. <http://www.CLIMB.org.uk>.

Foundation Fighting Blindness. Executive Plaza 1, 11350 McCormick Road, Suite 800, Hunt Valley, MD 21031-1014. (410) 785-1414 or (888) 394-3937. jchader@blindness.org. <http://www.blindness.org>.

Retinitis Pigmentosa International. 23241 Ventura Boulevard, Suite 117, Woodland Hills, CA 91364. (818) 992-0500. <http://groups.yahoo.com/group/Abetalipoproteinemia>.

Bryan Richard Cobb, PhD

Batten disease

Definition

Batten disease is a disorder of the nervous system that begins in childhood. Symptoms of the disorder include mental impairment, **seizures**, and loss of sight and motor skills.

Description

Batten disease was named after the British pediatrician who first described it in 1903. The disease is characterized by an abnormal buildup of lipopigments—substances made up of fats and proteins—in bubble-like compartments within cells. The compartments, called lysosomes, normally take in and break down waste products and complex molecules for the cell. In Batten disease, this process is disrupted, and the lipopigments accumulate. This breakdown is genetic. It is marked by vision failure and the loss of intellect and neurological functions, which begin in early childhood.

Batten disease is a form of a family of progressive neurological disorders known as neuronal ceroid lipofuscinoses

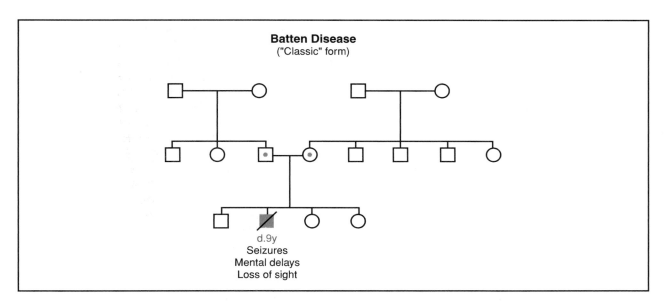

Batten Disease
("Classic" form)

d.9y
Seizures
Mental delays
Loss of sight

See Symbol Guide for Pedigree Charts. *(Gale Group.)*

(or NCLs). The disease is also known as Spielmeyer-Vogt-Sjögren-Batten disease, or juvenile NCL. There are three other disorders in the NCL family: Jansky-Bielchowsky disease, late infantile neuronal ceroid lipofuscinosis, and Kufs disease (a rare adult form of NCL). Although these disorders are often collectively referred to as Batten disease, Batten disease is a single disorder.

Demographics

Batten disease is relatively rare, occurring in two to four of every 100,000 births in the United States. NCLs appear to be more common in children living in Northern Europe and Newfoundland, Canada.

Causes and symptoms

Batten disease is an autosomal recessive disorder. This means that it occurs when a child receives one copy of the abnormal gene from each parent. Batten disease results from abnormalities in gene CLN3. This specific gene was identified by researchers in 1995.

Individuals with only one abnormal gene are known as carriers; they do not develop the disease but can pass the gene on to their own children. When both parents carry one abnormal gene, their children have a one in four chance of developing Batten disease.

Early symptoms of Batten disease include vision difficulties and seizures. There may also be personality and behavioral changes, slow learning, clumsiness, or stumbling. These signs typically appear between ages five and eight. Over time, the children experience mental impairment, worsening seizures, and the complete loss of vision and motor skills.

Batten disease, like other childhood forms of NCL, may first be suspected during an eye exam that displays a loss of certain cells. Because such cell loss can occur in other eye diseases, however, the disorder cannot be diagnosed by this sign alone. An eye specialist who suspects Batten disease may refer the child to a **neurologist**, who will analyze the medical history and information from various laboratory tests.

Diagnosis

Diagnostic tests used for Batten disease and other NCLs include:

• blood or urine tests that detect abnormalities that may indicate Batten disease

• skin or tissue sampling, which can detect the buildup of lipopigments in cells

• electroencephalogram, which displays electrical activity within the brain that suggests a person has seizures

• electrical studies of the eyes, which further detect various eye problems common in childhood NCLs

• brain scans, which spot changes in the brain's appearance

Treatment team

Patients suspected of having Batten disease will be diagnosed and then treated by an ophthalmologist and neurologist. Physical and occupational therapists will be consulted to help the patient maintain optimal functioning.

Key Terms

Lipopigments Substances made up of fats and proteins found in the body's tissues.

Lysosome Membrane-enclosed compartment in cells, containing many hydrolytic enzymes; where large molecules and cellular components are broken down.

Neuronal ceroid lipofuscinoses A family of four progressive neurological disorders.

Treatment

There is no known treatment to prevent or reverse the symptoms of Batten disease or other NCLs. Anticonvulsant drugs are often prescribed to reduce or control seizures. Other medicines may be prescribed to manage other symptoms associated with the disorder. Physical and occupation therapy may also help people retain function for a longer period of time. Scientists' recent discovery of the genes responsible for NCLs may help lead to effective treatments.

There have been reports of the slowing of the disease among children who were given vitamins C and E and diets low in vitamin A. However, the fatal outcome of the disease remained the same.

Prognosis

People with Batten disease may become blind, confined to bed, and unable to communicate. Batten disease is typically fatal by the late teens or 20s. Some people with the disorder, however, live into their 30s.

Resources

ORGANIZATIONS

Batten Disease Support and Research Association. 2600 Parsons Ave., Columbus, OH 43207. (800) 448-4570. <http://www.bdsra.org>.

Children's Brain Disease Foundation. 350 Parnassus Ave., Suite 900, San Francisco, CA 94117. (415) 566-5402.

Children's Craniofacial Association. PO Box 280297, Dallas, TX 75243-4522. (972) 994-9902 or (800) 535-3643. contact cca@ccakids.com. <http://www.ccakids.com>.

JNCL Research Fund. PO Box 766, Mundelein, IL 60060. <http://www.jnclresearch.org>.

National Organization for Rare Disorders (NORD). PO Box 8923, New Fairfield, CT 06812-8923. (203) 746-6518 or (800) 999-6673. Fax: (203) 746-6481. <http://www.rarediseases.org>.

WEBSITES

"Batten Disease Fact Sheet." (June 2000). *National Institute of Neurological Disorders and Stroke.* <http://www.ninds.nih.gov/health_and_medical/pubs/batten_disease.htm>.

"Gene for Last Major Form of Batten Disease Discovered." (September 18, 1997). *National Institute of Diabetes and Digestive and Kidney Disorders.* <http://www.niddk.nih.gov/welcome/releases/9_18_97.htm>.

Michelle Lee Brandt
Rosalyn Carson-DeWitt, MD

Behçet disease

Definition

Behçet disease (BD), also known as Behçet syndrome, is a chronic form of **vasculitis** (inflammation of the blood vessels) involving four primary symptoms: oral and genital ulcers, ocular inflammation, and arthritis.

Description

Behçet disease was first described in the 1930s by Turkish dermatologist Hulusi Behçet. His observations of the three classic symptoms (oral and genital ulcers and eye inflammation) now define this complex condition. BD also has a unique ability to affect all sizes of blood vessels, including arteries and veins. Symptoms related to vasculitis, such as inflammation of joints, gastrointestinal areas, or the **central nervous system**, are also common.

Demographics

Incidence of BD is very rare in the United States with approximately five in 100,000 people developing the syndrome. In Middle Eastern and Asian countries between Iran and Japan (known as the "Old Silk Route"), BD is quite prevalent. Incidence in these countries is double that of the United States.

More than twice as many females are diagnosed with BD than males in the United States. However, in Middle Eastern and Asian areas, significantly more men are affected than females.

Causes and symptoms

Behçet disease is caused by an autoimmune response that triggers inflammation of the blood vessels. Researchers have discovered a gene, HLA-B51, which predisposes an individual to BD. However, not all individuals with this gene develop the disease. The specific event leading to onset of BD is not known, but there are speculations that it may be related to the following:

Key Terms

Neuopathy   Disease or disorder, especially a degenerative one, that affects the nervous system.

Vasculitis   Inflammation of the blood vessels.

- herpes simplex virus infections
- frequent infections of *Streptococcus* bacteria
- environmental factors

The four primary symptoms of BD are recurring complications that rarely present simultaneously. These include:

- Oral ulcers (aphthous ulcers). Usually the first sign of disease, these sores resemble common canker sores, but are present in greater number, larger size, and occur more frequently. They may be painful and persist for up to two weeks.
- Genital ulcers. Similar in appearance to oral ulcers, genital sores typically occur on the scrotum in males and in the vulva in females. These ulcers are painful.
- Ocular inflammation (uveitis). May affect the front of or behind the eye, or both together. Inflammation of the middle eye area leads to blurred vision, light sensitivity, and possibly loss of sight.
- Arthritis. Temporary inflammation of the joints develops intermittently.

A large number of secondary symptoms are also associated with BD. These affect the following areas:

- Skin. Acne-like outbreaks of red skin sores develop on the legs and parts of the upper body.
- Vascular system. Formation of blood clots may lead to **aneurysms** or inflammation of veins (thrombosis). This is more frequent in men.
- Gastrointestinal system. Less often, patients may develop ulcers along the digestive tract.
- Central nervous system. Inflammation of the blood vessels in the brain can result in a variety of conditions such as **headache**, confusion, **stroke**, or seizures.

Diagnosis

Behçet disease is diagnosed based on a set of guidelines established by an international group of physicians. A physician observes clinical signs and symptoms during patient examination. The most recent and accepted guidelines for a positive diagnosis include the presence of recurring oral ulcers (three or more times in one year) and at least two of four secondary symptoms, including recurring genital ulcers, uveitis, skin lesions, a positive pathergy test.

A pathergy test is a skin-prick test to see if a red bump will form at the injection site. If there is a reaction, the test is positive. This test may be given to patients suspected of BD, but it is not an indicator for the disease. Only a small percentage of patients diagnosed with BD actually test positive.

Treatment team

Patients diagnosed with Behçet disease require a diverse treatment team due to the variety of symptoms and complications. The primary specialist is usually a physician who specializes in arthritis (rheumatologist). In addition, the team includes a dermatologist (skin), an ophthalmologist (eyes), a gynecologist or urologist (genital), a gastroenterologist (digestive system), and a **neurologist** (nervous system).

Treatment

Treatment is focused on the symptoms. Several medications are available to minimize discomfort caused by these symptoms.

Most treatment efforts attempt to reduce **pain** and inflammation. Corticosteroids such as Prednisone are prescribed since they are effective at regulating inflammatory responses. These may be administered as injections, pills, or creams. Immunosuppresant drugs such as cyclosporine, azathioprine or cyclophosphamide help suppress the immune system's response to a less-active state. Both corticosteroids and immunosuppressants can have serious side effects. Patients must be closely monitored by a physician while using these medications.

The use of interferon alpha 2a and 2b has been an effective treatment for ulcers and arthritis in patients who were less responsive to standard treatment regimens. Thalidomide has also shown potential as a treatment for BD. A complication of thalidomide is neuropathy. Thalidomide should not be used by women since it causes severe birth defects in fetuses.

Recovery and rehabilitation

Unlike most diseases, BD has symptoms that periodically flare up and then disappear for a period of time. As a result, patients may have long intervals with no complications. After treatment for active symptoms, patients usually require rest due to **fatigue**. Moderate **exercise** is also recommended to improve circulation and muscle strength.

Clinical trials

As of early 2004, the National Eye Institute was sponsoring two studies and recruiting patients with Behçet disease.

"Evaluation and Treatment of Patients with Inflammatory Eye Diseases" (study number 000204) evaluates patients with inflammatory eye diseases and the success of current therapies. "Biological Markers in Retinal Vasculitis" (study number 030068) is attempting to isolate biological markers related to primary retinal vasculitis by evaluating patients with differing initial causes of the disease.

Additional information on either of these studies can be found at the National Eye Institute (NEI), Patient Recruitment and Public Liaison Office, 9000 Rockville Pike, Bethesda, Maryland, 20892, (800) 411-1222, TTY (866) 411-1010.

Prognosis

For most patients, the prognosis of Behçet disease is good. Individuals typically experience periods of active symptoms followed by periods of remission in which there are no symptoms. The length of these intervals varies, with ulcerous outbreaks lasting a few weeks and other symptoms occurring for longer durations. With proper treatments and medication, patients can continue to lead active lifestyles in most cases.

Development of vascular or neurological complications often indicates a poorer prognosis. Blindness due to ocular inflammation is also prevalent in patients with BD.

Special concerns

In cases in which a patient becomes visually impaired, major lifestyle changes take place. The patient will have to learn adaptive behaviors and new forms of communication. Leader dog assistance or additional caregiver support are also considerations.

Resources

BOOKS

Lee, Sungnack. *Behçet's Disease: A Guide to Its Clinical Understanding.* New York: Springer Verlag, 2001.

Zeis, Joanne. *Essential Guide to Behçet's Disease.* Uxbridge, MA: Central Vision Press, 2003.

PERIODICALS

Okada, A. A. "Drug Therapy in Behçet's Disease." *Ocular Immunology and Inflammation* (June 2001): 85–91.

WEBSITES

Lee, Sungnack. "Behçet Disease." *EMedicine.* February 18, 2004 (May 17, 2004). <http://www.emedicine.com/derm/topic49.htm>.

"Types of Vasculitis: Behçet's Disease." *The Johns Hopkins Vasculitis Center Website.* The Johns Hopkins University. 2002 (May 17, 2004). <http://vasculitis.med.jhu.edu/typesof/behcets.html>.

ORGANIZATIONS

American Behçet's Disease Association. P.O. Box 19952, Amarillo, TX 79114. (800) 724-2387. jbadillo@behcets.com. <http://www.behcets.com>.

Behçets Organisation Worldwide. P.O. Box 27, Watchet, Somerset TA23 0YJ, United Kingdom. information@behcetsuk.org. <http://behcets.org>.

National Arthritis and Musculoskeletal and Skin Diseases Information Clearinghouse. 1AMS Circle, Bethesda, MD 20892. (301) 495-4484 or (877) 226-4267; Fax: (301) 718-6366. niamsinfo@mail.nih.gov. <http://www.niams.nih.gov>.

Stacey L. Chamberlin

Bell's palsy

Definition

Bell's palsy describes the acute onset of an unexplained weakness or paralysis of the muscles on one side of the face. Afflicted individuals may be unable to close the eye on the affected side of the face, and may also experience tearing, drooling, and hypersensitive hearing on the same side. The onset can be quite sudden, sometimes occurring overnight. The weakness and paralysis resolve completely in the majority of cases. Although it cannot be considered a serious condition from a health standpoint, it can cause extreme stress, embarrassment, and inconvenience for those affected.

Description

Bell's palsy has been described as a diagnosis of exclusion because several other disorders exhibit similar symptoms. Facial palsies have been linked to conditions such as **Lyme disease**, ear infection, meningitis, syphilis, German measles (rubella), mumps, chicken pox (varicella), and infection with Epstein-Barr virus (e.g., infectious mononucleosis). True Bell's palsy is an idiopathic facial palsy, meaning the root cause cannot be identified. Although Bell's palsy is not life-threatening, it can present symptoms similar to serious conditions such as **stroke**, ruptured aneurysm, or tumors.

Demographics

Every year, approximately 40,000–65,000 Americans are stricken with Bell's palsy. Worldwide, there is an annual incidence of 20–30 cases per 100,000 individuals. An

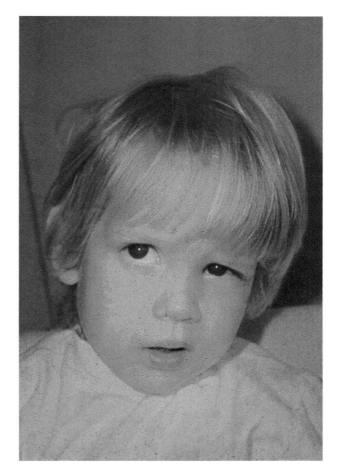

This boy's facial paralysis was caused by a tick-borne meningopadiculitis. *(Photo Researchers, Inc. Reproduced by permission.)*

individual can be affected at any age, but young and middle-aged adults are the most likely to be affected. It is unusual to see Bell's palsy in people less than 10 years old. Bell's palsy can affect either side of the face. Gender does not seem to factor into risk, though pregnant women and individuals with diabetes, influenza, a cold, or an upper respiratory infection seem to be at a greater risk.

In the large majority of cases (80–85%), the facial weakness or paralysis is temporary. However, individuals who experience complete paralysis seem to have a poorer recovery rate with only 60% returning to normal. Approximately 4–6% of all Bell's palsy cases result in permanent facial deformity, and another 10–15% experience permanent problems with spasms, twitching, or contracted muscles. Between 2% and 7.3% of individuals who have had Bell's palsy could experience a recurrence: on average, the first recurrence happens 9.8 years after the first episode; the second, 6.7 years later. One recurrence is very infrequent, and a second is extremely rare.

Causes and symptoms

The symptoms of Bell's palsy arise from an inflammation of the seventh cranial nerve, otherwise called the facial nerve. Each side of the face has a facial nerve that controls the muscles on that side of the face. Inflammation leads to the interference with conduction of nerve signals, and that in turn results in the loss of muscle control and tone.

Why the facial nerve becomes inflamed in Bell's palsy is a matter of considerable debate. Some evidence implicates the herpes simplex virus (HSV), which is responsible for cold sores and fever blisters. HSV infection has been suggested in up to 70% of Bell's palsy cases. Most people harbor this virus, although they may not exhibit symptoms. A number of other conditions have also been associated with the development of Bell's palsy, including facial or head injuries, **headache**, repeated middle ear infections, high blood pressure, diabetes, sarcoidosis, tumors, influenza, and other viral infections, as well as Lyme disease.

The major symptom of Bell's palsy is one-sided facial weakness or paralysis. Muscle control is either inadequate or completely missing. Patients frequently have difficulty shutting the affected eye and may not be able to close it at all.

Other symptoms can include **pain** in the jaw or behind the ear on the affected side, ringing in the ear, headache, decreased sense of taste, hypersensitivity to sound on the affected side, difficulty with speech, **dizziness**, and problems eating and drinking.

Diagnosis

Although Bell's palsy is not life-threatening, it has similar symptoms to serious conditions such as stroke. The fact that Bell's palsy is a diagnosis of exclusion becomes apparent in the course of the medical examination—it is imperative to rule out other disorders. Disorders that need to be excluded include demyelinating disease (e.g., **multiple sclerosis**), stroke, tumors, bacterial or viral infection, and bone fracture. Therefore, emergency medical attention is a wise and necessary precaution.

During the evaluation, the affected individual is asked about recent illnesses, accidents, infections, and any other symptoms. A visual exam of the ears, throat, and sinus is done, and hearing is tested. The extent of the symptoms is assessed by grading the symmetry of the face at rest and during voluntary movements such as wrinkling the forehead, puckering the lips, and closing the affected eye. Involuntary movements are assessed in combination with the voluntary movements. Neurologic exam is done to rule out involvement of other parts of the nervous system.

Blood tests and sometimes a cerebrospinal fluid (CSF) analysis may be needed. The results of these tests help determine the presence of a bacterial or viral infection or an inflammatory disease. Electrophysiological tests such as **electromyography** and **nerve conduction study**, in which a muscle or nerve is artificially stimulated, may be used to assess the condition of facial muscles and the facial nerve. Radiological tests may also be included, such as an x ray, **magnetic resonance imaging (MRI)**, and computed tomography (CT).

Once all other possibilities are exhausted, a diagnosis of Bell's palsy is made. During the next few weeks, the patient is carefully assessed. If facial movement, even a small amount, has not returned within 3–4 months, the diagnosis of Bell's palsy may need to be reevaluated.

Treatment team

The patient's primary care provider may be the initial contact; further consultation may be obtained from a **neurologist** and/or an ophthalmologist. Physical therapists may help with pain issues and regaining function.

Treatment

Many doctors prescribe an antiviral drug and/or a steroid for Bell's palsy, but there is some controversy about whether these drugs actually help. The consensus opinion seems to be that, although drugs might not be necessary, they are not dangerous, and they may help in

some cases. If drugs are used, they need to be taken as soon as possible following the onset of symptoms. The use of **antiviral drugs** such as acyclovir, famciclovir, or valacyclovir is recommended to destroy actively replicating herpes viruses. Steroids such as prednisone are thought to be useful in reducing inflammation and swelling.

In the past, surgery was performed to relieve the compression on the nerve. However, this treatment option is now used very infrequently because its benefits are uncertain, and it carries the risk of permanent nerve damage.

The need to protect the affected eye is universally promoted. Since the individual may not be able to lower the affected eyelid, the eye may become dry, particularly at night. Excessive dryness can damage the cornea. Daytime treatment includes artificial tears and may include an eye patch or other protective measures. Nighttime treatment involves a more intense effort at keeping the eye protected. Eye lubricants or viscous ointments, along with taping the eye shut, are frequently recommended.

In cases of permanent nerve damage, cosmetic treatment options such as therapeutic injections of **botulism** toxin or surgery may be sought or suggested.

Prognosis

Most individuals with Bell's palsy begin to notice improvement in their condition within 2–3 weeks of the symptoms' onset. At least 80% of them will be fully recovered within three months. Among the other 20% of afflicted individuals, symptoms may take longer to resolve or they may be permanent. Individuals suffering permanent nerve damage may not regain control of the muscles on the affected side of the face. These muscles may remain weak or paralyzed. As the nerve recovers, muscles may experience involuntary facial twitches or spasms that accompany normal facial expressions.

Resources

PERIODICALS

Billue, Joyce S. "Bell's Palsy: An Update on Idiopathic Facial Palsy." *The Nurse Practitioner* 22, no. 8 (1997): 88.

Kakaiya, Ram. "Bell's Palsy: Update on Causes, Recognition, and Management." *Consultant* 37, no. 8 (1997): 2217.

ORGANIZATIONS

Bell's Palsy Research Foundation. 9121 E. Tanque Verde, Suite 105-286, Tucson, AZ 85749. (520) 749-4614.

Julia Barrett
Rosalyn Carson-DeWitt, MD

Benign essential blepharospasm *see* **Blepharospasm**

Benign focal amyotrophy *see* **Monomelic amyotrophy**

Benign intracranial hypertension *see* **Pseudotumor cerebri**

Benign positional vertigo

Definition

Benign positional vertigo (BPV) is the most common cause of **dizziness** due to an impairment of the balance center in the ear.

Description

BPV was first described by Adler in 1987. Dix and Hallpike named the disorder benign paroxysmal positional vertigo. The disorder can also be called canalithiasis or positional vertigo or "top shelf vertigo" (affected persons tip their heads back to look up when having an attack).

The internal ear consists of sacs, ducts, and bone. The internal portion of the ear can be divided into the bony labyrinth and membranous labyrinth. The bony labyrinth is a cave-like area composed of three parts: the cochlea, vestibule, and semicircular canals. The shell-shaped cochlea is the organ for hearing. The vestibule is a small oval chamber that contains two structures, the utricle and the saccule, responsible for balance. A membrane within the utricle and saccule normally contains particles called otoliths (calcium carbonate particles). The semicircular canals that occupy three planes in space contain the semi-circular ducts for fluid (endolymph) flow.

The Canalolithiasis Theory, the most widely accepted explanation for the cause of BPV, explains the actual mechanism that causes BPV. The theory is that otoliths can become displaced from the utricle and enter a portion of the semicircular ducts. Changing head position can cause free otoliths to gravitate longitudinally through the canal. The endolymph fluid contained in the semicircular canal will flow abnormally, causing stimulation of special sensors (hair cells) of the affected posterior semicircular canal duct. This stimulation causes vertigo or dizziness.

Demographics

In the United States, the number of new cases (incidence) is 64 cases per 100,000 populations per year. The incidence is greater in patients older than 40 years, and women are affected twice more often than men. Several studies indicate that an average age of onset in the mid-50s. Approximately 20% of all falls by the elderly, resulting in hospitalization for serious injuries, are due to vertigo (dizziness). No information is available concerning predilection to race. Approximately 25–40% of patients with BPV express dizziness as their chief complaint. The incidence among the elderly is estimated to be about 8%.

Causes and symptoms

The most common cause of BPV is head trauma (21% of cases) with a secondary concussion. The force of head trauma is thought to displace otolith particles in the semicircular canal. Approximately 39% of cases do not have a cause (idiopathic), and 29% of patients with BPV usually present with an existing ear disease. Other common causes include alcoholism, **central nervous system** (CNS) disease (approximately 11%), major surgery, and chronic ear infections such as chronic otitis media (approximately 9% of cases).

The severity of cases varies. Some patients may experience nausea and vomiting even with the slightest head movement, whereas some patients may be minimally bothered by the dizziness. As the name implies, symptoms of BPV are typically dependent on head position. Head movement, rolling in bed, leaning forward or backward, or changing posture can cause an attack. The symptoms start abruptly and disappear with 20–30 seconds.

Diagnosis

In addition to a detailed history, the physical examination is important for detection of characteristic physical signs such as nystagmus (involuntary rhythmic oscillation of the eyes). The examination is also necessary to exclude other neurological diseases that may mimic benign positional vertigo. A physician familiar with the condition may perform the Hallpike test. Also, in patients with vertigo, hearing tests are generally necessary. Further testing may be necessary to evaluation other conditions that can cause vertigo or dizziness.

Treatment team

The treatment team can consist of an emergency room physician, ear, nose, and throat (ENT) specialist-surgeon, **neurologist**, and audiologist. A primary care practitioner can initiate symptomatic management. Patients typically require follow-up care and monitoring. Surgical candidates require specialty care from an ENT surgeon, as well as and a surgical team in a hospital that is equipped for such an intervention.

Treatment

There are three types of treatment given to patients with BPV: medical care, surgery, and home treatment. Medical care (office treatment) consists of either the Semont maneuver (also referred to as the Liberaroty maneuver) or the Epley maneuver, named after their inventors. The Semont maneuver (a series of head-turning exercises) involves a rapid shift from lying on one side to lying on the opposite side. The Epley maneuver involves sequentially moving the head in four different positions and waiting for 30 seconds on each turn. These maneuvers are effective in approximately 80% of patients who are diagnosed with BPV, although symptoms may reoccur after initial improvement in a substantial percentage of patients. If office medical treatment fails, patients can continue treatment at home with the Brandt-Daroff Exercises, which are difficult to perform, but effective in 95% of cases. These exercises are time consuming and done in three sets per day for two weeks. Medical treatment with medications is not recommended since they do not help relieve symptoms.

A surgical procedure called posterior canal plugging can be utilized in patients who had no response to any other form of treatment. With this procedure, there is a small risk of hearing deficit (usually less than 20%), but it is effective in most patients. The posterior semicircular canal is excised, exposing the membranous labyrinth with floating otoliths. The canal is patched off with tissue so otolith particles cannot move into the canal to stimulate the hair cells within this area. The canal is sealed and the incision sutured. Typically, the patient will stay in the hospital overnight and return one week later for suture removal.

Recovery and rehabilitation

Recovery and rehabilitation is favorable. Most patients recover well with head-tilting exercises. Patients who have recurrence of symptoms will undergo further exercises or surgical correction, which is successful for resolution of symptoms in more than 90% of surgical candidates.

Clinical trials

A large study is currently active concerning the treatment of BPV in family practice at McMaster University Department of Family Medicine in Hamilton, Ontario, Canada. Contact is Shawn Ling at (905) 521-2100 ext. 75451; fax: (905) 521-5010; e-mail: lingfpu@yahoo.ca. **Clinical trials** as of 2001 reported good results using the Epley canalith repositioning maneuver. In 86 patients studied, 70% had resolution of symptoms within two days after treatment.

Prognosis

The overall prognosis for patients who suffer from BPV is good. Spontaneous remission can occur within six weeks, but some cases never remit. Once treated, the recurrence rate is between 5% and 15%.

Resources

BOOKS

Goldman, Lee, et al. *Cecil's Textbook of Medicine*, 21st ed. Philadelphia: WB. Saunders Company, 2000.

PERIODICALS

Chang, Andrew K. "Benign Positional Vertigo." *eMedicine Series* (April 2002).

Haynes, D. S. "Treatment of Benign Positional Vertigo Using the Semont Maneuver: Efficacy in Patients Presenting without Nystagmus." *Laryngoscope* 112:5 (May 2002).

Li, John. "Benign Positional Vertigo." *eMedicine Series* (December 2001).

WEBSITES

"Benign Positional Vertigo." (May 17, 2004.) <http://search.allrefer.com/cgi-bin/allrefer-health.cgi?q=Benign+positional+vertigo&ul=http%3A%2F%2Fhealth.allrefer.com%2F>.

"Benign Positional Vertigo." (May 17, 2004.) <http://www.4medstudents.com/students/BPPV.PPT>.

ORGANIZATIONS

American Hearing Research Association Foundation. 8 South Michigan Avenue, Suite 814, Chicago, IL 60603-4539. (312) 726-9670; Fax: (312) 726-9695.

Laith Farid Gulli, MD
Robert Ramirez, DO
Nicole Mallory, MS,PA-C

Benzodiazepines

Definition

Benzodiazepines are medicines that help relieve nervousness, tension, and other symptoms by slowing the **central nervous system**.

Purpose

Benzodiazepines are a type of antianxiety drugs. While anxiety is a normal response to stressful situations, some people have unusually high levels of anxiety that can interfere with everyday life. For these people, benzodiazepines can help bring their feelings under control. The medicine can also relieve troubling symptoms of anxiety, such as pounding heartbeat, breathing problems, irritability, nausea, and faintness.

Physicians may sometimes prescribe these drugs for other conditions, such as muscle spasms, **epilepsy** and other seizure disorders, phobias, panic disorder, withdrawal from alcohol, and sleeping problems. However, this medicine should not be used every day for sleep problems that last more than a few days. If used this way, the drug loses its effectiveness within a few weeks.

Benzodiazepines should not be used to relieve the nervousness and tension of normal everyday life.

Description

The family of antianxiety drugs known as benzodiazepines includes alprazolam (Xanax), chlordiazepoxide (Librium), **diazepam** (Valium), and lorazepam (Ativan). These medicines take effect fairly quickly, starting to work within an hour after they are taken. Benzodiazepines are available only with a physician's prescription and are available in tablet, capsule, liquid, or injectable forms.

Recommended dosage

The recommended dosage depends on the type of benzodiazepine, its strength, and the condition for which it is being taken. Doses may be different for different people. Check with the physician who prescribed the drug or the pharmacist who filled the prescription for the correct dosage.

Always take benzodiazepines exactly as directed. Never take larger or more frequent doses, and do not take the drug for longer than directed. If the medicine does not seem to be working, check with the physician who prescribed it. Do not increase the dose or stop taking the medicine unless the physician says to do so. Stopping the drug suddenly may cause withdrawal symptoms, especially if it has been taken in large doses or over a long period. People who are taking the medicine for seizure disorders may have **seizures** if they stop taking it suddenly. If it is necessary to stop taking the medicine, check with a physician for directions on how to stop. The physician may recommend tapering down gradually to reduce the chance of withdrawal symptoms or other problems.

Precautions

Seeing a physician regularly while taking benzodiazepines is important, especially during the first few months of treatment. The physician will check to make sure the medicine is working as it should and will note unwanted side effects.

People who take benzodiazepines to relieve nervousness, tension, or symptoms of panic disorder should check

with their physicians every two to three months to make sure they still need to keep taking the medicine.

Patients who are taking benzodiazepines for sleep problems should check with their physicians if they are not sleeping better within 7-10 days. Sleep problems that last longer than this may be a sign of another medical problem.

People who take this medicine to help them sleep may have trouble sleeping when they stop taking the medicine. This effect should last only a few nights.

Some people, especially older people, feel drowsy, dizzy, lightheaded, or less alert when using benzodiazepines. The drugs may also cause clumsiness or unsteadiness. When the medicine is taken at bedtime, these effects may even occur the next morning. Anyone who takes these drugs should not drive, use machines, or do anything else that might be dangerous until they have found out how the drugs affect them.

Benzodiazepines may also cause behavior changes in some people, similar to those seen in people who act differently when they drink alcohol. More extreme changes, such as confusion, agitation, and **hallucinations**, also are possible. Anyone who starts having strange or unusual thoughts or behavior while taking this medicine should get in touch with his or her physician.

Because benzodiazepines work on the central nervous system, they may add to the effects of alcohol and other drugs that slow down the central nervous system, such as antihistamines, cold medicine, allergy medicine, sleep aids, medicine for seizures, tranquilizers, some **pain** relievers, and muscle relaxants. They may also add to the effects of anesthetics, including those used for dental procedures. These effects may last several days after treatment with benzodiazepines ends. The combined effects of benzodiazepines and alcohol or other CNS depressants (drugs that slow the central nervous system) can be very dangerous, leading to unconsciousness or, rarely, even death. Anyone taking benzodiazepines should not drink alcohol and should check with his or her physician before using any CNS depressants. Taking an overdose of benzodiazepines can also cause unconsciousness and possibly death. Anyone who shows signs of an overdose or of the effects of combining benzodiazepines with alcohol or other drugs should get immediate emergency help. Warning signs include slurred speech or confusion, severe drowsiness, staggering, and profound weakness.

Some benzodiazepines may change the results of certain medical tests. Before having medical tests, anyone taking this medicine should alert the health care professional in charge.

Children are generally more sensitive than adults to the effects of benzodiazepines. This sensitivity may increase the chance of side effects.

Key Terms

Anxiety   Worry or tension in response to real or imagined stress, danger, or dreaded situations. Physical reactions, such as fast pulse, sweating, trembling, fatigue, and weakness may accompany anxiety.

Asthma   A disease in which the air passages of the lungs become inflamed and narrowed.

Bronchitis   Inflammation of the air passages of the lungs.

Central nervous system   The brain, spinal cord, and the nerves throughout the body.

Chronic   A word used to describe a long-lasting condition. Chronic conditions often develop gradually and involve slow changes.

Emphysema   An irreversible lung disease in which breathing becomes increasingly difficult.

Epilepsy   A brain disorder with symptoms that include seizures.

Glaucoma   A condition in which pressure in the eye is abnormally high. If not treated, glaucoma may lead to blindness.

Myasthenia gravis   A chronic disease with symptoms that include muscle weakness and sometimes paralysis.

Panic disorder   A disorder in which people have sudden and intense attacks of anxiety in certain situations. Symptoms such as shortness of breath, sweating, dizziness, chest pain, and extreme fear often accompany the attacks.

Phobia   An intense, abnormal, or illogical fear of something specific, such as heights or open spaces.

Porphyria   A disorder in which porphyrins build up in the blood and urine.

Porphyrin   A type of pigment found in living things.

Seizure   A sudden attack, spasm, or convulsion.

Sleep apnea   A condition in which a person temporarily stops breathing during sleep.

Withdrawal symptoms   A group of physical or mental symptoms that may occur when a person suddenly stops using a drug to which he or she has become dependent.

Older people are more sensitive than younger adults to the effects of this medicine and may be at greater risk for side effects. Older people who take these drugs to help them sleep may be drowsy during the day. Older people also increase their risk of falling and injuring themselves when they take these drugs.

Special conditions

People with certain medical conditions or who are taking certain other medicines can have problems if they take benzodiazepines. Before taking these drugs, be sure to let the physician know about any of these conditions:

ALLERGIES Anyone who has had unusual reactions to benzodiazepines or other mood-altering drugs in the past should let his or her physician know before taking the drugs again. The physician should also be told about any allergies to foods, dyes, preservatives, or other substances.

PREGNANCY Some benzodiazepines increase the likelihood of birth defects. Using these medicines during pregnancy may also cause the baby to become dependent on them and to have withdrawal symptoms after birth. When taken late in pregnancy or around the time of labor and delivery, these drugs can cause other problems in the newborn baby, such as weakness, breathing problems, slow heartbeat, and body temperature problems.

Women who are pregnant or who may become pregnant should not use benzodiazepines unless their anxiety is so severe that it threatens their pregnancy. Any woman who must take this medicine while pregnant should be sure to thoroughly discuss its risks and benefits with her physician.

BREAST-FEEDING Benzodiazepines may pass into breast milk and cause problems in babies whose mothers take the medicine. These problems include drowsiness, breathing problems, and slow heartbeat. Women who are breast-feeding their babies should not use this medicine without checking with their physicians.

OTHER MEDICAL CONDITIONS Before using benzodiazepines, people with any of these medical problems should make sure their physicians are aware of their conditions:

• current or past drug or alcohol abuse

• **depression**

• severe mental illness

• epilepsy or other seizure disorders

• **swallowing disorders**

• chronic lung disease such as emphysema, asthma, or chronic bronchitis

- kidney disease
- liver disease
- brain disease
- glaucoma
- hyperactivity
- **myasthenia gravis**
- porphyria
- **sleep apnea**

USE OF CERTAIN MEDICINES Taking benzodiazepines with certain other drugs may affect the way the drugs work or may increase the chance of side effects.

Side effects

The most common side effects are **dizziness**, lightheadedness, drowsiness, clumsiness, unsteadiness, and slurred speech. These problems usually go away as the body adjusts to the drug and do not require medical treatment unless they persist or they interfere with normal activities.

More serious side effects are not common, but may occur. If any of the following side effects occur, check with the physician who prescribed the medicine as soon as possible:

- behavior changes
- memory problems
- difficulty concentrating
- confusion
- depression
- seizures (convulsions)
- hallucinations
- sleep problems
- increased nervousness, excitability, or irritability
- involuntary movements of the body, including the eyes
- low blood pressure
- unusual weakness or tiredness
- skin rash or itching
- unusual bleeding or bruising
- yellow skin or eyes
- sore throat
- sores in the mouth or throat
- fever and chills.

Patients who take benzodiazepines for a long time or at high doses may notice side effects for several weeks after they stop taking the drug. They should check with their physicians if these or other troublesome symptoms occur:

- irritability
- nervousness
- sleep problems.

Other rare side effects may occur. Anyone who has unusual symptoms during or after treatment with benzodiazepines should get in touch with his or her physician.

Interactions

Benzodiazepines may interact with a variety of other medicines. When this happens, the effects of one or both of the drugs may change or the risk of side effects may be greater. Anyone who takes benzodiazepines should let the physician know all other medicines he or she is taking. Among the drugs that may interact with benzodiazepines are:

- central nervous system (CNS) depressants such as medicine for allergies, colds, hay fever, and asthma
- sedatives
- tranquilizers
- prescription pain medicine
- muscle relaxants
- medicine for seizures
- sleep aids
- barbiturates
- anesthetics

Medicines other than those listed above may interact with benzodiazepines. Be sure to check with a physician or pharmacist before combining benzodiazepines with any other prescription or nonprescription (over-the-counter) medicine.

Resources

OTHER

"Medications." *National Institute of Mental Health Page.* 1995 <http://www.nimh.nih.gov>.

Nancy Ross-Flanigan

Beriberi

Definition

Beriberi is a condition caused by severe prolonged deficiency of vitamin B1 (also known as thiamine). Beriberi refers to a constellation of heart, gastrointestinal, and nervous system problems from thiamine deficiency.

Description

Thiamine is found in a variety of foods, particularly whole grains, legumes, and pork. Thiamine serves as a coenzyme in the chemical pathway responsible for the metabolism of carbohydrates. Thiamine deficiency interferes with the metabolism of glucose and the production of energy.

Four major types of beriberi exist: wet beriberi, which affects primarily the cardiovascular system; dry beriberi, which affects primarily the nervous system; shoshin, which is a rapidly evolving and frequently fatal form of cardiovascular beriberi; and infantile beriberi, which tends to strike babies between the ages of one and four months who are breastfed by mothers who are severely thiamine deficient.

Demographics

Because so many foods in the United States and other western countries are vitamin enriched, beriberi is extremely rare. In developed countries, beriberi is primarily a complication of malnutrition secondary to alcoholism or gastrointestinal disorders. Because alcoholism affects more males than females, rates of beriberi in developed countries are higher among males. The syndrome of symptoms caused by thiamine deficiency in alcoholism is called Wernicke-Korsakoff syndrome.

In developing countries, where diets are more limited, beriberi is endemic. In some areas of Asia, people subsist on polished rice, in which the outer, more nutritious husk is removed. The rates of beriberi in these areas are quite high. In certain parts of Indonesia, the prevalence of beriberi among low-income families is as high as 66%. The majority of patients with beriberi are infants (ages 1–4 months) and adults.

Causes and symptoms

Symptoms of beriberi are caused by abnormal metabolism of carbohydrates throughout the body, resulting in a decreased production of energy, and particular injury to the heart muscle and the nervous system.

Symptoms of dry beriberi include:

- numbness, tingling, burning **pain** in extremities
- pain and cramping in the leg muscles
- difficulty with speech
- problems walking
- disturbed sense of balance

Symptoms of wet beriberi include:

- fast heart rate
- swollen feet and legs

- enlarged heart
- enlarged, tender liver
- shortness of breath
- congestion in the lungs

Symptoms of shoshin beriberi are the same as those of wet beriberi, but the onset is sudden, the progression is rapid, and the risk of death is very high.

Symptoms of infantile beriberi include:

- restlessness
- difficulty sleeping
- diarrhea
- swollen arms and legs
- muscle wasting in arms and legs
- silent cry
- heart failure

Symptoms may coexist with other disorders due to thiamine deficiency such as Wernicke-Korsakoff **encephalopathy**. In such cases, confusion, memory loss, difficulty with eye movements, and even coma may occur.

Diagnosis

The first step to diagnosis includes taking a careful history to uncover a possible underlying cause for thiamine deficiency. Physical examination will demonstrate some of the expected signs of beriberi, such as swelling, decreased reflexes, decreased sensation, problems with walking or balance, etc.

Laboratory testing to demonstrate thiamine deficiency includes measurements of thiamine in the blood; tests of the activity of thiamine in whole blood or red blood cells (called transketolase activity), both before and after the administration of thiamine; measurements of the chemicals lactate and pyruvate in the blood (these will be increased in beriberi); and measurements of the amount of thiamine passed into the urine (this will be decreased in beriberi).

In some cases, the diagnosis of beriberi is made only after thiamine supplementation results in a resolution of the patient's symptoms.

Treatment team

Depending on how a patient enters the health care system, an emergency room physician, internal medicine physician, family practitioner, **neurologist**, gastroenterologist, or cardiologist may treat a patient for beriberi. A nutritionist should be consulted to develop a nutritional plan. If alcoholism is an underlying problem, the patient may need to enter an alcohol rehabilitation program. Physical therapy may help patients recover from the neurological complications of beriberi.

Treatment

When a patient has serious symptoms of thiamine deficiency, supplementation is usually started by giving thiamine through an IV or by intramuscular shots. Because magnesium is required for the proper functioning of thiamine, magnesium is usually administered through injections as well. After several days of this therapy, a multivitamin containing 5–10 times the usually recommended daily allowance of all the water-soluble vitamins, including thiamine, should be given for several weeks. Ultimately, the patient will be advised to follow a lifelong regimen of nutritious eating, with the regular diet supplying 1–2 times the recommended daily allowance of the water-soluble vitamins, including thiamine.

Recovery and rehabilitation

Recovery from the cardiovascular effects of beriberi is nearly always complete. Some of the neurological problems, however, may remain even after thiamine supplementation has been accomplished.

Prognosis

The longer a patient lives with a thiamine deficiency, the more severe the symptoms of beriberi. If untreated, beriberi is fatal. When treated with thiamine supplementation and a healthy diet, most of the symptoms of beriberi can be resolved.

Special concerns

Although beriberi is readily avoided with a healthy diet or successfully treated with thiamine supplementation and the initiation of a healthy diet, this is not always possible in developing countries where resources are scarce.

Resources

BOOKS

Brust, John C. "Nutritional Disorders of the Nervous System." In *Cecil Textbook of Medicine*, edited by Thomas E. Andreoli, et al. Philadelphia: W.B. Saunders Company, 2000.

Kinsella, Laurence A., and David E. Riley. "Nutritional Deficiencies and Syndromes Associated with Alcoholism." In *Textbook of Clinical Neurology*, edited by Christopher G. Goetz. Philadelphia: W.B. Saunders Company, 2003.

Russell, Robert M. "Vitamin and Trace Mineral Deficiency and Excess." In *Harrison's Principles of Internal Medicine*, edited by Eugene Braunwald, Anthony Fauci, et al. New York: McGraw-Hill, 2001.

Rosalyn Carson-DeWitt, MD

Bernhardt-Roth syndrome *see* **Meralgia paresthetica**

Binswanger disease

Definition

Binswanger disease is a rare form of progressive **dementia** that develops after age 60 and involves degeneration of the brain's white matter.

Description

Also known as subcortical arteriosclerotic **encephalopathy**, Binswanger disease is a form of subcortical dementia. Dementia is a general term used to describe a generalized deterioration of thinking and reasoning skills. In the case of Binswanger disease, the deterioration is due to physiological problems (i.e., organic factors). While many dementias result from damage to cortical areas of the brain, some diseases, including Binswanger disease, **Alzheimer's disease**, **Parkinson's disease**, **Huntington disease**, and dementia associated with **AIDS**, result from damage to subcortical areas of the brain (specifically, to subcortical connections).

Alternate names for Binswanger disease include Binswanger-type **multi-infarct dementia**, Binswanger encephalopathy, and Binswanger-type vascular dementia.

As with other individuals suffering subcortical dementia, people with Binswanger experience difficulties in maintaining attention to tasks and show depressed levels of motivation often accompanied by mood swings or apathy.

Demographics

Although Binswanger disease may occur in younger groups, the symptoms usually become pronounced in patients over 60 years of age.

Causes and symptoms

The exact cause of Binswanger disease is unknown, however, lesions in cerebrovascular tissue located in the inner white matter of the brain cause most of the symptoms. Prominent symptoms include rapid mood changes, loss of the ability to focus on tasks, a deterioration in thought processes (e.g., loss of memory and cognition), and mood changes.

Key Terms

Dementia Usually a long-lasting (chronic), often progressive, deterioration of the ability to think and reason due to an organic cause (an underlying illness or disorder).

Subcortical The neural centers located below (inferior to) the cerebral cortex.

Individuals with Binswanger disease may also have elevated blood pressure or suffer from **stroke**. Binswanger disease is found to be associated with blood (hematological) abnormalities with regard to the types and numbers of cells present, diseases of large blood vessels (especially in the upper chest and neck regions), and diseases of the heart. Abnormal electrical disturbances in the brain may cause **seizures**.

Binswanger's symptoms may be elusive in both appearance and degree. Not all people experience all the symptoms normally associated with the disease, and patients may experience symptoms for a period of time, followed by brief periods in which they are relatively symptom free.

As with other dementias, patients often present evidence of forgetfulness, memory loss, confusion and/or confabulation of events in terms of time and space (e.g., having a memory of two events that occur on different days as a combined memory of one event).

People with Binswanger disease often suffer **depression** and withdraw from family, friends, and co-workers (social withdrawal). Although clinical depression is a psychiatric term and requires a separate diagnosis, Binswanger patients suffering depression show a marked loss of interest in activities they once found pleasurable.

As the dementia progresses, people with Binswanger disease may initially lose the ability to perform tasks involving fine motor coordination, such as tying shoes or writing by hand, followed by a loss of broader function. Loss of bladder control (urinary incontinence) may develop, as well as generalized clumsiness or difficulty in walking. Later, patients often develop a blank-like stare and may have difficulty speaking or swallowing.

Diagnosis

Binswanger disease is identified by detection and characterization of lesions in the cerebrovascular tissue located in the inner white matter of the brain, which are usually visible on computed tomography (**CT**) **scan** or **magnetic resonance imaging (MRI)**.

A tentative diagnosis of Binswanger disease is made upon an evaluation of patient history and symptoms. A definitive diagnosis is made upon autopsy that reveals lesions in cerebrovascular tissue lying in the subcortical regions of the brain. Lesions are not always confined to subcortical areas and additional lesions also may extend into cortical areas.

Treatment team

The treatment team for patients suffering from dementia, either cortical or subcortical, usually includes physicians, nurses, and physical, speech, and occupational therapists.

The diagnosis of Binswanger disease is often made by a **neurologist**. Physical therapists evaluate deficits in strength, movement, and gait, and supervise exercises to improve these deficits. Speech-language pathologists evaluate deficits in the ability to eat and speak, and provide adaptive strategies to minimize their effects. Occupational therapists evaluate a person's ability to maintain posture and focus while executing normal activities of daily living (such as reaching for and using a toothbrush) and devise strategic movements and equipment to adapt to deficits.

An expanded network of professionals, including mental health counselors and social service workers, may be beneficial. Caregivers are often required for personal care during the late stages of the disease.

Treatment

There is no known cure or specific treatment for Binswanger disease. Patients are treated symptomatically, i.e., treated for the symptoms such as high blood pressure, seizures, or heart disease often associated with Binswanger disease.

In most cases, specialized treatment plans include medications to control mood swings and depression, blood pressure (both elevated and low), seizures, and rhythm irregularities in the heart. Treatment is designed to reduce the adverse effects of these associated conditions.

Recovery and rehabilitation

Although currently no cure exists for dementias such as the Binswanger type, the goal of therapy is to maintain the highest state of physical health by managing the symptoms, along with maintaining the highest possible state of functional activity and well being. In addition to physical and occupational therapy, treatment for mood swings or depression helps the person with Binswanger disease to remain active, socially engaged, and mobile for as long as possible.

When the disease progresses and mobility, along with mental ability, decreases, the person with Binswanger or

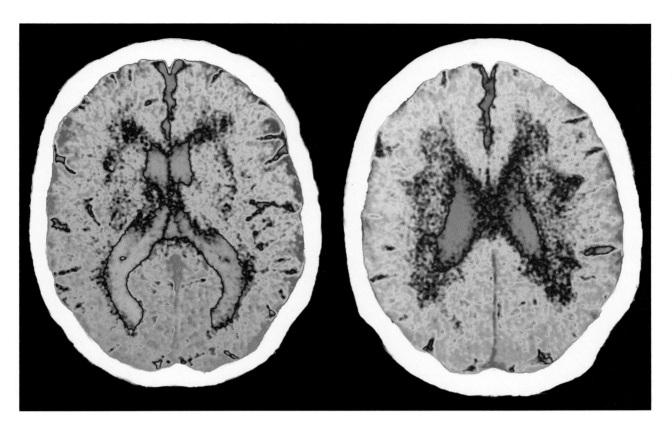

CT scans of a patient with Binswanger disease. The CT scans show the presence of periventricular white matter hypodensities. *(Phototake, Inc. All rights reserved.)*

other dementias will likely require a nurturing environment that provides for medical care and safety. Whether at home or in a care facility, personal care assistance may be necessary for many or all hours of the day.

Many communities have adult daycare centers with targeted, stimulating activities for persons with dementia in the early stages. Long-term care facilities that specialize in dementia can provide an environment that fosters mobility in a soothing environment, where staff provides cues to orient the person with dementia to memories and surroundings.

Clinical trials

Research on a wide range of neurological diseases, including dementias, is conducted by agencies of the National Institutes of Health such as the National Institute of Neurological Disorders and Stroke (NINDS), and other institutes and research organizations such as the National Institute on Aging and the National Institute of Mental Health. As of November 2003, scientists at the National Institute of Neurological Disorders and Stroke are reevaluating the definitions for many forms of dementia, including Binswanger disease.

Prognosis

Because there is no known specific cure for Binswanger disease, in most cases the disease follows a slowly progressing course during which a patient may suffer progressive strokes interspersed with periods of partial recovery. Once symptoms become visible (manifest), persons with Binswanger disease often die within five years of the onset of the disease.

Resources

OTHER

BBC News: Health and Medical Notes. "Binswanger's Disease." April 12, 1999. (November 13, 2003 [June 1, 2004].) <http://news.bbc.co.uk/1/hi/health/medical_notes/317488.stm>.

National Institute of Neurological Disorders and Stroke (NINDS)/National Institutes of Health. "Binswanger's Disease." November 8, 2002. (November 13, 2003 [June 1, 2004].) <http://www.ninds.nih.gov/health_and_medical/disorders/binswang_doc.htm>.

ORGANIZATIONS

Alzheimer's Association. 919 North Michigan Avenue, Suite 1100, Chicago, IL 60611-1676. (312) 335-8700 or (800)

272-3900; Fax: (312) 335-1110. info@alz.org.
<http://www.alz.org>.

Alzheimer's Disease Education and Referral Center (ADEAR).
P.O. Box 8250, Silver Spring, MD 20907-8250. (301)
495-3311 or (800) 438-4380; Fax: (301) 495-3334.
adear@alzheimers.org. <http://www.alzheimers.org>.

Family Caregiver Alliance. 690 Market Street / Suite 600, San
Francisco, CA 94104. (415) 434-3388 or (800) 445-8106;
Fax: (415) 434-3508. info@caregiver.org.
<http://www.caregiver.org>.

National Institute of Neurological Disorders and Stroke
(NINDS) at the National Institutes of Health.
P.O. Box 5801, Bethesda, MD 20824; (301)
496-5751 or (800) 352-9424; TTY (301) 468-5981.
braininfo@ninds.nih.gov. <http://www.ninds.nih.gov/>.

National Organization for Rare Disorders (NORD). 55 Kenosia
Avenue, Danbury, CT 06813-1968. (203) 744-0100 or
(800) 999-NORD; Fax: (203) 798-2291. orphan@
rarediseases.org. <http://www.rarediseases.org>.

Paul Arthur

Biopsy

Definition

A biopsy is the removal of a small portion of tissue
from the body for microscopic examination.

Description

When a physician diagnoses the nature of an ailment,
various examinations provide information that is vital to accurately determining the nature of the problem. Blood and
urine samples can be examined to determine the amounts
of various compounds. As useful as this information can be,
it reveals little about the state of tissues. In diseases such as
cancer, knowledge of the affected tissue is crucial for diagnosis and the formulation of treatment strategies.

Examination of tissues can be accomplished without
obtaining a sample, using techniques like ultrasound and
magnetic resonance imaging (MRI). However, the information gained may not be detailed enough for a definitive diagnosis. For example, a physician may be interested
in the activity of a particular enzyme in the tissue, as a
marker of a disease process, or the presence of a toxin. For
such determinations, a tissue sample that can be analyzed
in the laboratory is needed.

Similarly, for certain diseases and conditions that involve nerve abnormalities, the ability to directly examine
nerves can be advantageous in diagnosis and treatment.
For instance, direct microscopic examination of a nerve
sample can reveal whether or not the protective myelin

sheath that surrounds a nerve is intact or is in the process
of degrading. Obtaining a nerve via a biopsy is a valuable
aid to these examinations.

Muscle biopsies can serve a similar purpose, since
maladies that affect the structure and/or functioning of
nerves will ultimately affect the muscles into which the
nerve passes. The loss of muscle function or strength can
be the direct consequence of nerve damage.

Biopsy

A biopsy describes the procedure that is used to obtain a very small piece of the target tissue. For some tissues, like the lining of the cheek, cells can be obtained just
by scrapping the tissue surface. Other samples are collected using forceps that are positioned at the end of an op-
tical device called an endoscope. The physician can view
the tissue surface (such as the wall of the large intestine)
through the endoscope and use the forceps to pluck tissue
from the desired region of the surface. In other cases, the
tissue sample needs to be collected as a "plug," using a
large hypodermic needle. Examples of the latter include
liver or kidney biopsy samples. Samples of muscles and
nerves can also be obtained by cutting out a small piece of
the target once an incision has been made.

When a biopsy is obtained using a needle, the retrieval
of a sample relies on the design of the needle and the energy of its insertion into the tissue. The needle used is a hollow tube with a sharp point capable of puncturing tissue.
As the needle is driven deeper into a tissue following puncture, tissue will accumulate in the hollow tube. When the
needle is withdrawn from the tissue, the plug of tissue remains in the needle tube and can be retrieved for analysis.

Many biopsy samples are examined using a light microscope to look for abnormalities in the tissues cells. This
examination can involve the staining of the sample to
specifically detect target molecules. As well, samples can
be used for various biochemical tests, and even to test for
the presence and activity of particular genes.

A biopsy can remove the entire target region (excisional biopsy) or can remove just a small portion of the
target region (incisional biopsy). The latter can be done in
three different ways, depending on the sample. A shave
biopsy slices off surface tissue. Samples collected by
piercing the tissue with a needle represent a punch biopsy.
Finally, in fine needle aspiration, a needle is inserted and
tissue is subsequently withdrawn into the needle using a
syringe.

Muscle biopsy

A muscle biopsy can represent the punch type, in
which a plug of tissue is obtained using an inserted needle.
Or, in an open biopsy procedure, a small incision is made
and a piece of tissue is removed. This biopsy is done for a

Key Terms

Excisional biopsy Removal of an entire lesion for microscopic examination.

Incisional biopsy Removal of a small part of a sample tissue area for microscopic examination.

variety of reasons: to distinguish between nerve and muscle disorders, to identify specific muscular disorders such as **muscular dystrophy**, to probe muscle metabolic activities, and to detect muscle infections such as trichinosis and toxoplasmosis. Biopsy of a muscle necessarily involves nerves, as muscle is highly infused by nerves. The small amount of muscle that is extracted during a muscle biopsy does not damage nerves to such an extent that muscle function is affected.

Brain biopsy

A brain biopsy is performed following the drilling of a hole in the skull, through which the biopsy needle is subsequently introduced. An MRI or computed tomography (**CT**) **scan** is performed prior to the procedure in order to identify the area where the biopsy will be performed. As of the mid-1990s, the patient's head is no longer immobilized during the procedure by a frame device. Instead, the precise location is located by a computer-guided system that is designed to avoid damage to other regions of the brain. In contrast to a skin biopsy, for example, where the sample scraping may affect few nerves, a brain biopsy is a delicate and potentially problematic procedure. Rarely, nerve damage may result, and the puncture site may form scar tissue, causing **seizures**.

Nerve biopsy

Nerves such as the sural nerve in the ankle and the superficial radial nerve in the wrist are most often used for a nerve biopsy. A nerve biopsy is performed to detect nerve-damaging conditions, including leprosy, necrotizing **vasculitis** (an inflammation of the blood vessels), other nerve inflammation, and damage or loss of the nerve's protective myelin sheath (demyelination). A nerve biopsy can also be done to try to identify nerve abnormalities that are generically called neuropathies, or to confirm a specific diagnosis relating to a nerve. An example is the progressive wasting away of muscle tissue in the feet and legs that is known as Charcot-Marie-Tooth disease.

When a nerve biopsy is performed, local anesthetic is used. Then a small incision is made and a small piece of the target nerve is removed. Usually, a biopsy of the adjacent muscle is done at the same time. The biopsy procedure carries minimal risks, including allergic reaction to

the anesthetic, infection, and permanent numbness. A small degree of persistent numbness is to be expected, however, because a portion of nerve has been removed. As a nerve biopsy is generally performed in the ankle or wrist, the numbness is typically not debilitating and is seldom recognized during normal activities.

Biopsy sample processing and examination

Biopsy specimens are often sliced into thin slices, stained, mounted on a glass slide, and examined using a light microscope. Newer sample preparation techniques involve the rapid freezing of the sample and slicing of the still-frozen material. The latter technique has the advantage of avoiding the removal of water, which can alter the structure of the tissue cells. Microscopic examination focuses on the general appearance of the cells, including their structure, presence of abnormalities, and specific molecules that have been revealed by the use of specialized stains or antibodies. This interpretation can be subjective, and relies on the expertise of the experienced examiner.

Resources

BOOKS

Zaret, B. L. *The Yale University School of Medicine Patient's Guide to Medical Tests.* New Haven: Yale University School of Medicine and G.S. Sharpe Communications Inc., 1997.

OTHER

National Library of Medicine. "Muscle Biopsy." *Medline Plus.* May 5, 2004 (May 27, 2004). <http://www.nlm.nih.gov/medlineplus/ency/article/003924.htm>.

National Library of Medicine. "Nerve Biopsy." *Medline Plus.* May 5, 2004 (May 27, 2004). <http://www.nlm.nih.gov/medlineplus/ency/article/003928.htm>.

"What Is a Biopsy?" *Netdoctor.co.uk.* May 6, 2004 (May 27, 2004). <http://www.netdoctor.co.uk/health_advice/examinations/biopsy.htm>.

ORGANIZATIONS

American Academy of Neurology. 1080 Montreal Avenue, Saint Paul, MN 55116. (651) 695-2717 or (800) 879-1960; Fax: (651) 695-2791. memberservices@aan.com. <http://www.aan.com>.

Brian Douglas Hoyle, PhD

Blepharospasm

Definition

Blepharospasm is an involuntary closure of the eyelids.

Description

"Blepharo" refers to the eyelids, and "spasm" to involuntary muscle contraction. In blepharospasm, the eyelids close involuntarily due to an unknown cause within the brain. Blepharospasm is a form of **dystonia**, a disorder characterized by sustained muscle contraction. The most common form of blepharospasm is called "benign essential blepharospasm," meaning it is not life threatening and is not due to some other identifiable disorder. A condition called **hemifacial spasm** causes similar symptoms, but affects only one side of the face, and is caused by an irritation of the facial nerve outside of the brain.

Demographics

Blepharospasm is estimated to affect approximately 15,000 people in the United States. Onset is most commonly between the ages of 40 and 60, but can begin in childhood or old age. Women are affected approximately twice as often as men.

Causes and symptoms

The cause of benign essential blepharospasm is unknown. Evidence suggests it may be genetic in some cases, although genes have not been identified. A person with blepharospasm often has dystonia in another region of the body such as the mouth or the hands (i.e., writer's cramp). Other forms of dystonia or tremor may affect other family members. Blepharospasm is not caused by a problem with the eyes themselves, but rather with the brain regions controlling the muscles of the eyelids.

Secondary blepharospasm occurs due to some identifiable cause. The most-common cause of secondary blepharospasm is a reaction to antipsychotic medications, and is called tardive dystonia. Damage to the brain, either through **stroke**, **multiple sclerosis**, or trauma, may also cause blepharospasm.

Blepharospasm often begins with increased frequency of blinking, which may be accompanied by a feeling of irritation in the eyes or "dry eye." It progresses to intermittent, and then sustained, forceful closure of the eyelids. Symptoms are usually worse when the patient is tired, under stress, or exposed to bright light. Symptoms may become severe enough to interfere with activities of daily living, and can render the patient functionally blind.

Diagnosis

Blepharospasm is diagnosed by a careful clinical exam. A detailed medical history is taken to determine exposure to drugs or other possible causative agents, and a family history is used to determine if other family members are affected by other forms of dystonia or tremor.

Key Terms

Dystonia Painful involuntary muscle cramps or spasms.

Treatment team

The treatment team consists of a **neurologist** and possibly a neurosurgeon.

Treatment

The most effective treatment for blepharospasm is injection of **botulinum toxin** (BTX) into the muscles controlling the eyelids. BTX temporarily prevents the muscles from contracting, allowing patient to keep their eyes open. BTX is a safe and effective treatment for this condition. Usually the effects are seen within several days of injection, have their maximum effect for 6–8 weeks, and last between 12 and 16 weeks, at which time reinjection is performed. Side effects of BTX injection include mild discomfort at the injection site(s), and occasional double vision or inability to lift the eyelids due to local spread of the toxin to other muscles. Dry eyes or excessive tearing may also occur. Development of resistance to BTX injections is possible if the patient's immune system creates antibodies against the toxin. While this has not been reported in blepharospasm as the injected dose is very low, it has occurred in other conditions in which the doses are higher.

Oral medications are rarely effective for blepharospasm. Among the most widely used are **anticholinergics** (trihexyphenidyl, benztropine), baclofen, and **benzodiazepines** (**diazepam**, clonazepam). Surgery is an option for patients who do not respond to BTX injections. The surgical procedures are performed to remove part of the overactive muscles, or to sever the nerve leading to them, or both. Unfortunately, surgery is rarely completely successful, and there is a high rate of recurrence of blepharospasm.

Clinical trials

There are no current **clinical trials** for blepharospasm since effective treatment is available.

Prognosis

Blepharospasm is a chronic condition, which tends to worsen over time. Many patients with blepharospasm develop other dystonias in other body regions.

Resources

WEBSITES

Benign Essential Blepharospasm Research Foundation.
(April 19, 2004.) <http://www.blepharospasm.org/>.
WE MOVE. (April 19, 2004.) <http://www.wemove.org>.

Richard Robinson

Bloch-Sulzberger syndrome *see*
Incontinentia pigmenti

Blood-brain barrier *see* **Cerebral circulation**

▍Bodywork therapies

Definition

Bodywork therapies is a general term that refers to a group of body-based approaches to treatment that emphasize manipulation and realignment of the body's structure in order to improve its function as well as the client's mental outlook. These therapies typically combine a relatively passive phase, in which the client receives deep-tissue bodywork or postural correction from an experienced instructor or practitioner, and a more active period of movement education, in which the client practices sitting, standing, and moving about with better alignment of the body and greater ease of motion.

Bodywork should not be equated with massage simply speaking. Massage therapy is one form of bodywork, but in massage therapy, the practitioner uses oil or lotion to reduce the friction between his or her hands and the client's skin. In most forms of body work, little if any lubrication is used, as the goal of this type of hands-on treatment is to warm, relax, and stretch the fascia (a band or sheath of connective tissue that covers, supports, or connects the muscles and the internal organs) and underlying layers of tissue.

Purpose

The purpose of bodywork therapy is the correction of problems in the client's overall posture, connective tissue, and/or musculature in order to bring about greater ease of movement, less discomfort, and a higher level of energy in daily activity. Some forms of bodywork have as a secondary purpose the healing or prevention of repetitive stress injuries, particularly for people whose occupations require intensive use of specific parts of the body (e.g., dancers, musicians, professional athletes, opera singers, etc.). Bodywork may also heal or prevent specific musculoskeletal problems, such as lower **back pain** or neck **pain**.

Bodywork therapies are holistic in that they stress increased self-awareness and intelligent use of one's body as one of the goals of treatment. Some of these therapies use verbal discussion, visualization, or guided imagery along with movement education to help clients break old patterns of moving and feeling. Although most bodywork therapists do not address mental disorders directly in their work with clients, they are often knowledgeable about the applications of bodywork to such specific emotions as depession, anger, or fear.

Although some bodywork therapies, such as Rolfing or Hellerwork, offer programs structured around a specific number or sequence of lessons, all therapies of this type emphasize individualized treatment and respect for the uniqueness of each individual's body. Bodywork instructors or practitioners typically work with clients on a one-to-one basis, as distinct from a group or classroom approach.

Precautions

Persons who are seriously ill, acutely feverish, or suffering from a contagious infection should wait until they have recovered before beginning a course of bodywork. As a rule, types of bodywork that involve intensive manipulation or stretching of the deeper layers of body tissue are not suitable for persons who have undergone recent surgery or have recently suffered severe injury. In the case of Tragerwork, shiatsu, and trigger point therapy, clients should inform the therapist of any open wounds, bruises, or fractures so that the affected part of the body can be avoided during treatment. Craniosacral therapy, the Feldenkrais method, and the Alexander technique involve gentle touch and do not require any special precautions.

Persons who are recovering from abuse or receiving treatment for any post-traumatic syndrome or dissociative disorder should consult their therapist before undertaking bodywork. Although bodywork is frequently recommended as an adjunctive treatment for these disorders, it can also trigger flashbacks if the bodywork therapist touches a part of the patient's body associated with the abuse or trauma. Many bodywork therapists, however, are well informed about post-traumatic symptoms and disorders, and able to adjust their treatments accordingly.

Description

The following are brief descriptions of some of the more popular bodywork therapies.

Alexander technique

The Alexander technique was developed by an Australian actor named F. Matthias Alexander (1869-1955), who had voice problems that were not helped by any available medical treatments. Alexander decided to set up a number of mirrors so that he could watch himself during

Key Terms

Bodywork   Any technique involving hands-on massage or manipulation of the body.

Endorphins   A group of peptide compounds released by the body in response to stress or traumatic injury. Endorphins react with opiate receptors in the brain to reduce or relieve pain sensations. Shiatsu is thought to work by stimulating the release of endorphins.

Fascia (plural, fasciae)   A band or sheath of connective tissue that covers, supports, or connects the muscles and the internal organs.

Ki   The Japanese spelling of qi, the traditional Chinese term for vital energy or the life force.

Meridians   In traditional Chinese medicine, a network of pathways or channels that convey qi (also sometimes spelled "ki"), or vital energy, through the body.

Movement education   A term that refers to the active phase of bodywork, in which clients learn to

move with greater freedom and to maintain the proper alignment of their bodies.

Repetitive stress injury (RSI)   A type of injury to the musculoskeletal and nervous systems associated with occupational strain or overuse of a specific part of the body. Bodywork therapies are often recommended to people suffering from RSIs.

Somatic education   A term used in both Hellerwork and the Feldenkrais method to describe the integration of bodywork with self-awareness, intelligence, and imagination.

Structural integration   The term used to describe the method and philosophy of life associated with Rolfing. Its fundamental concept is the vertical line.

Tsubo   In shiatsu, a center of high energy located along one of the body's meridians. Stimulation of the tsubos during a shiatsu treatment is thought to rebalance the flow of vital energy in the body.

a performance from different angles. He found that he was holding his head and neck too far forward, and that these unconscious patterns were the source of the tension in his body that was harming his voice. He then developed a method for teaching others to observe the patterns of tension and stress in their posture and movement, and to correct these patterns with a combination of hands-on guidance and visualization exercises. As of 2002, the Alexander technique is included in the curricula of the Juilliard School of Music and many other drama and music schools around the world, because performing artists are particularly vulnerable to repetitive stress injuries if they hold or move their bodies incorrectly.

In an Alexander technique session, the client works one-on-one with an instructor who uses verbal explanations as well as guided movement. The sessions are usually referred to as "explorations" and last about 30 minutes. Although most clients see positive changes after only two or three sessions, teachers of the technique recommend a course of 20–30 sessions so that new movement skills can be learned and changes maintained.

Rolfing

Rolfing, which is also called Rolf therapy or structural integration, is a holistic system of bodywork that uses deep manipulation of the body's soft tissue to realign and balance the body's myofascial (muscular and connective tissue) structure. It was developed by Ida Rolf (1896-1979),

a biochemist who became interested in the structure of the human body after an accident damaged her health. She studied with an osteopath as well as with practitioners of other forms of alternative medicine, and developed her own technique of body movement that she called structural integration. Rolfing is an approach that seeks to counteract the effects of gravity, which tends to pull the body out of alignment over time and cause the connective tissues to stiffen and contract.

Rolfing treatment begins with the so-called "Basic Ten," a series of ten sessions each lasting 60–90 minutes, spaced a week or longer apart. After a period of integration, the client may undertake advanced treatment sessions. "Tune-up" sessions are recommended every six months. In Rolfing sessions, the practitioner uses his or her fingers, hands, knuckles, or elbows to rework the connective tissue over the client's entire body. The deep tissues are worked until they become pliable, which allows the muscles to lengthen and return to their proper alignment. Rolfing treatments are done on a massage table, with the client wearing only undergarments.

Hellerwork

Hellerwork is a bodywork therapy developed by Joseph Heller, a former NASA engineer who became a certified Rolfer in 1972 and started his own version of structural integration, called Hellerwork, in 1979. Heller describes his program as "a powerful system of somatic education and structural bodywork" based on a series of eleven sessions. Hellerwork is somewhat similar to Rolfing in that it begins with manipulation of the deep tissues of the body. Heller, however, decided that physical realignment of the body by itself is insufficient, so he extended his system to include movement education and "self-awareness facilitated through dialogue."

The bodywork aspect of Hellerwork is intended to release the tension that exists in the fascia, which is the sheath or layer of connective tissue that covers, supports, or connects the muscles and internal organs of the body. Fascia is flexible and moist in its normal state, but the effects of gravity and ongoing physical stresses lead to misalignments that cause the fascia to become stiff and rigid. The first hour of a Hellerwork session is devoted to deep connective tissue bodywork in which the Hellerwork practitioner uses his or her hands to release tension in the client's fascia. The bodywork is followed by movement education, which includes the use of video feedback to help clients learn movement patterns that will help to keep their bodies in proper alignment. The third component of Hellerwork is verbal dialogue, which is intended to help clients become more aware of the relationships between their emotions and attitudes and their body.

Tragerwork

Trager psychophysical integration, which is often called simply Tragerwork, was developed by Milton Trager (1908-1977), a man who was born with a spinal deformity and earned a medical degree in his middle age after working out an approach to healing chronic pain. Tragerwork is based on the theory that many illnesses are caused by tension patterns that are held in the unconscious mind as much as in the tissues of the body; clients are advised to think of Tragerwork sessions as "learning experiences" rather than "treatments." Tragerwork sessions are divided into bodywork, which is referred to as tablework, and an **exercise** period. Trager practitioners use their hands during tablework to perform a variety of gentle motions—rocking, shaking, vibrating, and gentle stretching—intended to help the client release their patterns of tension by experiencing how it feels to move freely and effortlessly on one's own. Following the tablework, clients are taught how to perform simple dance-like exercises called Mentastics, for practice at home. Tragerwork sessions take between 60–90 minutes, while clients are advised to spend 10–15 minutes three times a day doing the Mentastics exercises.

Feldenkrais method

The Feldenkrais method, like Hellerwork, refers to its approach as "somatic education." Developed by Moshe Feldenkrais (1904-1984), a scientist and engineer who was also a judo instructor, the Feldenkrais method consists of two major applications—Awareness Through Movement (ATM) lessons, a set of verbally directed exercise lessons intended to engage the client's intelligence as well as physical perception; and Functional Integration (FI), in which a Feldenkrais practitioner works with the client one-on-one, guiding him or her through a series of movements that alter habitual patterns and convey new learning directly to the neuromuscular system. Functional Integration is done with the client fully clothed, lying or sitting on a low padded table.

Perhaps the most distinctive feature of the Feldenkrais method is its emphasis on new patterns of thinking, attention, cognition, and imagination as byproducts of new patterns of physical movement. It is the most intellectually oriented of the various bodywork therapies, and has been described by one observer as "an unusual melding of motor development, biomechanics, psychology, and martial arts." The Feldenkrais method is the form of bodywork that has been most extensively studied by mainstream medical researchers.

Trigger point therapy

Trigger point therapy, which is sometimes called myotherapy, is a treatment for pain relief in the musculoskeletal system based on the application of pressure to trigger points in the client's body. Trigger points are defined as hypersensitive spots or areas in the muscles that cause pain when subjected to stress, whether the stress is an occupational injury, a disease, or emotional stress. Trigger points are not necessarily in the same location where the client feels pain.

Myotherapy is a two-step process. In the first step, the therapist locates the client's trigger points and applies pressure to them. This step relieves pain and also relaxes the muscles associated with it. In the second part of the therapy session, the client learns a series of exercises that progressively stretch the muscles that have been relaxed by the therapist's pressure. Most clients need fewer than 10 sessions to benefit from myotherapy. One distinctive feature of trigger point therapy is that clients are asked to bring a relative or trusted friend to learn the pressure technique and the client's personal trigger points. This "buddy system" helps the client to maintain the benefits of the therapy in the event of a relapse.

Shiatsu

Shiatsu is the oldest form of bodywork therapy, having been practiced for centuries in Japan as part of traditional medical practice. As of 2002, it is also the type of bodywork most commonly requested by clients in Western countries as well as in East Asia. The word *shiatsu* itself is a combination of two Japanese words that mean "pressure" and "finger." Shiatsu resembles **acupuncture** in its use of the basic concepts of ki, the vital energy that flows throughout the body, and the meridians, or 12 major pathways that channel ki to the various organs of the body. In Asian terms, shiatsu works by unblocking and rebalancing the distribution of ki in the body. In the categories of Western medicine, shiatsu may stimulate the release of endorphins, which are chemical compounds that block the receptors in the brain that perceive pain.

A shiatsu treatment begins with the practitioner's assessment of the client's basic state of health, including posture, vocal tone, complexion color, and condition of hair. This evaluation is used together with ongoing information about the client's energy level gained through the actual bodywork. The shiatsu practitioner works with the client lying fully clothed on a futon. The practitioner seeks out the meridians in the client's body through finger pressure, and stimulates points along the meridians known as tsubos. The tsubos are centers of high energy where the ki tends to collect. Pressure on the tsubos results in a release of energy that rebalances the energy level throughout the body.

Craniosacral therapy

Craniosacral therapy, or CST, is a form of treatment that originated with William Sutherland, an American osteopath of the 1930s who theorized that the manipulative techniques that osteopaths were taught could be applied to the skull. Sutherland knew from his medical training that the skull is not a single piece of bone, but consists of several bones that meet at seams; and that the cerebrospinal fluid that bathes the brain and spinal cord has a natural rise-and-fall rhythm. Sutherland experimented with gentle manipulation of the skull in order to correct imbalances in the distribution of the cerebrospinal fluid. Contemporary craniosacral therapists practice manipulation not only of the skull, but of the meningeal membranes that cover the brain and the spinal cord, and sometimes of the facial bones. Many practitioners of CST are also osteopaths, or DOs.

In CST, the patient lies on a massage table while the therapist gently palpates, or presses, the skull and spine. If the practitioner is also an osteopath, he or she will take a complete medical history as well. The therapist also "listens" to the cranial rhythmic impulse, or rhythmic pulsation of the cerebrospinal fluid, with his or her hands. Interruptions of the normal flow by abnormalities caused by tension or by injuries are diagnostic clues to the practitioner. Once he or she has identified the cause of the abnormal rhythm, the skull and spinal column are gently manipulated to restore the natural rhythm of the cranial impulse. Craniosacral therapy appears to be particularly useful in treating physical disorders of the head, including migraine headaches, ringing in the ears, sinus problems, and injuries of the head, neck, and spine. In addition, patients rarely require extended periods of CST treatments.

Preparation

Bodywork usually requires little preparation on the client's or patient's part, except for partial undressing for Rolfing, trigger point therapy, and Hellerwork.

Aftercare

Aftercare for shiatsu, trigger point therapy, and craniosacral therapy involves a brief period of rest after the treatment.

Some bodywork approaches involve various types of long-term aftercare. Rolfing clients return for advanced treatments or tune-ups after a period of integrating the changes in their bodies resulting from the Basic Ten sessions. Tragerwork clients are taught Mentastics exercises to be done at home. The Alexander technique and the Feldenkrais approach assume that clients will continue to practice their movement and postural changes for the rest of their lives. Trigger point therapy clients are asked to involve friends or relatives who can help them maintain the benefits of the therapy after the treatment sessions are over.

Risks

The deep tissue massage and manipulation in Rolfing and Hellerwork are uncomfortable for many people, particularly the first few sessions. There are, however, no serious risks of physical injury from any form of bodywork that is administered by a trained practitioner of the specific treatment. As mentioned, however, bodywork therapies that involve intensive manipulation or stretching of the deeper layers of body tissue are not suitable for persons who have undergone recent surgery or have recently suffered severe injury.

Normal results

Normal results from bodywork include deep relaxation, improved posture, greater ease and spontaneity of movement, greater range of motion for certain joints, greater understanding of the structures and functions of the body and their relationship to emotions, and release of negative emotions.

Many persons also report healing or improvement of specific conditions, including migraine headaches, repetitive stress injuries, osteoarthritis, insomnia, sprains and bruises, sports injuries, stress-related illnesses, **sciatica**, postpregnancy problems, menstrual cramps, temporomandibular joint disorders, lower back pain, **whiplash** injuries, disorders of the immune system, asthma, **depression**, digestive problems, chronic **fatigue**, and painful scar tissue. The Alexander technique has been reported to ease the process of childbirth by improving the mother's postural alignment prior to delivery.

Some studies of the Feldenkrais method have found that its positive effects on subjects' self-esteem, mood, and anxiety sympoms are more significant than its effects on body function.

Abnormal results

Abnormal results from bodywork therapies would include serious physical injury or trauma-based psychological reactions.

Resources

BOOKS

Pelletier, Kenneth R., MD. *The Best Alternative Medicine.* New York: Simon and Schuster, 2002.

PERIODICALS

Dunn, P. A., and D. K. Rogers. "Feldenkrais Sensory Imagery and Forward Reach." *Perception and Motor Skills* 91 (December 2000): 755-757.

Hornung, S. "An ABC of Alternative Medicine: Hellerwork." *Health Visit* 59 (December 1986): 387-388.

Huntley, A., and E. Ernst. "Complementary and Alternative Therapies for Treating Multiple Sclerosis Symptoms: A Systematic Review." *Complementary Therapies in Medicine* 8 (June 2000): 97-105.

Johnson, S. K., and others. "A Controlled Investigation of Bodywork in Multiple Sclerosis." *Journal of Alternative and Complementary Medicine* 5 (June 1999): 237-243.

Mackereth, P. "Tough Places to be Tender: Contracting for Happy or 'Good Enough' Endings in Therapeutic Massage/Bodywork?" *Complementary Therapies in Nursing and Midwifery* 6 (August 2000): 111-115.

Perron, Wendy. "Guide to Bodywork Approaches." *Dance Magazine* 74 (November 2000): 12-15.

Stallibrass, C., and M. Hampson. "The Alexander Technique: Its Application in Midwifery and the Results of Preliminary Research Into Parkinson's." *Complementary Therapies in Nursing and Midwifery* 7 (February 2001): 13-18.

ORGANIZATIONS

Bonnie Prudden Pain Erasure Clinic and School for Physical Fitness and Myotherapy. P.O. Box 65240. Tucson, AZ 85728. (520) 529-3979. Fax: (520) 529-6679. <www.bonnieprudden.com>.

Cranial Academy. 3500 DePauw Boulevard, Indianapolis, IN 46268. (317) 879-0713.

Craniosacral Therapy Association of the United Kingdom. Monomark House, 27 Old Gloucester Street, London, WC1N 3XX. Telephone: 07000-784-735. <www.craniosacral.co.uk/>.

Feldenkrais Guild of North America. 3611 S.W. Hood Avenue, Suite 100, Portland, OR 97201. (800) 775-2118 or (503) 221-6612. Fax: (503) 221-6616. <www.feldenkrais.com>.

The Guild for Structural Integration. 209 Canyon Blvd. P.O. Box 1868. Boulder, CO 80306-1868. (303) 449-5903. (800) 530-8875. <www.rolfguild.org>.

Hellerwork. 406 Berry St. Mt. Shasta, CA 96067. (530) 926-2500. <www.hellerwork.com>.

International School of Shiatsu. 10 South Clinton Street, Doylestown, PA 18901. (215) 340-9918. Fax: (215) 340-9181. <www.shiatsubo.com>.

The Society of Teachers of the Alexander Technique. <www.stat.org.uk>.

The Trager Institute. 21 Locust Avenue, Mill Valley, CA 94941-2806. (415) 388-2688. Fax: (415) 388-2710. <www.trager.com>.

OTHER

National Certification Board for Therapeutic Massage and Bodywork. 8201 Greensboro Drive, Suite 300. McLean, VA 22102. (703) 610-9015.

NIH National Center for Complementary and Alternative Medicine (NCCAM) Clearinghouse. P. O. Box 8218, Silver Spring, MD 20907-8218. TTY/TDY: (888) 644-6226; Fax: (301) 495-4957. Web site: <http://www.nccam.nih.gov>.

Rebecca Frey
Rosalyn Carson-DeWitt, MD

Botulinum toxin

Definition

Botulinum toxin is the purified form of a poison created by the bacterium *Clostridium botulinum*. These bacteria grow in improperly canned food and cause **botulism** poisoning. Minute amounts of the purified form can be injected into muscles to prevent them from contracting; it is used in this way to treat a wide variety of disorders and cosmetic conditions.

Purpose

Botulinum toxin was developed to treat strabismus (cross-eye or lazy eye), and was shortly thereafter discovered to be highly effective for many forms of **dystonia**. **Spasticity** can also be effectively treated with botulinum toxin. Injected into selected small muscles of the face, it can reduce wrinkling. Other conditions treated with botulinum toxin include:

• achalasia

• anismus

• **back pain**

• bruxism

• excess saliva production

- eyelid spasm
- **headache**
- **hemifacial spasm**
- hyperhidrosis
- **migraine**
- palatal **myoclonus**
- spastic bladder
- **stuttering**
- tics
- **tremor**
- uncontrollable eye blinking
- vaginismus

It is important to note that as of early 2004, the only Food and Drug Administration-approved uses for botulinum toxin are for certain forms of dystonia, hemifacial spasm, strabismus, **blepharospasm** (eyelid spasms), and certain types of facial wrinkles. While there is general recognition that certain other conditions can be effectively treated with botulinum toxin, other uses, including for headache or migraine, are considered experimental.

Description

A solution of botulinum toxin is injected into the overactive muscle. The toxin is taken up by nerve endings at the junction between nerve and muscle. Once inside the cell, the toxin divides a protein. The normal job of this protein is to help the nerve release a chemical, a neurotransmitter, which stimulates the muscle to contract. When botulinum toxin divides the protein, the nerve cannot release the neurotransmitter, and the muscle cannot contract as forcefully.

The effects of botulinum toxin begin to be felt several days after the injection. They reach their peak usually within two weeks, and then gradually fade over the next 2–3 months. Since the effects of the toxin disappear after several months, reinjection is necessary for continued muscle relaxation.

Recommended dosage

In the United States, purified botulinum toxin is available in two commercial forms: Botox and MyoBloc. The recommended doses of the two products are quite different, owing to the differing potencies of the two products. The size of the muscle and the degree of weakening desired also affect the dose injected. For Botox, the maximum recommended dose for adults is 400–600 units in any three-month period, while for MyoBloc it is 10,000–15,000 units. The maximum dosage may be reached in the treatment of spasticity or cervical dystonia,

---

Key Terms

Achalasia An esophageal disease of unknown cause, in which the lower sphincter or muscle is unable to relax normally, resulting in obstruction, either partial or complete.

Bruxism Habitual clenching and grinding of the teeth, especially during sleep.

Hyperhidrosis Excessive sweating. Hyperhidrosis can be caused by heat, overactive thyroid glands, strong emotion, menopause, or infection.

Migraine A throbbing headache that usually affects only one side of the head. Nausea, vomiting, increased sensitivity to light, and other symptoms often accompany a migraine.

Stuttering Speech disorder characterized by speech that has more dysfluencies than is considered average.

Tic A brief and intermittent involuntary movement or sound.

Tremor Involuntary shakiness or trembling.

Vaginismus An involuntary spasm of the muscles surrounding the vagina, making penetration painful or impossible.

---

while much smaller amounts are used in the treatment of facial lines, strabismus, and hemifacial spasm.

Precautions

When injected by a trained physician, botulinum toxin is very safe. The toxin remains mainly in the muscle injected, spreading only slightly to surrounding muscles or beyond. Botulism poisoning, which occurs after ingesting large amounts of the toxin, is due to the effects of the poison on the breathing muscles. In medical use, far less toxin is injected, and care is taken to avoid any chance of spread to muscles needed for breathing. Injection into the shoulders or neck may weaken muscles used for swallowing, which patients need to be aware of. Some patients may need to change to a softer diet to make swallowing easier during the peak effect of their treatment.

Repeated injections of large amounts of botulinum toxin can lead to immune system resistance. While this is not a dangerous condition, it makes further treatment ineffective.

Patients with neuromuscular disease should not receive treatment with botulinum toxin without careful consultation with a **neurologist** familiar with its effects.

Side effects

Botulinum toxin can cause a mild flu-like syndrome for several days after injection. Injection of too much toxin causes excess weakness, which may make it difficult to carry on normal activities of daily living. In some patients, toxin injection may cause blurred vision and dry mouth. This is more common in patients receiving MyoBloc than with Botox.

Interactions

Patients taking aminoglycoside antibiotics may be cautioned against treatment with botulinum toxin. These antibiotics include gentamicin, kanamycin, and tobramycin, among others.

Resources

BOOKS

Brin, M. F., M. Hallett, and J. Jankovic, editors. *Scientific and Therapeutic Aspects of Botulinum Toxin.* Philadelphia: Lippincott, 2002.

WEBSITES

WE MOVE. December 4, 2003 (February 18, 2004). <http://www.wemove.org>.

MD Virtual University. December 4, 2003 (February 18, 2004). <www.mdvu.org>.

Richard Robinson

▍ Botulism

Definition

Botulism is a neuroparalytic disease caused by the potent toxin of the *Clostridium botulinum* bacterium. There are three main types of botulism: foodborne botulism, infant botulism, and wound botulism.

Description

Botulism was first identified in Wildbad, Germany, in 1793, when six people died after consuming a locally produced blood sausage. In 1829, Jutinius Kerner, a health official, described 230 cases of sausage poisoning. Thereafter, the illness became known as "botulism," which is derived from the Latin "botulus," meaning sausage. In 1897, E. Van Ermengem identified the bacterium and its toxin while investigating an outbreak of the disease among musicians in Elezells, Belgium.

C. botulinum is a spore-forming, anaerobic, gram-positive bacilli found globally in soil and honey. The toxin has recently gain notoriety. It is a potential bioterrorism agent, and it is used as a beauty aid to eliminate frown lines.

Clinically, food-borne botulism is dominated by neurological symptoms, including dry mouth, blurred vision and diplopia, caused by the blockade of neuromuscular junctions.

In wound botulism the neurologic findings are similar to the food-borne illness, but the gastrointestinal symptoms are absent. Infants suffering from the intestinal colonization of spores of *C. botulinum* suffer first from constipation, and later develop neurological paralysis, which can lead to respiratory distress.

There are seven distinct neurotoxic serotypes, all of which are closely related to the tetanus toxin. Types A and B are most commonly implicated, but types E and, more rarely, F have been associated with human disease.

Demographics

Botulism is rare, but its incidence does vary by geographic region. The food-borne version remains highest among people who can their own foods. In 1995, only 24 cases of food-borne botulism were reported to the Centers for Disease Control and Prevention.

About 90% of global cases of infant botulism are diagnosed in the US, where the annual incidence is about 2 per 100,000 live births. It is the most common form of human botulism in the United States, with over 1,400 cases diagnosed between 1976 and 1996.

Between 1943 and 1985, 33 cases of wound botulism were diagnosed in the United States, mainly associated with deep and avascular wounds. However, between 1986 and 1996, 78 cases of wound botulism were diagnosed, many the result of illicit drug use, occurring at injection sites or at nasal or sinus sites associated with chronic cocaine snorting.

Causes and symptoms

Botulism is caused by the protein toxin released by the microorganism *C. botulinum*. After the toxin is absorbed into the bloodstream, it irreversibly binds to the acetylcholine receptors on the motor nerve terminals at neuromuscular junctions. After the toxin is internalized, it cleaves the apparatus in the neuron that is responsible for acetylcholine release, making the neuron unresponsive to action potentials. The blockade is irreversible and may last for months, until new nerve buds grow.

FOOD-BORNE BOTULISM The symptoms can range from mild to life threatening, depending on the toxin dose. Generally, symptoms appear within 36 hours of consuming food containing the toxin. Paralysis is symmetric and

Key Terms

Acetylcholine A chemical called a neurotransmitter that functions primarily to mediate activity of the nervous system and skeletal muscles.

Action potential The wave-like change in the electrical properties of a cell membrane, resulting from the difference in electrical charge between the inside and outside of the membrane.

Anaerobic Pertaining to an organism that grows and thrives in an oxygen-free environment.

Bacillus A rod-shaped bacterium, such as the diphtheria bacterium.

Congenital myopathy Any abnormal condition or disease of muscle tissue that is present at birth; it is characterized by muscle weakness and wasting.

Diplopia A term used to describe double vision.

Dysarthria Slurred speech.

Dysphagia Difficulty in swallowing.

ELISA protocols ELISA is an acronym for "enzyme-linked immunosorbent assay"; it is a highly sensitive technique for detecting and measuring antigens or antibodies in a solution.

Gram-positive Refers to a bacteria that takes on a purplish color when exposed to the Gram stain. Common examples of gram-positive bacteria include several species of streptococci, staphylococci, and clostridia.

Guillain-Barré syndrome Progressive and usually reversible paralysis or weakness of multiple muscles usually starting in the lower extremities and often

ascending to the muscles involved in respiration. The syndrome is due to inflammation and loss of the myelin covering of the nerve fibers, often associated with an acute infection. Also called acute idiopathic polyneuritis.

Myasthenia gravis A chronic, autoimmune, neuromuscular disease with symptoms that include muscle weakness and sometimes paralysis.

Polymerase chain reaction (PCR) A process by which numerous copies of DNA or a gene can be made within a few hours. PCR is used to evaluate false-negative results to the ELISA and Western blot tests for HIV and to make prenatal diagnoses of genetic disorders.

Reye syndrome A serious, life-threatening illness in children, usually developing after a bout of flu or chicken pox, and often associated with the use of aspirin. Symptoms include uncontrollable vomiting, often with lethargy, memory loss, disorientation, or delirium. Swelling of the brain may cause seizures, coma, and in severe cases, death.

Sepsis A severe systemic infection in which bacteria have entered the bloodstream or body tissues.

Spore A dormant form assumed by some bacteria, such as anthrax, that enable the bacterium to survive high temperatures, dryness, and lack of nourishment for long periods of time. Under proper conditions, the spore may revert to the actively multiplying form of the bacteria. Also refers to the small, thick-walled reproductive structure of a fungus.

descending. The first symptoms to appear include dysphagia, **dysarthria**, and diplopia, a reflection of cranial nerve involvement. Neck and limb weakness, nausea, vomiting, and **dizziness** follow. Respiratory muscle paralysis can lead to ventilatory failure and death unless support is provided.

WOUND BOTULISM The in vivo production of toxin by *C. botulinum* spores, leads to the neurologic symptoms seen in food-borne botulism. Gastrointestinal symptoms are absent.

INFANT BOTULISM Peak incidence occurs between 2 and 3 months of age. *C. botulinum* spores colonize the gastrointestinal tract and produce the toxin. Most infants show signs of constipation, followed by neuromuscular weakness that results in decreased sucking, lack of muscle tone and characteristic "floppy head." Symptoms may

range from mild to severe, and may lead to respiratory failure.

Diagnosis

Physicians should consider a diagnosis of botulism in a patient who presents with neuromuscular impairment, but remains mentally alert. The disease is often mistaken for other more common conditions, including **stroke**, encephalitis, **Guillain-Barré syndrome**, **myasthenia gravis**, tick paralysis, chemical or mushroom poisoning, and adverse reactions to antibiotics or other medication. Sepsis, electrolyte imbalances, **Reye syndrome**, congenital **myopathy**, Werdnig-Hoffman disease and **Leigh disease** should be considered in infants.

A definitive diagnosis can be made by detecting the toxin in serum samples, or isolating *C. botulinum* from stool or wound specimens. Toxins can be detected with a mouse neutralization assay, or using PCR or ELISA protocols.

Treatment

Because of the threat of respiratory complications, patients should be hospitalized immediately and closely monitored. Mechanical ventilation should begin when the vital capacity falls below 30% of predicted. Trivalent (types A, B and E) equine antitoxin should be administered as soon as botulism is suspected to slow the progression of the illness and limit the duration of respiratory failure in critical cases. Caution should be exercised as approximately 9% of patients experience a hypersensitivity reaction. Due to the high incidence of side effects and anaphylaxis, infants should not receive equine antitoxin.

In 2003, the FDA approved an intravenously administered human botulism immune globulin for types A and B infant botulism.

Patients suffering from wound botulism should receive equine antitoxin and antibiotics such as penicillin.

Clinical Trials

As of early 2004, there was one open clinical trial for infant botulism at the National Institutes of Health (NIH), to assess the safety and efficacy of human botulism immune globulin.

Prognosis

Prompt diagnosis and treatment coupled with improved respiratory care have decreased mortality from food-borne botulism. Severe cases often call for prolonged respiratory support. The case-fatality rate is 7.5%, although mortality is greater in patients older than 60 years. Infant botulism has an excellent prognosis, although relapse can occur following hospital discharge. The case-fatality rate for infant botulism is 2%. Because toxin binding is irreversible, acetylocholine release and strength return only after the nerve terminals sprout new endings.

Resources

BOOKS

Ashbury, A. K., G. M. McKhann, W. I. McDonald, et al., eds. *Diseases of the Nervous System: Clinical Neuroscience and Therapeutic Principles,* Third Edition. Cambridge University Press, 2002.

Ford, M. D., D. A. Delaney, L. J. Ling, and T. Erickson, eds. *Clinical Toxicology.* New York: W. B. Saunders Company, 2001.

PERIODICALS

Cox, M., and R. Hinkle. "Infant Botulism." *American Family Physician* 65 (April 1, 2002): 1388-92.

Shapiro, R. L., C. Hatheway, and D. L. Swerdlow. "Botulism in the United States: A Clinical and Epidemiologic Review." *Annals of Internal Medicine* 129 (August 1988): 221-228.

OTHER

Abrutyn, Elias. "Chapter 144: Botulism." *Harrison's Online.* McGraw Hill, 2001. <http://www.harrisonsonline.com>.

"Gastroenteritis Topics: Botulism," Section 3, chapter 28. In *The Merck Manual of Diagnosis and Therapy*, edited by TK. Merck & Co. Inc. 2004. <http://www.merck.com>.

World Health Organization. *Botulism.* Fact Sheet No. 270. <http://www.who.int/mediacentre/facsheets/who270.html>.

Hannah M. Hoag, MSc

Braces *see* **Assistive mobile devices**

Brachial plexitis neuritis *see* **Parsonage-Turner syndrome**

Brachial plexus injuries

Definition

Brachial plexus injuries affect the nerves that originate from the spinal cord behind the head and neck (cervical nerves).

Description

The brachial plexus are nerves that leave the cervical vertebrae (but originate in the brain) and extend to peripheral structures (muscles/organs) to transmit motor and sensory nerve impulses. The brachial plexus consists of several cervical nerve roots, which include: C4, sending fibers to the shoulder and trapezius muscle; C5, sending fibers to the deltoid muscle and sides of upper arm or distal radius and involved with shoulders abduction; C6, involved with elbow flexion and fibers in the biceps and lateral forearm and thumb; C7, fibers to the triceps muscle, index and middle finger tips and involved with elbow extension; and C8, involved with extension of thumb and 4th and 5th fingers. Injury to the brachial plexus can involve avulsion injuries (nerve torn from attachment to the spinal cord), which are the most serious type of injury; neuroma injuries, due to injury causing scar formation tissue, which compresses nerves; rupture injuries, nerve is torn, but not at the spinal cord; and stretch injuries, nerve is damaged, but not torn.

Sports related injuries to the the cervical spine are common, especially injury to cervical vertebra 5 (C5) and

Key Terms

Axonotmesis   Loss of the protective sheet of tissue that covers the axon (the part of the nerve cell which carries a transmission).

Biceps muscle   Muscle in the arm which helps to flex the arm.

Breech presentation   Buttocks presentation during delivery.

Deltoid muscle   A muscle near the clavicle bone which is responsible for arm movement.

Dysesthesias   A burning pain sensation.

Elbow extension   Movement away from the body at a jointed point.

Erb point   A point 2–3 centimeters above the clavicle.

Flail   To swing freely.

Lateral flexion   To flex toward a side.

Paresthesias   Abnormality of sensation (e.g., numbness, burning, tingling).

Pronation   The motion of the forearm to turn the palm downwards.

Shoulder dystocia   Difficult shoulder delivery.

Trapezius muscle   Muscle in the scapula, which helps in elevation of the scapula.

Vertex presentation   Head presentation during delivery.

C6. Erb described this condition with paralysis in 1874. Other names for the disorder include "burner" or "stinger" syndrome and cervical nerve pinch syndrome. Traumatic sports injury to the brachial plexus is characterized by a classical symptom—burning sensation that radiates down an upper extremity. The sensation may be short lived (2 minutes) or in chronic cases may last as long as two weeks. There are three common mechanisms that cause BPI, which include: direct impact to Erb point resulting in brachial plexus compression; traction caused by lateral flexion opposite from affected side; and **nerve compression** caused by hyperextension of the neck.

Obstetrical brachial plexus paralysis (OBPP) refers to injury to all or part of the brachial plexus during delivery. The condition was first described by Smellie in 1764 who described bilateral (both arms) paralysis in the newborn. Klumpke described paralysis (of the lower plexus) in 1885. Erb described paralysis of the upper brachial plexus (upper C5-C6 nerve damage) in 1874. Lower brachial plexus injuries are called Klumpke palsies and upper brachial plexus injury are termed Erb palsies. Injury is rare but is more prevalent in neonates born by cesarean delivery.

Demographics

In the United States a true measurement of new and existing cases is undetermined largely due to the significant underreporting of injuries. Approximately 5% of all peripheral nerve injuries results from trauma to the brachial plexus. Research studies conducted on college football players reported approximately 45% to 65% experience BPI during their collegiate careers. Additionally,

it is estimated that there is an 87% recurrence rate. Estimates in other countries are not possible due to significant underreporting.

The incidence (number of new cases) of OBPP ranges from 0.2–4% of live births globally. The World Health Organization estimates the worldwide incidence is approximately 1–2%. In the United States it is rare and the incidence is 0.2% of live births. Every year 1–2 babies per 1000 live births are affected by obstetrical brachial nerve injury.

Causes and symptoms

BPI typically occurs as a result of a blow to the head, shoulder, and/or Erb point in an athlete during a contact sport. There are two grades of BPI. Grade 1 occurs when there is an interruption of nerve function due to demyelination. Muscle weakness is often detected soon after injury. Grade 2 describes more extensive damage to deeper and vital nerve areas (axons). Muscle weakness is often present and if persistent could mean a higher-grade lesion. Further tests for grade 2 BPI are indicated to fully assess the extent of nerve degeneration.

The causes of OBPP include shoulder dystocia, large birth weight, and breech delivery (vertex presentation accounts for 94–97% of cases). Maternal diabetes (mother has diabetes) is associated as a risk factor. Mothers who have had several children who were recorded to be large babies have an increased risk for delivering neonates with OBPP.

Commonly, affected athletes complain and describe burning and/or numbness in the neck, shoulder, or upper extremity (affected arm). Symptoms typically occur after a blow to the head or shoulder. These symptoms include burning sensation in the neck, **pain** in the neck, (also called **dysesthesias**), and a feeling of weakness or "heaviness" in the affected arm. Bilateral (on both arms) numbness possibly indicates a more severe form of cervical cord injury. Symptoms can last from a few seconds to weeks.

Infants affected by OBPI may present with flail arms at birth. The affected arm may be internally rotated and pronated and devoid of elbow and shoulder movement (Erb palsy). If brachial plexus paralysis is present the entire hand and arm is flail with no movement ability.

The symptoms of OBPP can be grouped according to Sunderland's classification, which was proposed in 1951. A first-degree injury (also called neuropraxia or "stretch injuries") involves nerve injury that can completely resolve within 12 weeks. A second-degree injury results in severe trauma and nerve compression, but essential nerve elements are still intact and complete recovery is expected. A third-degree nerve injury is more severe, and essential nerve structures have been damaged as well as possible muscle damage. Some nerves and muscles may be permanently damaged. A fourth-degree injury results from extensive nerve damage that affects muscles, and typically it requires corrective surgical repair. The most severe form of obstetrical brachial plexus injury is fifth-degree injury, which is complete transaction of the nerve (the nerve is completely cut).

Diagnosis

A careful history, physical examination, and testing are essential for diagnosis. The clinician must suspect cervical fracture and/or **spinal cord injury** in an athlete presenting with altered consciousness. If the patient is awake and alert a complete neurological examination is indicated. The patient's mental status should be immediately assessed. Cervical nerve root assessment for detection of motor and sensory deficits is essential. A special test called the Spurling test is performed. During the Spurling test, the cervical spine is extended and head rotated toward the affected shoulder while loading axial weight. The purpose of manipulating the neck in this fashion is to reproduce the symptoms of the BPI. A positive Spurling test will reproduce symptoms. Clinical examination on-site at the time of injury typically includes; grip strength, identification of specific symptoms, duration of symptoms; assessment of motor impairment; assessment of cervical range of motion (only if no cervical fracture is present). Lab tests are generally not required and imaging studies are routinely limited to radiographic (x-ray) studies, taken from different views. Higher resolution studies such as **MRI** and **CT scans** can be utilized in cases where cervical spine or cervical nerve root damage is suspected. Use of a special test

to detect the extent of muscle damage (**electromyography**) can help to localize lesions and confirm the diagnosis. No specific lab tests are useful in the diagnostic process.

For infants with BPI due to delivery complications an assessment scale called the Active Movement Scale (7-point scale) can determine impairment from no contraction to full motion in the absence of or against gravity. This scale can help to assess arm movement impairment caused by nerve damage. The extent of nerve damage can be classified according to Sunderland. Typically, a lack of clinical evidence of elbow flexion by the 3rd or 4th month of life is indication for surgical repair of damaged nerves.

Treatment team

The treatment team for sports-related BPI typically includes the immediate responders (coach, team physician). Further consults from a comprehensive team can include a primary care practitioner, **neurologist**, physical therapist, and possibly a medical pain specialist.

For patients with OBPP a complete team of special nursing care and specialists is usually indicated. For surgical candidates, a specialist in neurosurgery or an orthopedic spine surgeon is essential. The pediatrician and pediatric neurologist play a vital role in assessment and provide information to parents. Long-term rehabilitation may be necessary in severe cases.

Treatment

On-site treatment for sports-related BPI typically includes mobilization and icing of the affected region. Treatment of BPI can be divided into three phases: the acute phase, recovery phase, and maintenance phases. Treatment during the acute phase typically involves physical therapy and medical issues (i.e., further imaging studies). Surgery may be required. During the recovery phases, physical therapy continues and the patient is monitored to continue follow-up care. During the maintenance phase of treatment physical therapy continues. The goal for medication is to prevent complications and help alleviate pain. Typically analgesics such as the anti-inflammatory type or an opiate narcotic are recommended. Analgesia may also help the affected person to cope better with physical therapy sessions. Typical opiate-narcotics include Lortab, Norcet, or Vicodin. Nonsteroidal anti-inflammatory drugs (NSAIDs, e.g., Motrin, Ibuprin) have both anti-inflammatory and analgesic effects.

For infants with OBPI medical treatment initially focuses on protection of ligaments, joints, and tendons from stress. Physical therapy may be indicated for movement exercises. Surgical intervention may be necessary if patients do not show recovery of neurological function by four months of age. Some controversy exists in the United States, with some surgeons advocating surgery on patients younger than 4 months.

Recovery and rehabilitation

Rehabilitation for BPI primarily entails physical therapy (PT) during the entire treatment course (acute, recovery, and maintenance treatment phases). The focus of PT during the acute phases primarily involves early mobilization and icing. Patients attempt to improve cervical range of motion to strengthen cervical muscles. During the recovery phases, special PT programs attempt to strengthen cervical muscles to a level of performance prior to injury. Special focus on muscles supporting the injured brachial plexus nerve (i.e., cervical and shoulder regions) is emphasized. Treatment for the maintenance phases primarily focuses on continuation of cervical muscle strength and conditioning. Clinical findings during examination and testing are key factors for determining return to play and recovery. A full recovery of affected muscle is necessary to prevent recurrence of burner syndrome and further injury. An athlete in a contact sport, who has fully recovered, is capable of supporting his or her weight at the neck leaning at a 45 degree angle. Some athletes may have some asymmetry of affected muscles that persists, and care should be taken as the athlete returns to contact sport participation.

Most infants with OBPI spontaneously recover (92-95% of reported cases) because the nerve injury is usually minor. Initial rehabilitation can include physical therapy to maintain passive range of movement. Surgery may be necessary for severe cases that require special postoperative care, monitoring, and physical therapy. Recovery for children with OBPP depends on the severity of nerve injury. Recovery after surgery is variable given that results depend on extent of damage to nerves and successful repair if surgery is indicated.

Prognosis

Prognosis for sports-related BPI is generally good. Some athletes develop a chronic complicated condition with symptoms called chronic burner syndrome. Most cases of nerve injury in infants are self-limiting and spontaneously resolve. Severe cases may require surgery. Surgical candidates typically have severe nerve injury and must undergo microsurgery to repair nerve damage.

Special concerns

In sports-related injury medical/legal problems can exist because cervical spine injury is sometimes not considered the cause of symptoms. Overlooking BPI can result in further damage to peripheral nerves.

Resources

PERIODICALS

Clancy, W. G. "Upper Trunk brachial plexus injuries in contact sports." *American Journal of Sport Medicine* 5, no. 5 (1977).

WEBSITES

Brachial plexus injury. <http://www.mayoclinic.org>.
Brachial plexus injury. <http://www.cincinnatichildrens.org>.

Laith Farid Gulli, M.D.
Robert Ramirez, D.O.

Brain aneurysm *see* **Aneurysm**

Brain biopsy *see* **Biopsy**

Brain injury *see* **Traumatic brain injury, Spinal cord injury**

Brain surgery *see* **Craniotomy**

Brain tumors *see* **Brain and spinal tumors**

Brain anatomy

Definition

The brain is a large mass of soft nervous tissue made up of both neurons and supporting glial cells lying within the cranium of the skull. The brain contains both gray and white matter. Gray matter is primarily nerve cell bodies, whereas white matter contains myelinated nerve cell processes, giving it a white appearance. White matter is mostly found in the cortex (shell) of the cerebral hemispheres. The brain has a highly complex appearance, with convolutions referred to as gyri and valleys referred to as sulci. These convolutions create a greater surface area within the same size skull.

Description

Central nervous system

The **central nervous system** is made up of the brain and spinal cord. The major divisions of the human brain are the brainstem, **cerebellum**, **diencephalon**, and cerebral hemispheres. The **meninges** cover and protect the brain and spinal cord.

BRAINSTEM The brainstem, made up of the midbrain, pons, and medulla, sits at the base of the brain. The brainstem is involved in sensory input and motor output. Sensory input enters the brainstem from the head, neck, and face area, while motor output from the brainstem controls muscle movements in these areas as well. The brainstem also receives sensory input from specialized cranial

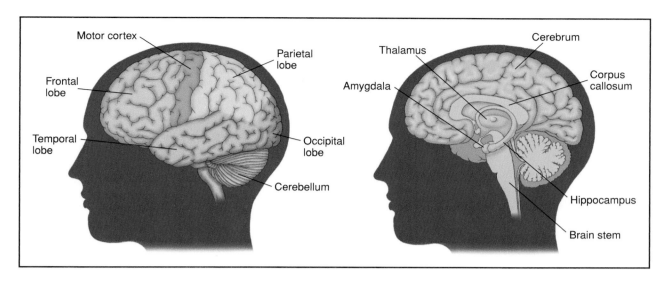

Anatomy of the brain. The exterior view on the left shows the lobes, and the interior view on the right shows other major areas and structures. *(Illustration by Frank Forney.)*

nerves for olfaction (smell), vision, hearing, gustation (taste), and balance. The brainstem contains ascending and descending nerve pathways that carry sensory input and motor output information to and from higher brain regions, like a relay center. Ascending nerve pathways bring information through the brainstem into the rest of the brain, and descending nerve pathways send information back that coordinates many activities, including motor function. The brainstem also plays a role in vital functions such as cardiovascular and respiratory activity and consciousness.

The medulla is a structure in the brainstem closest to the spinal cord. It is vaguely scoop shaped, with longitudinal grooves indicating the presence of many nerve tracts. It is responsible for maintaining vital body functions such as breathing and heart rate.

The pons is named after the Latin word for bridge. In appearance, the pons seems to be a bridge connecting the two hemispheres, but in reality the connection is indirect through a complicated nerve pathway. The pons is involved in motor control, sensory analysis, and levels of consciousness and sleep. Some structures within the pons are linked to the cerebellum, involving them in movement and posture.

The midbrain, also called the mesencephalon, is the smallest and most anterior part of the brainstem with a tubular appearance. It is involved in functions such as vision, hearing, movement of the eyes, and body motor function. The anterior part of the midbrain contains the cerebral peduncle, a large bundle of axons traveling from the cerebral cortex through the brainstem. These nerve fibers (along with other structures) are important for voluntary motor function.

CEREBELLUM The cerebellum, or "little brain," wraps around the brainstem. It is similar to the cerebrum in that it has two hemispheres with a highly folded surface (cortex). The cerebellum is involved in regulation and coordination of movement, posture, balance, and also some cognitive function.

DIENCEPHALON The diencephalon, or "between brain," lies between the cerebral hemispheres and the midbrain. It is formed by the thalamus and hypothalamus, and has connections to the limbic system and cerebral hemispheres.

The thalamus is a large body of gray matter at the top of the diencephalon, positioned deep within the forebrain. The thalamus has sensory and motor functions. Almost all sensory information enters this structure, where it is relayed to the cortex. Axons, or nerve endings, from every sensory system except olfaction come together (synapse) here as the last relay site before the information reaches the cerebral cortex. The synapse is the junction where nerve endings meet and communicate with each other using chemical messengers that cross the junction.

The hypothalamus is a part of the diencephalon lying next to the thalamus. The hypothalamus is involved in homeostasis, emotional responses, coordinating drive-related behavior such as thirst and hunger, circadian rhythms, control of the autonomic nervous system, and control of the pituitary gland.

MENINGES AND VENTRICULAR SYSTEMS The meninges are membranes that cover and protect the central nervous system (CNS) along with a fluid called cerebrospinal fluid (CSF) that buoys up the brain. The brain is very soft and mushy; without the meninges and CSF, it

Key Terms

Dorsal Pertaining in direction to the back or upper surface of an organ.

Endothelium A layer of cells called endothelial cells that lines the inside surfaces of body cavities, blood vessels, and lymph vessels.

Glial cell Nerve tissue of the central nervous system other than the signal-transmitting neurons. Glial cells are interspersed between neurons and providing support and insulation. There are three main types of neuroglia: astrocytes, oligodendrocytes, and microglia.

Myelin A white, fatty substance that covers and protects nerves.

Neuron A cell specialized to conduct and generate electrical impulses and to carry information from one part of the brain to another.

Ventral Pertaining in direction to the front or lower surface of an organ.

would be easily distorted and torn under the effects of gravity. The meninges are divided into three membranes: the thick external dura mater provides mechanical strength; the middle web-like, delicate arachnoid mater forms a protective barrier and a space for CSF circulation; and the internal pia mater is continuous with all the contours of the brain and forms CSF. The dura mater contains six major venous sinuses that drain the cerebral veins and several smaller sinuses.

Dural venous sinuses are formed in areas where the two layers of the dura mater separate, forming spaces. The sinuses are triangular in cross-section and lined with endothelium. There are six major dural sinuses that receive cerebral veins. The superior sagittal sinus, straight sinus, and right and left transverse sinuses meet in a structure known as the confluence of the sinuses. Venous blood circulation follows a pathway through the superior sagittal and straight sinuses into the confluence, and then through the transverse sinuses. Each transverse sinus then continues as a sigmoid sinus, carrying the venous blood flow along an S-shaped course until it empties into the internal jugular vein. The major dural sinuses also connect with several smaller sinuses. The inferior sagittal sinus, occipital sinus, and superior and inferior petrosal sinuses all empty into different parts of the major sinus system.

The arachnoid mater follows the general shape of the brain, creating a space between the two membranes. The space between the arachnoid and pia mater is called the

subarachnoid space and contains CSF. CSF enters venous circulation through small protrusions into the venous sinus called arachnoid villi. The pia mater forms part of the choroid plexus, a highly convoluted and vascular membranous material that lies within the **ventricular system** of the brain and is responsible for most CSF production.

The brain contains four ventricles. A pair of long, C-shaped lateral ventricles lies within the cerebral hemispheres. The lateral ventricles communicate with the narrow, slit-shaped third ventricle of the diencephalon. The third ventricle then communicates with the tent-shaped fourth ventricle of the pons and medulla, which protrudes into the cerebellum. The CSF of the brain flows in a specific pattern that allows newly formed CSF to replace the old CSF several times a day. The basic pattern of circulation is formation in lateral ventricles, flow into the third and then fourth ventricles, into basal cisterns, up and over the cerebral hemispheres, into the arachnoid villi, where drainage occurs into a venous sinus to return to the venous system. Some CSF diverts from the basal cisterns into the subarachnoid space of the spinal cord. Blockage of the circulation of CSF can cause a condition called **hydrocephalus**, where the CSF pressure rises high enough to expand the ventricles at the sacrifice of the surrounding brain. Blockage of CSF circulation can occur at any point in the pathway. Hydrocephalus conditions are divided into two types, communicating and noncommunicating. The classification depends on whether both lateral ventricles are in communication with the subarachnoid space. Non-communicating hydrocephalus involves blockage in the ventricular system, which prevents the flow of CSF to the subarachnoid space. Tumors sometimes cause hydrocephalus, through instigating either overproduction or physical obstruction of CSF. CSF circulation may also be obstructed in the subarachnoid space by adhesions that form as a result of meningitis.

CEREBRAL HEMISPHERES The cerebral hemispheres are made up of the cerebral cortex, hippocampus, and basal ganglia containing the amygdala of the limbic system. The cerebral hemispheres are divided by the inter-hemispheric fissure and are involved in higher motor functions, perception, cognition (pertaining to thought and reasoning), emotion, and memory. The cerebral cortex is divided into four major lobes. The frontal lobe contains the primary motor cortex and premotor area involved in voluntary movement, Broca's area involved in writing and speech, and the prefrontal cortex involved in personality, insight, and foresight. The parietal lobe contains the primary somatosensory cortex involved in tactile and positioning information, while remaining sections are involved in spatial orientation and language comprehension. The temporal lobe contains the primary auditory cortex, Wernicke's area involved in language comprehension, and areas involved in the higher processing of visual input, along with aspects of learning and memory associated with the limbic system. The occipital lobe contains the primary visual cortex and the visual association cortex.

The limbic lobe is a subdivision consisting of portions of the frontal, parietal, and temporal lobes that form a continuous band called the limbic system.

The limbic system, buried within the cerebrum, is also referred to as the "emotional brain." It includes the thalamus, hypothalamus, amygdala, and hippocampus. Through these structures, the limbic system is involved in drive-related behavior, memory, and emotional responses such as feeding, defense, and sexual behavior. The thalamus and hypothalamus are parts of the diencephalon, while the amygdala and hippocampus are parts of the cerebral hemispheres.

The left and right cerebral hemispheres are not equal in their functionality. In the human brain, the left hemisphere is more important for the production and comprehension of language than the right hemisphere. Damage to the left hemisphere is more likely to cause language deficits than damage to the right hemisphere. Because of this variation in hemisphere contribution, the left hemisphere is most commonly referred to as the dominant hemisphere and the right hemisphere is referred to as the nondominant hemisphere. Nearly all right-handed people and most left-handed people have a left-dominant brain. However, some people have a right-dominant brain or comparable language representation in both hemispheres.

The hippocampus is a curved sheet of cortex folded in the basal medial part of the temporal lobe. It is divided into three multilayered sections, the dentate gyrus, hippocampus proper, and the subiculum acting as a transitional zone between the two. The dentate gyrus receives input from the cortex, and sends output to the hippocampus proper. The hippocampus proper then sends output to the subiculum, which is the principal source of hippocampal output. The hippocampus, referred to as the gateway to memory, is involved in learning and memory functions. The hippocampus converts short-term memory to more permanent memory, is involved in the storage and retrieval of long-term memory, and recalling learned spatial associations.

The basal ganglia are masses of gray matter located deep in the cerebral hemispheres. The basal ganglia contain the corpus striatum, which is involved mostly in motor activity. The striatum is the major point of entry into basal ganglia circuitry, receiving input from almost all cortical areas. It is subdivided into three further divisions called the caudate nucleus, putamen, and globus pallidus. The caudate nucleus is involved more with cognitive function than with motor function. Of all the striatum subdivisions, the putamen is the most highly associated with motor functions of the basal ganglia. The globus pallidus is a wedge-shaped section of the striatum responsible for most basal

ganglia output. The basal ganglia also contain the amygdala, a portion of the limbic system involved in memory, emotion, and fear. The amygdala lies beneath the surface of the temporal lobe where it causes a bulge called the uncus. The basal ganglia collectively modulate the output of the frontal cortex involving motor function, but also cognition and motivation.

SPINAL CORD The spinal cord is a cord-like bundle of nerves comprising a major part of the central nervous system, which conducts sensory and motor nerve impulses to and from the brain and the periphery. It is a long tube-like structure extending from the base of the brain, through a string of skeletal vertebrae, to the small of the back. The spinal cord is continuous with the brainstem, and like the brain, it is encased in a triple sheath of membranes. Thirty-one pairs of spinal nerves belonging to the **peripheral nervous system** (PNS) arise from the sides of the spinal cord and branch out to both sides of the body. In addition to carrying impulses to and from the brain, the spinal cord regulates reflexes. Reflexes produce a rapid motor response to a stimulus because the sensory neuron synapses directly with the motor neuron in the spinal cord, so the impulse does not need to travel to and from the brain.

NERVOUS TRACTS Tracts are groups or bundles of nerve fibers that constitute an anatomical and functional unit. Commissural tracts such as the corpus callosum connect the two cerebral hemispheres. Association tracts make connections within the same hemisphere. Projection tracts connect the brain with the spinal cord. Sensory tracts project upward from the spinal cord into regions of the brain, bringing sensory input from the periphery via ascending pathways. Motor tracts project down from the brain into the spinal cord, bringing motor output information to the periphery via descending pathways. The internal capsule is the major structure carrying ascending and descending nerve projection fibers to and from the cerebral cortex. It is a curved, funnel-shaped group of cortical projection fibers divided into five regions, based on each region's relationship to the putamen and globus pallidus of the striatum.

Peripheral nervous system

The peripheral nervous system (PNS) is all of the nervous system outside the brain and spinal cord, including the spinal and cranial nerves. The PNS is divided into the somatic and autonomic subdivisions. The somatic nervous system, regulating activities that are under conscious control such as the voluntary movement of skeletal muscles, includes the spinal and cranial nerves and peripheral sensory receptors. Peripheral neurons that transmit information from the periphery toward the CNS are called afferent neurons, whereas those that transmit information away from the CNS toward the periphery are called efferent neurons.

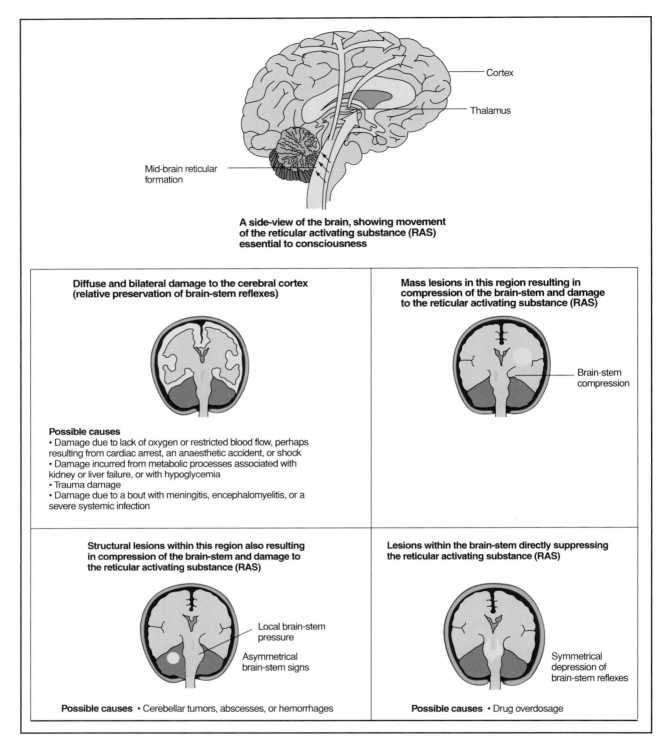

Cortex

Thalamus

Mid-brain reticular formation

A side-view of the brain, showing movement of the reticular activating substance (RAS) essential to consciousness

Diffuse and bilateral damage to the cerebral cortex (relative preservation of brain-stem reflexes)

Possible causes
• Damage due to lack of oxygen or restricted blood flow, perhaps resulting from cardiac arrest, an anaesthetic accident, or shock
• Damage incurred from metabolic processes associated with kidney or liver failure, or with hypoglycemia
• Trauma damage
• Damage due to a bout with meningitis, encephalomyelitis, or a severe systemic infection

Mass lesions in this region resulting in compression of the brain-stem and damage to the reticular activating substance (RAS)

Brain-stem compression

Structural lesions within this region also resulting in compression of the brain-stem and damage to the reticular activating substance (RAS)

Local brain-stem pressure

Asymmetrical brain-stem signs

Possible causes • Cerebellar tumors, abscesses, or hemorrhages

Lesions within the brain-stem directly suppressing the reticular activating substance (RAS)

Symmetrical depression of brain-stem reflexes

Possible causes • Drug overdosage

Diagram of the brain indicating sites and causes of possible damage. *(Illustration by Electronic Illustrators Group.)*

The 31 pairs of spinal nerves are each named according to the location of their respective vertebrae. Each spinal nerve consists of a dorsal root and a ventral root. The dorsal roots contain afferent neurons transmitting information to the CNS from various kinds of sensory neurons. The ventral roots contain the axons of efferent motor neurons transmitting information to the periphery. Information travels great distances via interneurons, which are neurons that connect neurons to each other. Spinal nerves have sensory fibers and motor fibers. The sensory fibers supply nerves to specific areas of skin, while the motor fibers supply nerves to specific muscles. A dermatome, which means "skin-cutting," is an area of skin supplied by nerve fibers originating from a single dorsal nerve root. The dermatomes are named with respect to the spinal nerves that supply them. Dermatomes form bands around the body. In the limbs, dermatome organization is more complex as a result of being "stretched out" during embryological development. There is a high degree of overlap of nerves between adjacent dermatomes. If one spinal nerve loses sensation from the dermatome that it supplies, compensatory overlap from adjacent spinal nerves occurs with reduced sensitivity. In addition to dermatomes supplying the skin, each muscle in the body is supplied by a particular level or segment of the spinal cord and by its corresponding spinal nerve. The muscle, in conjunction with its nerve, makes up a myotome. Although slight variations do exist, dermatome and myotome patterns of distribution are relatively consistent from person to person.

Cranial nerves also carry sensory information from the periphery to the brain, and motor information away from the brain to the periphery. Humans have 12 pairs of cranial nerves numbered by the level at which they enter the brain. Seven of the cranial nerves specialize in information about olfaction, vision, hearing, gustation, and balance. The other cranial nerves control eye and mouth movements, swallowing, and facial expressions. Cranial nerve X is called the vagus nerve; it has effects on visceral gut function and has the ability to slow the heart when stimulated through the parasympathetic nervous system.

The autonomic nervous system includes further sympathetic, parasympathetic, and enteric subdivisions. The autonomic nervous system regulates activities that are not under conscious control but rather are involuntary, such as contractions of the heart and digestion of food. The autonomic nervous system is involved in maintaining homeostasis in the body. The sympathetic and parasympathetic subdivisions of the autonomic nervous system have opposite effects on the organs they control. Most organs controlled by the autonomic nervous system are under the influence of both the sympathetic and parasympathetic nervous systems, which strike a balance with each other to maintain proper body function. The sympathetic nervous system generally stimulates organs, whereas the parasympathetic nervous system generally suppresses organ function or slows it down. An example of this coordination of activity is seen in the fight-or-flight response, which is the body's response to a sudden threatening or stressful situation in which excessive energy is needed to either deal with such an attack or run from it. In the fight-or-flight response, both the sympathetic and parasympathetic nervous

systems work in coordination with each other to produce the appropriate results. The sympathetic and parasympathetic nervous systems increase blood pressure and heart rate and slow digestion to enable the physical exertion necessary to respond to the threatening circumstance.

The digestive system contains its own, local nervous system referred to as the enteric, or intrinsic, nervous system. The enteric nervous system is extremely complex and contains as many neurons as does the spinal cord. The enteric nervous system is divided into two networks, or plexuses, of neurons, both of which are embedded in the walls of the digestive tract and extend from the esophagus to the anus. The myenteric plexus is located between the longitudinal and circular layers of muscle in the tunica muscularis and is involved in digestive tract motility. The submucous plexus lies buried in the submucosa. Its principal role is regulating gastrointestinal blood flow and controlling epithelial cell function in response to the environment within the lumen. In regions where these functions are minimal, such as the esophagus, the submucous plexus is sparse. The enteric nervous system functions independently from other nervous systems, but normal digestive function requires communication between the enteric system, other PNS systems, and the CNS. Stimulation of the sympathetic nervous system causes inhibition of gastrointestinal secretions and motor activity, while the parasympathetic nervous system stimulates the same functions. Parasympathetic and sympathetic fibers connect either the central and enteric nervous systems or connect the CNS directly within the digestive tract. In this manner, the digestive system provides sensory information to the CNS, and the CNS is involved in gastrointestinal function. The CNS can also relay input from outside of the digestive system to the digestive system. An example is the sight or smell of food stimulating stomach secretions.

Resources

BOOKS

Nolte, John, PhD. *The Human Brain: An Introduction to Its Functional Anatomy.* St. Louis, MO: Mosby, Inc., 2002.

Thomas, Clayton L., MD, MPH, ed. *Taber's Cyclopedic Medical Dictionary.* Philadelphia, PA: F. A. Davis Company, 1993.

Zigmond, Michael J., PhD, Floyd E. Bloom, MD, Story C. Landis, PhD, James L. Roberts, PhD, and Larry R. Squire, PhD, eds. *Fundamental Neuroscience.* New York: Academic Press, 1999.

WEBSITES

Serendip. *Brain Structures and Their Functions.* (March 30, 2004.) <http://serendip.brynmawr.edu>.

Adjunct College Waguespack Seminars and Workshops. *Brain Functions.* (March 30, 2004.) <http://www.adjunct college.com>.

Maria Basile, PhD

Brain and spinal tumors

Definition

A brain tumor is an abnormal growth of cells (neoplasm) in the skull. A spinal tumor is a growth associated with the spinal cord. Tumors are classified as noncancerous tumors (benign tumors) or cancerous tumors (malignant tumors).

Description

Because the skull is a rigid structure that limits expansion, tumors (both benign and malignant) can exert destructive pressure on neural and support tissues. Although all brain tumors are contained within the rigid skull, tumors can exist within brain tissue (intracranial tumors) or as tumors associated with the outer surface of the brain.

Primary tumors

Tumors that initially arise and grow within the brain are termed primary tumors. Most adult brain cancers are not primary tumors, but are the result of primary cancer that has spread from other areas of the body. Most brain tumors in children, however, are primary tumors. The cells that nourish and support the neurons that compose the brain are most often those cells that exhibit the uninhibited division and growth that results in primary tumor formation. A glioma is a tumor that originates in the cells supporting and nourishing brain neural tissue (glial cells). The most common primary brain tumors include gliomas such as astrocytomas, ependymomas, and oligodendrogliomas.

Primary tumors are sometimes associated with specific genetic diseases such as **tuberous sclerosis** or **neurofibromatosis**. Tumors can also arise following exposure to a sufficient dosage to carcinogens (cancer-causing chemical substances) or nuclear **radiation**.

The most observed form of primary brain tumor found in adults within the general population are diffuse fibrillary astrocytomas that are then divided on the basis of microscopic examination of the tissue (histopathologic diagnosis) into three specific WHO (World Health Organization) grades of malignancy: grade II astrocytomas, grade III anaplastic astrocytomas, and grade IV glioblastoma multiform.

Pilocytic astrocytomas are the most common astrocytic tumors found in children. Desmoplastic cerebral astrocytoma of infancy (DCAI) and desmoplastic infantile ganglioglioma (DIGG) are present as large, superficial, usually benign astrocytomas that most commonly affect children under the age of two years.

Other gliomas and astrocytomas include brainstem gliomas (usually found in children) that are a form of diffuse, fibrillary astrocytoma that often follow a malignant course. The pleomorphic xanthoastrocytomas (PXA) are low-grade astrocytic tumors that are often found in young adults.

Subependymal giant cell astrocytomas (SEGA) are a form of periventricular, astrocytic tumor that are usually benign or low grade.

Other benign tumors include meningioma tumors (a fairly common, usually benign class of intracranial tumor affecting the **meninges**), epidermoid tumors, dermoid tumors, hemangioblastomas (usually benign tumors that occur most frequently in the **cerebellum** and spinal cord of young adults), colloid cysts, pleomorphic xanthoastrocytomas, craniopharyngiomas, and schwannomas. Schwannomas are not strictly a brain or spinal tumor because they arise on peripheral nerves—but they do grow on cranial nerves, particularly the vestibular portion of the acoustic nerve.

Other tumor forms related to diffuse, fibrillary astrocytomas include oligodendrogliomas and oligoastrocytomas. These cerebral tumors are, however, less common than astrocytomas.

Ependymoma tumors are gliomas that are unpredictable. Ependymomas found in the ventricles can be aggressive and highly destructive; other ependymomas are benign spinal cord tumors. Transformation of ependymomas to more malignant forms is rare.

Key Terms

Benign Non-cancerous.

Carcinogen A substance known to cause cancer.

Glioma A tumor that originates in the cells supporting and nourishing brain neural tissue (glial cells).

Neoplasm An abnormal growth of tissue or cells (a tumor) that may be either malignant (cancerous) or benign.

Metastasis The spread of cancer from one part of the body to another. Cells in the metastatic (secondary) tumor are like those in the original (primary) tumor.

Myelogram An x-ray exam of the spinal cord, nerves, and other tissues within the spinal cord that are highlighted by injected contrast dye.

Primary tumor Abnormal growths that originated in the location where they have are diagnosed.

Tumorigenesis Formation of tumors.

Tumors of the choroid plexus tumors are also unpredictable. Occurring in the choroids plexus that line most of the **ventricular system**, they can result in the overproduction of cerebrospinal fluid. As with ependymomas, some are malignant, while others are benign.

Other tumors that are usually malignant include medulloblastomas (a highly malignant tumor usually found in children), atypical meningiomas, and hemangiopericytomas (tumors of the dura that may become aggressive and metastasize.)

Brain and spinal tumors are sometimes associated with diseases or disorders. For example, multiple hemangioblastomas are associated with **von Hippel-Lindau disease** (VHL), an inherited tumor syndrome. Neurological tumor syndromes are those in which patients are genetically predisposed and, therefore, at an increased risk for developing multiple tumors of the nervous system.

Demographics

Brain and spinal tumors occur in people of all races and sexes, but are slightly more common in Caucasian people than other races. About 40,000 people are diagnosed with a brain tumor each year in the United States. Overall, brain tumors tend to occur more frequently in males than females. Meningiomas, however, occur more frequently in females. Most brain tumors occur in people over 70 years of age, and most brain tumors in childhood occur before age eight. Brain and spinal cord tumors in children are the second most common form of childhood cancer, with about 1,500 children developing these tumors each year. Family history may be predictive, especially with regard to chromosomal abnormalities or changes that may result in the loss of tumor suppressor genes. People with family members who have glioma may be at higher risk of developing a brain tumor.

Long-term exposure to certain chemicals may increase the risk of developing a brain tumor. People exposed to acrylonitrile and vinyl chloride while manufacturing some textiles and plastics, pathologists exposed to formaldehyde, and workers in the nuclear industry may all be at higher risk of developing malignant brain tumors.

Almost 10,000 Americans are diagnosed each year with a spinal cord tumor. Primary spinal cord tumors are rare; most are the result of metastasis (spread) from another site of primary cancer in the body. Most primary spinal tumors are not malignant, but as they occupy space surrounding the spinal cord, they may cause **pain** and disability.

Causes and symptoms

With the exception of a few genetic syndromes associated with tumors of the brain and spinal cord, the cause of primary nervous system tumors remains a mystery. As most malignant brain tumors are secondary tumors that result from primary cancer that has spread from elsewhere in the body, factors known to influence the development of other cancers, such as smoking, may be considered related causes.

Although not all of the molecular mechanisms are fully understood, there have been dramatic advances in understanding the causes of the cellular transformations of normal healthy cells into tumor cells (tumorigenesis) within the brain.

Present molecular models identify specific genes that play a role regulating the cell cycle and that data indicate that they play a role suppressing tumor growth (tumor suppressor genes such as the p53 gene). Damage to the gene or loss of the chromosome on which it resides (chromosome 17) correlates to the initiation of astrocytoma tumorigenesis. Oncogenic viruses that interfere with tumor suppressor genes have also been linked to tumor formation. More research is needed into the mechanisms of tumor cell transformation before a definitive link can be established.

Other potential causes of brain or spinal cord tumor development under investigation include head injury, occupational exposure to chemicals, and viruses. Additionally, scientists continue to research the possibility of a relationship between cell phone use and malignant tumors of the **central nervous system**. As of mid-2004, no relationship has yet been established between cell phone use and increased rates of brain cancer.

Symptoms of brain tumors include headaches, nausea, vomiting, **seizures**, and disturbances in vision and hearing that cannot be related to a disorder of the external sensory organs. Changes in personality and developmental problems, motor problems, and balance problems are also characteristic of tumors.

Spinal cord tumor symptoms often include pain, invalid sensory inputs such as numbness in the toes, feet, or legs, and motor coordination problems.

Diagnosis

Brain and spinal tumors may be diagnosed by a combination of neurological examination and imaging such as **magnetic resonance imaging (MRI)** scans, computed tomography (**CT**) **scans**, and **positron emission tomography (PET)**. Other diagnostic tests include laboratory tests (including blood and spinal fluid analysis), myelography, radionucleotide bone scan, **biopsy**, and microscopic examination of tissues.

Brain and spinal tumors are usually confirmed by computerized axial tomography (CAT) scan, or via the more accurate MRI or PET scans.

MRI scans provide the ability to image and anatomically pinpoint tumors of the brain and spinal cord and thus

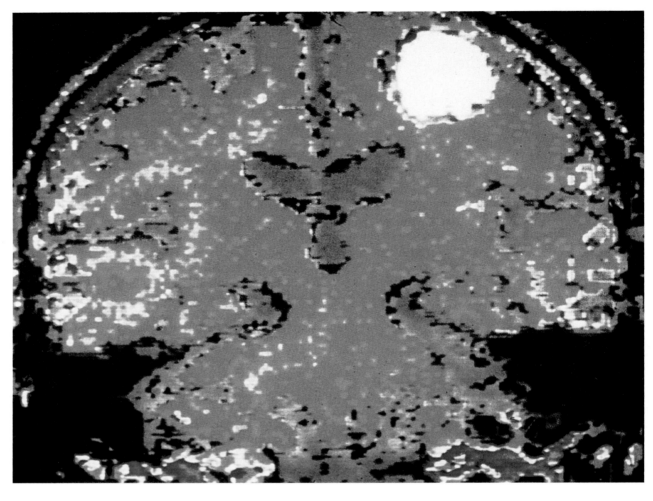

MRI of a brain tumor (the roundish white area). *(© Visuals Unlimited. Reproduced by permission.)*

provide accurate diagnosis without surgery. Both the MRI and CAT scans produce segmental images of the brain that allow physicians to determine the location and extent of tumors, as well as the extent of damage to neural or surrounding tissue. PET scans use a glucose-and-tracer mixture that is injected into the bloodstream to form a picture of metabolic activity of the brain. As tumor tissue uses more glucose than normal tissue, the tumor presents a brighter image than normal tissue in the picture generated by the scan.

At the tissue level, the presence of cell division at the time of histological examination (tissue exam) is indicative of a higher grade tumor. The greater the rate of mitotic activity (cell division), usually the greater potential for a tumor to advance to a higher and more dangerous type.

GBM tumors are characterized by densely packed cells and the highest high rates of mitotic division. Other tumors such as other gliomas and astrocytomas are diagnosed on the bases of histological examination.

Tumors of the human brain and spinal cord can also be differentiated based on molecular genetic studies that link specific changes in tumors to underlying chromosomal and gene changes (e.g., inactivation of a particular tumor suppressor gene).

Treatment team

In addition to the primary physician, neurologists, and neurosurgeons, treatment often involves oncologists, chemotherapists, and radiation oncologists who can assist the patient and family with treatment decisions. Physical, occupational, and respiratory therapists provide specialized care, as do nurses. Social service consultants coordinate hospital care and community support services.

Treatment

Treatment for brain and spinal tumors is specific to the type of tumor, location of the tumor, and general health of the patient. Surgery, radiation therapy, and chemotherapy, used alone or in combination, are the three procedures used most to combat brain and spinal cord tumors.

Surgery involves removing as much of the tumor as possible without damage to the surrounding tissues of the brain or spinal cord. Many benign tumors are encapsulated in sac-like membranes or are single structures that can be completely removed. Surgeons use specialized instrumentation and techniques to remove tumors that are irregularly shaped, near vital structures, or are almost inaccessible.

Stereotactic surgery allows surgeons access to tumors in areas of the brain that are difficult to reach. Using computer-assisted instrumentation, surgeons are guided by a three-dimensional map of the brain to remove tissue or implant radiation pellets into the tumor site. Ultrasonic aspirators break up tumor tissue using sound wave pulses, and the tumor fragments are then removed from the brain by suction.

Microsurgery involves a microscope that gives the surgeon a large view of the operative field in the brain or spinal cord. This reduces the possibility of removing surrounding tissue and injuring critical structures. Electrodes inserted into nerves during surgery evoke the potential, or demonstrate the role of specific nerves, thus guiding the surgeon to avoid damage.

Shunting devices are also placed to divert the blocked or excess flow of cerebrospinal fluid that sometimes occurs with a brain tumor. The ventriculoperitoneal shunt is most often used, and is placed in the ventricles of the brain to divert cerebrospinal fluid to the abdomen. Shunting is frequently required with brain tumors in children.

If the tumor is malignant or is in an area of the brain or spinal cord that would cause critical damage to the nervous system, radiation therapy, chemotherapy, or experimental therapies may be recommended. Radiation therapy involves beams of radiation that are aimed at tumor cells to kill them. Traditional radiation therapy is usually given in six-week courses, and involves some damage to surrounding tissues. Radiation therapy using gamma knife technology, also called stereotactic radiosurgery, is much more precise, and focuses approximately 200 beams of gamma radiation guided by MRI at precise points in the tumor simultaneously. Gamma knife technology reduces damage to surrounding tissues.

Chemotherapy drugs are usually given orally or are injected intravenously, and work to kill rapidly dividing cells. As cancer cells divide more rapidly than normal cells, chemotherapy drugs are effective in killing cancer cells. The side effects most associated with chemotherapy, including nausea, hair loss, and skin problems, result from normally dividing cells that are killed along with the cancer cells. Combination chemotherapy drugs are often prescribed for the treatment of brain tumors, such as BCNU and CCNU. Some of the latest chemotherapy modalities use wafers and pumps to deliver chemotherapy drugs directly into tumor tissue.

Steroids are also prescribed in treating brain or spinal cord tumors to reduce swelling the brain tissues. **Anticonvulsants** are given to control seizures. A number of other supportive measures are used to relieve pain and combat unwanted side effects of treatment such as medications used to reduce irritation and relieve nausea during radiation and chemotherapy.

Recovery and rehabilitation

After surgery and other treatments for a brain or spinal cord tumor, patients are monitored for recurrence of the tumor or new tumor growth on a regular basis. Initially, CT or MRI scans are done in periods ranging from one to three months. Later, scans are usually decreased to every six months.

Counseling and cognitive therapy can help with the memory problems and personality changes that some people experience after treatment for a brain tumor. Physical therapy and occupational therapy are useful after treatment for a spinal cord tumor to help with any deficits in mobility, reaching, and positioning. Speech therapists can help with challenges in communication. Physical changes in the structure of the brain after treatment may affect the way a child learns, and a **neuropsychologist** is often helpful in identifying weaknesses and compensation strategies to ease a child's return to school.

Clinical trials

Persons with recurrent tumors or tumors resistant to treatment are often offered participation in an experimental protocol or clinical trial. Experimental treatments include **gene therapy** that introduces substances into the brain tumor, changing the genetic makeup of the tumor cells. Another experimental therapy involves new forms of brachytherapy, where radioactive pellets are implanted directly into the tumor.

The scientific community continually conducts **clinical trials** in the effort to find new drugs and treatments that are effective against cancer, including those types most often occurring in the brain and spinal cord. As of mid-2004, the National Institutes of Health (NIH) and related agencies were sponsoring more than 200 ongoing studies and trials specific for the treatment of brain and spinal cord tumors. Updated information on these and other trials can be found at the NIH website for clinical trials at <http://www.clinicaltrials.gov>.

Prognosis

Symptoms of malignant brain and spinal cord tumors are usually progressive over time. Symptoms become more pronounced and troublesome as tumors invade or otherwise obstruct healthy tissue. Benign tumors can also cause severe dysfunction by placing pressure on surrounding vital structures, but with treatment, they have a more favorable prognosis.

The slowest growing and least serious of these tumor types, grade II astrocytomas (a "low grade" tumor) can still infiltrate surrounding tissue and thus hold a potential for malignancy. Grade III anaplastic astrocytomas are more malignant than type II tumors. This increase in malignancy translates into lower long-term survival rates. Many persons with grade III anaplastic astrocytomas die within two to three years, while may people with the grade II astrocytoma show long-term survival beyond five years.

Patients with the most severe form of astrocytoma (glioblastoma multiforme, or GBH) usually show survival times of less than two years. Patients with oligodendrogliomas and oligoastrocytomas have generally better prognoses than the diffuse astrocytomas. Brainstem gliomas (a form of pediatric diffuse, fibrillary astrocytoma) have a tendency toward malignancy, and survival beyond two years is unusual. Because PXA tumors are usually slow growing and superficial, they are therefore more likely to be successfully treated by surgical removal.

Primary tumors of the spinal cord are often benign, and surgical removal results in a favorable prognosis. With metastatic spinal tumors, prognosis depends on the type of primary cancer.

Resources

BOOKS

Goetz C. G., et al. *Textbook of Clinical Neurology.* Philadelphia: W.B. Saunders Company, 1999.
Guyton & Hall. *Textbook of Medical Physiology*, 10th ed. Philadelphia: W.B. Saunders Company, 2000.
Roloff, Tricia Ann. *Navigating through a Strange Land: A Book for Brain Tumor Patients and Their Families.* Minneapolis, MN: Fairview Press, 2001.
Shiminski-Maher, Tania. *Childhood Brain & Spinal Cord Tumors: A Guide for Families, Friends & Caregivers.* Sebastopol, CA: O'Reilly & Associates, 2001.
Stark-Vance, Virginia. *100 Q & A about Brain Tumors.* Sudbury, MA: Jones & Bartlett, 2003.

OTHER

"Brain and Spinal Cord Tumors—Hope through Research." *National Institute of Neurological Disorders and Stroke.* May 2, 2004 (May 22, 2004). <http://www.ninds.nih.gov/ health_and_medical/pubs/brain_tumor_hope_through_ research.htm#What_Research_is_Being_Done>.
"Facts About Brain Tumors." *National Brain Tumor Foundation.* May 2, 2004 (May 22, 2004).
<http://www.braintumor.org/newsroom/quick_facts/ index.html>.
Francavilla, Thomas L. "Intramedullary Spinal Cord Tumors." *eMedicine* May 2, 2004 (May 22, 2004). <http://www.emedicine.com/med/topic2995.htm>.
"Living with a Brain Tumor: A Guide for Brain Tumor Patients." American Brain Tumor Association. May 2, 2004 (May 22, 2004). <http://www.abta.org/ Livingwi.pdf>.
"NINDS Brain and Spinal Tumors Information Page." *National Institute of Neurological Disorders and Stroke.* May 4, 2004 (May 22, 2004). <http://www.ninds.nih. gov/health_and_medical/disorders/brainandspinal tumors.htm>.
"What You Need To Know about Brain Tumors." *National Cancer Institute.* May 2, 2004 (May 22, 2004). <http://www.cancer.gov/cancerinfo/wyntk/brain>.

ORGANIZATIONS

American Brain Tumor Association (ABTA). 2720 River Road, Des Plaines, IL 60018-4110. (847) 827-9910; Fax: (847) 827-9918. info@abta.org. <http://www.abta.org>.
National Cancer Institute (NCI), National Institutes of Health. Bldg. 31, Rm. 10A31, Bethesda, MD 20892-2580. (301) 435-3848 or (800) 4CANCER (422-6237); Fax: (847) 827-9918. cancermail@icicc.nci.nih.gov. <http://cancer net.nci.nih.gov>.

Paul Arthur

Brown-Séquard syndrome

Definition

Brown-Séquard syndrome (BSS), also known as hemisection of the spinal cord or partial spinal sensory syndrome, is a rare condition caused by an incomplete lesion of the spinal cord. This damage, most often from physical trauma, results in a contralateral (opposite side of the body) loss of sensation and temperature and ipsilateral (same side of the body) paralysis or extreme weakness.

Description

In 1849, French physiologist Charles Edouard Brown-Séquard published a document discussing the condition that now bears his name. Using information gathered through animal experimentation and human autopsies, he identified and described the hallmark signs of BSS: paralysis affecting only one side of the body (ipsilateral paralysis) and loss of sensation on the opposite side of the body.

Injury or damage to one side of the spinal cord, typically in the cervical (neck) region, results in BSS. The severity of the condition depends on the amount of damage to the spinal cord and associated neurons. The onset of symptoms may also vary depending on the cause.

Demographics

Information on the prevalence of Brown-Séquard syndrome is collected from 16 **spinal cord injury** centers in the United States. According to The University of Alabama's National Spinal Cord Injury Statistical Center (NSCISC), which compiles the data, approximately 11,000 spinal cord injuries (SCIs) occur each year (as of 2003). Although specific incidence is unknown, BSS is estimated to occur in 200–400 of these injuries.

The average age of a patient sustaining a spinal cord injury is 32 years, with injuries most commonly occurring in individuals between 16 and 30 years. Men account for more than 80% of reported SCIs.

Within the United States, approximately 70% of individuals with BSS are white, nearly 20% are African American, and the remaining 10% comprise other origins, according to NSCISC reports. Little data is known regarding SCIs in countries outside the United States.

Causes and symptoms

In most cases, Brown-Séquard syndrome is caused by severe physical trauma such as a puncture wound or gunshot wound, which partially severs or damages the spinal cord. Nontraumatic conditions that compress the spinal cord may also cause BSS. Examples include tumors, **multiple sclerosis**, **epidural hematoma** (swelling in the area between the brain and skull), meningitis, myelitis (spinal cord inflammation), and tuberculosis.

Physical trauma usually causes a more rapid onset of symptoms than nontraumatic conditions. The two primary symptoms of BSS are loss of sensation and paralysis. The side of the body that sustained injury typically loses touch and vibration senses. The opposite side of the body tends to lose its sense of **pain** and temperature. In both cases, these symptoms occur below the site of the SCI. Paralysis or muscle weakness occurs on the same side of the body as the injury.

Loss of bladder and bowel control may result, but the majority of patients will regain control. Horner syndrome, a condition resulting from damage to the sympathetic facial nerves, has also been known to develop.

Diagnosis

Brown-Séquard syndrome is diagnosed based on the patient's medical history and a physical examination. Imaging studies may be performed to isolate the extent

Key Terms

Corticosteroids A group of anti-inflammatory drugs similar to the natural corticosteroid hormones produced by the adrenal glands.

Lesion A change in tissue due to injury or disease.

Paralysis The inability to use a muscle because of injury to or disease of the nerves leading to the muscle.

and location of the SCI. These include **magnetic resonance imaging (MRI)**, computed tomography (CT) scans, or x rays. Additional testing may be required for secondary conditions or symptoms.

Several neurological disorders have symptoms similar to BSS, making differential diagnosis very important, especially in those cases related to nontraumatic conditions. The incomplete lesion of the spinal cord in conjunction with the unique presentation of ipsilateral sensory loss and paralysis are key for identifying BSS.

Treatment team

The team of specialists needed to treat a patient with BSS will vary. Primary members include:

- a **neurologist** to evaluate brain and nerve function

- an orthopedic specialist to monitor the spine and assist with walking therapy

- a physical therapist to help regain muscle strength and walking ability

- an occupational therapist to facilitate adaptation of new physical limitations

Treatment

In cases of physical trauma, treatment begins at the accident site with proper immobilization and emergency medical care to prevent further spinal cord damage. Surgery may be required in these or nontraumatic cases to eliminate the cause, whether a bullet or a fluid-filled cyst.

Treatment of symptoms is the typical focus for this condition. Several studies have shown increased success with early administration of high-dose steroids such as corticosteroids, but this is not yet a standard practice. Other medications are prescribed as needed for secondary symptoms.

Physical therapy should begin immediately in order to maintain muscle strength and agility since most patients with BSS will regain mobility. Specialized devices, including wheelchairs or braces, may be necessary during this transition.

Recovery and rehabilitation

The recovery time for each patient depends on the extent of nerve damage and underlying cause of the syndrome. The NSCISC reports that individuals with SCIs spend an average of 16 days in the hospital and 44 days in rehabilitation. Rehabilitation may be required outside the hospital for several months or years.

Extensive physical therapy should take place immediately. Initial therapy focuses on respiratory exercises, upright positioning, and range of motion in affected muscles. Progressive therapy gradually helps the patient with the strength and control necessary to be mobile or begin walking again.

Occupational therapy is also important for helping patients return to their daily activities. This therapist provides methods for modifying everyday tasks, evaluates progress, and facilitates the necessary changes to restore independence when possible.

Clinical trials

The National Institute of Child Health and Human Development is currently conducting a clinical trial to evaluate the effectiveness of walking on a treadmill by individuals with incomplete SCIs. As of early 2004, this five-year study was in Phase II and III **clinical trials** and still recruiting patients. The proposed end date for the study is January 2005. For additional information contact: Andrea L. Behrman, PhD (Principal Investigator), University of Florida, "Retraining Walking after Spinal Cord Injury" (Study ID: K01HD01348); Telephone: (352) 273-6117; E-mail: abehrman@hp.ufl.edu.

Prognosis

Patients with Brown-Séquard syndrome usually have a good prognosis. The extent to which a patient recovers depends on the cause of injury and secondary conditions or complications. According to the National Organization for Rare Disorders, more than 90% of affected individuals successfully regain the ability to walk. Additional studies have found that the majority of a patient's motor skills return within the first two months after injury. The recovery period is usually two years, but will vary by patient.

Special concerns

Not all patients with BSS make a full recovery. In these instances, long-term care options need to be considered. By working with the treatment team, individuals can determine their level of activity and recognize areas where adaptation may be required. Some patients and their caregivers could benefit from psychological therapy to discuss the variety of changes that occur after traumatic injury.

Resources

BOOKS

The Official Patient's Sourcebook on Brown-Séquard Syndrome: A Revised and Updated Directory for the Internet Age. San Diego: Icon Health Publications, 2002.

PERIODICALS

Bateman, D. E., and I. Pople. "Brown-Séquard at Disney World." *The Lancet* 352, no. 9144 (December 12, 1998): 1902.

Lim, E., Y. S. Wong, Y. L. Lo, et al. "Traumatic Atypical Brown-Séquard Syndrome: Case Report and Literature Review." *Clinical Neurology and Neurosurgy* 105 (2003): 143–45.

Pollard, Matthew E., and David F. Apple. "Factors Associated with Improved Neurologic Outcomes in Patients with Incomplete Tetraplegia." *Spine* 28, no. 1 (January 1, 2003): 33–39.

Tattersall, Robert, and Benjamine Turner. "Brown-Séquard and His Syndrome." *The Lancet* 356, no. 9223 (July 1, 2000): 61.

WEBSITES

Beeson, Michael S, and Scott Wilber. "Brown-Séquard Syndrome." *eMedicine*. July 30, 2003 (May 20, 2004). <http://www.emedicine.com/pmr/topic70.htm>.

"Retraining Walking after Spinal Cord Injury." *ClinicalTrials.gov.* March 19, 2004 (May 20, 2004). <http://www.clinicaltrails.gov/ct/show/NCT00059553?order=1>.

Vandenakker, Carol. "Brown-Séquard Syndrome." *eMedicine*. July 29, 2002 (May 20, 2004). <http://www.emedicine.com/pmr/topic17.htm>.

ORGANIZATIONS

Christopher Reeve Paralysis Foundation. 500 Morris Avenue, Springfield, NJ 07081. (800) 225-0292. info@paralysis.org. <http://www.christopherreeve.org>.

National Organization for Rare Disorders. 55 Kenosia Avenue, P.O. Box 1968, Danbury, CT 06813. (203) 744-0100 or (800) 999-6673; Fax: (203) 798-2291. orphan@rarediseases.org. <http://www.rarediseases.org>.

National Spinal Cord Injury Association. 6701 Democracy Blvd. #300-9, Bethesda, MD 20817. (301) 214-4006 or (800) 962-9629; Fax: (301) 881-9817. info@spinalcord.org. <http://www.spinalcord.org>.

Stacey L. Chamberlin

Bruit *see* **Hearing disorders**

Bulbospinal muscular atrophy *see* **Kennedy's disease**

C

Canavan disease

Definition

Canavan disease, which results when the body produces less than normal amounts of a protein called aspartoacylase, is a fatal inherited disorder characterized by progressive damage to the brain and nervous system.

Description

Canavan disease is named after Dr. Myrtelle Canavan who described a patient with the symptoms of Canavan disease but mistakenly diagnosed this patient with **Schilder's disease**. It was not until 1949, that Canavan disease was recognized as a unique genetic disease by Van Bogaert and Betrand. The credit went to Dr. Canavan, however, whose initial description of the disease dominated the medical literature.

Canavan disease, which is also called aspartoacylase deficiency, spongy degeneration of the brain, and infantile spongy degeneration, results from a deficiency of the enzyme aspartoacylase. This deficiency ultimately results in progressive damage to the brain and nervous system and causes **mental retardation**, **seizures**, **tremors**, muscle weakness, blindness and an increase in head size. Although most people with Canavan disease die in their teens, some die in childhood and some live into their twenties and thirties.

Canavan disease is sometimes called spongy degeneration of the brain since it is characterized by a sponginess or swelling of the brain cells and a destruction of the white matter of the brain. Canavan disease is an autosomal recessive genetic condition that is found in all ethnic groups, but is most common in people of Ashkenazi (Eastern European) Jewish descent and people of Saudi Arabian descent.

Demographics

Although Canavan disease is found in people of all ethnicities, it is most common in Ashkenazi Jewish individuals. Approximately one in 40 Ashkenazi Jewish individuals are carriers for Canavan disease and approximately one in 6,400 Ashkenazi Jewish people are born with Canavan disease. People of Saudi Arabian descent also have a relatively high risk of Canavan disease.

Causes and symptoms

Canavan disease is an autosomal recessive genetic disease. A person with Canavan disease has changes (mutations) in both of the genes responsible for producing the enzyme aspartoacylase and has inherited one changed gene from his or her mother and one changed gene from his or her father.

Reduced production of aspartoacylase results in lower than normal amounts of this enzyme in the brain and nervous system. Aspartoacylase is responsible for breaking down a substance called N-acetylaspartic acid (NAA). When the body produces decreased levels of aspartoacylase, a build-up of NAA results. This results in the destruction of the white matter of the brain and nervous system and causes the symptoms of Canavan disease.

Parents who have a child with Canavan disease are called carriers, since they each possess one changed ASPA gene and one unchanged ASPA gene. Carriers usually do not have any symptoms since they have one unchanged gene that can produce enough aspartoacylase to prevent the build-up of NAA. Each child born to parents who are both carriers for Canavan disease, has a 25% chance of having Canavan disease, a 50% chance of being a carrier and a 25% chance of being neither a carrier nor affected with Canavan disease.

Most infants with Canavan disease appear normal for the first month of life. The onset of symptoms, such as a lack of head control and poor muscle tone, usually begins by two to three months of age, although some may have an onset of the disease in later childhood. Children with Canavan disease usually experience sleep disturbances, irritability, and swallowing and feeding difficulties after the first or second year of life. In many cases, irritability resolves by the third year. As the child with Canavan disease grows older there is a deterioration of mental and physical functioning. The speed at which this deterioration occurs will vary for each affected person. Children with Canavan disease are mentally retarded and most will never be able to sit, stand, walk or talk, although they may learn to laugh and smile and reach for objects. People with Canavan disease have increasing difficulties in controlling their muscles. Initially they have poor muscle tone but eventually their muscles become stiff and difficult to move and may exhibit spasms. Canavan disease can cause vision problems and some people with Canavan disease may eventually become blind. People with Canavan disease typically have disproportionately large heads and may experience seizures.

Diagnosis

Diagnostic testing

Canavan disease should be suspected in a person with a large head who has poor muscle control, a lack of head control and a destruction of the white matter of the brain, which can be detected through a computed tomography (**CT**) **scan** or **magnetic resonance imaging (MRI)**. A diagnosis of Canavan disease can usually be confirmed by measuring the amount of NAA in a urine sample since a person with Canavan disease typically has greater than five to ten times the normal amount of NAA in their urine. Canavan disease can be less accurately diagnosed by measuring the amount of aspartocylase enzyme present in a sample of skin cells.

Once a biochemical diagnosis of Canavan disease is made, DNA testing may be recommended. Detection of an ASPA gene alteration in a person with Canavan disease can confirm an uncertain diagnosis and help facilitate prenatal diagnosis and carrier testing of relatives. Although there are a number of different ASPA gene changes responsible for Canavan disease, most clinical laboratories typically test for only two to three common gene changes. Two of the ASPA gene changes are common in Ashkenazi Jews with Canavan disease and the other ASPA gene change is common in those of other ethnic backgrounds. Testing for other types of changes in the ASPA gene is only done on a research basis.

Carrier testing

DNA testing is the only means of identifying carriers of Canavan disease. If possible, DNA testing should be first performed on the affected family member. If a change in the ASPA gene is detected, then carrier testing can be performed in relatives such as siblings, with an accuracy of greater than 99%. If the affected relative does not possess a detectable ASPA gene change, then carrier testing will be inaccurate and should not be performed. If DNA testing of the affected relative cannot be performed, carrier testing of family members can still be performed but will

be less accurate. Carrier testing for the three common ASPA gene mutations identifies approximately 97–99% of Ashkenazi Jewish carriers and 40–55% of carriers from other ethnic backgrounds.

Carrier testing of individuals without a family history of Canavan disease is only recommended for people of Ashkenazi Jewish background since they have a higher risk of being carriers. As of 1998, both the American College of Obstetricians and Gynecologists and the American College of Medical Genetics recommend that DNA testing for Canavan disease be offered to all Ashkenazi Jewish couples who are planning children or who are currently pregnant. If only one member of the couple is of Ashkenazi Jewish background than testing of the Jewish partner should be performed first. If the Jewish partner is a carrier, than testing of the non-Jewish partner is recommended.

Prenatal testing

Prenatal testing through chorionic villus sampling (CVS) and amniocentesis is available to parents who are both carriers for Canavan disease. If both parents possess an ASPA gene change, which is identified through DNA testing, then DNA testing of their baby can be performed. Some parents are known to be carriers for Canavan disease since they already have a child with Canavan disease, yet they do not possess ASPA gene changes that are detectable through DNA testing. Prenatal diagnosis can be performed in these cases by measuring the amount of NAA in the amniotic fluid obtained from an amniocentesis. This type of prenatal testing is less accurate than DNA testing and can lead to misdiagnoses.

Treatment team

A child with Canavan disease will require treatment from a pediatric **neurologist**, pediatric ophthalmologist, and a pediatric surgeon for the installation of certain kinds of feeding tubes. Physical and occupational therapists can and educational specialists can provide supportive treatment.

Treatment

There is no cure for Canavan disease and treatment largely involves the management of symptoms. Seizures and irritability can often be controlled through medication. Children with loss of head control will often benefit from the use of modified seats that can provide full head support. When feeding and swallowing becomes difficult, liquid diets and/or feeding tubes become necessary. Feeding tubes are either inserted through the nose (nasogastric tube) or through a permanent incision in the stomach (gastrostomy). Patients with a later onset and slower progression of the disease may benefit from special education

Key Terms

Amniocentesis A procedure performed at 16-18 weeks of pregnancy in which a needle is inserted through a woman's abdomen into her uterus to draw out a small sample of the amniotic fluid from around the baby. Either the fluid itself or cells from the fluid can be used for a variety of tests to obtain information about genetic disorders and other medical conditions in the fetus.

Amniotic fluid The fluid which surrounds a developing baby during pregnancy.

Amniotic sac Contains the fetus which is surrounded by amniotic fluid.

Biochemical testing Measuring the amount or activity of a particular enzyme or protein in a sample of blood or urine or other tissue from the body.

Carrier A person who possesses a gene for an abnormal trait without showing signs of the disorder. The person may pass the abnormal gene on to offspring.

Chorionic villus sampling (CVS) A procedure used for prenatal diagnosis at 10-12 weeks gestation. Under ultrasound guidance a needle is inserted either through the mother's vagina or abdominal wall and a sample of cells is collected from around the early embryo. These cells are then tested for chromosome abnormalities or other genetic diseases.

Chromosome A microscopic thread-like structure found within each cell of the body and consists of a complex of proteins and DNA. Humans have 46 chromosomes arranged into 23 pairs. Changes in either the total number of chromosomes or their shape and size (structure) may lead to physical or mental abnormalities.

Deoxyribonucleic acid (DNA) The genetic material in cells that holds the inherited instructions for growth, development, and cellular functioning.

DNA testing Analysis of DNA (the genetic component of cells) in order to determine changes in genes that may indicate a specific disorder.

Enzyme A protein that catalyzes a biochemical reaction or change without changing its own structure or function.

Gene A building block of inheritance, which contains the instructions for the production of a particular protein, and is made up of a molecular sequence found on a section of DNA. Each gene is found on a precise location on a chromosome.

Poor muscle tone Muscles that are weak and floppy.

Prenatal testing Testing for a disease such as a genetic condition in an unborn baby.

Protein Important building blocks of the body, composed of amino acids, involved in the formation of body structures and controlling the basic functions of the human body.

White matter A substance found in the brain and nervous system that protects nerves and allows messages to be sent to and from the brain to the various parts of the body.

---

programs and physical therapy. Research trials of **gene therapy** are ongoing and involve the transfer of an unchanged ASPA gene into the brain cells of a patient. The goal of gene therapy is to restore normal amounts of aspartoacylase in the brain and nervous system and prevent the build-up of NAA and the symptoms of Canavan disease. The initial results of these early **clinical trials** have been somewhat promising but it will take time for gene therapy to become a viable treatment for Canavan disease.

Prognosis

The life span and progression of Canavan disease is variable and may be partially dependent on the type of medical care provided and other genetic risk factors. Most people with Canavan disease live into their teens, although some die in infancy or survive into their 20's and 30's.

There can be a high degree of variability even within families; some families report having one child die in infancy and another die in adulthood. Although different ASPA gene changes are associated with the production of different amounts of enzyme, the severity of the disease does not appear to be related to the type of ASPA gene change. It is, therefore, impossible to predict the life span of a particular individual with Canavan disease.

Resources

BOOKS

Scriver, C. R., et al., eds. *The Metabolic and Molecular Basis of Inherited Disease.* New York: The McGraw Hill Companies, 1995.

PERIODICALS

ACOG committee opinion. "Screening for Canavan disease." Number 212, November 1998. Committee on Genetics.

American College of Obstetricians and Gynecologists. *International Journal of Gynaecology and Obstetrics* 65, no. 1 (April 1999): 91–92.

Besley, G. T. N., et al. "Prenatal Diagnosis of Canavan Disease–Problems and Dilemmas." *Journal of Inherited Metabolic Disease* 22, no. 3 (May 1999): 263–66.

Matalon, Reuben, and Kimberlee Michals-Matalon. "Chemistry and Molecular Biology of Canavan Disease." *Neurochemical Research* 24, no. 4 (April 1999): 507–13.

Matalon, Reuben, and Kimberlee Michals-Matalon. "Recent Advances in Canavan Disease." *Advances In Pediatrics* 46 (1999): 493–506.

Matalon, Reuben, Kimberlee Michals-Matalon, and Rajinder Kaul. "Canavan Disease." *Handbook of Clinical Neurology* 22, no. 66 (1999): 661–69.

Traeger, Evelyn, and Isabelle Rapin. "The clinical course of Canavan disease." *Pediatric Neurology* 18, no. 3 (1999): 207–12.

ORGANIZATIONS

Canavan Foundation. 320 Central Park West, Suite 19D, New York, NY 10025. (212) 877-3945.

Canavan Research Foundation. Fairwood Professional Building, New Fairwood, CT 06812. (203) 746-2436. canavan_research@hotmail.com. <http://www.canavan.org>.

National Foundation for Jewish Genetic Diseases, Inc. 250 Park Ave., Suite 1000, New York, NY 10017. (212) 371-1030. <http://www.nfjgd.org>.

National Tay-Sachs and Allied Diseases Association. 2001 Beacon St., Suite 204, Brighton, MA 02135. (800) 906-8723. ntasd-Boston@worldnet.att.net. <http://www.ntsad.org>.

WEBSITES

American College of Medical Genetics. Position Statement on Carrier Testing for Canavan Disease. FASEB. (January 1998). <http://www.faseb.org/genetics/acmg/pol-31.htm>.

Matalon, Reuben. "Canavan disease." *GeneClinics.* (20 July 1999). <http://www.geneclinics.org/profiles/canavan/details.html?>.

Matalon, Reuben and Kimberlee Michals-Matalon. "Spongy Degeneration of the Brain, Canavan Disease: Biochemical and Molecular Findings." *Frontiers in Biosience.* (March 2000) . <http://www.bioscience.org/2000/v5/d/matalon/fulltext.htm>.

McKusick, Victor A. "Canavan disease." *OMIM—Online Mendelian Inheritance in Man.* (December 8, 1999). <http://www.ncbi.nlm.nih.gov/htbin-post/Omim/dispmim?271900>.

Lisa Maria Andres, MS, CGC
Rosalyn Carson-DeWitt, MD

Carbamazepine

Definition

Carbamazepine is an antiepileptic drug used to reduce or suppress **seizures**. The medication is also commonly prescribed to relieve certain neurogenic **pain** such as **trigeminal neuralgia**. This drug decreases abnormal electrical impulses through nerve cell pathways by inhibiting the activity of sodium channels in neurons. Consequently, it blocks the repetitive impulses that trigger seizures. In the United States, brand names for carbamazepine include Tegretol, Carbatrol, and Epitol. This medication is classified into the following categories: anticonvulsant, antimanic, and antineuralgic.

Purpose

Due to its high efficacy, carbamazepine is in many cases a first-line treatment for **epilepsy**, and is also frequently prescribed to treat acute neuralgias such as trigeminal neuralgia. Sometimes the drug is also used to improve bipolar disorder symptoms, especially during the manic phase of this disease.

Description

Carbamazepine is a lipid-soluble substance metabolized in the liver by enzymes of the P-450 family and therefore, its chronic administration may induce liver toxicity, especially in patients with reduced liver function. In contrast, persons whose P-450 enzymes are very efficient and metabolize the drug rapidly tend to have decreased carbamazepine half-life and therefore, reduced efficacy of the medication. The body slowly absorbs carbamazepine and the drug easily passes through the blood-brain barrier. It is rapidly transported into the **central nervous system** (CNS), where it exerts a depressant effect.

Recommended dosage

For treatment of seizures, the usual initial dose of carbamazepine for adults and children over 12 years of age is 200 milligrams, taken twice daily. The prescribing physician may increase the dosage in weekly intervals until optimum seizure control is achieved. Dosages generally do not exceed a range of 1000–1200 milligrams (mg) per day. For the treatment of trigeminal neuralgia, daily dosages usually range from 800–1200 mg per day during the stage of acute pain and 400–800 mg per day for preventative therapy.

Precautions

The ingestion of alcoholic drinks during carbamazepine therapy is contraindicated because both substances may potentiate (increase) the effects of the other.

Key Terms

Epilepsy A disorder associated with disturbed electrical discharges in the central nervous system that cause seizures.

Neurogenic pain Pain originating in the nerves or nervous tissue.

Trigeminal neuralgia A disorder affecting the trigeminal nerve (the 5th cranial nerve), causing episodes of sudden, severe pain on one side of the face.

Other depressants of the central nervous system such as antihistamines, analgesic drugs, muscle relaxants, and tranquilizers, are also potentiated when used with carbamazepine or other antiepileptic medications. Diabetic patients should be monitored during the administration of this drug since it interferes with glucose blood levels. The drug should not be taken during pregnancy due to the absence of safety clinical studies for pregnant women. Tests in animals have shown that carbamazepine causes developmental defects in embryos when administered in high doses. As the drug is found in breast milk, the use of this medication is also contraindicated during breast-feeding. Carbamazepine may interfere with several biomarkers used in medical laboratory tests, and persons taking the medication should report its intake before blood or urine samples are collected for analysis.

Side effects

The intensity of side effects (or adverse effects) of carbamazepine is dose-dependant. Among the mild adverse effects observed during chronic administration of this medication are drowsiness, vertigo, **fatigue**, blurred vision, gastritis, constipation, aching muscles or joints, skin sensitivity to solar **radiation**, loss of appetite, and dry mouth. In most patients, these side effects are mild and tend to decrease in intensity or to completely disappear within a few days of treatment. However, if they are particularly intense or do persist for two or more weeks they should be reported to the physician.

Nevertheless, elderly patients or patients exhibiting one or more severe symptoms in association with carbamazepine intake such as chest pain, blurred vision, mental confusion or hallucinations, numbness, tachycardia, **depression** or marked mood changes, urinary retention or excessive diuresis, peripheral edema, severe diarrhea or vomiting, should report such symptoms to their physicians as soon as possible.

Moreover, immediate medical attention may be required in the presence of one or more of the following adverse effects: presence of blood in the urine or urine with a dark color, black tarry stools or pale stools, unusual bleeding or bruising, skin rashes, ulcers or white spots in the mouth or lips, chills and fever, shallow or uneasy breathing or wheezing chest, jaundice, arrhythmia, sudden blood pressure fall or unusual high blood pressure, cough and/or sore throat. These side effects could indicate the presence of a potentially serious blood disorder.

Interactions

The use of carbamazepine reduces the effectiveness of oral contraceptives and also reduces the effects of corticosteroids. The concomitant use of one of the following drugs inhibits the metabolism of carbamazepine, thereby decreasing its effectiveness: cimetidine, erythromycin, isoniazid, diltiazem, and propoxyphene. Conversely, carbamazepine decreases the plasma levels of phenytoin, another antiepileptic drug. Clarithromycin, an antibiotic, increases the blood levels of carbamazepine and thus, increases the risk of adverse effects.

The use of particular antidepressant medicines known as monoamine oxidase (MAO) inhibitors during carbamazepine therapy, or within the previous two weeks before initiating carbamazepine therapy may increase the risk of fever, severe high blood pressure, **stroke**, and convulsions. Therefore, an interval of at least two weeks is recommended between the administration of these two classes of drugs.

Resources
BOOKS

Champe, Pamela C., and Richard A. Harvey, eds. *Pharmacology,* 2nd ed. Philadelphia, PA: Lippincott Williams & Wilkins, 2000.

OTHER

"Carbamazepine." *Medline Plus.* National Library of Medicine. (January 1, 2003) (March 20, 2004). <http://www.nlm.nih.gov/medlineplus/druginfo/medmaster/a682237.html>.

National Institute of Neurological Disorders and Stroke. *NINDS Trigeminal Neuralgia Information Page.* (May 29, 2001) (March 20, 2004). <http://www.ninds.nih.gov/health_and_medical/disorders/trigemin_doc.htm>.

ORGANIZATIONS

Epilepsy Foundation. 4351 Garden City Drive, Landover, MD 20785-7223. (800) 332-1000. <http://www.epilepsyfoundation.org>.

National Institute of Neurological Disorders and Stroke. P.O. Box 5801, Bethesda, MD, 20892-2540. (301) 496-5751 or (800) 352-9424. <http://www.ninds.nih.gov/>.

contact_us.htm> or <http://www.ninds.nih.gov/index.htm>.

Sandra Galeotti

Carotid endarterectomy

Definition

Carotid endarterectomy is a surgical procedure to treat obstruction of the carotid artery caused by atherosclerotic plaque formation.

Purpose

The purpose of surgical therapy for vascular disease is to prevent **stroke**. Stroke can be caused by atherosclerosis of the carotid arteries located in the neck. Atherosclerosis is a degenerative disease of the cardiovascular system, which can occur in the carotid arteries in the neck, resulting in plaques of lipids, cholesterol crystals, and necrotic cells. The plaques in the carotid arteries can result in disease by embolizing, thrombosing, or causing stenosis (narrowing of artery). The plaques in the carotid arteries can cause disease if they obstruct a vessel or get dislodged and obstruct another area.

Precautions

The procedure is contraindicated in patients with an occluded carotid artery and in cases of severe neurologic deficit resulting from cerebral infarction. Additionally, the procedure is not performed in persons with concurrent medical illness severe enough to limit life expectancy. During the operation, precautions should be taken to prevent intraoperation movement of the atherosclerotic plaque. This can occur by excessive manipulation of the carotid bifurcation (the anatomical point where the internal and external carotid is joined together). The internal carotid will extend from the neck and penetrate the brain (to provide the brain with blood), whereas the external carotid will form other smaller arteries to provide blood to structures within the neck region. Atherosclerotic plaques are fragile especially if they are ulcerated. During the operation the surgeon must carefully dissect free other attached vessels such as the common carotid, internal carotid, and external carotid arteries with minimal physical manipulation of the affected carotid vessel.

Description

The first successful carotid endarterectomy was performed by DeBakey in 1953. During the past 40 years the procedure has been optimized and has become the most frequently performed peripheral vascular operation in the United States. There are more than 130,000 cases of carotid endarterectomy performed annually in the United States. Several randomized prospective **clinical trials** have conclusively established both the safety and efficacy of carotid endarterectomy and its superiority for favorable outcomes when compared to the best medical management. Largely due to credible scientific and clinical research, there has been a very large increase in the performance of this procedure over the past ten years. It is understandable that the procedure is common since it is utilized for the treatment of stroke, which is a condition that is associated with high morbidity (death rates) and is frequent. Carotid endarterectomy is the most common surgical procedure in the United States utilized to treat stenosis (narrowing) of the carotid artery. There are approximately more than 700,000 incident strokes annually and 4.4 million stroke survivors. There are 150,000 annual deaths from stroke. Approximately 30% of stroke survivors die within the first 12 months. Within 12 years approximately 66% will eventually die from stroke, making this condition the third leading cause of death in the United States. The cause of atherosclerosis is unknown, but injury to the arteries can occur from infectious agents, hyperlipidemia, cigarette smoking, and hypertension. The aggregate cost associated with approximately 400,000 first strokes in 1990 was $40.6 billion. Among those who have experienced one stroke, the incidence of stroke within five years is 40–50%. Research as of 2002 concludes that carotid endarterectomy remains the standard of care for the treatment of carotid artery atherosclerosis.

Surgical Description

A vertical incision is made in front of the sternocleidomastoid muscle providing optimal exposure of the surgical field. The line of the incision (10 cm in length) begins at the mastoid process and extends to approximately one to two fingerbreadths above the sternal notch. The exact location of carotid bifurcation can be determined before operation by ultrasound studies or arteriography. Muscles and nerves within the area are carefully displaced to allow access to the diseased area (plaque). When the surgical field is cleared of adjacent anatomical structures the endarterectomy portion of the procedure is carried out. This is accomplished by an incision in the common carotid artery at the site below the atherosclerotic plaque. The surgeon then uses an angled scissor (called a Potts scissor) to incise the common carotid artery through the plaque into the normal internal carotid artery. It is vital to extend the arterial incision (arteriotomy) above and below the atherosclerotic plaque. The surgeon utilizes a blunt dissecting instrument called a Penfield instrument to dissect the atherosclerotic plaque from the attachment to the arterial wall.

Arterial Reconstruction

After removing the atherosclerotic plaque, primary closure with sutures, or closure with a vein or prosthetic patch, is performed. Research indicates that utilization of a prosthetic patch is more favorable than suture closing. During this stage of the operation flushing is important to remove debris and air. Vein patch is advantageous because this type of closure reduces the risk of thrombus accumulation and possibly prevents perioperative stroke.

Preparation

As part of the preoperative preparation, routine laboratory tests for blood chemistry (complete blood count, electrolytes), kidney function tests, lipid profiles, and special blood tests to monitor clotting times are ordered by the clinician. Measurement of clotting times is important because blood thinner medications are typically given to patients preoperatively. Neuroimaging studies of the head are important in symptomatic patients to identify old or new cerebral infarcts. Carotid ultrasound studies are the screening test of choice accepted by surgeons to evaluate for **carotid stenosis**. An electrocardiogram (ECG) is important for evaluating past myocardial infarction and ischemic cardiac changes. The importance of ECG monitoring cannot be overemphasized given that the most common cause of postoperative mortality (death) is cardiac arrest. Positioning of the patient is also important. The operating table should be horizontal without head elevation. The head should be partially turned to the opposite side of the surgical field. It may be advantageous to place a rolled towel under the patient's shoulders to exaggerate neck extension. Gentle preparation and cleaning of operative fields should ensure minimal physical manipulation and pressure to avoid dislodging fragments of atherosclerotic plaque. The goals for anesthetic management include control of blood pressure and heart rate, protection of the brain and heart from ischemic insult, and relief of surgical **pain** and operative stress responses. Routine monitors (ECG and pulse oximetry to measure blood oxygen levels) and oxygen face mask are placed prior to anesthetic induction. Typically, any commonly utilized anesthetic and muscle relaxants (nondepolarizing) can be administered for carotid endarterectomy.

Aftercare

Aspirin therapy should be initiated at the time of diagnosis of **transient ischemic attack** (TIA), amaurosis fugax (transient visual loss), or stroke. Recent research from the prospective Aspirin and Carotid Endarterectomy (ACE) trial suggests that low dose (80 to 325 mg per day) of aspirin is optimal in preventing thromboembolic events after carotid endarterectomy. After carotid endarterectomy the patient's blood should be tested (complete blood count and electrolytes). Cardiac function can be monitored with ECG recordings. Frequent neurologic assessment is essential as well as hemodynamic monitoring (with the goal of maintaining blood pressure at its prior range). The patient should be observed for hemotoma formation which could cause airway obstruction. Antiplatelet therapy is necessary. About two weeks postoperatively patients are evaluated for neurologic and wound complications. Carotid ultrasound studies are performed after six months postoperatively and annually scheduled.

Risks

There are several important complications that can occur after carotid endarterectomy. Stroke or transient neurologic deficit can occur within 12 to 24 hours after operation. These conditions are usually caused by thromboembolic complications, which typically originate from the endarterectomy site or damaged vessels that were involved during the operative procedure (internal, common, and external carotid arteries). In approximately 33–50% of patients, hypertension or hypotension can occur. Wound complications such as hemotoma formation can cause pain and tracheal (wind pipe) deviation, which can impair normal breathing. During surgery, damage to vital nerves can occur, such as cervical nerves which supply sensation to the neck region. Patients may complain of numbness in the lower ear, lower neck, and upper face regions. Damage to the hypoglossal nerve (which provides innervations of the tongue), can produce deviation of the tongue to the paralyzed side and speech impairment. Additionally, the problem can reoccur, resulting in stenosis and symptoms.

Normal results

The normal progression of results following carotid endarterectomy is the prevention of stroke which is approximately 1.6% (two-year stroke risk), compared to 12.2% for patients who are medically treated. The results of the Asymptomatic Carotid Atherosclerosis Study (ACAS) reveal that the incidence of stroke for the postsurgical group (those receiving carotid endarterectomy) was 5.1%; for the group treated medically, the incidence was 11%. As with all surgical procedures, it is important for patients to select a surgeon who has expertise in the particular procedure and in the management of the condition. Some studies indicate that surgeons should perform 10 to 12 carotid endarterectomies every year in order to maintain surgical expertise and management skills.

Resources
BOOKS
Miller, Ronald D., et al, eds. *Anesthesia.* 5th ed. Churchill Living Stone, Inc. 2000.

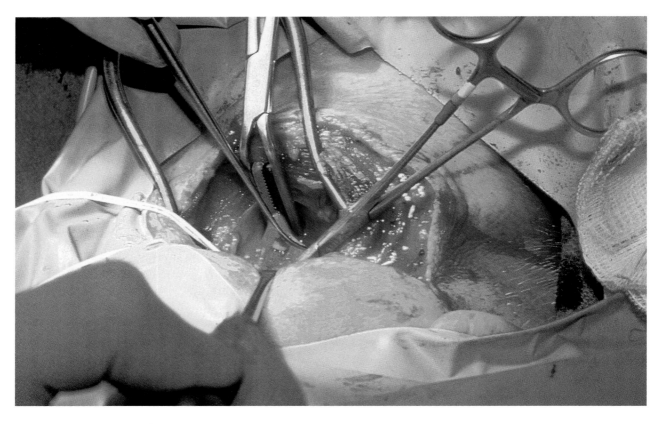

Carotid endarterectomy. *(Custom Medical Stock Photo. Reproduced by permission.)*

Key Terms

Atherosclerotic plaque   A deposit of fatty and calcium substances that accumulate in the lining of the artery wall, restricting blood flow.

Cerebral infarction   Brain tissue damage caused by interrupted flow of oxygen to the brain.

Electrolytes   Salts and minerals that produce electrically charged particles (ions) in body fluids. Common human electrolytes are sodium chloride, potassium, calcium, and sodium bicarbonate. Electrolytes control the fluid balance of the body and are important in muscle contraction, energy generation, and almost all major biochemical reactions in the body.

Hyperlipidemia   A condition characterized by abnormally high levels of lipids in blood plasma.

Hypertension   Abnormally high arterial blood pressure that if left untreated can lead to heart disease and stroke.

Mastoid process   The protrusions of bone behind the ears at the base of the skull.

Myocardial infarction   Commonly known as a heart attack, a myocardial infarction is an episode in which some of the heart's blood supply is severely cut off or restricted, causing the heart muscle to suffer and die from lack of oxygen.

Sternocleidomastoid muscle   A muscle located in front of the neck that functions to turn the head from side to side.

Stroke   Interruption of blood flow to a part of the brain with consequent brain damage. A stroke may be caused by a blood clot or by hemorrhage due to a burst blood vessel. Also known as a cerebrovascular accident.

Transient ischemic attack   A brief interruption of the blood supply to part of the brain that causes a temporary impairment of vision, speech, or movement. Usually, the episode lasts for just a few moments, but it may be a warning sign for a full-scale stroke.

Townsend, Courtney M. *Sabiston Textbook of Surgery*. 16th ed. W. B. Saunders Company, 2001.

PERIODICALS

Barnett, Henry J. M. "The appropriate use of carotid endarterectomy." *Canadian Medical Association Journal* 166 (April 2002): 9.

Gross, Cary, P. "Relation between prepublication release of clinical trial results and the practice of carotid endarterectomy." *Journal of the American Medical Association* 284 (December 2000): 22.

Mullenix, Philip. "Carotid Endarterectomy remains the gold standard." *American Journal of Surgery* 183, no. 59 (May 2002).

Perler, Bruce A. "Carotid Endarterectomy: The 'gold standard' in the endovascular era." *Journal of the American College of Surgeons* 194, no. 1 (January 2002).

Walker, Paul M. "Carotid Endarterectomy: applying trial results in clinical practice." *Canadian Medical Association Journal* 157 (1997).

ORGANIZATIONS

National Stroke Association. 9707 E. Easter Lane, Englewood, Colarado 80112. 303-649-9299 or 1-800-strokes; Fax: 303-649-1328. <http://www.stroke.org>.

Laith Farid Gulli, M.D.
Robert Ramirez, D.O.

∎ Carotid stenosis

Definition

Carotid stenosis is the medical description of the narrowing or constriction of the carotid artery. The artery is located in the neck, and the narrowing of the artery is caused by the buildup of plaque (fatty deposits). The process of atherosclerosis causes a hardening of the walls of the arteries and, in the case of atherosclerosis in the carotid artery, results in a carotid stenosis that reduces the flow of blood and nutrients to the brain.

Description

The carotid arteries run up the sides of the neck. They are vital arteries, and are a route of blood to the anterior part of the brain and, via branches, to the eyes, forehead, and nose. The deposition of plaque along the inner wall of an artery narrows its diameter. This makes the clogged artery less efficient in transporting blood. Plaque formation can become so severe that an artery is effectively blocked.

Carotid stenosis poses another danger when bits of the plaque dislodge. These pieces, which are referred to as blood clots or emboli, can move upward with the flow of blood towards the brain and can become lodged, blocking blood flow. This blockage interrupts the supply of nutrients and oxygen to the brain, and is one of the causes of cerebral vascular accidents, known as **stroke**. Carotid stenosis is a form of cerebral vascular disease and atherosclerosis.

Demographics

Stroke is the third leading cause of death in the United States after coronary artery disease and cancer, with approximately 750,000 strokes and more than 150,000 deaths occurring each year in the United States. Approximately 50% of these strokes are thought to be the result of carotid stenosis.

Causes and symptoms

The cause of carotid stenosis is the buildup of plaque on the inner wall of the carotid artery. The reduced blood flow to the brain and the blockage of other arteries following the release of emboli can cause a stroke. Increased risk of carotid stenosis is associated with smoking, hypertension, elevated levels of cholesterol, obesity, and a sedentary lifestyle. Some of these factors such as hypertension and cholesterol level may also be related to a person's physiology. Another risk factor is diabetes. Older, less active people are more prone to carotid stenosis. Additionally, the older a person is, the greater the risk posed by carotid stenosis.

Sometimes, prior to a major stroke, a person can be temporarily affected by the arterial blockage or release of a small embolus. The interrupted flow of blood to the brain, which can be very brief or last a few hours, does not persist longer than 24 hours. Symptoms of this transient event, called a **transient ischemic attack** (TIA), include weakness, as well as visual and speech difficulties. The exact symptoms of carotid stenosis depend on the area of the brain that is affected. Symptoms can also be absent, with the stenosis discovered only incidentally during a clinical examination.

In the event of a stroke, if the blocked blood flow is not restored, brain cells can die, causing permanent brain damage.

Diagnosis

Although not as accurate as other methods, a physician can listen to the pulsing of blood through the carotid artery by means of a stethoscope. The weaker pulse that is a result of stenosis will be evident in the form of altered sounds (bruits) as the blood flows past the area of disturbance.

Sometimes, carotid stenosis is suspected if a person has a transient malfunction of blood flow to the brain, or a TIA. A TIA can last anywhere from a few seconds to several hours. The temporary blockage of the artery can

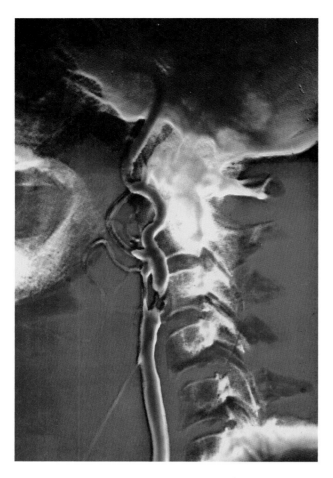

False-color angiogram showing stenosis in the carotid artery. *(Photograph by Alfred Pasteka. (c) CNRI/ Science Photo Library, National Audubon Society Collection/Photo Researchers, Inc. Reproduced by permission.)*

cause a momentary loss of vision in one eye, a weak or numb sensation on one side of the body, slurred speech, or inability to speak. A TIA can be a warning to a physician of the potential presence of carotid stenosis.

Three main diagnostic tests aid in the diagnosis of carotid stenosis. The first is known as a duplex sonogram, or a carotid duplex. The procedure involves the use of high-frequency sound waves (ultrasound). The ultrasonic waves echo off of the carotid artery to produce a two-dimensional image on a monitor. If narrowing or obstruction of the carotid artery is present, it is often apparent in the image.

Another powerful imaging technique is **magnetic resonance imaging (MRI)** or magnetic resonance **angiography** (MRA). Both rely on the use of magnetism. Pulses of magnetic energy can be used to image the targeted area of the body, based on the interruption of the flow of the electrons in the magnetic field. This information is then converted to a visual image.

The third technique is known as an angiogram or arteriogram. An angiogram is an examination that utilizes x rays after a small tube (catheter) is inserted into the base of the carotid artery. An x-ray dye is then injected. The dye reveals the areas of the regions of the artery that are narrowed or blocked.

Treatment team

Diagnosis and treatment of carotid stenosis involves the primary care physician, nurses, **neurologist**, neurosurgeons, neuroradiologists, and specialists who are skilled in performing angioplasty.

Treatment

Carotid stenosis is treated surgically or medically. One of two surgical treatments is typically used. The first approach is known as microsurgical **carotid endarterectomy**. The second approach is termed endovascular angioplasty and stenting.

Carotid endarterectomy is the surgical exposure of the carotid artery and the removal of the plaque. This re-establishes the uninterrupted flow of blood to the brain. This approach is the method of choice for most patients. However, the technique does itself carry a risk of stroke (stroke can be caused in up to 3% of surgeries).

For patients who are unable to undergo surgery, the angioplasty and stenting approach is used. In this approach a catheter that contains an expandable region at one end is inserted into the carotid artery. The end of the catheter is then expanded. This "balloon" squeezes the plaque against the arterial wall, increasing the effective diameter of the artery. Then, a stent is placed inside the artery. A stent is a tubular arrangement of fibers somewhat similar visually to wire fencing rolled up into a tube. The stent reinforces the carotid artery to prevent its collapse and to keep the plaque tightly against the arterial wall.

Surgery and the associated risks may not be warranted in patients whose arterial blockage is less than 50%.

Anticoagulant medications such as aspirin can be used instead to reduce the tendency of blood clots to form. Treatment can also consist of lifestyle modifications such as stopping smoking, limiting cholesterol intake, or use of cholesterol-lowering medications.

Clinical trials

As of February 2004, a clinical trial designed to investigate the relative effectiveness of carotid angioplasty with stenting versus carotid endarterectomy in preventing stroke, myocardial infarction, and death was recruiting patients in the United States and Canada. Participants should have symptoms of carotid stenosis. The trial, called "Carotid Revascularization Endarterectomy versus Stent Trial (CREST)," was being coordinated by the National Institute for Neurological Diseases and Stroke.

Another clinical trial was designed to examine the role of diet (specifically high doses of vitamin E) on the metabolism of low-density lipoprotein, which is critical in plaque formation. This trial was being coordinated by the National Institute of Health's National Center for Complimentary and Alternative Medicine. Information on both **clinical trials** may be found at the National Institute of Health Clinical Trials website: www.clinicaltrials.gov.

Prognosis

With prompt medical treatment, including surgery, recovery from carotid stenosis can be complete with no residual effects. However, if treatment is delayed or if a stroke occurs, damage can be permanent.

If carotid stenosis is dealt with promptly by surgery, medicine, or lifestyle modifications, prognosis is good. For example, at the Johns Hopkins Medical School, carotid stenosis corrective surgery has a mortality rate of 0.8% (80 in 1,000 people) and a morbidity rate (the person survives, but with some complication) of 1.8% (18 in 1,000 people).

However, undiagnosed stenosis can result in stroke. Depending on the severity of the stroke, prognosis is variable. An estimated 325,000 strokes and 75,000 deaths occur each year in the United States due to carotid stenosis.

Special concerns

Even if there are no symptoms associated with the presence of carotid stenosis, the malady is often a warning sign of possible blockage of the arteries of the heart, or coronary artery disease. Thus, people diagnosed with carotid stenosis should be carefully monitored for coronary artery disease.

Resources

BOOKS

Wiebers, David. *Stroke-Free for Life: The Complete Guide to Stroke Prevention and Treatment.* 2nd. ed. Mayo Clinic. New York: Harper Resource, 2002.

PERIODICALS

Biller, J., and W. H. Thies. "When to operate in carotid artery disease." *American Family Physician* (January 2000): 400–406.

OTHER

Johns Hopkins Department of Neurosurgery. "What is Carotid Stenosis?" *Johns Hopkins University School of Medicine.* (February 1, 2004).<http://www.neuro.jhmi.edu/cerebro/cs.html>.

"Risk Reduction through Surgery: Carotid Endarterectomy." *National Stroke Association.* (March 1, 2004). <http://209.107.44.93/NationalStroke/StrokePrevention/Risk+Reduction+through+Surgery.htm>.

Toronto Brain Vascular Malformation Study Group. "Carotid Stenosis. What is Carotid Stenosis?" University of Toronto. (February 1, 2004).<http://brainavm.uhnres.utoronto.ca/malformations/content/carotid_stenosis.htm>.

ORGANIZATIONS

American Stroke Association, a division of the American Heart Association. 7272 Greenville Avenue, Dallas, TX 75231. (888) 4-STROKE. <http://www.strokeassociation.org>.

Centers for Disease Control and Prevention (CDC). 1600 Clifton Road, Atlanta, GA 30333. (404) 639-3311 or (800) 311-3435. <http://www.cdc.gov>.

National Institute for Neurological Diseases and Stroke (NINDS). 6001 Executive Boulevard, Bethesda, MD 20892. (301) 496-5751 or (800) 352-9424. <http://www.ninds.nih.gov>.

Brian Douglas Hoyle, PhD

Carpal tunnel syndrome

Definition

Carpal tunnel syndrome is an entrapment neuropathy of the wrist. It occurs when the median nerve, which runs through the wrist and enervates the thumb, pointer finger, middle finger and the thumb side of the ring finger, is aggravated because of compression. Symptoms include numbness, tingling and **pain** in the fingers the median nerve sensitizes. Some people have difficulty grasping items and may have pain radiating up the arm. Carpal tunnel syndrome is common in people who work on assembly lines, doing heavy lifting and packing involving repetitive motions. Other repetitive movements such as typing; are often implicated in cause carpal tunnel syndrome, however some clinical evidence contradicts this association. Additional causes of the syndrome include pregnancy, diabetes, obesity or simply wrist anatomy in which the carpal tunnel is narrow. Treatment includes immobilization with a splint or in severe cases surgery to release the compression of the median nerve.

Description

Carpal tunnel syndrome (CTS) is caused by a compression of the median nerve in the wrist, a condition known as nerve entrapment. Nerve entrapments occur when a nerve that travels through a passage between bones and cartilage becomes irritated because a hard edge presses against it. In almost every case of nerve entrapment, one side of the passage is moveable and the repetitive rubbing exacerbates the injury.

Three sides of the carpal tunnel are made up of three bones that form a semicircle around the back of the wrist. The fourth side of the carpal tunnel is made up of the transverse carpal tunnel ligament also called the palmar carpal ligament, which runs across the wrist on the same side as the palm. This ligament is made of tissue that cannot stretch or contract, making the cross sectional area of the carpal tunnel a fixed size. Running through the carpal tunnel are nine tendons that assist the muscles that move the hand and the median nerve. The median nerve enervates the thumb, forefinger, middle finger, and the thumb side of the ring finger. The ulnar nerve that serves the little finger side of the ring finger and the little finger runs outside of the transverse carpal tunnel ligament and is therefore less likely to become entrapped in the wrist.

The tendons that run through the carpal tunnel are encased in a lubricating substance called tensynovium. This substance can become swollen when the tendons rub quickly against one another, as occurs when the finger muscles are used repeatedly. When this happens, there is less space within the carpal tunnel for the median nerve and it becomes compressed or pinched.

When a nerve is compressed, the blood supply to the nerve is interrupted. In an attempt to alleviate the problem, the body's immune system sends new cells called fibroblasts to the area to try to build new tissue. This eventually results in scar tissue around the nerve. In an area that cannot expand this only worsens the situation and puts more pressure on the nerve. A compressed nerve can be likened to an electrical wire that has been crimped. It cannot transmit electrical signals to the brain properly and the result is a feeling of numbness, tingling or pain in the areas that the nerve enervates.

Compression of the median nerve causes tingling and numbness in the thumb, forefinger, middle finger and on

Key Terms

Median nerve   A nerve that runs through the wrist and into the hand. It provides sensation and some movement to the hand, the thumb, the index finger, the middle finger, and half of the ring finger.

Neuropathy   A disease or abnormality of the peripheral nerves (the nerves outside the brain and spinal cord). Major symptoms include weakness, numbness, paralysis, or pain in the affected area.

the thumb-side of the fourth finger. It may also cause pain in the forearm and occasionally into the shoulder. Some persons have a difficult time gripping and making a fist.

People who suffer from CTS range from those who are mildly inconvenienced and must wear a splint at night to relieve pressure on the median nerve to those who are severely debilitated and lose use of their hands. Problems associated with CTS can invade a person's life making even simple tasks such as answering the phone, reading a book or opening a door extremely difficult. In severe cases, surgery to release the median nerve is often suggested by an orthopedist. The carpal tunnel ligament is cut, relieving the pressure within the carpal tunnel. Rates of success are quite high with the surgical procedure.

Demographics

Carpal tunnel syndrome is more common in women than in men, perhaps because the carpal tunnel generally has a smaller cross section in women than in men. The ratio of women to men who suffer from CTS is about three to one. CTS is most often diagnosed in people who are between 30 and 50 years old. It is more likely to occur in people whose professions require heavy lifting and repetitive movements of the hands such as manufacturing, packing, cleaning and finishing work on textiles.

Causes and symptoms

Carpal tunnel syndrome may occur when anything causes the size of the carpal tunnel to decreases or when anything puts pressure on the median nerve. Often the cause is simply the result of an individual's anatomy; some people have smaller carpal tunnels than others. Trauma or injury to the wrist, such as bone breakage or dislocation can cause CTS if the carpal tunnel is narrowed either by the new position of the bones or by associated swelling. Development of a cyst or tumor in the carpal tunnel will also result in increased pressure on the median nerve and likely CTS. Systemic problems that result in swelling may also cause CTS such as hypothyroidism, problems with the pituitary gland, and the hormonal imbalances that occur during pregnancy and menopause. Arthritis, especially rheumatoid arthritis, may also cause CTS. Some patients with diabetes may be more susceptible to CTS because they already suffer from nerve damage. Obesity and cigarette smoking are thought to aggravate symptoms of CTS.

Much evidence suggests that one of the more common causes of CTS involves performing repetitive motions such as opening and closing of the hands or bending of the wrists or holding vibrating tools. Motions that involve weights or force are thought to be particularly damaging. For example, the types of motions that assembly line workers perform such as packing meat, poultry or fish, sewing and finishing textiles and garments, cleaning, and manufacturing are clearly associated with CTS. Other repetitive injury disorders such as data entry while working on computers are also implicated in CTS. However, some clinical data contradicts this finding. These studies show that computer use can result in bursitis and tendonitis, but not CTS. In fact, a 2001 study by the Mayo Clinic found that people who used the computer up to seven hours a day were no more likely to develop CTS than someone who did not perform the type of repetitive motions required to operate a keyboard.

The two major symptoms of carpal tunnel syndrome include numbness and tingling in the thumb, forefinger, middle finger and the thumb side of the fourth finger and a dull aching pain extending from the wrist through the shoulder. The pain often worsens at night because most people sleep with flexed wrists, which puts additional pressure on the median nerve. Eventually the muscles in the hands will weaken, in particular, the thumb will tend to lose strength. In severe cases, persons suffering from CTS are unable to differentiate between hot and cold temperatures with their hands.

Diagnosis

Diagnosis of carpal tunnel syndrome begins with a physical exam of the hands, wrists and arms. The physician will note any swelling or discoloration of the skin and the muscles of the hand will be tested for strength. If the patient reports symptoms in the first four fingers, but not the little finger, then CTS is indicated. Two special tests are used to reproduce symptoms of CTS: the Tinel test and the Phalen test. The Tinel test involves a physician taping on the median nerve. If the patient feels a shock or a tingling in the fingers, then he or she likely has carpal tunnel syndrome. In the Phalen test, the patient is asked to flex his or her wrists and push the backs of the hands together. If the patient feels tingling or numbness in the hands within one minute, then carpal tunnel syndrome is the likely cause.

A variety of electronic tests are used to confirm CTS. Nerve conduction velocity studies (NCV) are used to measure the speed with which an electrical signal is transferred along the nerve. If the speed is slowed relative to normal, it is likely that the nerve is compressed. **Electromyography** involves inserting a needle into the muscles of the hand and converting the muscle activity to electrical signals. These signals are interpreted to indicate the type and severity of damage to the median nerve. Ultrasound imaging can also be used to visualize the movement of the median nerve within the carpal tunnel. X rays can be used to detect fractures in the wrist that may be the cause of carpal tunnel syndrome. **Magnetic resonance imaging (MRI)** is also a useful tool for visualizing injury to the median nerve.

Treatment team

Treatment for carpal tunnel syndrome usually involves a physician specializing in the bones and joints (orthopedist) or a **neurologist**, along with physical and occupational therapists, and if necessary, a surgeon.

Treatment

Lifestyle changes are often the first type of treatment prescribed for carpal tunnel syndrome. Avoiding activities that aggravate symptoms is one of the primary ways to manage CTS. These activities include weight-bearing repetitive hand movements and holding vibrating tools. Physical or occupational therapy is also used to relieve symptoms of CTS. The therapist will usually train the patient to use exercises to reduce irritation in the carpal tunnel and instruct the patient on proper posture and wrist positions. Often a doctor or therapist will suggest that a patient wear a brace that holds the arm in a resting position, especially at night. Many people tend to sleep with their wrists flexed, which decreases the space for the median nerve within the carpal tunnel. The brace keeps the wrist in a position that maximizes the space for the nerve.

Doctors may prescribe non-steroidal anti-inflammatory medications to reduce the swelling in the wrist and relieve pressure on the median nerve. Oral steroids are also useful for decreasing swelling. Some studies have shown that large quantities of vitamin B-6 can reduce symptoms of CTS, but this has not been confirmed. Injections of corticosteroids into the carpal tunnel may also be used to reduce swelling and temporarily provide some extra room for the median nerve.

Surgery can be used as a final step to relieve pressure on the median nerve and relieve the symptoms of CTS. There are two major procedures in use, both of which involve cutting the transverse carpal tunnel ligament. Dividing this ligament relieves pressure on the median nerve and allows blood flow to the nerve to increase. With time,

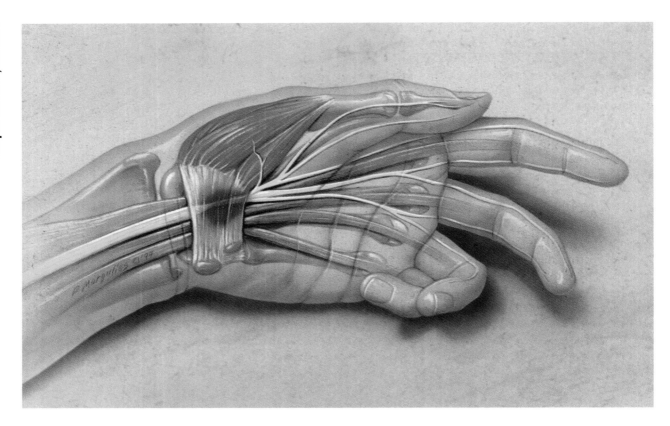

Medical illustration of left wrist and hand showing carpel tunnel syndrome. The yellow lines represent the median nerve, the blue bands the tendons. Repetitive motion of the wrist and hand causes swelling, and the resulting compression of the nerve results in pain and sometimes nerve damage. (© R. Margulies. Custom Medical Stock Photo. Reproduced by permission.)

the nerve heals and as it does so, the numbness and pain in the arm are reduced.

Open release surgery is the standard for severe CTS. In this procedure, a surgeon will open the skin down the front of the palm and wrist. The incision will be about two inches long stretching towards the fingers from the lowest fold line on the wrist. Then next incision is through the palmar fascia, which is a thin connective tissue layer just below the skin, but above the transverse carpal ligament. Finally, being careful to avoid the median nerve and the tendons that pass through the carpal tunnel, the surgeon carefully cuts the transverse carpal ligament. This releases pressure on the median nerve.

Once the transverse carpal tunnel ligament is divided, the surgeon stitches up the palma fascia and the skin, leaving the ends of the ligament loose. Over time, the space between the ends of the ligament will be joined with scar tissue. The resulting space, which studies indicate is approximately 26% greater than prior to the surgery, is enlarged enough so that the median nerve is no longer compressed.

A second surgical method for treatment of CTS is endoscopic carpal tunnel release. In this newer technique, a surgeon makes a very small incision below the crease of the wrist just below the carpal ligament. Some physicians will make another small incision in the palm of the hand, but the single incision technique is more commonly used. The incision just below the carpal ligament allows the surgeon to access the carpal tunnel. He or she will then insert a plastic tube with a slot along one side, called a cannula, into the carpal tunnel along the median nerve just underneath the carpal ligament. Next an endoscope, which is a small fiber-optic cable that relays images of the internal structures of the wrist to a television screen, is fed through the cannula. Using the endoscope, the surgeon checks that the nerves, blood vessels and tendons that run through the carpal tunnel are not in the way of the cannula. A specialized scalpel is fed through the cannula. This knife is equipped with a hook on the end that allows the surgeon to cut as he or she pulls the knife backward. The surgeon positions this knife so that it will divide the carpal ligament as he pulls it out of the cannula. Once the knife is pulled through the cannula, the carpal ligament is severed, but the palma fascia and the skin are not cut. Just as in the open release surgery, cutting the carpal ligament releases the pressure on the median nerve. Over time, scar tissue will form between the ends of the carpal ligament. After the cannula is removed from the carpal tunnel, the surgeon will stitch the small incision in patient's wrist and the small incision in the palm if one was made.

The two different surgical techniques for treating CTS have both positive and negative attributes and the technique used depends on the individual case. In open release, the surgeon has a clear view of the anatomy of the wrist and can make sure that the division of the transverse ligament is complete. He or she can also see exactly which structures to avoid while making the incision. On the other hand, because the incision to the exterior is much larger than in endoscopic release, recovery time is usually longer. While the symptoms of CTS usually improve rapidly, the pain associated with the incision may last for several months. Many physicians feel that the recovery time associated with endoscopic release is faster than that for open release because the incision in the skin and palma fascia are so much smaller. On the other hand, endoscopic surgery is more expensive and requires training in the use of more technologic equipment. Some believe that are also risks that the carpal ligament may not be completely released and the median nerve may be damaged by the cannula, or the specialized hooked knife. Research is ongoing in an attempt to determine whether open or endoscopic release provides the safest and most successful results.

Success rates of release surgery for carpal tunnel syndrome are extremely high, with a 70–90% rate of improvement in median nerve function. There are complications associated with the surgery, although they are generally rare. These include incomplete division of the carpal ligament, pain along the incisions and weakness in the hand. Both the pain and the weakness are usually temporary. Infections following surgery for CTS are reported in less than 5% of all patients.

Recovery and rehabilitation

One day following surgery for carpal tunnel syndrome, a patient should begin to move his or her fingers, however gripping and pinching heavy items should be avoided for a month and a half to prevent the tendons that run through the carpal tunnel from disrupting the formation of scar tissue between the ends of the carpal ligament.

After about a month and a half, a patient can begin to see an occupational or physical therapist. Exercises, massage and stretching will all be used to increase wrist strength and range of motion. Eventually, the therapist will prescribe exercises to improve the ability of the tendons within the carpal tunnel to slide easily and to increase dexterity of the fingers. The therapist will also teach the patient techniques to avoid a recurrence of carpal tunnel syndrome in the future.

Clinical trials

There are a variety of **clinical trials** underway that are searching for ways to prevent and treat carpal tunnel syndrome. The National Institute of Arthritis and Musculoskeletal and Skin Diseases (NIAMS) supports this research on CTS. Their website is <http://clinicaltrials.gov/search/term=Carpal+Tunnel+Syndrome>.

One trial seeks to determine which patients will benefit from surgical treatments compared to non-surgical treatments using a new magnetic resonance technique. The study is seeking patients with early, mild to moderate carpal tunnel syndrome. Contact Brook I. Martin at the University of Washington for more information. The phone number is (206) 616–0982 and the email is bim@u.washington.edu.

A second trial compares the effects of the medication amitriptyline, **acupuncture**, and placebos for treating repetitive stress disorders such as carpal tunnel syndrome. The study is located at Harvard University. For information contact Ted Kaptchuk at (617) 665–2174 or tkaptchu@caregroup.harvard.edu.

A third study is evaluating the effects of a protective brace for preventing carpal tunnel syndrome in people who use tools that vibrate in the workplace. The brace is designed to absorb the energy of the vibrations while remaining unobtrusive. For information on this study contact Prosper Benham at the UCLA Hand Center. The phone number is (310) 206–4468 and the email address is pbenhaim@mednet.ucla.edu.

Prognosis

Persons with carpal tunnel syndrome can usually expect to gain significant relief from prescribed surgery, treatments, exercises, and positioning devices.

Resources

BOOKS

Johansson, Phillip. *Carpal Tunnel Syndrome and Other Repetitive Strain Injuries*. Brookshire, TX: Enslow Publishers, Inc. 1999.

Shinn, Robert, and Ruth Aleskovsky. *The Repetitive Strain Injury Handbook*. New York: Henry Holt and Company. 2000.

OTHER

"Carpal Tunnel Syndrome." *American Association of Orthopaedic Surgeons.* (February 11, 2004).

<http://orthoinfo.aaos.org/brochure/thr_report.cfm? Thread_ID=5&topcategory=Hand>.

"Carpal Tunnel Syndrome Fact Sheet." *National Instititute of Neurological Disorders and Stroke.* (February 11, 2004). <http://www.ninds.nih.gov/healt_and_medical/disorders/ carpal_tunnel.htm>.

ORGANIZATIONS

American Chronic Pain Association (ACPA). P.O. Box 850, Rocklin, CA 95677. (916) 632-0922 or (800) 533-3231. ACPA@pacbell.net. <http://www.theacpa.org>.

National Chronic Pain Outreach Association (NCPOA). P.O. Box 274, Millboro, VA 24460. (540) 862-9437; Fax: (540) 862-9485. ncpoa@cfw.com. <http://www.chronic pain.org>.

National Institute of Arthritis and Musculoskeletal and Skin Dieseases (NIAMS). National Institutes of Health, Bldg. 31, Rm. 4C05, Bethesda, MD 20892. (301) 496-8188; Fax: (540) 862-9485. ncpoa@cfw.com. <http://www.niams.nih.gov/index.htm>.

Juli M. Berwald, Ph.D.

Catechol-O-methyltransferase inhibitors

Definition

Catechol-O-methyltransferase (COMT) inhibitors are a class of medication used in combination with levodopa and carbidopa in the treatment of symptoms of **Parkinson's disease** (PD). COMT inhibitors such as tolcapone and entacapone optimize the active transport of levodopa to the **central nervous system** (CNS) and allow the administration of lower doses of both levodopa and carbidopa, which decreases or even prevents the side effects related to these two drugs.

Purpose

Levodopa is a drug that helps to supplement dopamine, a neurotransmitter, to the brain of persons with PD. A neurotransmitter is a chemical that is released during a nerve impulse that transmits information from one nerve cell to another. In PD, levels of the neurotransmitter dopamine progressively decrease as the disease evolves. Drug therapy with levodopa also leads to dopamine formation in tissues outside the brain and in the gastrointestinal tract, causing undesirable side effects and reduced availability of levodopa to the nerve cells. The addition of carbidopa to the treatment regimen inhibits this action and thus, increases levodopa uptake into the brain. However, the inhibition of dopamine results in activation of certain enzymes (including catechol-O-methyltransferase) that compete with levodopa for transport to the

---

Key Terms

Ataxia Loss of muscle coordination due to nerve damage.

Carbidopa A drug combined with levodopa to slow the breakdown of the levodopa, used to treat the symptoms of Parkinson's disease.

Levodopa A precursor of dopamine which is converted to dopamine in the brain, and the drug most commonly used to treat the symptoms of Parkinson's disease.

---

brain. By giving drugs that reduce these enzymes, competition is reduced, and more levodopa is utilized by the brain. The administration of a COMT inhibitor drug prolongs the duration of each levodopa dose, and allows the reduction of doses of both levodopa and carbidopa by approximately 30%.

Description

Tolcapone was the first COMT inhibitor approved by the United States Food and Drug Administration to be taken orally in association with the levodopa/carbidopa regimen. Tolcapone is readily absorbed through the gastrointestinal tract and has a fairly rapid action. The drug is metabolized in the liver and eliminated from the body through the feces and urine. However, its COMT inhibitory activity lasts much longer, due to the high affinity of tolcapone with the enzyme.

Entacapone, another COMT inhibitor, was first approved in the European Union and its effects are similar to those obtained with tolcapone when added to levodopa/carbidopa regimen.

Recommended dosage

The physician will adjust the dose of either tolcapone or entacapone to each patient in accordance with other individual clinical characteristics.

Precautions

The use of tolcapone requires a reduction of levodopa/carbidopa to prevent the occurrence of levodopa-related side effects, such as low blood pressure and **dizziness** when rising, loss of appetite, nausea, drowsiness, and hallucinations. Patients with liver disorders or reduced liver function should not receive tolcapone due to its high toxicity to the liver cells. All patients using tolcapone should be regularly monitored by their physician and laboratory blood tests to determine the concentrations of liver enzymes should be periodically performed. As the chronic use of tolcapone may cause irreversible liver injury, any signs of dark urine, pale stools, unusual **fatigue**, fever, jaundice, persistent nausea or vomiting, and tenderness in the upper right side of the abdomen should be reported to the physician. Tolcapone is contraindicated in pregnant women and during breast-feeding, or to patients already suffering from low blood pressure. Kidney deficiency reduces the elimination rate of tolcapone metabolites and increases the severity of adverse effects.

Entacapone is metabolized in the liver and a pre-existing reduced liver function or chronic deficiency should be reported to the physician to allow for adjustments in dosage. Dosage adjustments or special precautions may be also necessary when entacapone is administered to patients under treatment with one or more of the following medications: isoproterenol, epinephrine, apomorphine, isoetherine, or bitolterol. Except for selegiline, all monoamine oxidase (MAO) inhibitors are contraindicated when using entacapone.

Side effects

The more common tolcapone-related side effects are abdominal **pain**, nausea, vomiting, diarrhea, drowsiness, sleep disorders, **headache**, and dizziness, especially in the first few days of treatment. Elderly patients may have hallucinatory episodes (sensations of seeing, hearing or feeling something that does not exist). Some patients report irritability, aching joints and neck, muscle cramps, agitation, **ataxia**, difficulty in concentrating, and increased urination. Severe episodes of diarrhea may occur after the second month of treatment.

Common side effects with entacapone are abdominal discomfort (constipation, nausea, diarrhea, abdominal pain) and fatigue, which tend to disappear as the body adapts to the medication. Some patients may experience gastritis, heartburns, belching, sleep disorders, increased perspiration, drowsiness, agitation, irritation and mood changes, and fatigue.

Interactions

Patients should inform the physician of any other medication in use when tolcapone prescription is being considered. The concomitant use of entacapone and methyldopa may cause heart rhythm disturbances and abrupt changes in blood pressure.

Resources
BOOKS
Champe, Pamela C., and Richard A. Harvey, eds. *Pharmacology,* 2nd ed. Philadelphia, PA: Lippincott Williams & Wilkins, 2000.

Weiner, William J., M.D., *Parkinson's Disease: A Complete Guide for Patients and Families.* Baltimore: Johns Hopkins University Press, 2001.
OTHER
Hubble, Jean Pintar, M.D., Richard C. Berchou, Pharm.D. "CATECHOL-O-METHYL TRANSFERASE (COMT) INHIBITORS." *The National Parkinson Foundation, Inc.* (April 25, 2004). <http://www.parkinson.org/med18.htm>.
"Entacapone and Tolcapone." *We Move.* July 25, 1999. (April 24, 2004). <http://www.wemove.org/emove/article.asp?ID=91>.
ORGANIZATIONS
National Parkinson Foundation. 1501 N.W. 9th Avenue, Bob Hope Research Center, Miami, FL 33136-1494. (305) 243-6666 or (800) 327-4545; Fax: (305) 243-5595. mailbox@parkinson.org. <http://www.parkinson.org/>.

Sandra Galeotti

Causalgia *see* **Reflex sympathetic dystrophy**

Cavernous angioma *see* **Cerebral cavernous malformation**

Cavernous malformation *see* **Cerebral cavernous malformation**

Central cervical cord syndrome *see* **Central cord syndrome**

Central cord syndrome
Definition

Central cord syndrome is an "incomplete lesion," a condition in which only part of the spinal cord is affected. In central cord syndrome, there is greater weakness or outright paralysis of the upper extremities, as compared with the lower extremities. Unlike a complete lesion, that causes loss of all sensation and movement below the level of the injury, an incomplete lesion causes only a partial loss of sensation and movement.

Description

Central cord syndrome specifically affects the central part of the spinal cord, also known as the "grey matter." The segment of spinal cord affected by central cord syndrome is the cervical segment, the part of the spinal cord that is encased within the first seven vertebrae, running from the base of the brain and into the neck. The central part of the cervical spinal cord is responsible for carrying information to and from the upper extremities and the brain, resulting in movement. Because the outer (peripheral) areas of the cervical spinal cord are spared, information going to and from the brain and the lower extremities is not as severely affected.

The specific degree of impairment depends on the severity of the injury. More mild impairment may result in problems with fine motor control of the hands, while more severe impairment may cause actual paralysis of the upper limbs. While the lower limbs are less severely affected in central cord syndrome, in more serious injuries the lower extremities may demonstrate some degree of weakness, loss of sensation, or discoordination. Loss of bladder control may be evident as well.

Central cord syndrome often strikes people who are already suffering from a degenerative spinal disease called spondylosis or spinal stenosis. In spondylosis, a progressive narrowing of the spinal canal puts increasing pressure on the spinal cord, resulting in damage and debilitation. Often, a fall or other injury that causes a person with spondylosis to extend his or her neck will cause the already-narrowed spinal canal to injure the spinal cord, resulting in central cord syndrome.

Demographics

As with other types of spinal cord injuries, men are more frequently affected by central cord syndrome than women. Because central cord syndrome can result from either injury or as a sequelae to the spinal disease spondylosis, there are two age peaks for the condition: in younger individuals (secondary to trauma) or in older individuals (secondary to spondylosis).

Causes and symptoms

Any injury or condition that preferentially damages the central, gray matter of the cervical spinal cord can lead to central cord syndrome. The most common causes include complications of the progressive, degenerative spinal disease called spondylosis, as well as traumatic injury to the cervical spine, such as fractures or dislocations. Injuries to a cervical spine that is already abnormally narrow due to disease is a particularly common cause of central cord syndrome. Tumors or **syringomyelia** (a chronic disease involving abnormal accumulations of fluid within the spinal column) may also lead to central cord syndrome.

Individuals with central cord syndrome may first notice neck **pain** and shooting or burning pains in the arms and hands. Tingling, numbness, and weakness may also be evident. Fine motor control of the upper extremities may be significantly impaired. Sensation in the upper limbs may be dulled or completely lost. Sensation from the legs may be lost, as well, and the lower extremities may demonstrate some degree of weakness and impaired movement. Bladder control may be weakened or lost.

Diagnosis

Diagnosis is usually accomplished through imaging of the cervical spine, with plain x rays, **CT scans**, and/or **MRI** imaging.

Treatment team

The treatment team for central cord syndrome will consist of a **neurologist** and a neurosurgeon, as well as multiple rehabilitation specialists, including physiatrists, physical therapists, and occupational therapists.

Treatment

Usually, intravenous steroids are immediately administered to patients suspected of suffering from central cord syndrome, to decrease swelling and improve outcome. Surgery may be performed in certain cases, in order to stabilize the spine or in order to decompress the spinal cord.

Prognosis

Many patients will be able to rehabilitate their less-severely affected lower extremities and will continue walking, although sometimes with a permanently abnormal, stiff, spastic gait. Many individuals also regain some strength and function of their upper extremities. Upper extremity fine motor coordination, however, usually remains impaired.

Resources

BOOKS

Hammerstad, John P. "Strength and Reflexes." In *Textbook of Clinical Neurology*, edited by Christopher G. Goetz. Philadelphia: W. B. Saunders Company, 2003.

Mercier, Lonnie R. "Spinal Cord Compression." In *Ferri's Clinical Advisor: Instant Diagnosis and Treatment*, edited by Fred F. Ferri. St. Louis: Mosby, 2004.

Morris, Gabrielle, F., William R. Taylor, and Lawrence F. Marshall. "Spine and Spinal Cord Injury." In *Cecil Textbook of Internal Medicine*, edited by Lee Goldman, et al. Philadelphia: W. B. Saunders Company, 2000.

WEBSITES

National Institute of Neurological Disorders and Stroke (NINDS). *NINDS Central Cord Syndrome Information Page.* November 6, 2002. (June 4, 2004). <http://www.ninds.nih.gov/health_and_medical/disorders/central_cord.htm>.

ORGANIZATIONS

National Spinal Cord Injury Association. 6701 Democracy Blvd. #300-9, Bethesda, MD 20817. 301-214-4006 or 800-962-9629; Fax: 301-881-9817. info@spinalcord.org. <http://www.spinalcord.org>.

Rosalyn Carson-DeWitt, MD

Central nervous system

Definition

The central nervous system (CNS) is composed of the brain and spinal cord. The brain receives sensory information from the nerves that pass through the spinal cord, as well as other nerves such as those from sensory organs involved in sight and smell. Once received, the brain processes the sensory signals and initiates responses. The spinal cord is the principle route for the passage of sensory information to and from the brain.

Information flows to the central nervous system from the **peripheral nervous system**, which senses signals from the environment outside the body (sensory-somatic nervous system) and from the internal environment (autonomic nervous system). The brain's responses to incoming information flow through the spinal cord nerve network to the various effector organs and tissue regions where the target responsive action will take place.

Description

Brain

The brain is divided into three major anatomical regions, the prosencephalon (forebrain), mesencephalon (midbrain), and the rhombencephalon (hindbrain). The brain also contains a **ventricular system**, which consists of four ventricles (internal cavities): two lateral ventricles, a third ventricle, and a fourth ventricle. The ventricles are filled with cerebrospinal fluid and are continuous with the spinal canal. The ventricles are connected via two interventricular foramen (connecting the two lateral ventricles to the third venticle), and a cerebral aqueduct (connecting the third ventricle to the fourth ventricle).

The brain and spinal cord are covered by three layers of **meninges** (dura matter, arachnoid matter, and pia mater) that dip into the many folds and fissures. The meninges are three sheets or layers of connective tissue that cover all of the spinal cord and the brain. Infections of the meninges are called meningitis. Bacterial, viral, and protozoan meningitis are serious and require prompt medical attention. Between the arachnoid and the pia matter is a fluid called the cerebrospinal fluid. Bacterial infections of the cerebrospinal fluid can occur and are life-threatening.

GROSS ANATOMY OF THE BRAIN The prosencephalon is divided into the **diencephalon** and the telencephalon (also known as the cerebrum). The cerebrum contains the two large bilateral hemispherical cerebral cortex that are responsible for the intellectual functions and house the neural connections that integrate, personality, speech, and the interpretation of sensory data related to vision and hearing.

The midbrain, or mesencephalon region, serves as a connection between higher and lower brain functions, and contains a number of centers associated with regions that create strong drives to certain behaviors. The midbrain is involved in body movement. The so-called pleasure center is located here, which has been implicated in the development of addictive behaviors.

The rhombencephalon, consisting of the medulla oblongata, pons, and **cerebellum**, is an area largely devoted to lower brain functions, including autonomic functions involved in the regulation of breathing and general body coordination. The medulla oblongata is a cone-like knot of tissue that lies between the spinal cord and the pons. A median fissure (deep, convoluted fold) separates swellings (pyramids) on the surface of the medulla. The pons (also known as the metencephalon) is located on the anterior surface of the cerebellum and is continuous with the superior portion of the medulla oblongata. The pons contains large tracts of transverse fibers that serve to connect the left and right cerebral hemispheres.

The cerebellum lies superior and posterior to the pons at the back base of the head. The cerebellum consists of left and right hemispheres connected by the vermis. Specialized tracts (peduncles) of neural tissue also connect the

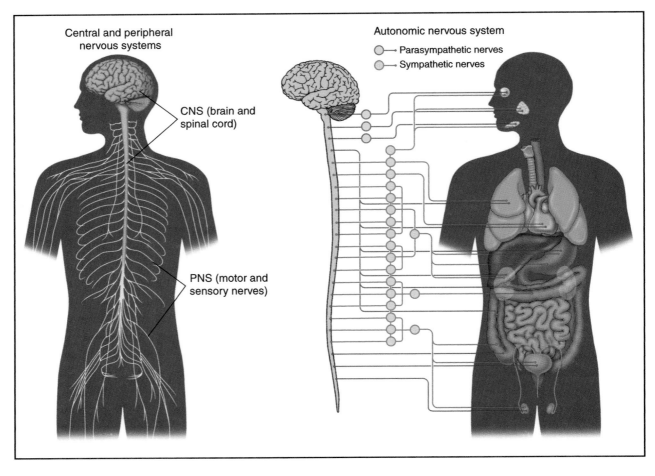

Central and peripheral
nervous systems

CNS (brain and
spinal cord)

PNS (motor and
sensory nerves)

Autonomic nervous system

○—→ Parasympathetic nerves
○—→ Sympathetic nerves

(Illustration by Frank Forney.)

Key Terms

Central nervous system (CNS)   Composed of the
brain and spinal cord.

cerebellum with the midbrain, pons, and medulla. The surface of the cerebral hemispheres (the cortex) is highly
convoluted into many folds and fissures.

The midbrain serves to connect the forebrain region to
the hindbrain region. Within the midbrain a narrow aqueduct connects ventricles in the forebrain to the hindbrain.
There are four distinguishable surface swellings (colliculi)
on the midbrain. The midbrain also contains a highly vas-
cularized mass of neural tissue called the red nucleus that
is reddish in color (a result of the vascularization) compared to other brain structures and landmarks.

Although not visible from an exterior inspection of
the brain, the diencephalon contains a dorsal thalamus
(with a large posterior swelling termed the pulvinar) and
a ventral hypothalamus that forms a border of the third
ventricle of the brain. In this third ventral region lies a
number of important structures, including the optic chiasma (the region where the ophthalmic nerves cross) and
infundibulum.

Obscuring the diencephalon are the two large, well-
developed, and highly convoluted cerebral hemispheres
that comprise the cerebrum. The cerebrum is the largest of
the regions of the brain. The corpus callosum is connected
to the two large cerebral hemispheres. Within each cerebral hemisphere lies a lateral ventricle. The cerebral hemispheres run under the frontal, parietal, and occipital bones
of the skull. The gray matter cortex is highly convoluted
into folds (gyri) and the covering meninges dip deeply into
the narrow gaps between the folds (sulci). The divisions of
the superficial anatomy of the brain use the gyri and sulci

as anatomical landmarks to define particular lobes of the cerebral hemispheres. As a rule, the lobes are named according to the particular bone of the skull that covers them. Accordingly, there are left and right frontal lobes, parietal lobes, an occipital lobe, and temporal lobes.

In a reversal of the pattern found within the spinal cord, the cerebral hemispheres have white matter tracts on the inside of the hemispheres and gray matter on the outside or cortex regions. Masses of gray matter that are present within the interior white matter are called basal ganglia or basal nuclei.

Spinal cord

The spinal cord is a long column of neural tissue that extends from the base of the brain, downward (inferiorly) through a canal created by the spinal vertebral foramina. The spinal cord is between 16.9 and 17.7 inches (43 and 45 centimeters) long in the average woman and man, respectively. The spinal cord usually terminates at the level of the first lumbar vertebra.

The spinal cord is enclosed and protected by the vertebra of the spinal column. There are four regions of vertebrae. Beginning at the skull and moving downward, there are the eight cervical vertebrae, 12 thoracic vertebrae, five lumbar vertebrae, five sacral vertebrae, and one set of fused coccygeal vertebra.

Along the length of the spinal cord are positioned 31 pairs of nerves. These are known as mixed spinal nerves, as they convey sensory information to the brain and response information back from the brain. Spinal nerve roots emerge from the spinal cord that lies within the spinal canal. Both dorsal and ventral roots fuse in the intervertebral foramen to create a spinal nerve.

Although there are only seven cervical vertebra, there are eight cervical nerves. Cervical nerves one through seven (C1–C7) emerge above (superior to) the corresponding cervical vertebrae. The last cervical nerve (C8) emerges below (inferior to) the last cervical vertebrae from that point downward the spinal nerves exit below the corresponding vertebrae for which they are named.

In the spinal cord of humans, the myelin-coated axons are on the surface and the axon-dendrite network is on the inside. In cross-section, the pattern of contrasting color of these regions produces an axon-dendrite shape that is reminiscent of a butterfly.

The nerves of the spinal cord correspond to the arrangement of the vertebrae. There are 31 pairs of nerves, grouped as eight cervical pairs, 12 thoracic pairs, five lumbar pairs, five sacral pairs, and one coccygeal pair. The nerves toward the top of the cord are oriented almost horizontally. Those further down are oriented on a progressively upward slanted angle toward the bottom of the cord.

Toward the bottom of the spinal cord, the spinal nerves connect with cells of the sympathetic nervous system. These cells are called pre-ganglionic and ganglionic cells. One branch of these cells is called the gray ramus communicans and the other branch is the white ramus communicans. Together they are referred to as the rami. Other rami connections lead to the pelvic area.

The bi-directional (two-way) communication network of the spinal cord allows the reflex response to occur. This type of rapid response occurs when a message from one type of nerve fiber, the sensory fiber, stimulates a muscle response directly, rather than the impulse traveling to the brain for interpretation. For example, if a hot stove burner is touched with a finger, the information travels from the finger to the spinal cord and then a response to move muscles away from the burner is sent rapidly and directly back. This response is initiated when speed is important.

Development and histology of the CNS

Both the spinal cord and the brain are made up of structures of nerve cells called neurons. The long main body extension of a neuron is called an axon. Depending on the type of nerve, the axons may be coated with a material called myelin. Both the brain and spinal cord components of the central nervous system contain bundles of cell bodies (out of which axons grow) and branched regions of nerve cells that are called dendrites. Between the axon of one cell body and the dendrite of another nerve cell is an intervening region called the synapse. In the spinal cord of humans, the myelin-coated axons are on the surface and the axon-dendrite network is on the inside. In the brain, this arrangement is reversed.

The brain begins as a swelling at the cephalic end of the neural tube that ultimately will become the spinal cord. The neural tube is continuous and contains primitive cerebrospinal fluids. Enlargements of the central cavity (neural tube lumen) in the region of the brain become the two lateral, third, and forth ventricles of the fully developed brain.

The embryonic brain is differentiated in several anatomical regions. The most cephalic region is the telencephalon. Ultimately, the telencephlon will develop the bilateral cerebral hemispheres, each containing a lateral ventricle, cortex (surface) layer of gray cells, a white matter layer, and basal nuclei. Caudal (inferior) to the telencephalon is the diencephalon that will develop the epithalamus, thalamus, and hypothalamus

Caudal to the diencephalon is the mesencephalon, the midbrain region that includes the cerebellum and pons. Within the myelencephalon region is the medulla oblongata.

Neural development inverts the gray matter and white matter relationship within the brain. The outer cortex is composed of gray matter, while the white matter (myelinated axons) lies on the interior of the developing brain.

The meninges that protect and help nourish neural tissue are formed from embryonic mesoderm that surrounds the axis established by the primitive neural tube and notochord. The cells develop many fine capillaries that supply the highly oxygen-demanding neural tissue.

Diseases and disorders of the CNS

Diseases that affect the nerves of the central nervous system include rabies, polio, and sub-acute sclerosing panencephalitis. Such diseases affect movement and can lead to mental incapacitation. The brain is also susceptible to disease, including toxoplasmosis and the development of empty region due to prions. Such diseases cause a wasting away of body function and mental ability. Brain damage can be so compromised as to be lethal.

Resources

BOOKS

Bear, M., et al. *Neuroscience: Exploring the Brain.* Baltimore: Williams & Wilkins, 1996.

Goetz, C. G., et al. *Textbook of Clinical Neurology.* Philadelphia: W.B. Saunders Company, 1999.

Goldman, Cecil. *Textbook of Medicine*, 21st ed. New York: W.B. Saunders Co., 2000.

Guyton & Hall. *Textbook of Medical Physiology*, 10th ed. New York: W.B. Saunders Company, 2000.

Tortora, G. J., and S. R. Grabowski. *Principles of Anatomy and Physiology*, 9th ed. New York: John Wiley and Sons Inc., 2000.

Brian Douglas Hoyle, PhD
Paul Arthur

Central nervous system stimulants

Definition

Central nervous system (CNS) stimulants are drugs that increase activity in certain areas of the brain. These drugs are used to improve wakefulness in patients that have **narcolepsy**. CNS stimulants are also used to treat patients that have **attention deficit hyperactivity disorder** (ADHD). There are four different types of central nervous system stimulants available in the United States: mixed amphetamine salts (brand name Adderall); dextroamphetamine (Dexedrine and Dextrostat); methylphenidate (Ritalin, Metadate, Methylin, and Concerta); and pemoline (Cylert).

Purpose

Central nervous system stimulants are used to keep patients who suffer from narcolepsy from falling asleep. Narcolepsy is a disorder that causes people to fall asleep during daytime hours.

These drugs are also used to treat behavioral symptoms associated with attention deficit hyperactivity disorder. Although it seems contradictory to give patients with ADHD drugs that are stimulants, these medications are often effective at treating symptoms of impulsivity, inattention, and hyperactivity, which are hallmark features of the disorder.

Description

The exact way that CNS stimulants work in treating narcolepsy and ADHD is not understood. The drugs' mechanism of action appears to involve enhanced activity of two **neurotransmitters** in the brain, norepinephrine and dopamine. Neurotransmitters are naturally occurring chemicals that regulate transmission of nerve impulses from one cell to another. A proper balance between the various neurotransmitters in the brain is necessary for healthy mental well-being.

Central nervous system stimulants increase the activities of norepinephrine and dopamine in two different ways. First, the CNS stimulants increase the release of norepinephrine and dopamine from brain cells. Second, the CNS stimulants may also inhibit the mechanisms that normally terminate the actions of these neurotransmitters. As a result of the dual activities of central nervous system stimulants, norepinephrine and dopamine have enhanced effects in various regions of the brain. Some of these brain areas are involved with controlling wakefulness and others are involved with controlling motor activities. It is believed that CNS stimulants restore a proper balance of neurotransmitters, which alleviates symptoms and features associated with narcolepsy and ADHD.

Although the intended actions of central nervous system stimulants are in the brain, their actions may also affect norepinephrine in other parts of the body. This can cause unwanted side effects such as increased blood pressure and heart arrhythmias due to reactions of norepinephrine on the cardiovascular system.

Recommended dosage

The usual dosage of amphetamine salts is 5–60 mg per day taken two or three times a day, with at least 4–6 hours between doses. The extended release form of amphetamine salts is taken as 10–30 mg once a day. Like amphetamine salts, the dose of immediate-release methylphenidate tablets is also 5–60 mg per day taken two or three times a day. Additionally, methylphenidate is

Key Terms

Attention deficit hyperactivity disorder (ADHD) A mental disorder characterized by impulsiveness, lack of attention, and hyperactivity.

Milligram One thousandth of a gram; the metric measure equals 0.035 ounces.

Narcolepsy An extreme tendency to fall asleep when surroundings are quiet or monotonous.

Neurotransmitter Naturally occurring chemicals that regulate transmission of nerve impulses from one cell to another.

available in sustained-release dosage forms and extended-release dosage forms, which are typically taken only once a day.

The usual dosage of dextroamphetamine is 5–60 mg per day given two or three times a day, with at least 4–6 hours between doses. A sustained-release form of dextroamphetamine is also available, which may be given once a day. The recommended dose of pemoline is 37.5–112.5 mg per day taken only once a day. However, due to pemoline's association with life-threatening liver dysfunction, pemoline is rarely used at the present time.

The therapeutic effects of central nervous system stimulants are usually apparent within the first 24 hours of taking the drugs. If effects are not evident, the dosages of CNS stimulants may be slowly increased at weekly intervals. CNS stimulants should always be used at the lowest effective dosages to minimize unwanted side effects. When the drugs are used for treating ADHD in children, therapy should be interrupted occasionally to determine whether symptoms reoccur and whether the drug is still necessary.

Precautions

Central nervous system stimulants are widely abused street drugs. Abuse of these drugs may cause extreme psychological dependence. As a result, new hand-written prescriptions must be obtained from physicians each month and any time a dosage adjustment is made. These drugs are best avoided in patients with a prior history of drug abuse.

CNS stimulants may cause anorexia and weight loss. Additionally, these drugs slow growth rates in children. Height and weight should be checked every three months in children who need to use these medications on a long-term basis.

The use of CNS stimulants should be avoided in patients with even mild cases of high blood pressure since the drugs may elevate blood pressure further.

Side effects

Central nervous system stimulants may increase heart rates and cause irregular heart rhythms, especially at high doses.

Symptoms of excessive stimulation of the central nervous system include restlessness, difficulty sleeping, tremor, **headaches**, and even psychotic episodes.

Loss of appetite and weight loss may also occur with central nervous system stimulants. It is necessary to monitor liver function regularly in patients who take pemoline since this drug has been associated with life-threatening liver disease.

Interactions

CNS stimulants should not be administered with certain types of antidepressant medications, including monoamine oxidase inhibitors (MAOIs) and selective serotonin reuptake inhibitors (SSRIs). Patients taking CNS stimulants should avoid MAOIs since the combination may elevate blood pressure to dangerously high levels, while SSRIs are best avoided since they may increase the central nervous system effects of CNS stimulants if the drugs are taken together.

Antacids may prevent CNS stimulants from being eliminated by the body and can increase the side effects associated with use of the stimulants.

Resources

BOOKS

Dipiro, J. T., R. L. Talbert, G. C. Yee, et al., eds. *Pharmacotherapy: A Pathophysiologic Approach*, 4th edition. Stamford, CT: Appleton and Lange, 1999.

Facts and Comparisons Staff. *Drug Facts and Comparisons*, 6th edition. St. Louis, MO: A Wolter Kluwer Company, 2002.

Kelly Karpa, PhD, RPh

Central pain syndrome

Definition

Central **pain** syndrome is a type of pain that occurs because of injuries to the brain or spinal cord.

Description

Central pain syndrome can occur in conjunction with a number of conditions involving the brain or spinal cord, including **stroke**; traumatic injury to, or tumors involving, the brain or spinal cord; **Parkinson's disease**; **multiple sclerosis**; or **epilepsy**.

The pain of central pain syndrome is an extremely persistent, intractable type of pain that can be quite debilitating and depressing to the sufferer. The pain may be localized to a particular part of the body (such as the hands or feet), or may be more widely distributed. The quality of the pain may remain the same or may change. Some of the types of pain experienced in central pain syndrome include sensations of crampy muscle spasms; burning; an increased sensitivity to painful stimuli; pain brought on by normally unpainful stimuli (such as light touch or temperature changes); shooting, lightening, or electric shock–like pains; tingling, pins-and-needles, stinging, numbness, or burning pain; sense of painful abdominal or bladder bloating and burning sensations in the bladder.

Central pain syndrome can be divided into two categories: pain related to prior **spinal cord injury** and pain related to prior brain injury. Spinal cord–related pain occurs primarily after traumatic injury, usually due to motor vehicle accidents. Other reasons for spinal cord–related pain include complications of surgery, tumors, congenital disorders (conditions present at birth), blood vessel–related injury (such as after a **spinal cord infarction** or stroke), and inflammatory conditions involving the spinal cord. Brain-related central pain usually follows a stroke, although tumors and infection may also lead to brain-related central pain.

Demographics

Eight percent of all stroke patients will experience central pain syndrome; 5% will experience moderate to severe pain. The risk of developing central pain syndrome is higher in older stroke patients, striking about 11% of patients over the age of 80. Spinal cord–related pain occurs in a very high percentage; research suggests a range of 25-85% of all individuals with spinal cord injuries will experience central pain syndrome.

Causes and symptoms

In general, central pain syndrome is thought to occur either because the transmission of pain signals in the nerve tracts of the spinal cord is faulty, or because the brain isn't processing pain signals properly. Although details regarding the origin of central pain syndrome remain cloudy, some of the mechanisms that may contribute to its development include muscle spasm; **spasticity** of muscles (chronically increased muscle tone); instability of the vertebral column (due to vertebral fracture or damage to ligaments); compression of nerve roots; the development of a fluid-filled area of the spinal cord (called a **syringomyelia**), which puts pressure on exiting nerves; and overuse syndrome (muscles that are used to compensate for those that no longer function normally are overworked, resulting in muscle strain).

The pain of central pain syndrome can begin within days of the causative insult, or it can be delayed for years (particularly in stroke patients). While the specific symptoms of central pain syndrome may vary over time, the presence of some set of symptoms is essentially continuous once they begin. The pain is usually moderate to severe in nature and can be very debilitating. Symptoms may be made worse by a number of conditions, such as temperature change (especially exposure to cold), touching the painful area, movement, and emotions or stress. The pain is often difficult to describe.

Diagnosis

Diagnosis is usually based on the knowledge of a prior spinal cord or brain injury, coupled with the development of a chronic pain syndrome. Efforts to delineate the cause of the pain may lead to neuroimaging (**CT** and **MRI** scanning) of the brain, spinal cord, or the painful anatomical area (abdomen, limbs); electromyographic and nerve conduction studies may also be performed. In many cases of central pain syndrome, no clear-cut area of pathology will be uncovered, despite diagnostic testing. In fact, this is one of the frustrating and confounding characteristics of central pain syndrome; the inability to actually delineate an anatomical location responsible for generating the pain, which creates difficulty in addressing the pain.

Treatment team

Neurologists will usually be the mainstay for treating central pain syndrome. Physical and occupational therapists may help an individual facing central pain syndrome obtain maximal relief and regain optimal functioning. Psychiatrists or psychologists may be helpful for supportive psychotherapy, particularly in patients who develop **depression** related to their chronic pain.

Treatment

A variety of medications may be used to treat central pain syndrome. Injection of IV lidocaine can significantly improve some aspects of central pain syndrome, but the need for intravenous access makes its chronic use relatively impractical. Tricyclic antidepressants (such as nortriptyline or amitriptyline) and antiepileptic drugs (such as **lamotrigine**, **carbamazepine**, **gabapentin**, **topiramate**) have often been used for neurogenic pain syndromes (pain due to abnormalities in the nervous system), and may be helpful to sufferers of central pain syndrome. When muscle spasms or spasticity are part of the central pain syndrome, a variety of medications may be helpful, including baclofen, tizanidine, **benzodiazepines**, and dantrolene sodium. In some cases, instilling medications (such as baclofen) directly into the cerebrospinal fluid around the spinal cord may improve spasms and spasticity. Newer therapy with injections of **botulinum toxin** may help relax painfully spastic muscles. Chronically spastic, painful muscles may also be treated surgically, by cutting through tendons (tendonotomy).

Severe, intractable pain may be treated by severing causative nerves or even severing certain nervous connections within the spinal cord. However, while this seems to provide pain relief in the short run, over time, about 60-80% of patients develop the pain again.

Counterstimulation uses electrodes implanted via needles in the spinal cord or specific nerves. These electrodes stimulate the area with electric pulses in an effort to cause a phenomenon referred to as "counter-irritation," which seems to interrupt the transmission of painful impulses. **Deep brain stimulation** requires the surgical implanatation of an electrode deep in the brain. A pulse generator that sends electricity to the electrode is implanted in the patient's chest, and a magnet passed over the pulse generator by the patient activates the brain electrode, stimulating the thalamic area.

Prognosis

Although central pain syndrome is never fatal, it can have serious consequences for an individual's level of functioning. Severe, chronic pain can be very disabling and have serious psychological consequences. Furthermore, central pain syndrome remains difficult to completely resolve; treatments may provide relief, but rarely provide complete cessation of pain.

Resources
BOOKS
Braunwald, Eugene, et al., eds. *Harrison's Principles of Internal Medicine.* NY: McGraw-Hill Professional, 2001.
Frontera, Walter R., ed. *Essentials of Physical Medicine and Rehabilitation,* 1st ed. Philadelphia: Hanley and Belfus, 2002.
Goldman, Lee, et al., eds. *Cecil Textbook of Internal Medicine.* Philadelphia: W. B. Saunders Company, 2000.

PERIODICALS
Nicholson, Bruce D. "Evaluation and treatment of central pain syndromes." *Neurology* 62, no. 5 (March 2004): 30–36.

WEBSITES
National Institute of Neurological Disorders and Stroke (NINDS). *Central Pain Syndrome Fact Sheet.* <http://disabilityexchange.org/upload/files/150_Central_Pain_Syndrome.doc>.

ORGANIZATIONS
American Chronic Pain Association (ACPA). P.O. Box 850, Rocklin , CA 95677-0850. 916-632-0922 or 800-533-3231; Fax: 916-632-3208. ACPA@pacbell.net. <http://www.theacpa.org>.

American Pain Foundation. 201 North Charles Street Suite 710, Baltimore , MD 21201-4111. 410-783-7292 or 888-615-PAIN (7246); Fax: 410-385-1832. info@pain foundation.org. <http://www.painfoundation.org>.
National Foundation for the Treatment of Pain. P.O. Box 70045, Houston , TX 77270. 713-862-9332 or 800-533-3231; Fax: 713-862-9346. markgordon@paincare.org. <http://www.paincare.org>.

Rosalyn Carson-DeWitt, MD

Cerebellar dysfunction *see* **Ataxia**

Cerebellar-pontine angle tumors *see* **Vestibular Schwanomma**

Cerebellum
Definition
The cerebellum is a cauliflower-shaped brain structure located just above the brainstem, beneath the occipital lobes at the base of the skull.

Description
The word cerebellum comes from the Latin word for "little brain." The cerebellum has traditionally been recognized as the unit of motor control that regulates muscle tone and coordination of movement. There is an increasing number of reports that support the idea that the cerebellum also contributes to non-motor functions such as cognition (thought processes) and affective state (emotion).

The cerebellum comprises approximately 10% of the brain's volume and contains at least half of the brain's neurons. The cerebellum is made up of two hemispheres (halves) covered by a thin layer of gray matter known as the cortex. Beneath the cortex is a central core of white matter. Embedded in the white matter are several areas of gray matter known as the deep cerebellar nuclei (the fastigial nucleus, the globise-emboliform nucleus, and the dentate nucleus). The cerebellum is connected to the brainstem via three bundles of fibers called peduncles (the superior, middle, and inferior).

Anatomy
The cerebellum is a complex structure. At the basic level, it is divided into three distinct regions: the vermis, the paravermis (also called the intermediate zone), and the cerebellar hemispheres. Fissures, deep folds in the cortex that extend across the cerebellum, further subdivide these regions into 10 lobules, designated lobules I–X. Two of

Cerebellum

Key Terms

Autoantibodies Antibodies that attack the body's own cells or tissues.

Axon A long, threadlike projection that is part of a neuron (nerve cell).

Gray matter Areas of the brain and spinal cord that are comprised mostly of unmyelinated nerves.

Multiple sclerosis A progressive, autoimmune disease of the central nervous system characterized by damage to the myelin sheath that covers nerves. The disease, which causes progressive paralysis, is marked by periods of exacerbation and remission.

White matter A substance, composed primarily of myelin fibers, found in the brain and nervous system that protects nerves and allows messages to be sent to and from the brain and various parts of the body. Also called white substance.

these fissures in particular, the posterolateral fissure and the primary fissure, separate the cerebellum into three lobes that have different functions: the flocculonodular lobe, or the vestibulocerebellum (lobule X); the anterior lobe (lobules I–V); and the posterior lobe (lobules VI–IX).

The cerebellum plays an important role in sending and receiving messages (nerve signals) necessary for the production of muscle movements and coordination. There are both afferent (input) and efferent (output) pathways. The major input pathways (also called tracts) include:

- dorsal spinocerebellar pathway
- ventral spinocerebellar pathway
- corticopontocerebellar pathway
- cerebo-olivocerebellar pathway
- cerebroreticulocerebellar pathway
- cuneocerebellar pathway
- vestibulocerebellar pathway

The major output pathways include the following:

- globose-emboliform-rubral pathway
- fastigial reticular pathway
- dentatothalamic pathway
- fastigial vestibular pathway

There is a network of fibers (cells) within the cerebellum that monitors information to and from the brain and the spinal cord. This network of neural circuits links the input pathways to the output pathways. The Purkinje

fibers and the deep nuclei play key roles in this communication process. The Purkinje fibers regulate the deep nuclei, which have axons that send messages out to other parts of the **central nervous system**.

Function

The flocculonodular lobe helps to maintain equilibrium (balance) and to control eye movements. The anterior lobe parts of the posterior lobe (the vermis and paravermis) form the spinocerebellum, a region that plays a role in control of proximal muscles, posture, and locomotion such as walking. The cerebellar hemispheres (part of the posterior lobe) are collectively known as the cerebrocerebellum (or the pontocerebellum); they receive signals from the cerebral cortex and aid in initiation, coordination, and timing of movements. The cerebrocerebellum is also thought to play a role in cognition and affective state.

The cerebellum has been reported to play a role in psychiatric conditions such as **schizophrenia**, **autism**, mood disorders, **dementia**, and **attention deficit hyperactivity disorder** (ADHD). Currently, the relationship between the cerebellum and psychiatric illness remains unclear. It is hoped that further research will reveal insights into the cerebellar contribution to these conditions.

Disorders

There are a variety of disorders that involve or affect the cerebellum. The cerebellum can be damaged by factors including:

- toxic insults such as alcohol abuse
- paraneoplastic disorders; conditions in which autoantibodies produced by tumors in other parts of the body attack neurons in the cerebellum
- structural lesions such as strokes, **multiple sclerosis**, or tumors
- inherited cerebellar degeneration such as in **Friedreich ataxia** or one of the spinocerebellar ataxias
- congenital anomalies such as cerebellar hypoplasia (underdevelopment or incomplete development of the cerebellum) found in **Dandy-Walker syndrome**, or displacement of parts of the cerebellum such as in **Arnold-Chiari malformation**

Typical symptoms of cerebellar disorders include **hypotonia** (poor muscle tone), movement decomposition (muscular movement that is fragmented rather than smooth), dysmetria (impaired ability to control the distance, power, and speed of an act), gait disturbances (abnormal pattern of walking), abnormal eye movement, and **dysarthria** (problems with speaking).

208

GALE ENCYCLOPEDIA OF NEUROLOGICAL DISORDERS

Resources

BOOKS

Manto, Mario U., and Massimo Pandolfo, eds. *The Cerebellum and its Disorders*. Cambridge, England: Cambridge University Press, 2001.

De Zeeuw, C. I., P. Strata, and J. Voogd, eds. *The Cerebellum: From Structure to Control*. St Louis, MO: Elsevier Science, 1997.

PERIODICALS

Daum, I., B. E. Snitz, and H. Ackermann. "Neuropsychological Deficits in Cerebellar Syndromes." *International Review of Psychiatry* 13 (2001): 268–275.

Desmond, J. E. "Cerebellar Involvement in Cognitive Function: Evidence from Neuroimaging." *International Review of Psychiatry* 13 (2001): 283–294.

Leroi, I., E. O'Hearn, and R. Margolis. "Psychiatric Syndromes in Cerebellar Degeneration." *International Review of Psychiatry* 13 (2001): 323–329.

O'Hearn, E., and M. E. Molliver. "Organizational Principles and Microcircuitry of the Cerebellum." *International Review of Psychiatry* 13 (2001): 232–246.

Rapoport, M. "The Cerebellum in Psychiatric Disorders." *International Review of Psychiatry* 13 (2001): 295–301.

Schmahmann, J. D. "The Cerebrocerebellar System: Anatomic Substrates of the Cerebellar Contribution to Cognition and Emotion." *International Review of Psychiatry* 13 (2001): 247–260.

Shill, H. A., and M. Hallett. "Cerebellar Diseases." *International Review of Psychiatry* 13 (2001): 261–267.

WEBSITES

"BrainInfo Web Site." *Cerebellum Information Page*. Neuroscience Division, Regional Primate Research Center, University of Washington, 2000. (May 22, 2004.) <http://braininfo.rprc.washington.edu>.

The Cerebellum Database Site. (May 22, 2004). <http://www.cerebellum.org/8home/>.

The National Institute of Neurological Disorders and Stroke (NINDS). *Cerebellar Degeneration Information Page*. PO Box 5801 Bethesda, MD, 2003. (May 22, 2004). <http://www.ninds.nih.gov/health_and_medical/disorders/cerebellar_degeneration.htm>.

The National Institute of Neurological Disorders and Stroke (NINDS). *Cerebellar Hypoplasia Information Page*. PO Box 5801 Bethesda, MD, 2003. (May 22, 2004). <http://www.ninds.nih.gov/health_and_medical/disorders/cerebellar_hypoplasia.htm>.

ORGANIZATIONS

National Institute of Mental Health. 6001 Executive Boulevard, Room 8184, MSC 9663, Bethesda, MD 20892-9663. (301) 443-4513 or (866) 615-6464; TTY: (301) 443-8431; Fax: (301) 443-4279. nimhinfo@nih.gov. <http://www.nimh.nih.gov/>.

National Institute of Neurological Disorders and Stroke (NINDS), NIH Neurological Institute. P.O. Box 5801, Bethesda, MD 20824. (301) 496-5751 or (800) 352-9424; TTY: (301) 468-5981. <http://www.ninds.nih.gov/>.

Dawn Cardeiro, MS

Cerebral aneurysm *see* **Aneurysm**

Cerebral arteriosclerosis *see* **Stroke**

Cerebral gigantism *see* **Hypoxia, Sotos syndrome**

Cerebral angiitis

Definition

Cerebral angiitis is an inflammation of the small arteries in the brain.

Description

Cerebral angiitis is a type of **vasculitis** in which an aberrant immune response results in inflammation and destruction of the small arteries that feed brain tissue. As a result of the inflammation, blood clots form within the arteries, compromising blood flow and resulting in decreased oxygen delivery to vulnerable brain tissue. Two types of cerebral angiitis have been recognized. The first type is considered to be an encephalopathic type, which results in wide-spread, slowly progressive damage to the brain. The second type causes abrupt, acute damage to a focal area of the brain, similar to a **stroke**.

Demographics

While cerebral angiitis can affect people of all ages, it is most common in the middle aged. Cerebral angiitis affects slightly more males than females. It may also be responsible for the unusual presentation of vasculitis in children, often following a simple chicken pox infection. Cerebral angiitis can also occur as a rare complication of allogeneic bone marrow transplant (bone marrow transplant received from a donor).

Causes and symptoms

Cerebral angiitis may occur spontaneously, with no known cause, or in conjunction with, or as a sequela to (an aftereffect of) a variety of viral infections, including herpes zoster (shingle), varicella zoster (chicken pox), and HIV/AIDS.

Symptoms can include slowly progressive **headache**, nausea, vomiting, stiff neck, confusion, irritability, loss of memory, **seizures**, and **dementia**. Cerebral angiitis may also cause the sudden onset of more acute and focal loss

Key Terms

Encephalopathic Widespread brain disease or dysfunction.

Vasculitis A condition characterized by inflammation of blood vessels.

of function, such as sudden loss of the use of one side of the body or the inability to speak.

Diagnosis

Cerebral angiitis may be diagnosed by examining a sample of cerebrospinal fluid, which will likely reveal increased levels of protein and abnormal white cell activity. **MRI** scanning of the brain will usually show a diffuse pattern of lesions throughout the white matter of the brain, although the stroke-like type of cerebral angiitis may reveal a more focal area of damage. **Biopsy** of a sample of brain tissue is the most definitive diagnostic test; it will reveal inflammation and immune system activity affecting the damaged small arteries of the brain.

Treatment team

Individuals with cerebral angiitis may be treated by a **neurologist** or a rheumatologist.

Treatment

Treatment for cerebral angiitis addresses the inflammation and the immune response, both of which are responsible for the complications of the condition. Corticosteroids (to quell inflammation) and cyclophosphamide (to dampen the immune system) may be given in tandem, often at high doses for about six weeks, and then at lower doses for up to a year. Occasionally, symptoms rebound after the dose is dropped, requiring that the higher dose be reutilized; even after supposed cure, relapse may supervene, necessitating another course of corticosteroids and cyclophosphamide.

Some patients with cerebral angiitis will also benefit from the administration of anticoagulant agents to thin the blood and prevent arterial obstruction by blood clots.

Recovery and rehabilitation

The type of rehabilitation program required will depend on the types of deficits caused by cerebral angiitis, but may include physical therapy, occupational therapy, and speech and language therapy.

Prognosis

Untreated cerebral angiitis will inevitably progress to death, often within a year of the onset of the disease. More research is needed to define the prognosis of treated cerebral angiitis; current research suggests that slightly more than half of all treated patients have a good outcome.

Resources

BOOKS

Sergent, John S. "Polyarteritis and related disorders." In *Kelley's Textbook of Rheumatology,* 6th edition, edited by Shaun Ruddy, et al. St. Louis: W. B. Saunders Company, 2001.

PERIODICALS

Rollnik, J. D., A. Brandis, K. Dehghani, J. Bufler, M. Lorenz, F. Heidenreich, and F. Donnerstag. "Primary angiitis of CNS (PACNS)." *Nervenarzt* 72, no. 10 (October 2001): 798–801.

Singh, S., S. John, T. P. Joseph, and T. Soloman. "Primary angiitis of the central nervous system: MRI features and clinical presentation." *Australasian Radiology* 47, no. 2 (June 2003): 127–134.

Singh, S., S. John, T. P. Joseph, and T. Soloman. "Prognosis of patients with suspected primary CNS angiitis and negative brain biopsy." *Neurology* 61, no. 6 (September 2003) 831–833.

Rosalyn Carson-DeWitt, MD

Cerebral cavernous malformation

Definition

Cerebral cavernous malformations (CCM) are tangles of malformed blood vessels located in the brain and/or spinal cord.

Description

The blood vessels composing a cerebral cavernous malformation are weak and lack supporting tissue, thus they are prone to bleed. If seen under a microscope, a cavernous malformation appears to be composed of fairly large blood-filled caverns. A characteristic feature of a CCM is slow bleeding, or oozing, as opposed to the dangerous sudden rupture of an aneurysm (a weak, bulging area of a blood vessel). However, depending on the size and location of the CCM, and the frequency of bleeding, a CCM can also create a dangerous health emergency. Cerebral cavernous malformations are also known as cavernomas or cavernous angiomas.

Key Terms

Aneurysm A weak, bulging area of a blood vessel.

Autosomal dominant inheritance A pattern of inheritance where only one parent must have the illness for it to be passed on to offspring. The risk of an affected parent passing the condition to an offspring is 50% with each pregnancy.

CCM is usually distinct from the surrounding brain tissue and resembles a mass or a blood clot. It can occur either sporadically or in a familial (inherited) pattern. Usually, only one or two lesions are present when the CCM occurs sporadically. Those with a familial pattern of CCM usually have multiple lesions of malformed blood vessels, along with a strong family history of **stroke** or related neurological difficulties. Familial CCM has a pattern of autosomal dominant inheritance, meaning that only one parent must have the illness for it to be passed on to offspring, and the risk of an affected parent passing the condition to an offspring is 50%. The first gene (CCM1) involved in this disease was recently identified and mapped to the long arm of chromosome 7. Additionally, two other genes responsible for CCM formation were also identified, one mapped to the short arm of chromosome 7 (the CCM2 gene) and the other mapped to the long arm of chromosome 3 (the CCM3 gene).

The size of the malformation varies greatly and can change depending on the amount and severity of each bleeding episode. Typically, they range from something microscopic to something the size of an orange. It is possible for a CCM not to bleed, and the ones that do so, may not necessarily bleed with the severity or intensity that requires surgery. Depending on the size and location of the lesion, the blood can reabsorb causing symptoms to disappear.

Demographics

Cavernous malformations occur in people of all races and both sexes. The male-female ratio is about equal. Family history may be predictive, especially in patients of Hispanic descent. CCM can be found in any region of the brain, can be of varying size, and present with varying symptoms. In a general population of one million people, 0.5% or 5,000 people may be found to have a cavernous malformation, although many are not symptomatic.

In the United States alone, 1.5 million people, or 1 in 200, are estimated to have some form of CCM. This translates to approximately 0.5% of the population. Approximately 20–30% of the diagnoses are made in children and 60% of affected adults are diagnosed in their 20s and 30s. It is estimated that approximately 20 million people worldwide have some kind of vascular malformation.

Causes and symptoms

Most familial cerebral cavernous malformations are present at birth (congenital). They are thought to arise between three and eight weeks of gestation, although the exact mechanism of CCM formation is not understood.

Vascular malformations can potentially occur many years after **radiation** therapy to the brain. Additionally, it is also assumed that severe or repeated head trauma can cause cerebral capillaries to bleed. Over time, the brain attempts to repair itself and control the bleeding by developing a lesion. Researchers assume that these theories may answer the question why some people develop the sporadic form of CCM.

Although these common neurovascular lesions affect almost 0.5% of the population, only 20–30% of these individuals experience symptoms. Symptoms include **seizures**, **dizziness**, stroke, vomiting, uncontrollable hiccups, periodic weakness, irritability and/or changes in personality, **headaches**, difficulty speaking, vision problems or, rarely, brain hemorrhage.

Symptoms are caused by the pressure of accumulated blood in and around the CCM on adjacent brain tissue. If the area of bleeding is small, it may take several subsequent bleeding episodes until enough pressure is built up in order for symptoms to be noticeable. The CCM could also bleed substantially, causing immediate problems and symptoms. Finally, the CCM could remain dormant without any evidence of bleeding.

Diagnosis

Cerebral cavernous malformations are usually diagnosed by computerized axial tomography (CAT) scan or, more accurately, a **magnetic resonance imaging (MRI)** scan with gradient echo sequencing.

MRI has provided the ability to image and localize otherwise hidden lesions of the brain and provide accuracy of diagnosis before surgery. Both the MRI and CAT scans produce images of slices through the brain. These tests help physicians to see exactly where the cavernoma is located. Cavernomas cannot be seen on a cerebral angiogram.

Often, CCMs are diagnosed when the person becomes symptomatic. However, it is common for CCMs to be diagnosed by accident when a CAT scan or MRI is conducted to investigate other health problems. Despite the presence of a CCM, it often remains inactive, meaning there is no evidence that the lesion produces bleeding.

Treatment team

Treatment for CCMs must be specific for each case. A team of cerebrovascular experts (neurologists, neurosurgeons, neuroradiologists, and radiation oncologists), together with the patient and families, decide on whether treatment is necessary and the best treatment option.

Treatment

There are three main treatment options for CCM, including observation, stereotactic radiosurgery, and surgery. If the person with CCM has no symptoms, the first treatment option is to simply observe the CCM with periodic MRI scans to assess for change. This option may be indicated if the lesion is discovered incidentally.

Stereotactic radiosurgery involves delivering highly-focused radiation in a single treatment to the CCM. This has been used almost exclusively for lesions causing repeated hemorrhages located in areas of the brain that are not surgically accessible. It is often difficult to determine if radiosurgery is effective unless the lesion never bleeds again. In certain cases, radiosurgery has likely decreased the repeat hemorrhage rate; however, radiosurgery has never been shown to completely eliminate the malformation.

Surgery is the most common option when treatment is necessary. Because these malformations are so distinct from the surrounding brain tissue, cavernous malformations often can be completely removed without producing any new problems. It is very important to remove the entire malformation as it can regenerate if a small piece is left behind. The risk of the operation depends on the size and location of the cavernous malformation and the general health of the patient.

Clinical trials

Although there are no **clinical trials** for treatment of CCM ongoing as of early 2004, much of the current research focuses on the genetics of the disorder. Duke University's Center for Inherited Neurovascular Diseases was recruiting individuals with familial CCM for participation in research designed to develop a blood test for detecting CCM. For information about participating in the study, contact Ms. Sharmila Basu at (410) 614–0729, or via email at sbasu4@jhmi.edu.

Prognosis

Persons experiencing CCM-related symptoms are likely to remain symptomatic or experience a worsening of symptoms without treatment. Frequent or uncontrolled seizures, increase in lesion size on MRI, or hemorrhage are indications for removal of surgically accessible CCM lesions. Persons treated surgically experience remission or a reduction of symptoms in most cases. Approximately half of patients experience elimination of seizures, and the remainder usually have fewer, less frequent seizures. Successfully excised CCM lesions are considered cured, and it is unusual for them to return.

Special concerns

There are differing opinions about activity restriction for a person diagnosed with CCM lesions. Some physicians encourage their patients to continue their usual activities; others advocate avoiding activities where the risk for head trauma is high, such as sports including football, soccer, hockey, skiing, or skating. It is important to discuss this issue with the physician, wear approriate protective equipment when particiapting in sports, and make decisions pertaining to activity level based on the current status of the CCM and general health. It is also helpful to keep an activity record, to document any relationship between activities and symptoms.

Resources

BOOKS

Klein, Bonnie Sherr, and Persimmon Blackbridge. *Out of the Blue: One Woman's Story of Stroke, Love, and Survival.* Berkeley, CA: Wildcat Press, 2000.

PERIODICALS

Labauge, P. et al. "Prospective follow-up of 33 asymptomatic patients with familial cerebral cavernous malformations." *Neurology* 57 (November 2001): 1825–1828.

Laurans, M. S., et al. "Mutational analysis of 206 families with cavernous malformations." *Journal of Neurosurgery* 99 (July 2003): 38–43.

Narayan, P., and D. L. Barrow. "Intramedullary spinal cavernous malformation following spinal irradiation." *Journal of Neurosurgery* 98 (January 2003): 68–72.

Reich, P. et al. "Molecular genetic investigations in the CCM1 gene in sporadic cerebral cavernomas." *Neurology* 60 (April 2003): 1135–1138.

OTHER

"NINDS Cavernous Malformation Information Page." National Institute of Neurological Disorders and Stroke. (March 1, 2004). <http://www.ninds.nih.gov/health_and_medical/disorders/cavernous_malformation.htm>.

"What Is Cavernous Angioma?" *Angioma Alliance.* (March 1, 2004). <http://www.angiomaalliance.org>.

ORGANIZATIONS

Brain Power Project. P.O. Box 2250, Agoura Hills Englewood, CA 91376. (818) 735-7335; Fax: (818) 706-8246. lee@thebrainpowerproject.org. <http://www.thebrain powerproject.org>.

National Organization for Rare Disorders (NORD). P.O. Box 1968 (55 Kenosia Avenue), Danbury, CT 06813-1968. (203) 744-0100 or (800) 999-NORD (6673); Fax: (203)

798-2291. orphan@rarediseases.org.
<http://www.rarediseases.org>.

Beatriz Alves Vianna
Iuri Drumond Louro, M.D., Ph.D.

Cerebral circulation

Definition

Cerebral circulation, the supply of blood to the brain

Understanding how the brain is supplied with blood is important because a significant number of neurological disorders that result in hospital admissions are due to problems with cerebral vascular disease. In some hospitals, nearly half the admissions due to neurologic disorders relate in some form to problems with cerebral circulation.

Insufficient supply of blood to the brain can cause **fainting** (syncope) or a more severe loss of consciousness. A continuous supply of highly oxygenated blood is critical to brain tissue function and a decrease in pressure or oxygenation (percentage of oxygen content) can cause tissue damage within minutes. Depending on a number of other physiological factors (e.g., temperature, etc.), brain damage or death may occur within two to 10 minutes of severe oxygen deprivation. Although there can be exceptions—especially when the body is exposed to cold temperatures—in general, after two minutes of oxygen deprivation, the rate of brain damage increases quickly with time.

Anatomy of cerebral circulation

Arterial supply of oxygenated blood

Four major arteries and their branches supply the brain with blood. The four arteries are composed of two internal carotid arteries (left and right) and two vertebral arteries that ultimately join on the underside (inferior surface) of the brain to form the arterial circle of Willis, or the circulus arteriosus.

The vertebral arteries actually join to form a basilar artery. It is this basilar artery that joins with the two internal carotid arteries and their branches to form the circle of Willis. Each vertebral artery arises from the first part of the subclavian artery and initially passes into the skull via holes (foramina) in the upper cervical vertebrae and the foramen magnum. Branches of the vertebral artery include the anterior and posterior spinal arteries, the meningeal branches, the posterior inferior cerebellar artery, and the medullary arteries that supply the medulla oblongata.

Key Terms

Cerebral collateral blood flow Anatomical and physiological mechanisms that allow blood destined for one hemisphere of the brain to crossover and nourish tissue on the other side of the brain when the supply to the other side of the brain is impaired.

Circle of Willis Also known as the circulus arteriosus; formed by branches of the internal carotid arteries and the vertebral arteries.

The basilar artery branches into the anterior inferior cerebellar artery, the superior cerebellar artery, the posterior cerebral artery, the potine arteries (that enter the pons), and the labyrinthine artery that supplies the internal ear.

The internal carotids arise from the common carotid arteries and pass into the skull via the carotid canal in the temporal bone. The internal carotid artery divides into the middle and anterior cerebral arteries. Ultimate branches of the internal carotid arteries include the ophthalmic artery that supplies the optic nerve and other structures associated with the eye and ethmoid and frontal sinuses. The internal carotid artery gives rise to a posterior communicating artery just before its final splitting or bifurcation. The posterior communicating artery joins the posterior cerebral artery to form part of the circle of Willis. Just before it divides (bifurcates), the internal carotid artery also gives rise to the choroidal artery (also supplies the eye, optic nerve, and surrounding structures). The internal carotid artery bifurcates into a smaller anterior cerebral artery and a larger middle cerebral artery.

The anterior cerebral artery joins the other anterior cerebral artery from the opposite side to form the anterior communicating artery. The cortical branches supply blood to the cerebral cortex.

Cortical branches of the middle cerebral artery and the posterior cervical artery supply blood to their respective hemispheres of the brain.

The circle of Willis is composed of the right and left internal carotid arteries joined by the anterior communicating artery. The basilar artery (formed by the fusion of the vertebral arteries) divides into left and right posterior cerebral arteries that are connected (anastomsed) to the corresponding left or right internal carotid artery via the respective left or right posterior communicating artery. A number of arteries that supply the brain originates at the circle of Willis, including the anterior cerebral arteries that originate from the anterior communicating artery.

In the embryo, the components of the circle of Willis develop from the embryonic dorsal aortae and the embryonic intersegmental arteries.

The circle of Willis provides multiple paths for oxygenated blood to supply the brain if any of the principal suppliers of oxygenated blood (i.e., the vertebral and internal carotid arteries) are constricted by physical pressure, occluded by disease, or interrupted by injury. This redundancy of blood supply is generally termed collateral circulation.

Arteries supply blood to specific areas of the brain. However, more than one arterial branch may support a region. For example, the **cerebellum** is supplied by the anterior inferior cerebellar artery, the superior cerebellar artery, and the posterior inferior cerebellar arteries.

Venous return of deoxygenated blood from the brain

Veins of the cerebral circulatory system are valve-less and have very thin walls. The veins pass through the subarachnoid space, through the arachnoid matter, the dura, and ultimately pool to form the cranial venous sinus.

There are external cerebral veins and internal cerebral veins. As with arteries, specific areas of the brain are drained by specific veins. For example, the cerebellum is drained of deoxygenated blood by veins that ultimately form the great cerebral vein.

External cerebral veins include veins from the lateral surface of the cerebral hemispheres that join to form the superficial middle cerebral vein.

Nourishing brain tissue

The cerebral arteries provide blood to the brain, but a sufficient arterial blood pressure is required to provide an adequate supply of blood to all brain tissue. Unlike the general body blood pressure, the cerebral blood pressure and cerebral blood flow remain relatively constant, a feat of regulation made possible by rapid changes in the resistance to blood flow within cerebral vessels. Resistance is lowered, principally through changes in the diameter of the blood vessels, as the cerebral arterial pressure lowers, and resistance increases as the incoming arterial pressure increases.

A complex series of nerves, including a branch of the glossopharyngeal nerve (the sinus nerve), relate small changes in the size of the carotid sinus (a dilation or enlargement of the internal carotid artery) such that if arterial pressure increases and causes the sinus to swell, the nervous impulses transmit signals to areas of the brain that inhibit the heart rate.

An oxygenated blood supply is critical to brain function

An adequate blood supply is critical to brain function and healthy neural tissue. Physiological studies utilizing radioisotopes and other traceable markers establish that the majority of the blood originally passing through the left vertebral and left internal carotid arteries normally supply the left side of the brain, with a similar situation found on the right with the right vertebral and right internal carotid arteries. Accordingly, the left half of the brain receives its blood supply from the left internal carotid and left vertebral artery. The right half of the brain receives its blood supply from the right internal carotid and right vertebral artery.

The two independent blood supplies do not normally mix or crossover except for a small amount in the posterior communicating artery (and in some cases, the arterial circle of Willis).

Compensating mechanisms

However, if there is some obstruction of blood flow (cerebral ischemia), there is a compensating mechanism. The two left and right supplies of blood normally do not mix in the posterior communicating artery because they are at roughly equal pressures. Even after the two vertebral arteries join to form the basilar artery prior to joining the arterial circle of Willis, the bloodstreams from the two vertebral arteries remain largely separated as though there were a partition in the channel.

If there is an obstruction on one side that reduces the flow of blood, the pressures of the two sides do not remain equal and so blood from the unaffected side (at a relatively higher pressure) is able to crossover and help nourish tissue on the occluded side of the brain.

The arterial circle of Willis can also permit crossover flow when the pressures are altered by an obstruction or constriction in an internal carotid or vertebral artery.

In addition to crossover flow, the size of the communicating arteries and the arteries branching from the circle of Willis is able to change in response to increased blood flow that accompanies occlusion or interruption of blood supply to another component of the circle.

Accordingly, oxygenated blood from either vertebral artery or either internal carotid may be able to supply vital oxygen to either cerebral hemisphere.

Vascular disorders

The disorders that result from an inadequate supply of blood to the brain depend largely on which artery is occluded (blocked) and the extent of the occlusion.

There are three general types of disorders that can result in inadequate blood flow to the brain. Although there are pressure-compensating mechanisms in the cerebral circulation, heart disease and diseases that affect blood pressure in the body can also influence cerebral blood pressure. Sometimes people get lightheaded or dizzy when they stand up suddenly after sitting for long periods. The **dizziness** is often due to postural hypotension, an inadequate supply of blood to the brain due to a lowered cerebral arterial blood pressure initially caused by an obstruction to the return of venous blood to the heart. Shock can also cause a lowering of cerebral blood pressure.

Disorders or diseases that result in the blockage of arteries can certainly have a drastic impact on the quality of cerebral circulation. A clot (thrombus) that often originates in plaque lining the carotid or vertebral arteries can directly obstruct blood flow in the cerebral circulation. Cerebral **aneurysms**, small but weakening dilations of the cerebral blood vessels, can rupture, trauma can cause hemorrhage, and a number of other disorders can directly impair blood flow.

Lastly, diseases that affect the blood vessels themselves, especially the arterial walls, can result in vascular insufficiency that can result in loss of consciousness, paralysis, or death.

Resources
BOOKS
Bear, M., et al. *Neuroscience: Exploring the Brain.* Baltimore: Williams & Wilkins, 1996.
Goetz, C. G., et al. *Textbook of Clinical Neurology.* Philadelphia: W. B. Saunders Company, 1999.

WEBSITES
Mokhtar, Yasser. *The Doctor's Lounge.net.* "Cerebral Circulation." May 5, 2004 (May 27, 2004). <http://www.thedoctorslounge.net/studlounge/articles/cerebcirc/>.

Paul Arthur

Cerebral dominance

Definition
Cerebral dominance refers to the dominance of one cerebral hemisphere over the other in the control of cerebral functions.

Description
Cerebral dominance is the ability of one cerebral hemisphere (commonly referred to as the left or right side of the brain) to predominately control specific tasks. Accordingly, damage to a specific hemisphere can result in an

Key Terms

Cerebral dominance The preeminence of one cerebral hemisphere over the other in the control of cerebral functions.

Handedness The preference of either the right or left hand as the dominant hand for the performance of tasks such as writing.

impairment of certain identifiable functions. For example, trauma to the left hemisphere can impair functions associated with speech, reading, and writing. Trauma to the right hemisphere can result in a decreased ability to perform such tasks as judging distance, determining direction, and recognizing tones and similar artistic functions.

Cerebral dominance and handedness
Cerebral dominance is also related to handedness—whether a person has a strong preference for the use of their right or left hand. More than 90% of people are right-handed and in the vast majority of these individuals, the left hemisphere controls language-related functions.

In left-handed individuals, however, only about 75% have language functions predominantly controlled by the left hemisphere. The remainder of left-handed individuals have language functions controlled by the right hemisphere, or do not have a dominant hemisphere with regard to language and speech.

A very small percentage of people are ambidextrous, having no preference for performing tasks with either hand.

One aspect of cerebral dominance theory that has received considerable research attention is the relationship between a lack of cerebral dominance and **dyslexia**. Some research data suggest that indeterminate dominance with regard to language—a failure of one hemisphere to clearly dominate language functions—results in dyslexia. Evidence to support this hypothesis is, however, not uniform or undisputed.

In general terms, for right-handed people the left side of the brain is usually associated with analytical processes while the right side of the brain is associated with intuitive or artistic abilities. The data to support such generalizations is, however, not uniform.

The cortex is divided into several cortical areas, each responsible for separate functions such as planning of complex movements, memory, personality, elaboration of thoughts, word formation, language understanding, motor coordination, visual processing of words, spatial orientation, and body spatial coordination. The association areas of the cortex receive and simultaneously analyze multiple sensations received from several regions of the brain. The brain is divided into two large lobes interconnected by a bundle of nerves, the corpus callosum. It is now known that in approximately 95% of all people, the area of the cortex in the left hemisphere can be up to 50% larger than in the right hemisphere, even at birth. Both Wernicke's and the Broca's areas (specific anatomical regions) are usually much more developed in the left hemisphere, which gave origin to the theory of left hemisphere dominance. The motor area for hand coordination is also dominant in nine of out 10 persons, accounting for the predominance of right-handedness among the population.

Studies also show that the non-dominant hemisphere plays an important role in musical understanding, composition and learning, perception of spatial relations, perception of visual and other esthetical patterns, understanding of connotations in verbal speeches, perception of voice intonation, identification of other's emotions and mood, and body language.

One hindrance to the acceptance of data relating to cerebral dominance is the fact that social pressure to conform to the norm can drive some left-handed people to adopt the predominant use of their right hand.

Resources

BOOKS

Bear, M., et al. *Neuroscience: Exploring the Brain.* Baltimore: Williams & Wilkins, 1996.

Tortora, G. J., and S. R. Grabowski. *Principles of Anatomy and Physiology*, 9th ed. New York: John Wiley and Sons Inc., 2000.

PERIODICALS

White, L. E., G. Lucas, A. Richards, and D. Purves. "Cerebral Asymmetry and Handedness." *Nature* 368 (1994): 197–198.

Sandra Galeotti
Brian Douglas Hoyle, PhD

Cerebral hematoma

Definition

Cerebral hematoma involves bleeding into the cerebrum, the largest section of the brain, resulting in an expanding mass of blood that damages surrounding neural tissue.

Description

A hematoma is a swelling of blood confined to an organ or tissue, caused by hemorrhaging from a break in one or more blood vessels. As a cerebral hematoma grows, it damages or kills the surrounding brain tissue by compressing it and restricting its blood supply, producing the symptoms of **stroke**. The hematoma eventually stops growing as the blood clots, the pressure cuts off its blood supply, or both.

Cerebral hematomas are categorized by their diameter and estimated volume as small, moderate, or massive. The neurologic effects produced by a cerebral hematoma are quite variable, and depend on its location, size, and duration (length of time until the body breaks down and absorbs the clot). Additional bleeding into the ventricles, which contain the cerebrospinal fluid (CSF), may occur. Blood in the CSF presents a risk for further neurologic damage.

Intracerebral hematoma (ICH) is another frequently used term for the condition. The initials "ICH" may also be seen in different places denoting several related conditions—an *intracerebral hematoma* is due to an *intracerebral hemorrhage*, which is one type of *intracranial hemorrhage*. However, the causes and symptoms of all three are roughly the same.

Demographics

The two basic types of stroke are hemorrhagic (including ICH) and ischemic (blockage in a blood vessel). Each year 700,000 people in the United States, or about 1 in 50 individuals, experience a new or recurrent stroke. Of these, about 12% are due to intracranial hemorrhage. Stroke kills an estimated 170,000 people each year in the United States, and is the leading cause of serious, long-term disability. Thirty-five percent of individuals suffering a hemorrhagic stroke die within 30 days, while the one-month mortality rate for ischemic stroke is 10%.

Stroke occurs somewhat more frequently in men than in women. Compared to whites, the incidence of first-occurrence strokes in most other ethnic groups in the United States is slightly higher, except African-Americans, whose rate is nearly twice as high. In adults, the risk of stroke increases with age. The highest risk for stroke in children is in the newborn period (especially in premature infants), with an incidence of 1 in 4000. The risk then decreases throughout childhood to a low of 1 in 40,000 in teen-agers. Twenty-five percent of strokes in children are due to intracranial hemorrhage.

Causes and symptoms

The most frequent causes of intracranial hemorrhage, including ICH, are:

• Hypertension-induced vascular damage

• Ruptured aneurysm or arteriovenous malformation (AVM)

Key Terms

Aneurysm   A weakened area in the wall of a blood vessel which causes an outpouching or bulge. Aneurysms may be fatal if these weak areas burst, resulting in uncontrollable bleeding.

Cerebrum   The largest section of the brain, which is responsible for such higher functions as speech, thought, vision, and memory.

Hematoma   A localized collection of blood, often clotted, in body tissue or an organ, usually due to a break or tear in the wall of blood vessel.

Hemorrhage   Severe, massive bleeding that is difficult to control. The bleeding may be internal or external.

Hypertension   Abnormally high arterial blood pressure that if left untreated can lead to heart disease and stroke.

Ischemia   A decrease in the blood supply to an area of the body caused by obstruction or constriction of blood vessels.

Stroke   Interruption of blood flow to a part of the brain with consequent brain damage. A stroke may be caused by a blood clot or by hemorrhage due to a burst blood vessel. Also known as a cerebrovascular accident.

- Head trauma
- Diseases that result in a direct or indirect risk for uncontrolled bleeding
- Unintended result from the use of anticoagulant (anticlotting) or thrombolytic (clot dissolving) drugs for other conditions
- Complications from arterial amyloidosis (cholesterol plaques)
- Hemorrhage into brain tumors

Preventable factors that increase the risk for stroke include chronic hypertension, obesity, high cholesterol (atherosclerosis), sedentary lifestyle, and chronic use of tobacco and/or alcohol. These factors primarily increase the risk for ischemic stroke, but play a role in ICH as well.

As previously noted, a massive ICH can result in sudden loss of consciousness, progressing to coma and death within several hours. For small and moderate hemorrhages, the usual symptoms are sudden **headache** accompanied by nausea and vomiting, and these may remit, recur, and worsen over time. Other, more serious symptoms of stroke include weakness or paralysis on one side of the body (hemiparesis/hemiplegia), difficulty speaking (**aphasia**), and pronounced confusion with memory loss. **Seizures** are not a common symptom of ICH. Hydrocephalus—increased fluid pressure in the brain—may result if pressure from the hematoma or a clot obstructs normal circulation of the CSF. Again, the severity and type of symptoms depend greatly on the location and size of the hematoma.

Diagnosis

Symptoms may indicate the possibility of an ICH, but the diagnosis can only be made by visualizing the hematoma using either a computed tomography (**CT**) or magnetic resonance imaging (**MRI**) scan. In some cases, more sophisticated imaging methods such as functional-MRI, SPECT, or **PET** scans can be used to visualize damaged areas of the brain.

Treatment team

An ICH producing mild symptoms might prompt a direct or referred visit to a **neurologist**, while individuals with more serious symptoms are first seen by hospital emergency room staff. Once the diagnosis of ICH is made, other specialists consulted or involved could include a neurosurgeon, radiologist, neurologist, and intensive care unit (ICU) staff. Long-term care might involve a psychiatrist/psychologist, dietitian, occupational/physical/speech therapists, rehabilitation specialists, and health professionals from assisted-living facilities or home-care agencies.

Treatment

Initial treatments in patients who have lost consciousness involve stabilizing any affected systems such as respiration, fluid levels, blood pressure, and body temperature. In many cases, monitoring intracranial pressure (ICP) is critical, since elevated ICP poses a serious risk for coma and death. Management of elevated ICP can be attempted with medication or manipulation of blood oxygen levels, but surgery is sometimes required. The possibility of further hemorrhaging in the brain poses a serious risk, and requires follow-up imaging scans.

If an ICH is detected very early, a neurosurgeon may attempt to drill through the skull and insert a small tube to remove (aspirate) the blood. Once the blood has clotted, however, aspiration becomes more difficult or impossible. Surgery to remove a hematoma is usually not advised unless it threatens to become massive, is felt to be life-threatening, or is causing rapid neurologic deterioration.

Recovery and rehabilitation

Recovery and rehabilitation centers around regaining as much neurologic function as possible, along with developing adaptive and coping skills for those neurologic problems that might be permanent. Recovery from neurologic injury caused by hemorrhagic stroke is frequently long and difficult, but there are many sources of information and support available.

Rehabilitation is most often done on an outpatient basis, but more serious cases may require nursing assistance at home or institutional care. Those who lapse into a coma or persistent vegetative state will need 24-hour professional care, and may take days, months, or years to recover, or they may never recover.

Clinical trials

Research is under way to develop effective, safer medications and methods to both stop a hemorrhage while it is occurring, and dissolve clots within the brain once they have formed. Direct injection of a local-acting clotting agent into an expanding hematoma, or of a thrombolytic drug, such as recombinant tissue plasminogen activator (rt-PA), into the clot are two avenues of research.

Prognosis

The prognosis after an ICH varies anywhere from excellent to fatal, depending on the size and location of the hematoma. However, ICH is the most serious form of stroke, with the highest rates of mortality and long-term disability, and the fewest available treatments. Only a small proportion of patients with an ICH can be given a good or excellent prognosis.

Resources

BOOKS

Bradley, Walter G., et al., eds. "Principles of Neurosurgery." In *Neurology in Clinical Practice,* 3rd ed., pp. 931-942. Boston: Butterworth-Heinemann, 2000.

Victor, Maurice and Allan H. Ropper. "Cerebrovascular Diseases." In *Adams' and Victor's Principles of Neurology,* 7th ed., pp. 881-903. New York: The McGraw-Hill Companies, Inc., 2001.

Wiederholt, Wigbert C. *Neurology for Non-Neurologists,* 4th ed. Philadelphia: W. B. Saunders Company, 2000.

PERIODICALS

Glastonbury, Christine M. and Alisa D. Gean. "Current Neuroimaging of Head Injury." *Seminars in Neurosurgery* 14 (2003): 79-88.

Mayer, Stephan A. "Ultra-Early Hemostatic Therapy for Intracerebral Hemorrhage." *Stroke* 34 (January 2003): 224-229.

Rolli, Michael L. and Neal J. Naff. "Advances in the Treatment of Adult Intraventricular Hemorrhage." *Seminars in Neurosurgery* 11 (2000): 27-40.

ORGANIZATIONS

Brain Aneurysm Foundation. 12 Clarendon Street, Boston, MA 02116. 617-723-3870; Fax: 617-723-8672. <http://www.bafound.org>.

Brain Injury Association. 8201 Greensboro Drive, Suite 611, McLean, VA 22102. 800-444-6443; Fax: 703-761-0755. <http://www.biausa.org>.

Brain Trauma Foundation. 523 East 72nd Street, 8th Floor, New York , NY 10021. 212-772-0608; Fax: 212-772-0357. <http://www.braintrauma.org>.

National Institute on Disability and Rehabilitation Research (NIDRR). 600 Independence Ave., S.W., Washington, DC 20013-1492. 202-205-8134. <http://www.ed.gov/offices/OSERS/NIDRR>.

National Rehabilitation Information Center (NARIC). 4200 Forbes Boulevard, Suite 202, Lanham, MD 20706-4829. 800-346-2742; Fax: 301-562-2401. <http://www.naric.com>.

National Stroke Association. 9707 East Easter Lane, Englewood, CO 80112-3747. 800-787-6537; Fax: 303-649-1328. <http://www.stroke.org>.

Scott J. Polzin, MS, CGC

Cerebral palsy

Definition

Cerebral palsy is a term used to describe a group of chronic conditions affecting body movements and muscle coordination. It is caused by damage to one or more specific areas of the brain, usually occurring during fetal development or during infancy.

Description

Cerebral palsy (CP) is an umbrella-like term used to describe a group of chronic disorders impairing movement control that appear in the first few years of life and generally do not worsen over time. The disorders are caused by faulty development or damage to motor areas in the brain that disrupt the brain's ability to control movement and posture. The causes of such cerebral insults include vascular, metabolic, infectious, toxic, traumatic, hypoxic (lack of oxygen) and genetic causes. The mechanism that originates cerebral palsy involves multi-factorial causes, but much is still unknown.

Cerebral palsy distorts messages from the brain to cause either increased muscle tension (hypertonus) or reduced muscle tension (hypotonus). Sometimes this tension will fluctuate, becoming more or less obvious.

Symptoms of CP include difficulty with fine motor tasks (such as writing or using scissors) and difficulty maintaining balance or walking. Symptoms differ from

Key Terms

Ataxic   Muscles that are unable to perform coordinated movements due to damage to one or more parts of the brain.

Contracture   Chronic shortening of muscle fibers resulting in stiffness and decrease in joint mobility.

Hypertonus   Increased tension of a muscle or muscle spasm.

Hypotonus   Decreased tension of a muscle, or abnormally low muscle tone.

Hypoxic   Oxygen deficient.

Ischemic   Having inadequate blood flow.

Orthotic device   Devices made of plastic, leather, or metal which provide stability at the joints or passively stretch the muscles.

Spasticity   Increased muscle tone, resulting in involuntary muscle movements, muscle tightness, and rigidity.

Teratogenic   Able to cause birth defects.

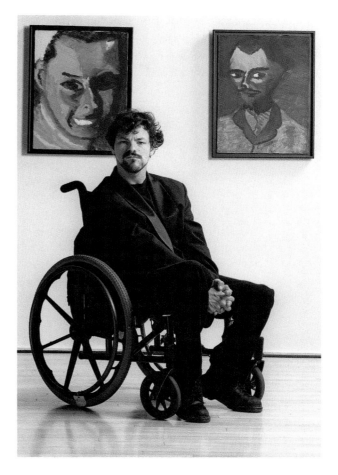

Dan Keplinger, author of the 1999 Oscar-winning documentary "King Gimp," sits in a wheelchair among his paintings on display at the Phillis Kind Gallery in New York. *(AP/Wide World Photos. Reproduced by permission.)*

person to person and may change over time. Some people with CP are also affected by other medical disorders, including **seizures** or mental impairment. Early signs of CP usually appear before three years of age. Infants with this disease are frequently slow to reach developmental milestones such as learning to roll over, sit, crawl, smile, or walk.

Causes of CP may be congenital (present at birth) or acquired after birth. Several of the causes that have been identified through research are preventable or treatable: head injury, jaundice, Rh incompatibility, and rubella (German measles). Cerebral palsy is diagnosed by testing motor skills and reflexes, examining the medical history, and employing a variety of specialized tests. Although its symptoms may change over time, this disorder by definition is not progressive. If a patient shows increased impairment, the physician considers an alternative diagnosis.

Demographics

Cerebral palsy is one of the most common causes of chronic childhood disability. About 3,000 babies are born with the disorder each year in the United States, and about 1,500 preschoolers are diagnosed with cerebral palsy during the first three years of life. In almost 70% of cases, CP is found with some other disorder, the most common being

mental retardation. In all, around 500,000–700,000 Americans have some degree of cerebral palsy.

The prevalence of CP has remained very stable for many years. The incidence increases with premature or very low-weight babies regardless of the quality of care. Twins are also four times more likely to develop CP than single births.

Despite medical advances, in some cases the incidence of CP has actually increased over time. This may be attributed to medical advances in areas related to premature babies or the increased usage of artificial fertilization techniques.

Causes and symptoms

CP is caused by damage to an infant's brain before, during or shortly after delivery. The part of the brain that is damaged determines what parts of the body are affected.

There are a number of factors which appear to predispose a child to CP including:

• Exposure of the expectant mother to certain infections like rubella, toxoplasmosis and cytomegalovirus,

• Exposure of the expectant mother to certain chemicals like alcohol, cigarettes, cocaine and teratogenic (capable of causing birth defects) agents,

• Severe physical trauma to the mother during pregnancy, multiple births or maternal illness,

• Children who are born prematurely (less than 32 weeks) or who are very low birth weight (less than 1,500 grams or about $3\frac{1}{3}$ pounds),

• Failure of the brain to develop properly or neurological damage to the infant's developing brain, including **hypoxia** (lack of oxygen) during birth,

• Bacterial meningitis and other infections, bleeding in the brain, lack of oxygen, severe jaundice, and head injury during the first few years of a child's life.

Cerebral palsy is categorized into four different groups that are characterized by different symptoms. Generally, babies that are severely affected may have obvious signs immediately following birth. Many infants do not display immediate CP symptoms. Parents are usually able to notice developmental delays, especially if they have another unaffected child. At the age of about three months, parents may notice a lack of facial expressions or that their baby does not respond to some sounds, or does not follow movement with their eyes. Certain other indicative symptoms may appear at around six months of age, including inability to lift the head or roll over and difficulty feeding. An affected child may be unable to crawl, sit, or stand without support and drooling is a common problem because of poor facial and throat muscle control. CP symptoms depend on the individual and the type of CP and, in particular, whether or not there is a mixed form of the condition.

The four main categories of cerebral palsy are:

• Spastic CP: Children with spastic CP have increased muscle tone. Their muscles are stiff and their movements can be awkward. Seventy to eighty percent of people with this disease have **spasticity**. Spastic CP is usually described further by what parts of the body are affected. In spastic diplegia, the main effect is found in both legs. In spastic hemiplegia, one side of the person's body is affected. Spastic quadriplegia affects a person's whole body (face, trunk, legs, and arms).

• Athetoid or dyskinetic CP: Children with athetoid CP have slow, writhing movements that they cannot control. The movements usually affect a person's hands, arms, feet, and legs. Sometimes the face and tongue are affected and the person has a hard time talking. Muscle tone can change from day to day and can vary even during a single day. Ten to twenty percent of people with CP have the athetoid form of the condition.

• Ataxic CP: Children with ataxic CP have problems with balance and depth perception. They might be unsteady when they walk. They might have a hard time with quick movements or movements that need a lot of control, like writing. Controlling their hands or arms when they reach for something is often difficult. People with ataxic CP can have increased or decreased muscle tone.

• Mixed CP: Some people have more than one type of CP, but this is most often a mixture of spasticity and athetoid movements, with tight muscle tone and involuntary reflexes.

Diagnosis

Diagnosing CP in an infant is often a difficult and slow process that takes time to establish with certainty, as there other health problems that can mimic the condition. The physician may suspect that the infant has CP because of a history of difficulties at birth, seizures, feeding problems or low muscle tone. Detailed medical and developmental history, including the history of the pregnancy and delivery, medications taken by the mother during fetal development, infections and fetal movement are all considered. A detailed family history, including the mother's history of miscarriage, relatives with similar conditions, ethnic background, and consanguinity (marriage between close blood relatives) can also prove helpful. The child's physician will perform a thorough physical examination and may order vision and hearing testing.

Infants suffering from brain injury are often slow to reach developmental milestones including rolling over, sitting up, crawling, walking and talking. Healthcare professionals are often hesitant to reach an early diagnosis because the child may recover and they may use other, less emotive terms in labeling the condition such as: neuromotor dysfunction, developmental delay, motor disability, static **encephalopathy** and **central nervous system** dysfunction.

Physicians must test the child's motor skills, using many of the techniques outlined above and looking for evidence of slow development, abnormal muscle tone, and unusual posture. Healthcare professionals will move slowly and carefully towards a positive diagnosis only after eliminating all other possible causes of the child's condition.

Neuroimaging studies can help to evaluate brain damage and to determine those at risk of developing CP. No study exists to support definitive diagnosis of CP. Computed tomography (**CT**) **scans** provide information to help diagnose congenital malformations and intracranial hemorrhages in the infant. **Magnetic resonance imaging**

(**MRI**) is most useful after two to three weeks of life, and is also used to detect brain disease in an older child.

Ultrasound in the neonate (newborn) provides information about the structures of the brain as well as diagnostic information on possible hemorrhage or hypoxic-ischemic (lack of oxygen) injury.

Evoked potentials are used to evaluate the anatomic pathways of the nerves responsible for hearing and vision. Electroencephalogram (EEG) is useful in evaluating severe hypoxic-ischemic injury.

Treatment team

A **neurologist** may help to differentiate cerebral palsy from other neurological disorders. Consultation with a neurologist also may be helpful in treatment of patients with seizures. Pulmonologists (lung specialists) may help treat the patient with bronchopulmonary dysplasia or frequent aspiration pneumonia. Orthopedic surgery consultation may be needed to help correct any structural deformities. An ophthalmologist may be indicated to follow up with any patient experiencing visual deficits. Audiologists help screen for hearing deficits. A gastroenterologist (specialist on digestive disorders) may help with reflux and constipation and may be helpful in coordinating feedings to regulate weight gain or weight loss if needed. A periodic nutrition consultation is important to make sure the child does not suffer from growth failure or nutritional deficiencies.

Treatment

Drug therapy is used for those who have seizures associated with CP. Anticonvulsant medications are usually very effective in preventing seizures associated with CP. Drugs are also used to control spasticity in some cases. Medications used most often are **diazepam**, a general relaxant of the brain and body, baclofen, which blocks signals sent from the spinal cord to contract the muscles, and datrolene, which interferes with the process of muscle contraction. These drugs are used for short periods, but long-term control of spasticity is more difficult to achieve.

Persons with athetoid CP are sometimes given drugs to help reduce abnormal movements, usually **anticholinergics**. Anticholinergics reduce the activity of acetylcholine, a chemical messenger that helps some brain cells communicate and trigger muscle contraction. Physicians may inject drugs directly into a muscle to reduce spasticity for a short period.

Surgery is used when muscle contractures are severe enough to create problems in movement. The surgeons lengthen the muscle that is too short. Lengthening a muscle usually makes it weaker, so surgery for contractures is usually followed by an extended recovery and therapy period. To reduce spasticity in the legs, surgery called selective dorsal root rhizotomy sometimes proves effective. It reduces the amount of stimulation that reaches leg muscles by the nerves.

Recovery and rehabilitation

Cerebral palsy cannot be cured. Treatment can, however, help a person take part in family, school, and work activities as much as possible. There are many treatments, including physical therapy, occupational therapy, medicine, operations, and orthotic devices that help maintain the highest possible state of wellness and activity.

Specialized Therapies

Physical therapy improves infant-caregiver interaction, gives family support, and supplies resources for parental education, as well as promoting motor and developmental skills. Physical therapists teach the parent or caregiver exercises or activities necessary to help the child reach his or her full potential.

Daily range of motion (ROM) exercises are important to prevent or delay contractures (fixed, rigid muscles) secondary to spasticity, and to maintain mobility of joints and soft tissues. Stretching exercises are performed to increase motion. Progressive resistance exercises also increase strength. Age-appropriate play and adaptive toys and games using the desired exercises are important to elicit the child's full cooperation. Strengthening knee extensor muscles helps to improve crouching and stride length. Postural and motor control training is important following the normal developmental sequence of children (i.e., achieve head and neck control if possible before advancing to trunk control).

Occupational therapists keep the child's developmental age in mind and use adaptive equipment as needed to help attain these milestones. For example, if a child is developmentally ready to stand and explore the environment, but is limited by lack of motor control, a stander or modified walker is used. Performance based upon previous success is encouraged to maintain the child's interest and cooperation. Assistive devices and durable medical equipment help attain function that may not be possible otherwise. Orthotic devives frequently are required to maintain functional joint position especially in persons who are non-ambulatory. Frequent reevaluation of orthotic devices is important as children quickly outgrow them and can develop skin irritation from improper use of orthotic devices.

Recreational therapy, especially hippotherapy (horseback riding therapy) is frequently a well-liked activity of parents and patients alike to help with muscle tone, range

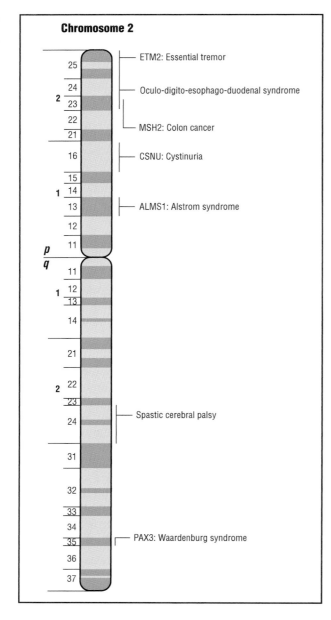

Chromosome 2

25 — ETM2: Essential tremor

24 — Oculo-digito-esophago-duodenal syndrome
2 23

22
   21 — MSH2: Colon cancer

16 — CSNU: Cystinuria

15
1 14
   13 — ALMS1: Alstrom syndrome

12

11

p
q

11

1 12
   13

14

21

2 22
   23
   24 — Spastic cerebral palsy

31

32

33
34
35 — PAX3: Waardenburg syndrome
36

37

Cerebral palsy, on chromosome 2. *(Gale Group.)*

of motion, strength, coordination, and balance. Hippotherapy also offers many potential cognitive, physical, and emotional benefits. Incorporation of play into all of a child's therapies is important. The child should view physical and occupational therapy as fun, not work. Caregivers should seek fun and creative ways to stimulate children, especially those who have decreased ability to explore their own environments.

Many children with dyskinetic CP have involvement of the face and oropharynx causing difficulty swallowing properly, drooling, and speech difficulties. Speech therapy can be implemented to help improve swallowing and communication. Those patients with athetoid CP may benefit the most from speech therapy, as most have normal intelligence and communication is an obstacle secondary to abnormal muscle movements that affect their speech. Adequate communication is probably the most important goal for enhancing function in the athetoid CP patient.

Clinical trials

As of mid-2004, there were numerous open **clinical trials** for the study and treatment of cerebral palsy, including:

- "Botulinum Toxin (BOTOX) for CP," "Relaxation Training to Decrease **Pain** and Improve Function in Adolescents with CP," and "Constraint-based Therapy to Improve Motor Function in Children with CP," sponsored by the National Institute of Child Health and Human Development (NICHD),

- "Classification of CP Subtypes," "Eye-Hand Coordination in Children with Spastic Diplegia," "Beneficial Effects of Antenatal Magnesium Sulfate (BEAM Trial)," and "Brain Control of Movements in CP," sponsored by National Institute of Neurological Disorders and Stroke (NINDS),

- Study of Tongue Pressures, sponsored by Warren G. Magnuson Clinical Center.

Updated information about these clinical trials can be found at the National Institutes of Health website for clinical trials at www.clinicaltrials.gov.

Prognosis

The prognosis of persons with CP varies according to the severity of the disorder. Some children have only mild problems in muscle tone and no problems with daily activities, while others are unable to purposefully move any part of the body. Regression, or worsening of long-term symptoms, is not characteristic of CP. If regression occurs, it is necessary to look for a different cause of the child's problems. In order for a child to be able to walk, a major cascade of events in motor control have to occur. A child must be able to hold up his head before he can sit up on his own, and he must be able to sit independently before he can walk on his own. It is generally assumed that if a child is not sitting up by himself by age four or walking by age eight, he will never be an independent walker. But a child who starts to walk at age three will certainly continue to walk unless he has a disorder other than CP.

In people with severe CP, motor problems often lead to medical complications, including more frequent and serious infections, severe breathing problems, feeding intolerance, and skin breakdown. These medical complications can lead to frequent hospitalizations and a shortened life expectancy.

Epilepsy also occurs in about a third of children with CP and is more frequent in patients with spastic quadriplegia or mental retardation. Cognitive impairment occurs more frequently in CP than in the general population, and mental delays or some form of learning disability has been estimated to occur in over two thirds of CP cases.

Resources

BOOKS

Anderson, Mery Elizabeth, Dineen Tom. *Taking Cerebral Palsy to School.* St. Louis: Jayjo Books, 2000.

Mechan, Merlin L. *Cerebral Palsy.* Austin, TX: Pro-Ed Publishers, 2002.

Pincus, Dion. *Everything You Need to Know About Cerebral Palsy (Need to Know Library).* New York: Rosen Publishing Group, 1999.

PERIODICALS

Darrah, J., et al. "Conductive education intervention for children with cerebral palsy: an AACPDM evidence report." *Dev Med Child Neurol* 46 (March 2004): 187–203.

OTHER

"Cerebral Palsy—Facts & Figures." *United Cerebral Palsy.* (May 1, 2004). <http://www.ucp.org/ucp_generaldoc.cfm/1/9/37/37-37/447>.

"NINDS Cerebral Palsy Information Page." National Institute of Neurological Disorders and Stroke. (May 1, 2004). <http://www.ninds.nih.gov/health_and_medical/disorders/cerebral_palsy.htm>.

ORGANIZATIONS

March of Dimes Birth Defects Foundation. 1275 Mamaroneck Avenue, White Plains, NY 10605. (914) 428-7100 or (888) 663-4637; Fax: (914) 428-8203. askus@marchofdimes.com. <http://www.marchofdimes.com>.

United Cerebral Palsy (UCP). 1600 L Street, NW, Suite 700, Washington, DC 20036. (202) 776-0406 or (800) USA-5UCP (872-5827); Fax: (202) 776-0414. national@ucp.org. <http://www.ucp.org>.

Francisco de Paula Careta
Iuri Drumond Louro

Cerebrovascular accident (CVA) *see* **Stroke**

Cervical disc herniation *see* **Disc herniation**

Cervical radiculopathy *see* **Radiculopathy**

Channelopathies

Definition

Channelopathies are inherited diseases caused by defects in cell proteins called ion channels.

Channelopathies include a wide range of neurologic diseases, including **periodic paralysis**, congenital myasthenic syndromes, malignant hypothermia, a form of Charcot-Marie-Tooth disease, and several other disorders. Cystic fibrosis and long Q-T syndrome, which are not neurological diseases, are also types of channelopathy.

Description

Cells of the body, including nerve and muscle cells, are surrounded by thin coverings called membranes. Embedded in these membranes are a large and varied set of proteins that control the movement of materials across the membrane, in and out of the cell. One major type of material that crosses through such proteins are called ions, and the proteins that transport them are called ion channels.

Ions perform many different functions in cells. In neurons (nerve cells), they help transmit the electrical messages that allow neurons to communicate with each other, and with muscle cells. In muscle cells, they allow the muscle to contract. When the ion channels are defective, these activities may be disrupted.

Inheritance

The proteins responsible for channelopathies are made by genes, and defects in genes are the cause for the diseases. Genes are inherited from both parents. If two defective copies of a gene are needed in order for a person to develop the disease, this is known as a recessive inheritance pattern. Two parents, each of whom carry one defective copy, have a 25% chance with each pregnancy of having a child with the disease.

If only one defective copy of the gene is needed in order to develop the disease, this is known as a dominant inheritance pattern. A single parent who carries the disease gene (and likely has the disease as well) has a 50% chance with each pregnancy of having a child with the disease.

Types of Channelopathies
Periodic paralysis

A person with periodic paralysis experiences sudden onset of weakness, which gradually subsides, only to return again later. Two forms of periodic paralysis exist, termed "hyperkalemic," referring to the excessively high levels of potassium in the blood which can trigger attacks, and "hypokalemic," in which excessively low levels of potassium are the culprit. Each is caused by different genetic mutations of a potassium ion channel, and both exhibit the dominant inheritance pattern. Onset is usually in childhood for the hyperkalemic form, and childhood to adulthood for the hypokalemic form. Dietary restrictions can reduce the frequency of attacks of both forms, with a high-carbohydrate, low-potassium diet for the hyperkalemic form, and a low-carbohydrate, high-potassium diet for the hypokalemic form.

Congenital myasthenic syndromes

Congenital myasthenic syndromes are a group of related disorders caused by inherited defects in the acetylcholine receptor. This protein sits on the surface of muscle cells; when a nearby neuron releases the chemical acetylcholine, it binds to the receptor, causing the muscle to contract. Defects cause myasthenia ("muscle weakness") and **fatigue**, and may be life-threatening in some individuals. Most forms display the recessive inheritance pattern. Onset is in infancy. Treatment usually includes the drug mestinon, which blocks the breakdown of the acetylcholine after it is released, prolonging its action, and another drug, called 3,4-DAP, which increases the amount of acetylcholine released.

Malignant hyperthermia

Malignant hyperthermia is caused by mutations in the gene for a membrane protein inside the muscle cell, called the ryanodine receptor, which controls calcium ion movement within the muscle. Another form is due to mutation in a different muscle protein controlling calcium. Malignant hyperthermia is usually triggered by exposure to certain kinds of anesthetics or muscle relaxants. It causes a dangerous increase in the rate of activity within the muscle, and a sharp rise in temperature, leading to a cascade of crises which may include severe damage to muscle cells, heart malfunction, swelling of tissues including the brain, and death. It is treated with dantrolene, an antispasticity medication that blocks calcium ion movement in the muscle. Awareness of the condition has led to better screening for it among anesthesia patients and a significant reduction in mortality.

X-linked Charcot-Marie-Tooth disease

X-linked Charcot-Marie-Tooth disease (CMTX) is caused by a defect in connexin 32. This protein forms connections between adjacent cells, allowing ions to flow between them. The cells affected are those that surround neurons and provide their electrical insulation. Outside the brain and spinal cord (together called the **central nervous system**, or CNS), this job is performed by Schwann cells.

Inside the CNS, the insulating cells are called oligodendrocytes. Like other forms of CMT, CMTX causes slowly progressing muscle weakness in the distal muscles (those furthest away from the body center), including the hands and feet. There may also be decreased sensation in the extremities. CMTX is inherited on the X chromosome, of which males have one and females have two. For this reason, CMTX usually affects males more severely than females because they have only one X chromosome, and therefore lack a second normal copy of the gene.

Resources
WEBSITES

Muscular Dystrophy Association. <www.mdausa.org>.
Charcot-Marie-Tooth Association. <www.cmta.org>.

Richard Robinson

Charcot-Marie-Tooth disorder

Definition

The name Charcot-Marie-Tooth disorder (CMT) refers to a group of hereditary diseases, all involving chronic motor and sensory neuropathies. Drs. Charcot and Marie of France, and Dr. Tooth of England first described the disorder in 1886 when they found patients with progressive muscle weakness and muscle loss in their feet and lower legs. Over time, this weakness progressed to their hands and forearms. More is now known about the numerous disease subtypes, including their complex genetics and inheritance patterns.

Description

Charcot-Marie-Tooth disorder is also known by the names hereditary motor and sensory neuropathy, and peroneal muscular atrophy. A person with CMT often has distal muscle weakness and atrophy that involves the feet, legs, and hands. Many people with CMT are diagnosed later in life as adults. However, diagnosis can happen as early as the first to third decade of life when there is a family history of CMT. The muscle weakness may begin painlessly, symmetrically, and slowly. Many CMT subtypes seem similar and may only be identified through further neurological or genetic testing.

Learning problems are not commonly associated with CMT, but psychological issues from living with progressive muscle weakness can occur. Only some rare X-linked forms of CMT involve **mental retardation** or deafness as

Key Terms

Atrophy Wasting or loss of tissue.

Biopsy Process of removal of tissue for study.

Chronic Ongoing and long-term.

Distal Situated away from the center of the body, like the legs and hands.

Duplication Extra genetic material due to a duplicate copy.

Electromyography Testing that shows the electrical activity associated with muscle movements and actions.

Gait The way in which one walks.

Motor Having to do with movement.

Mutation A change in the order of deoxyribonucleic acid (DNA) bases that make up genes.

Nerve conduction study Testing that shows electrical impulse activity along nerves.

Neuropathy Term for any disorder affecting the nervous system or cranial nerves.

Peroneal Related to the legs.

Pes cavus A highly arched foot.

Scoliosis Curving of the spine bones.

Sensory Related to the senses, or the ability to feel.

---

occasional symptoms, but these are not typical of classical CMT.

Demographics

CMT is the most common genetic cause of neuropathy. It is estimated to affect between one in 2,500 to one in 5,000 people, with most of them having CMT type 1 (CMT1). About 20% of people who come to neuromuscular clinics with a chronic **peripheral neuropathy** have some form of CMT. The condition affects people of all ethnic groups worldwide. Most forms affect males and females equally, with the exception of the X-linked form, which usually affects males more severely than females.

As of 2004, numerous genes have been found responsible for various subtypes of CMT. Genetic testing is available for some types. For other types, genetic testing is not yet available.

Causes and symptoms

Mutations in several genes cause the various types of CMT to occur. The most common form of the disorder, CMT1A, is caused by duplication in the peripheral myelin protein 22 (PMP22) gene. In these cases, the PMP22 gene is too active from the extra genetic material, so it makes too much myelin protein. The correct amount of myelin protein is important for normal muscle strength and movement, so the extra amount can cause these problems.

CMT is inherited in many ways, as seen by varying family histories of the condition. CMT1 and CMT2 are typically inherited in an autosomal dominant manner. This means that an affected individual has a 50/50 chance of passing a disease-causing mutation to his or her children,

regardless of gender. In these cases, a strong family history of the condition may be seen.

CMT4 and some forms of CMT2 are inherited in an autosomal recessive manner. This means that an affected individual has parents who each carry the CMT gene. These parents run the risk of having a child with CMT with every pregnancy.

CMT is also inherited in an X-linked manner, and the most common type is called CMTX. Women may be carriers of this type. They are usually more at risk to have affected sons. Daughters may be carriers and they may or may not show milder symptoms.

The neurological symptoms in CMT can progress slowly, but may become problematic over time. Muscle weakness is usually found first in the foot and lower leg muscles. It can eventually include the upper leg and hips in severely affected people. Since the middle of the legs are usually stronger, most people with CMT can still usually walk with the aid of ankle splints.

Some early signs of CMT may be gait abnormalities, or clumsiness in running. Many people with CMT develop *pes cavus* with very high arches in their feet, and this can be associated with curled-up toes. Loss of nerve functioning can lead to the inability to notice very hot and cold sensations, or the sensation of touch.

Upper limb muscles may become weaker, and this includes the hands and forearms. Due to this, people may have difficulty with fine motor tasks like writing. People with more advanced CMT may develop bone changes, like scoliosis. This may cause **back pain** if it is very severe.

A specific sign of CMT1A is the "onion bulb" formation in muscular nerves. Nerves with repeated myelination and demyelination (due to abnormalities in the

PMP22 gene) may eventually take on the shape of an onion bulb, which is how the finding was named.

Diagnosis

Until the discovery of the CMT genes, the diagnosis of the condition was made on a clinical basis. The difficulties lie in the similarities with other neuropathies like hereditary neuropathy with liability to pressure palsies (HNPP) and those associated with disorders like alcoholism, drug dependence, and diabetes.

An important first step to diagnosing CMT is taking a careful family history. A positive family history is an indicator that the neuropathy may be hereditary. Additionally, the pattern of affected individuals can give clues about the inheritance type in the family.

Carefully documenting the timing of symptoms is also important. Only a minority of people with CMT seek a medical opinion in childhood, since most are diagnosed later in life. An exception might be the highly informed family in which there is a strong history of the condition.

Skeletal signs like *pes cavus* and scoliosis occur in hereditary neuropathies, but tend to show up when the symptoms begin early. They may be absent when the onset is later in life, even in CMT. This may be an important clue when attempting to diagnose CMT. CMT may also include symptoms like mental retardation and hearing loss, as seen in some rarer X-linked forms.

A slow progression of symptoms is typical of CMT. Some hereditary neuropathies, like HNPP, may have periods of severe symptoms that get better and then worsen later. Again, careful documentation of symptoms is important to diagnose CMT.

Some signs of CMT are found through electrophysiological studies, like **electromyography** (EMG) and nerve conduction velocity (NCV) testing. EMG results are usually abnormal, and NCV studies may show slowed nerve conduction, a sign of muscle weakness. Those with CMT type 1 usually show severe slowing in NCV studies, and type 2 is associated with mild or no slowing.

EMG and NCV studies are very important tools for physicians to use when thinking of a hereditary neuropathy. These are often abnormal, with reduced NCV values. A nerve **biopsy** is rarely necessary to pinpoint a specific type of CMT, because onion-bulb abnormalities are a sign of CMT1A.

It may still be difficult to diagnose CMT with electrophysiological test results and clinical information. The results from testing may help to determine which genetic testing to pursue. Genetic testing is useful for confirming a clinical diagnosis or for family testing when there is an identified CMT gene mutation in the family. As of 2004, genetic testing for CMT type 1 is more available than testing for CMT type 2.

Genetic testing is not perfect and results can be tricky to interpret. An informative test result is one that identifies a known mutation in a CMT gene, and this confirms that the person has CMT. A negative test result means a mutation was not found in the gene. This either means that the tested individual does not have CMT, or has a mutation that cannot be found through testing. It may also mean the individual has a different type of CMT or another disorder altogether. Medical geneticists and genetic counselors can be very helpful in interpreting complex genetic test results.

Treatment team

Treatment for people with CMT is often dependent upon symptoms. A multi-disciplinary team and approach can be helpful. A treatment team may include a **neurologist**, medical geneticist, genetic counselor, orthopedic surgeon, otolaryngologist, physical therapist, occupational therapist, social worker, physiatrist, **neuropsychologist**, and a primary care provider. Oftentimes there are pediatric specialists in these fields who aid in the care for children. The key is good communication between the various specialists to coordinate medical care.

Treatment

There is no cure for Charcot-Marie-Tooth disorder. No specific treatment is known to reverse, slow, or stop the progressive nature of the disease.

In order to keep flexibility and muscle length in the ankles and feet, daily stretching of the heel cords can be helpful. Special shoes with ankle and orthopedic inserts may help to improve walking and movement. Corrective surgery by an orthopedic surgeon is required in some cases. Others need forearm crutches or canes to keep stable while walking, but fewer than 5% of people with CMT need wheelchair assistance. Splints, specific exercises, orthopedic devices, and sometimes surgery are needed to keep hands functioning well.

Certain medications can be helpful for people with CMT, while others should be avoided because they can cause nerve damage. Examples of drugs to be avoided include alcohol, high doses of vitamins A and D, penicillin, taxol, and certain chemotherapy medications (vincristine, cisplatin).

For overall health, a good diet and regular **exercise** are recommended. Exercise is particularly important because it keeps muscles functioning and maintains endurance levels.

Recovery and rehabilitation

Rehabilitation can be ongoing in CMT, particularly if the muscle weakness has progressed considerably. Since the disorder does not typically get better with time, physical therapy and strength maintenance is very important. The disease's early stages may not cause problems for walking or daily activities, but over time it can greatly impact a person's life. Physical therapy may be relatively infrequent early on, but may increase as time goes on.

Children may have difficulty with tasks in school, such as writing and other fine motor skills. Occupational therapists, often available at school, are helpful in these situations. Overall, a person's time spent in recovery and rehabilitation is variable. Specialists in physical medicine and rehabilitation can be helpful in coordinating a plan to help someone retain his or her strength for as long as possible.

Prognosis

Prognosis for someone with Charcot-Marie-Tooth disorder is unique to the person. The severity of the symptoms can vary greatly, even within the same family. Those who develop the disease as children may have more severe muscle weakness by the time others first see signs of the disease. However, only about 5% of people with CMT need wheelchairs at any point in their lives. CMT is not considered a fatal disease. Symptoms are chronic and progressive, and can negatively impact a person's life.

Genetic testing now helps identify people before they even develop symptoms, so personalized medical care can begin as early as possible. This has helped to reduce the risk of complications and increase the quality of life for many. Medical screening may be further tailored to the individual as scientific studies identify medical complications associated with specific CMT mutations in families.

Special concerns

Due to specific muscular weakness and difficulty with fine motor tasks, careful career and job consideration is helpful for people with CMT.

Resources

BOOKS

Parker, James N., and Philip M. Parker. *The Official Patient's Sourcebook on Charcot-Marie-Tooth Disorder: A Revised and Updated Directory for the Internet Age.* San Diego: Icon Health Publishers, 2002.

Parry, Gareth J. *Charcot-Marie-Tooth Disorders: A Handbook for Primary Care Physicians.* DIANE Publishing Co., 1995.

PERIODICALS

Bell, Christine, and Neva Haites. "Genetic Aspects of Charcot-Marie-Tooth Disease." *Archives of Disease in Childhood* (April 1998) 78: 296–300.

Benstead, Timothy J., and Ian A. Grant. "Charcot-Marie-Tooth Disease and Related Inherited Peripheral Neuropathies." *Canadian Journal of Neurological Sciences* (2001) 28: 199–214.

Berciano, Jose, and Onofre Combarros. "Hereditary Neuropathies." *Current Opinion in Neurology* (2003) 16: 613–622.

Pareyson, Davide. "Diagnosis of Hereditary Neuropathies in Adult Patients." *Journal of Neurology* (2003) 250: 148–160.

Vallat, Jean-Michel. "Dominantly Inherited Peripheral Neuropathies." *Journal of Neuropathology and Experimental Neurology* (July 2003) 62(7): 699–714.

WEBSITES

National Institute of Neurological Disorders and Stroke. (March 30, 2004). <http://www.ninds.nih.gov/index.htm>.

Online Mendelian Inheritance in Man. (March 30, 2004). <http://www.ncbi.nlm.nih.gov/omim/>.

ORGANIZATIONS

Charcot-Marie-Tooth Association. 2700 Chestnut Street, Chester, PA 19013-4867. (800) 606-CMTA; Fax: (610) 499-9267. CMTAssoc@aol.com. <www.charcot-marie-tooth.org>.

CMT World. P.O. Box 601, Hillsburgh, Ontario N0B 1Z0, Canada. (519) 855-6376; Fax: (519) 855-6746. info@cmtworld.org. <www.cmtworld.org/index.php>.

Muscular Dystrophy Campaign U.K. 7-11 Prescott Place, London SW4 6BS, U.K. +44 (0)171-720-8055; Fax: +44 (0)171-498-0670. info@muscular-dystrophy.org. <www.muscular-dystrophy.org>.

Deepti Babu, MS, CGC

Chiari malformation *see* **Arnold-Chiari malformation**

Cholinergic stimulants

Definition

Cholinergic stimulants are a class of drugs that produce the same effects as those of the body's parasympathetic nervous system. Cholinergic drugs are used for a variety of purposes, including the treatment of **myasthenia gravis** and during anesthesia.

Purpose

The parasymapthetic nervous system is responsible for conserving and restoring energy in the body by regulating day-to-day functions such as digestion, sphincter muscle relaxation, salivation, and reducing heart rate and blood pressure. Nerve impulses in the parasympathetic nervous system are transmitted from one nerve junction to another with the help of acetylcholine, the most common neurotransmitter in the parasympathetic nervous system. Cholinergic drugs are drugs that affect the levels of acetylcholine at the nerve junction.

Cholinergic stimulants result in increased acetylcholine accumulation at the neuromuscular junction and prolong its effect. Cholinergic stimulant drugs are used in the diagnosis and treatment of myasthenia gravis, a disorder of nerve impulse transmission at the neuromuscular junction, resulting in severe muscle weakness. Cholinergic stimulants are also used in surgery to reduce urinary retention and to counteract the effects of some muscle relaxant medications given during anesthesia.

Description

Cholinergic stimulant drugs include edrophonium chloride, (brand name, Tensilon), neostigmine (Prostigmine), piridogstimina (Mestinon), and ambenonium chloride (Mytelase). Cholinergic stimulants are available in tablet, syrup, time-release tablet, and injectable forms.

Recommended dosage

Cholinergic stimulants are given in varying dosages according to the reason for use. In the treatment of myasthenia gravis, cholinergic stimulant dosages are tailored to the individual person. Patients are encouraged to keep a diary and record their response to each dose during the initial treatment period, as well as during periods of increased muscle weakness, stress, and other illness, as these conditions frequently require adjustments in dosage.

Precautions

Cholinergic stimulant drugs may not be suitable for persons with asthma, heart block or slow heart rate, **epilepsy**, hyperactive thyroid gland, bladder obstruction, gastrointestinal tract obstruction, or stomach ulcer. Patients should notify their physicians if they have any of these conditions before taking these drugs.

Side effects

The adverse effects of cholinergic stimulants include mostly rash and digestive system complaints, including queasiness, loose stools, nausea, vomiting, abdominal cramps, muscle **pain**, increased salivation, increase in

---

Key Terms

Acetylcholine   The neurotransmitter, or chemical, that works in the brain to transmit nerve signals involved in regulating muscles, memory, mood, and sleep.

Myasthenia gravis   A chronic autoimmune disease characterized by fatigue and muscular weakness, especially in the face and neck, that results from a breakdown in the normal communication between nerves and muscles caused by the deficiency of acetylcholine at the neuromuscular junction.

Neuromuscular junction   The junction between a nerve fiber and the muscle it supplies.

Neurotransmitter   Chemical that allows the movement of information from one neuron across the gap between the adjacent neuron.

Parasympathetic nervous system   A branch of the autonomic nervous system that tends to induce secretion, increase the tone and contraction of smooth muscle, and cause dilation of blood vessels.

---

stomach acid production, and diarrhea. Rare and potentially more serious side effects include reduced heart rate, possibly leading to cardiac arrest, and weak, shallow breathing.

Interactions

Certain antibiotics, especially neomycin, streptomycin, and kanamycin, can exacerbate the effects of some cholinergic stimulants. These antibiotics should be used with caution by people with myasthenia gravis.

Resources

BOOKS

Henderson, Ronald E. *Attacking Myasthenia Gravis.* Seattle: Court Street Press, 2002.

Staff. *The Official Patient's Sourcebook on Myasthenia Gravis: A Revised and Updated Directory for the Internet Age.* San Diego: Icon Health Publications Group Int., 2002.

OTHER

"Myasthenia Gravis Fact Sheet." *National Institute of Neurological Disorders and Stroke.* February 11, 2004 (May 22, 2004). <http://www.ninds.nih.gov/ health_and_medical/pubs/myasthenia_gravis.htm>.

"Tensilon Test." *Medline Plus.* National Library of Medicine. May 14, 2004 (May 22, 2004). <http://www.nlm.nih.gov/ medlineplus/ency/article/003930.htm>.

ORGANIZATIONS

Myasthenia Gravis Foundation of America, Inc. 5841 Cedar Lake Road Suite 204, Minneapolis, MN 55416. (952)

545-9438 or (800) 541-5454; Fax: (952) 646-2028. myastheniagravis@msn.com. <http://www.myasthenia.org>.

Adrienne Wilmoth Lerner

Cholinesterase inhibitors

Definition

Cholinesterase inhibitors are a group of drugs prescribed to treat symptoms resulting from the early and middle stages of **Alzheimer disease**.

Purpose

Cholinesterase inhibitors are drugs that block the activity of an enzyme in the brain called cholinesterase. Cholinesterase breaks apart the neurotransmitter acetylcholine, which is vital for the transmission of nerve impulses. Cholinesterase inhibitors are used to reduce the action of cholinesterase, thereby making more acetylcholine available to nerve cells in the brain.

For normal nerve-to-nerve communication to occur, the excess acetylcholine must be dissolved following the transmission of a nerve impulse. This is the normal function of cholinesterase. This enzyme dissolves acetylcholine into its component molecules; acetate and choline. These building blocks can then be recycled to form more acetylcholine for the next round of nerve signal transmission.

In disorders such as Alzheimer disease, Lewy body disease, and vascular **dementia**, the production of acetylcholine is decreased. As a result, nerve communication is less efficient, with consequent problems of memory and other brain and body functions. The use of cholinesterase inhibitors impedes the normal enzymatic breakdown of the little acetylcholine that is present. Although improved nerve function results with the use of cholinesterase inhibitors, the damage to brain cells caused in Alzheimer disease cannot be halted or reversed.

Description

As of mid-2004, there are four types of cholinesterase inhibitors that are available. These include donepezil (Aricept®), rivastigmine (Exelon®), galantamine (Reminy®), and tacrine (Cognex®). Tacrine is not available for use in Canada.

Donepezil was approved for use in the United States by the U.S. Food and Drug Administration (USFDA) in 1996. It is marketed by Pfizer as Aricept®. Rivastigmine received USFDA approval in 2000 and is sold by Novartis Pharmaceuticals as Exelon®. Galatamine received its

Key Terms

Acetylcholine The neurotransmitter, or chemical that works in the brain to transmit nerve signals, involved in regulating muscles, memory, mood, and sleep.

Alzheimer disease A neurological disorder characterized by slow, progressive memory loss due to a gradual loss of brain cells.

Neurotransmitter Chemicals that allow the movement of information from one neuron across the gap between the adjacent neuron.

USFDA approval in 2001 and is marketed in the U.S. as Reminyl® by Jassen Pharmaceuticals and Ortho-McNeil. Pointing out the importance of the natural world in providing therapeutic compounds, galatamine is extracted from the bulbs of daffodils. Finally, the drug tacrine is the oldest of the cholinesterase inhibitors, having received USFDA approval in 1993. Its use has declined due to incidents of serious side effects that include reversible liver damage.

Cholinesterase inhibitors are typically used to treat the early and middle stage symptoms of diseases such as Alzheimer's. This is because the deterioration in the production of acetylcholine accelerates over time, as more and more brain cells become damaged. Thus, the best chance to achieve a benefit for a person lies at the beginning of the disease path.

The benefits of cholinesterase inhibitors are judged by three patterns of the symptoms. In the early stages of Alzheimer disease, cholinesterase inhibitors may improve a person's condition, resulting in improvement of symptoms. As the disease progresses, cholinesterase inhibitors may act to stabilize the symptoms. Finally, the symptoms continue to worsen, but at a rate that is slower than would occur if the drug(s) were not taken.

One symptom that benefits from the use of cholinesterase inhibitors is called cognition. Cognition encompasses memory, language, and orientation (knowing the date, time, and a proper sense of direction). By improving, or at least retarding the rate of loss of cognition, the drugs can improve a person's quality of life. The benefits bestowed by cholinesterase inhibitors last only as long as effective levels of the drugs are present. Discontinuing the drug leads the return of symptoms within weeks.

Studies that have charted the time course of cognitive changes after taking the various cholinesterase inhibitors have demonstrated that improvements tend to peak about three months after the particular drug is first taken. After that time, a person's mental condition slowly begins to decline back to their starting point over the next six to nine months. If the drug continues to be taken, the cognitive decline becomes slower than in people who do not take the medication.

Recommended dosage

The recommended dosage of cholinesterase inhibitors varies with the approving agency in a particular country. But, dosages tend not to vary appreciably. The maximum daily dose of donepezil is normally 5–10 milligram (mg). This dose is taken just once a day, either in the morning or in the evening. The maximum daily dose of rivastimine is 6–12 mg. The drug is taken twice a day with meals (typically breakfast and dinner). The maximum daily dose of galantamine is 16–24 mg, and it is also taken twice a day with meals.

Precautions

As with any prescription drug, the recommended daily dosage and schedule for the drugs should not be changed independent of a physician's notification. Neither should someone stop taking cholinesterase inhibitors without seeking advice from a physician.

Side effects

Cholinesterase inhibitors can cause side effects. These are usually relatively minor, and constitute problems in digesting food, loss of appetite, nausea, vomiting, abdominal **pain**, and diarrhea. Not everyone will experience each discomfort, and the severity of the side effects can vary from person to person, depending on their tolerance to the discomfort. The drugs can vary in the severity of side effects caused. For example, rivastigmine produces greater weight loss and degree of nausea that the other drugs.

Less commonly, cholinesterase inhibitors can slow the heartbeat, cause **dizziness**, **fainting**, insomnia, **fatigue**, and produce muscle cramps in the legs. In general, the side effects tend to be mild and lessen after a drug has been taken for a few weeks. A notable exception is tacrine, which can cause liver damage. Periodic blood testing in order to monitor enzymes that relate to liver function is usually part of therapy with tacrine.

Interactions

Some cholinesterase inhibitors should be used with caution in persons with asthma or lung disease, as cholinesterase inhibitors may interact with theophylline, a drug commonly used to treat both conditions.

Resources

BOOKS

Bird, T. D. "Memory loss and dementia." In *Harrison's Principles of Internal Medicine,* 15th edition, A. S. Franci, E. Daunwald, and K. J. Isrelbacher, eds. New York: McGraw Hill, 2001.

Castleman, Michael, et. al. *There's Still a Person in There: The Complete Guide to Treating and Coping with Alzheimer's.* New York: Perigee Books, 2000.

Fillit, Howard M. *Drug Discovery and Development for Alzheimer's Disease.* New York: Springer, 2001.

PERIODICALS

Cummings, J. L. "Cholinesterase inhibitors: a new class of psychotropic compounds." *American Journal of Psychiatry* (January 2000): 4–14.

Masterman, D. "Cholinesterase inhibitors in the treatment of Alzheimer's disease and related dementias." *Clinical and Geriatric Medicine* (February 2004): 59–68.

OTHER

"Cholinesterase Inhibitors: Current Drug Treatments for Alzheimer Disease." *Alzheimer Society of Canada.* (May 6, 2004). <http://www.alzheimer.ca/english/treatment/treatments-cholinhib.htm>.

National Institute of Neurological Disorders and Stroke. *NINDS Alzheimer's Disease Information Page.* (May 6, 2004). <http://www.ninds.nih.gov/health_and_medical/disorders/alzheimersdisease_doc.htm>.

ORGANIZATIONS

Alzheimer Society of Canada. 20 Eglinton Avenue W., Suite 1200, Toronto, ON M4R 1K8, CANADA. (416) 488-8772 or (800) 616-8816; Fax: (416) 488-3778. info@alzheimer.ca. <http://www.alzheimer.ca>.

Alzheimer's Association. 225 N. Michigan Avenue, Chicago, IL 60601. (312) 335-8700 or (800) 272-3900; Fax: (312) 335-1110. info@alz.org. <http://www.alz.org>.

Brian Douglas Hoyle, PhD

Chorea

Definition

Chorea refers to brief, repetitive, jerky, or dancelike uncontrolled movements caused by muscle contractions that occur as symptoms of several different disorders. The English word "chorea" itself comes from the Greek word *choreia,* which means "dance." The symptom takes its name from the rapid involuntary jerking or twitching movements of the patient's face, limbs, and upper body.

Description

A patient with chorea may appear restless, fidgety, or unable to sit still. The body movements are continually changing and may appear to move from one part of the

Key Terms

Athetosis A symptom of movement disorders that consists of slow, writhing, wavelike movements, usually in the hands or feet. It is also known as mobile spasm. It may occur together with chorea; the combined symptom is called choreoathetosis.

Ballismus Involuntary violent flinging movements that may take the form of uncontrollable flailing. It is also called ballism. Ballismus that occurs with chorea is known as choreoballismus or choreoballism.

Basal ganglia (singular, ganglion) Groups of nerve cell bodies located deep within the brain that govern movement as well as emotion and certain aspects of cognition (thinking).

Chorea gravidarum Chorea occurring in the early months of pregnancy.

Dopamine A neurotransmitter that acts within certain parts of the brain to help regulate movement and emotion.

Encephalitis Inflammation of the brain.

Hemichorea Chorea that affects only one side of the body.

Hyperthyroidism Abnormally high levels of thyroid hormone. About 2% of patients with this condition develop chorea.

Hypocalcemia Abnormally low levels of calcium in the blood.

Neurosyphilis Late-stage syphilis that affects the central nervous system.

Neurotransmitter Any of a group of chemicals that transmit nerve impulses across the gap (synapse) between two nerve cells.

body to another. Jerking or twitching of the hands and feet may resemble piano playing or dancing. The patient may assume strange postures or make clumsy or wide-swinging leg movements when trying to walk. If the chest muscles are affected, the patient may have difficulty speaking normally, or make grunting or groaning noises. Facial expressions may be distorted by twitching of the lips, cheeks, eyebrows, or jaw. In severe cases, involuntary movements of the arms and legs may result in falling on the ground or throwing objects placed in the hand.

Other symptoms that may occur together with chorea include athetosis, which refers to slow, sinuous, writhing movements of the hands and feet, and ballismus, which refers to violent flinging or flailing of the limbs. A patient with one of these symptoms in addition to chorea may be said to have choreoathetosis or choreoballismus.

In some cases, only one side of the patient's body is affected by the involuntary movements. This condition is known as hemichorea.

Causes and associated disorders

The basic cause of choreic movements is overactivity of a neurotransmitter called dopamine in a set of structures deep within the brain known as the basal ganglia. The basal ganglia belong to a larger part of the nervous system that controls the muscles responsible for normal movement.

Several different unrelated disorders and conditions may lead to imbalances of dopamine in the basal ganglia, including:

- **Huntington**'s chorea (HC), an incurable hereditary disorder caused by a mutation in a gene on the short arm of human chromosome 4. It is characterized by **dementia** and psychiatric disturbances as well as chorea.
- **Sydenham's chorea**, a treatable complication of rheumatic fever following a streptococcal throat infection. It occurs most often in children and adolescents.
- Chorea gravidarum or chorea occurring in the first three months of pregnancy. It is most likely to affect women who had rheumatic fever or Sydenham's chorea in childhood.
- Senile chorea, which is gradual in onset, is not associated with other causes of chorea, does not cause personality changes, and develops in people over the age of 60. At one time, senile chorea was thought to be a late-onset form of HC, but is presently considered to be the result of a different genetic mutation.
- Blockage or rupture of one of the arteries supplying the basal ganglia.
- Metabolic disorders. About 2% of patients with abnormally high levels of thyroid hormone (hyperthyroidism) develop chorea. Abnormally low levels of calcium (hypocalcemia) may also produce chorea.
- Infectious diseases that affect the **central nervous system**. Chorea may be a symptom of viral encephalitis or late-stage neurosyphilis.
- Medications. Some drugs, most commonly those used to treat psychotic disorders or **Parkinson's disease**, cause

chorea as a side effect. Other drugs that sometimes cause chorea include **anticonvulsants (antiepileptic drugs)**, lithium, amphetamines, and some antinausea medications.

Diagnosis

A doctor diagnosing the cause of chorea is guided by such factors as the patient's age and sex as well as medication history and family history. A patient with symptoms of Huntington's chorea is typically an adult over 35, whereas Sydenham's chorea most often occurs in children aged six to 14. Huntington's chorea affects both sexes equally, whereas Sydenham's chorea affects girls twice as often as boys. A patient with a family history of Huntington's can be given a blood test to detect the presence of the gene that causes HC. A history of a recent throat infection or rheumatic fever suggests Sydenham's chorea. Metabolic disorders can be detected by blood tests.

Hemichorea or chorea accompanied by ballismus may indicate a vascular disorder affecting the basal ganglia, particularly when the chorea is sudden in onset. The doctor will order imaging studies, usually computed tomography (**CT**) **scans** or **magnetic resonance imaging (MRI)** if an arterial blockage or rupture is suspected. Neurosyphilis and encephalitis are diagnosed by testing a sample of the patient's cerebrospinal fluid.

Treatment

In general, chorea is not treated by itself unless the movements are so severe as to cause embarrassment or risk injury to the patient. Drugs that are given to treat chorea suppress the activity of dopamine in the basal ganglia but may also produce such undesirable side effects as muscular rigidity or drowsiness. These drugs cannot be given to women with chorea gravidarum because they may harm the fetus; pregnant patients may be given a mild benzodiazepine tranquilizer instead. Drugs given to treat patients with HD may help to control chorea, but cannot stop the progression of the disease.

Prognosis

The prognosis of chorea depends on its cause. Huntington's chorea is incurable, leading to the patient's death 10–25 years after the first symptoms appear. Almost all children with Sydenham's chorea, however, recover completely within one to six months. Chorea gravidarum usually resolves by itself when the baby is born or shortly afterward. Chorea caused by a vascular disorder may last for six to eight weeks after the blockage or rupture is treated. Chorea associated with metabolic disorders usually goes away when the chemical or hormonal imbalance is corrected.

Resources
BOOKS

"Disorders of Movement." *The Merck Manual of Diagnosis and Therapy*, edited by Mark H. Beers, MD, and Robert Berkow, MD. Whitehouse Station, NJ: Merck Research Laboratories, 2002.

Martin, John H. *Neuroanatomy: Text and Atlas*, 3rd ed. New York: McGraw-Hill, 2003.

"Movement Disorders: Choreas." *The Merck Manual of Geriatrics*, edited by Mark H. Beers, MD, and Robert Berkow, MD. Whitehouse Station, NJ: Merck Research Laboratories, 2004.

"Sydenham's Chorea (Chorea Minor; Rheumatic Fever; St. Vitus' Dance)." *The Merck Manual of Diagnosis and Therapy*, edited by Mark H. Beers, MD, and Robert Berkow, MD. Whitehouse Station, NJ: Merck Research Laboratories, 2002.

PERIODICALS

Caviness, John M., MD. "Primary Care Guide to Myoclonus and Chorea." *Postgraduate Medicine* 108 (October 2000): 163–172.

Grimbergen, Y. A., and R. A. Roos. "Therapeutic Options for Huntington's Disease." *Current Opinion in Investigational Drugs* 4 (January 2003): 51–54.

Jordan, L. C., and H. S. Singer. "Sydenham Chorea in Children." *Current Treatment Options in Neurology* 5 (July 2003): 283–290.

Karageyim, A. Y., B. Kars, R. Dansuk, et al. "Chorea Gravidarum: A Case Report." *Journal of Maternal-Fetal and Neonatal Medicine* 12 (November 2002): 353–354.

Sanger, T. D. "Pathophysiology of Pediatric Movement Disorders." *Journal of Child Neurology* 18 (September 2003) (Supplement 1): S9–S24.

Stemper, B., N. Thurauf, B. Neundorfer, and J. G. Heckmann. "Choreoathetosis Related to Lithium Intoxication." *European Journal of Neurology* 10 (November 2003): 743–744.

OTHER

Herrera, Maria Alejandra, MD, and Nestor Galvez-Jiminez, MD. "Chorea in Adults." *eMedicine*, 1 February 2002 (April 27, 2004.) <http://www.emedicine.com/neuro/topic62.htm>.

National Institute of Neurological Disorders and Stroke (NINDS). *NINDS Chorea Information Page.* (April 27, 2004). <http://www.ninds.nih.gov/health_and_medical/disorders/chorea.htm>.

Ramachandran, Tarakad S., MD. "Chorea Gravidarum." *eMedicine*, 9 June 2002 (April 27, 2004). <http://www.emedicine.com/neuro/topic61.htm>.

ORGANIZATIONS

American Geriatrics Society (AGS). Empire State Building, 350 Fifth Avenue, Suite 801, New York, NY 10118. (212) 308-1414; Fax: (212) 832-8646. info@american geriatrics.org. <http://www.americangeriatrics.org>.

Huntington's Disease Society of America (HDSA). 158 West 29th Street, 7th Floor, New York, NY 10001-5300. (212)

242-1968 or (800) 345-HDSA; Fax: (212) 239-3430. hdsainfo@hdsa.org. <http://www.hdsa.org>.

National Institute of Neurological Disorders and Stroke (NINDS). 9000 Rockville Pike, Bethesda, MD 20892. (301) 496-5751 or (800) 352-9424. <http://www.ninds.nih.gov>.

Worldwide Education and Awareness for Movement Disorders (WE MOVE). 204 West 84th Street, New York, NY 10024. (212) 875-8389 or (800) 437-MOV2. wemove@wemove.org. <http://www.wemove.org>.

Rebecca Frey, PhD

Chronic inflammatory demyelinating polyneuropathy

Definition

Chronic inflammatory demyelinating polyneuropathy (CIDP) is a disorder that affects the nerves outside of the brain and spinal cord (peripheral nerves). Specifically, the fatty covering, or sheath, that is wrapped around the outside of a nerve cell is damaged. The covering is called myelin, and the damage is called demyelination. The nerve damage becomes apparent as weakness in the legs and arms increases in severity with time.

Description

The demyelination of peripheral nerves causes a weakness in the legs and arms that grows progressively more severe over time. The ability of the limbs to feel sensory impulses such as touch, **pain**, and temperature can also be impaired. Typically, the malady is first apparent as a tingling or numbness in the toes and the fingers. The symptoms can both spread and become more severe with time.

The symptoms, treatment, and prognosis of CIDP is very similar to another nerve disease known as **Guillain-Barré syndrome**. In fact, CIDP has been historically known as "chronic Guillain-Barré syndrome" (Guillain-Barré syndrome is an acute malady whose symptoms appear and clear up more rapidly). Despite their similarities, however, CIDP and Guillain-Barré are two distinct conditions. CIDP is also known as chronic relapsing polyneuropathy.

Demographics

CIDP can occur at any age. However, the malady is more common in young adults, and in men more than in women. The disorder is rare in the general population.

Causes and symptoms

CIDP is an immune system disorder. Specifically, the immune system mistakenly recognizes the myelin sheath of the peripheral nerve cells as foreign. Damage to the sheath occurs when the immune system attempts to rid the body of the invader. There is no evidence to support a genetic basis for the disease, such as a family history of CIDP or other, similar disorders. CIDP cannot be inherited.

As with Guillain-Barré syndrome, it is strongly suspected that CIDP is at least triggered by a recent viral infection. For example, critical immune cells can be damaged in viral infection such as occurs in acquired immunodeficiency syndrome (**AIDS**), leading to malfunction of the immune system. Whether viral or other microbial infections are the direct cause of CIDP is not clear.

CIDP is different from Guillain-Barré syndrome in that the viral infection often does not occur within several months of the first appearance of the symptoms. In Guillain-Barré syndrome, a viral or bacterial infection typically immediately precedes the appearance of the symptoms.

CIDP typically begins with a tingling or prickling sensation, or numbness in the fingers and toes. This can spread to the arms and legs (an ascending pattern of spread). Both sides of the body can be affected; this is described as a symmetrical pattern. Other symptoms that can develop over time include the loss of reflexes in some tendons (a condition referred to as areflexia), extreme tiredness, and muscle ache. In some people, these symptoms develop slowly, reach a peak over several weeks or months, and then resolve themselves over time. However, for the majority of people with CIDP, the symptoms do not improve without treatment, and the symptoms can persist for many months to years.

Diagnosis

An important part of the diagnosis of CIDP is the detection of muscle weakness by a neurological examination. One relevant neurological test is nerve conduction velocity. In this test, a patch that is attached to the skin's surface over the target muscle is stimulated. A very mild electrical current stimulates the nerves in the muscle. A measurement called the nerve conduction velocity is then calculated as the time it takes for the impulses to travel the known distance between electrodes.

In demyelinating diseases such as CIDP, the nerves are not capable of transmitting electrical impulses as speedily as normal, myelinated nerves. Thus, the damaged nerves will display a greater conduction velocity than that displayed by an unaffected person.

Another test called **electromyography** (EMG) is used to measure muscle response to electrical stimulation. In EMG, an electrode contained within a needle is pushed through the skin into the muscle; several electrodes may need to be inserted throughout a muscle to accurately measure the muscle's behavior. Stimulation of a muscle causes a visual or audio pattern. The pattern of wavelengths carries information about the muscle's response. The characteristic pattern of wavelengths produced by a healthy muscle, which is called the action potential, can be compared to a muscle in someone suspected of having CIDP. For a nerve-damaged muscle, the action potential's wavelengths are smaller in height and less numerous than displayed by a normal muscle.

An electrocardiogram can be used to record the electrical activity of the heart when paralysis of the heart muscle is suspected. Nerve damage will alter the normal pattern of the heartbeat.

Finally, an examination of the cerebrospinal fluid by a lumbar puncture (also known as a spinal tap) may detect a higher than normal level of protein in the absence of an increase in the number of white blood cells (WBCs). An increase in WBCs occurs when there is a microbial infection.

Treatment team

CIDP treatment typically involves neurologists, immunologists, and physical therapists. Support groups are a useful adjunct to treatment.

Treatment

The treatments for CIDP and Guillain-Barré syndrome are similar. The use of corticosteroids such as prednisone, which lessen the response of the immune system, can reduce the amount of demyelination that occurs. Corticosteroids can be prescribed alone or in combination with other immunosupressant drugs.

The medical procedure known as plasmapheresis, or plasma exchange, can be another useful treatment. In plasmapheresis, the liquid portion of the blood that is known as plasma is removed from the body. The red blood cells are retrieved from the plasma and added back to the body with antibody-free plasma or intravenous fluid. Although plasmapheresis can lessen the symptoms of CIDP, it is not known exactly why plasmapheresis works. Because the blood plasma withdrawn from the body of a CIDP patient can contain antibodies to the nerve myelin sheath, the subsequent removal of these antibodies may lessen the effects of the body's immune attack on the nerve cells.

Another procedure that produces similar results involves the administration of intravenous immunoglobulin (IVIG). IVIG is a general all-purpose treatment for immune system-related neuropathies. As with plasmapheresis, immunoglobulin may help reduce the amount of anti-myelin antibodies, and so suppress the immune response. As well, IVIG contains healthy antibodies from the donated blood. These antibodies can help neutralize the defective antibodies that are causing the demyelination. When more standard approaches fail, alternative forms of immunosuppressive therapies are sometimes considered, including the drugs azathioprine, cyclophosphamide, and cyclosporine.

Physical therapy is helpful. Caregivers can move a patient's arms and legs to help improve the strength and flexibility of the muscles, and minimize the shrinkage of muscles and tendons that are not being actively used.

Recovery and rehabilitation

Recovery from CIDP varies from person to person. Some people recover completely without a great deal of medical intervention, while others may relapse again and again. Because some people can display permanent muscle weakness or numbness, physical therapy can be a useful part of a rehabilitation regimen.

Clinical trials

The National Institutes of Health (NIH) sponsored four **clinical trials** for the study and treatment of CIDP, all completed by 2001. The National Institute of Neurological Disorders and Stroke supports continued broad research for demyelinating diseases, although no further clinical trials are ongoing as of March 2004.

Prognosis

A patient's prognosis can range from complete recovery to a pattern of a periodic reappearance of the symptoms and residual muscle weakness or numbness.

Special concerns

The potential exists that IVIG will increase the risk of kidney damage in older or diabetic patients. Enoxaparin, a drug that can be prescribed to reduce the risk of blood clotting in patients with high blood pressure, can make a patient more prone to bleeding. This risk can be greater when enoxaparin is given at the same time as aspirin or anti-inflammatory drugs. The use of corticosteroids can restrict the efficiency of the immune system, which can increase the risk that other microorganisms will establish a secondary, or opportunistic, infection. Medical staff regularly monitor people receiving these treatments for signs of complication.

Resources

BOOKS

PERIODICALS

Comi, G., A. Quattrini, R. Fazio, and L. Roveri. "Immunoglobulins in Chronic Inflammatory Demyelinating Polyneuropathy." *Neurological Science* (October 2003): S246–S250.

Fee, D. B., and J. O. Flemming. "Resolution of Chronic Inflammatory Demyelinating Polyneuropathy-associated Central Nervous System Lesions after Treatment with Intravenous Immunoglobulin." *Journal of the Peripheral Nervous System* (September 2003): 155–158.

Katz, J. S., and D. S. Saperstein. "Chronic Inflammatory Demyelinating Polyneuropathy." *Current Treatment Options in Neurology* (September 2003): 357–364.

OTHER

NINDS Chronic Inflammatory Demyelinating Polyneuropathy (CIDP) Information Page. National Institute of Neurological Disorders and Stroke. December 22, 2003 (March 30, 2004). <http://www.ninds.nih.gov/health_and_medical/disorders/cidp.htm>.

ORGANIZATIONS

American Autoimmune Related Diseases Association. 22100 Gratiot Avenue, Eastpointe, MI 48201-2227. (586) 776-3900 or (800) 598-4668; Fax: (586) 776-3903. aarda@aol.com. <http://www.aarda.com>.

Guillain-Barre Syndrome Foundation International. P.O. Box 262, Wynnewood, PA 19096. (610) 667-0131; Fax: (610) 667-7036. info@gbsfi.com. <http://www.aarda.org>.

National Organization for Rare Disorders. P.O. Box 1968, Danbury, CT 06813-1968. (203) 744-0100. orphan@rarediseases.org. <http://www.rarediseases.org>.

Neuropathy Association. 60 East 42nd Street, New York, NY 10165-0999. (212) 692-0662 or (800) 247-6968; Fax: (212) 696-0668. info@neuropathy.org. <http://www.neuropathy.org>.

Brian Douglas Hoyle, PhD

Circle of Willis *see* **Cerebral circulation**

Clinical trials

Definition

A clinical trial is a carefully designed research study that is carried out with human volunteers. The trial is designed to answer specific questions concerning the effectiveness of a drug, treatment, or diagnostic method, or to improve patients' quality of life.

Description

Qualification for a clinical trial involves the selection of various desirable criteria (inclusion criteria), as well as criteria by which volunteers are rejected (exclusion criteria). Typical criteria include age, gender, the type and severity of the disease, prior treatment, and other medical conditions.

Depending on the clinical trial, the volunteers that are recruited could be healthy or ill with the disease under study. There are a number of different types of clinical trials that utilize differing types of study plans (protocols). A treatment trial evaluates a new treatment, new drug combinations, new surgical strategies, or innovative **radiation** therapy. A prevention trial seeks to find better ways to prevent disease from occurring or prevent disease from returning. Medicines, vaccines, vitamins, and lifestyle changes can all be candidates for a prevention trial. A diagnostic trial is designed to find better means of diagnosis for a particular disease or medical condition. A screening trial is designed to determine the best way to detect a particular disease or medical condition. Finally, a quality of life trial (supportive care trial) seeks to improve the comfort and daily life of people with a chronic illness.

Clinical trials, particularly treatment and prevention trials, often have several components, or phases. The following phases (I-IV) relate to the scope of the trial:

• Phase I trial evaluates the new drug or treatment in a small group of people (less than 100). Humans do not necessarily need to participate in such a trial. Experiments in the lab using microbiological cultures or tissue cells may suffice. The trial's purpose is to provide early indications of a drug or treatment's safety, safe dosage range, and reveal any side effects.

• Phase II trial follows a phase I trial. A promising drug or treatment is tested on a larger group of people (100–300) to better determine the effectiveness and to monitor safety more critically. Use of a larger population can help reveal side effects that could be hidden by the use of only a few volunteers.

• Phase III trial evaluates a drug or treatment that has proven effective in the phase I and II trials and is tested

Key Terms

Double blind study A study or clinical trial designed to minimize any bias, in that neither participant or study director knows who is assigned to the control group and who is assigned to the test group until the end of the study.

Exclusion criteria A predetermined set of factors that make a potential participant not eligible for inclusion in a clinical trial or study.

Inclusion criteria A predetermined set of factors that make a potential participant eligible for inclusion in a clinical trial or study.

Placebo A drug containing no active ingredients, such as a sugar pill, that may be used in clinical trials to compare the effects of a given treatment against no treatment.

on a large population (1,000–3,000) to confirm its effectiveness, reveal any rarer side effects, and gather information that will allow the drug or treatment to be safely marketed.

• Phase IV trial occurs after a product has been released in the marketplace. Monitoring of a drug or treatment in very large numbers of people provides further information on benefits and risks.

A typical clinical trial involves medical doctors and nurses, although **social workers** and other health care workers may also contribute. The members of the clinical team monitor the health of each volunteer at the outset and during the trial, give instructions, and often provide follow-up after the trial is completed. For a clinical trial volunteer, this means more visits to the health care facility than would normally occur, although compensation such as transportation expense is sometimes provided.

A critical part of a clinical trial is obtaining the consent of volunteers for their participation. It is mandatory that a trial's risks (i.e., side effects, little or no effect of treatment) and benefits (i.e., more proactive role in health care, access to new therapies, advance medical care) be clearly explained to participants. Once this is done, volunteers provide their informed consent by signing a document. This document is not legally binding, so volunteers are not obligated to complete the trial. An ethical clinical trial will never reveal the identities of the volunteers.

In addition to the drug being studied, clinical trials of new drugs will typically use a pill, liquid, or powder that looks the same as the active compound, but that has no medicinal value. This inactive compound, known as a

placebo, is usually given to the control group of volunteers, who are compared to the test group that receives the active drug. Usually the volunteers do not know whether they receive a placebo or the active drug. A clinical trial can be designed so that the researchers are also unaware of which people receive the active drug. When volunteers and researchers are both unaware, the trial is described as being double blind. Volunteers are often assigned to the control or test groups at random. This action is designed to minimize any bias due to age, gender, race, or other factors.

Resources

OTHER

"An Introduction to Clinical Trials." *ClinicalTrials.gov.* January 21, 2004 (March 30, 2004). <http://www.clinicaltrials.gov/ct/info/whatis)>.

ORGANIZATIONS

National Institutes of Health, Clinical Center. 6100 Executive Blvd., Suite 3C01MSC 7511, Bethesda, MD 20892-7511. (301) 496-2563 or (800) 411-1222; Fax: (301) 402-2984. occc@cc.nih.gov. <http://www.cc.nih.gov/home.cgi>.

Brian Douglas Hoyle, PhD

Cluster headache *see* **Headache**

Complex regional pain syndrome *see* **Reflex sympathetic dystrophy**

Congenital facial diplegia *see* **Moebius syndrome**

Congenital vascular cavernous malformation *see* **Cerebral cavernous malformation**

Congenital myasthenia

Definition

Congenital myasthenia is an inherited condition present at birth that interferes with nerve messages to the muscles. Although some symptoms are similar (muscle weakness worsened by use), congenital myasthenia differs from **myasthenia gravis**, which usually presents in adulthood and is almost always due to an autoimmune disorder rather than an inherited genetic defect.

Description

Most cases of congenital myasthenia are noticeable at or shortly after birth. In rare cases, symptoms don't present themselves until some time later in childhood or in early adult life.

Normal muscle function requires a chemical messenger called acetylcholine (ACh) to travel from the nerve cell to a receptor on the muscle endplate, in order to stimulate muscle contraction and movement. After the ACh has initiated muscle contraction, it is degraded by an enzyme.

In congenital myasthenia, one of three problems occurs with this system:

• Too little ACh is produced, or its release from the nerve cell is impaired

• The enzyme that should degrade ACh is faulty, resulting in prolonged stimulation of the muscle by excess ACh and ultimately in muscle damage

• The area of the muscle that should be stimulated by the presence of ACh (called the endplate receptor) is defective, and therefore the muscle can not be sufficiently stimulated

Demographics

Figures regarding the frequency of congenital myasthenia are not available, but it is considered to be a very rare condition.

Causes and symptoms

Most cases of congenital myasthenia are inherited in a recessive fashion, meaning that a baby has to receive a defective gene from each parent to actually manifest the condition.

Babies with congenital myasthenia are often described as "floppy," with weak muscle tone, droopy eyelids, excessive **fatigue**, compromised eye movements, facial weakness, feeding problems and delayed developmental milestones (such as holding up head, sitting, crawling). In more severe conditions, the muscles that aid breathing are affected, resulting in respiratory difficulties.

The baseline degree of weakness is exacerbated by any activity, including feeding, crying, or moving. Episodes of more severe symptoms may be precipitated by illness, emotional upset, or fever. Some cases of congenital myasthenia progress over time, so that initially mild symptoms can become more severe as the individual ages.

Diagnosis

The diagnosis of congenital myasthenia will usually be suspected when a careful physical examination reveals muscle weakness that is worsened by use of a particular muscle. Certainly, a family history of congenital myasthenia heightens such a suspicion.

A test called **electromyography** measures muscle activity after stimulation. When muscle activity decreases

with repeated stimulation, congenital myasthenia is suspected. Testing the blood for the presence of specific antibodies can help distinguish between myasthenia gravis and congenital myasthenia. Very specific microelectrode testing of the muscle endplate receptors can help define whether faulty receptors are responsible for the impairment. Genetic testing and muscle **biopsy** examination are being researched, but are not currently used for routine diagnosis.

Treatment team

Children with congenital myasthenia will usually be treated by a team consisting of a pediatric **neurologist**, as well as a physical therapist, occupational therapist, and speech and language therapist. If respiratory problems ensue, a pulmonologist and respiratory therapist may need to be consulted.

Treatment

There are no treatments available to cure congenital myasthenia. A number of medications may improve symptoms in children with congenital myasthenia. The specific medication that will be most helpful depends on whether the impairment is due to decreased ACh production and release, impaired enzyme degradation of ACh, or faulty ACh receptors in the muscle endplates. Some of the types of medications available include:

• Anticholinesterase medications: Inhibit the degradation of ACh, allowing more to be available to stimulate muscles.

• 3,4, diaminopyridine: Increases the release of ACh from the nerve cells.

• Qunidine or fluoxetine: Prevents overstimulation of ACh receptors on muscle endplates, thus preventing muscles from damage secondary to prolonged stimulation.

Prognosis

The severity of symptoms, responsiveness to medication, and ultimate prognosis varies widely among congenital myasthenia patients.

Resources
BOOKS

"Nutritional Disorders of the Neuromuscular Transmission and of Motor Neurons." In *Nelson Textbook of Pediatrics*, edited by Richard E. Behrman, et al. Philadelphia: W. B. Saunders Company, 2004.

Rose, Michael, and Robert C. Griggs. "Congenital Myasthenias." In *Textbook of Clinical Neurology*, edited by Christopher G. Goetz. Philadelphia: W. B. Saunders Company, 2003.

ORGANIZATIONS

Muscular Dystrophy Association. 3300 East Sunrise Drive, Tucson, AZ 85718. (800) 572-1717. mda@mdausa.org. <http://www.mdausa.org>.

Rosalyn Carson-DeWitt, MD

Congenital myopathies

Definition

Myopathies are diseases that cause weakness and **hypotonia** (poor tone) in the muscles that control voluntary movements. Congenital myopathies are a group of myopathies, usually present from birth, that display structural changes in the skeletal muscles. The list of diseases defined as congenital myopathies varies. Three inherited conditions in particular are definitively known as congenital myopathies: central core disease, nemaline **myopathy**, and centronuclear (myotubular) myopathy. These myopathies lead to generalized muscle weakness, decreased muscle tone, weak muscle reflexes, poor muscle bulk, and often a characteristic facial and bodily appearance.

Description

Central core disease

First described in 1956, central core disease (CCD) is named for the abnormalities found in the muscle biopsies of affected people. The central parts, or cores, of certain muscle cells lack structures called mitochondria, the energy-producing parts of the cells. CCD is a variable disorder with onset in early infancy to childhood. Hip displacement is not uncommon. Some children with CCD show mildly delayed motor milestones and appear only slightly uncoordinated. Others have more significant delays, though they eventually walk and move about with some limitation. Some children use braces for walking, and a few use wheelchairs.

Nemaline myopathy

Also known as rod myopathy or rod body disease, nemaline myopathy (NM) was first described in two separate reports in 1963. NM is named for the thread-like structures known as nemaline bodies that are visible on muscle **biopsy**. The term "nemaline" comes from the Greek word *nema* meaning "thread." The main features of NM are muscle weakness, loss of muscle tone, and absent or weak deep tendon reflexes (for example, knee and ankle jerks). Based on the age of onset and severity of symptoms, NM has been classified into six forms: neonatal (severe congenital), Amish nemaline myopathy (a congenital form),

Key Terms

Congenital   Present at birth.

Fetal   Refers to the fetus. In humans, the fetal period extends from the end of the eighth week of pregnancy to birth.

Gene   A building block of inheritance, which contains the instructions for the production of a particular protein, and is made up of a molecular sequence found on a section of DNA. Each gene is found on a precise location on a chromosome.

Nerve conduction   The speed and strength of a signal being transmitted by nerve cells. Testing these factors can reveal the nature of nerve injury, such as damage to nerve cells or to the protective myelin sheath.

Serum   The fluid part of the blood that remains after blood cells, platelets, and fibrogen have been removed. Also called blood serum.

intermediate congenital form, typical congenital form, childhood-onset form, and adult-onset form. Most cases (over 80%) are one of the congenital forms. All six forms of NM are unified by the presence of nemaline rods, abnormal structures that are found in the sarcoplasm of the muscles.

Centronuclear (myotubular) myopathy

Centronucler myopathy, also known as myotubular myopathy (MTM), is an extremely variable condition characterized by a poor muscle tone and weakness. The centronuclear myopathies are called "myotubular myopathies" due to the presence of myotubes, immature muscle cells found in affected individuals. Myotubes have nuclei (structures that contain the chromosomes) that are central rather than peripheral (at the edge). Mature muscle cells have peripheral nuclei. Although MTM can lead to death in infancy, it can be a mildly progressive condition that begins as late as early adulthood. There are X-linked, autosomal dominant and autosomal recessive forms of the disorder. The X-linked form, also known as X-linked myotubular myopathy or XLMTM, is thought to be the most common form of the condition and typically is the most severe form of MTM.

Demographics

Although central core disease is thought to be rare, the incidence of this congenital myopathy remains unknown. Both males and females are affected. Due to the range of severity observed in CCD, it is possible that there are undiagnosed cases within CCD families and within the general population. The X-linked form of centronuclear myopathy affects approximately 1/50,000 newborn males. The autosomal recessive and autosomal dominant forms are apparently less common; however, the frequency of these forms remains unknown. Nemaline myopathy occurs in about 1/50,000 live births.

Causes and symptoms

Causes

CENTRAL CORE DISEASE Central core disease is inherited in an dominant manner, due to a mutation in one copy of the RYR1 (ryanodine receptor) gene on the long arm of chromosome 19. Researchers think that mutations in this receptor affect the way calcium flows out of the sarcoplasmic reticulum, a functional unit in the muscle. Mutations in the RYR1 gene are also known to cause malignant hyperthermia (MH), a genetic predisposition that makes an individual prone to serious reactions to certain general anesthetics. In fact, MH is a feature of CCD. An individual with CCD has a 50% chance of passing the disorder on to each child. There are also occurrences of sporadic inheritance, which means that a gene alters spontaneously to cause the disorder in a person with no family history of the disease.

NEMALINE ROD MYOPATHY Nemaline myopathy is caused by alterations in genes that affect filament proteins. When the filament proteins aren't working, muscles can't contract and there is a subsequent loss of tone and strength. Nemaline myopathy can be inherited as an autosomal dominant or an autosomal recessive condition. Autosomal dominant inheritance implies that the affected person has one altered or non-functioning copy and one normal copy of a particular NM gene. The changed gene may occur for the first time in that individual (*de novo*) or may be inherited from a parent (familial). When NM occurs as an autosomal recessive condition, the affected individual has two altered or non-functioning NM genes, one from each parent. As of March 2004, there were five genes known to cause NM abbreviated as ACT1, NEB, TNNT1, TMP2, and TMP3; each gene codes for protein components of thin filament, a type of muscle fiber.

MYOTUBULAR MYOPATHY The MTM1 gene on the long arm of the X chromosome encodes myotubularin, a protein thought to promote normal muscle development. As of 2004, the precise mechanisms by which MTM1 mutations cause XLMTM were unresolved. X-linked MTM primarily affects males because they have only one X chromosome and therefore lack a second, normal copy of the gene responsible for the condition. Female carriers of the X-linked MTM have one X chromosome with a normal MTM1 gene and one X chromosome with a non-working MTM1 gene. As of March 2004, researchers were working to identify the gene or genes responsible for the autosomal recessive form of centronuclear myopathy. One gene, the myogenic factor-6 gene (MYF6) has been shown to cause some cases of the autosomal dominant form. It is possible that other genes will be discovered in the future.

Symptoms

CENTRAL CORE DISEASE Central core disease is characterized by a mild, non-progressive muscle weakness. Signs of central core disease usually appear in infancy or early childhood and may present even earlier. There may be decreased fetal movements and breech (feet first) presentation *in utero*. The main features of CCD are poor muscle tone (hypotonia), muscle weakness, and skeletal problems including congenital hip dislocation, scoliosis (curvature of the spine), *pes cavus* (high-arched feet), and clubbed feet. Children with CCD experience delays in reaching motor milestones and tend to sit and walk much later than those without the disorder. A child with the disease usually cannot run easily, and may find that jumping and other physical activities are often impossible. Although central core disease may be disabling, it usually does not affect intelligence or life expectancy.

People who have central core disease are sometimes vulnerable to **malignant hyperthermia** (MH), a condition triggered by anesthesia during surgery. MH causes a rapid, and sometimes fatal, rise in body temperature, producing muscle stiffness.

NEMALINE MYOPATHY There is variability in age of onset, presence of symptoms, and severity of symptoms in nemaline myopathy. Most commonly, NM presents in infancy or early childhood with weakness and poor muscle tone. In some cases there may have been pregnancy complications such as polyhydramnios (excess amniotic fluid) and decreased fetal movements. Affected children with NM tend to have delays in motor milestones such as rolling over, sitting and walking. Muscle weakness commonly occurs in the face, neck and upper limbs. Over time, a characteristic myopathic face (a long face that lacks expression) develops. Skeletal problems including chest deformities, scoliosis, and foot deformities may develop. In the most severe cases of NM, feeding difficulties and potentially fatal respiratory problems may also occur. In those who survive the first two years of life, muscle weakness tends to progress slowly or not at all.

CENTRONUCLEAR MYOPATHY Typically the X-linked form of MTM (XLMTM) is the most severe of the three forms (X-linked, autosomal recessive, and autosomal dominant). XLMTM usually presents as a newborn male with poor muscle tone and respiratory distress. The pregnancy may have been complicated by polyhydramnios and decreased fetal movements. Of those who survive the newborn period, many will at least partially depend on a ventilator for breathing. Because of the risk of aspiration, many will also have a gastrostomy tube (G-tube). Boys with XLMTM can experience significant delays in achieving motor milestones and may not ever walk independently. They tend to be tall with a characteristic facial appearance (long, narrow face with a highly arched roof of the mouth and crowded teeth). Intelligence is generally not affected. Medical complications that may develop include: scoliosis, eye problems (eye muscle paralysis and droopy eyelids), and dental malocclusion (severe crowding). In X-linked MTM, other problems including undescended testicles, spherocytosis, peliosis, elevated liver enzymes, and gallstones may occur.

The autosomal recessive and autosomal dominant forms of MTM tend to have a milder course than the X-linked form. The autosomal recessive form can present in infancy, childhood, or early adulthood. Common features include generalized muscle weakness with or without facial weakness and ophthalmoplegia (paralysis of the eye muscles). Although feeding and breathing problems can occur, affected individuals usually survive infancy. Onset of the autosomal dominant form ranges from late childhood through early adulthood. It tends to be the mildest of the three forms of MTM. Unlike the X-linked form of the condition, problems with other organs (such as the liver, kidneys, and gall bladder) haven't been reported with the autosomal recessive and autosomal dominant forms of MTM.

Diagnosis

Diagnosis of a congenital myopathy generally includes evaluation of the patient's personal and family history, physical and neurological examinations that test reflexes and strength, and specialized tests. Since there is overlap between the symptoms of a congenital myopathy and other neuromuscular disorders, a number of tests may be performed to help narrow down the diagnosis. Serum CK (creatinine kinase) analysis, EMG (electromyelogram), nerve conduction studies, and muscle ultrasound tend to be of limited value in making this diagnosis. The definitive diagnosis of a congenital myopathy usually relies upon genetic testing and/or muscle biopsy. Also, muscle biopsy can be used to determine a patient's susceptibility to malignant hyperthermia.

Central core disease

The muscle biopsy from a person with CCD typically displays a metabolically inactive "core" or central region that appears blank when stained (tested) for certain metabolic enzymes (proteins) that should be there. These central regions also lack mitochondria, the energy producing "factories" of the cells. Genetic testing for RYR1 mutations is available on a research basis. The same genetic test may be used to determine the presence of the gene change

in family members who may have or be at-risk for the disease. For families in which a RYR1 mutation has been found, prenatal diagnosis may be possible using the DNA of fetal cells obtained from chorionic villus sampling (CVS) or amniocentesis.

Nemaline myopathy

The clinical diagnosis of NM is suspected in an infant under age one with muscle weakness and hypotonia (decreased muscle tone). Definitive diagnosis of nemaline myopathy is made by demonstration of nemaline bodies, rod-shaped structures characteristic of this disease, using a specific stain known as "Gomori trichrome" on a muscle biopsy sample. Muscle biopsy may also show predominance of structures known as type I fibers. As of 2004, genetic testing was available on a clinical basis for one gene, the ACTA1 gene located on the long arm of chromosome 1. About 15% of NM cases are due to mutations in this gene. Prenatal diagnosis is possible for families with known ACTA1 mutations. The DNA of a fetus can be tested using cells obtained from chorionic villus sampling (CVS) or amniocentesis.

Centronuclear (myotubular) myopathy

Diagnosis of X-linked MTM is usually made on muscle biopsy. Findings include: centrally located nuclei in muscle fibers that look like myotubules, absence of structures known as myofibrils, and possibly, persistence of certain proteins usually seen in fetal muscle cells. If timing is not an issue, genetic testing may be undertaken. Gene testing detects a mutation (disease-causing gene change) in up to 97-98% of people with the X-linked form. Though genetic testing is available, it tends to be time intensive and used to confirm a diagnosis, to screen potential carriers, or for prenatal testing.

Treatment team

Management of a congenital myopathy requires a multidisciplinary approach. In addition to the patient's primary health care professionals, medical professionals involved in the care of patients with may include specialists in neurology, neonatology, pulmonology, gastroenterology, orthopedics, ophthalmology, and orthodontistry. Additional specialists in physical therapy, speech therapy and occupational therapy may be needed. Patients with one of the congenital myopathies may receive comprehensive services through a **muscular dystrophy** association (MDA) clinic and/or a Shriner's Hospital for Children. Genetic evaluation and counseling may be helpful to the patient and family, especially at the time of diagnosis. Psychological counseling and support groups may also assist families in coping with this condition.

Treatment

As of 2004, there is no cure for the congenital myopathies. The purpose of treatment, which is largely supportive, is to help patients optimize function and to manage any medical complications associated with the disorder. Treatment measures for the congenital myopathies greatly depend on the severity of the individual's symptoms, and especially upon the degree of muscle weakness and presence of skeletal deformities. Treatment mainly consists of respiratory and feeding support, and orthopedic intervention. Ophthalmologic and dental care is also important to help manage problems that may arise such as dry eyes and dental crowding. In the case of X-linked MTM, management of associated complications including undescended testicles, spherocytosis, peliosis, elevated liver enzymes, and gallstones is also recommended.

Affected infants, especially those with X-linked myotubular myopathy or nemaline myopathy, usually require a feeding tube (a gastrostomy or G-tube) for nutrition and mechanical ventilation through a tracheostomy to help with breathing. Other means of ventilation such as BiPAP (bilevel positive airway pressure) may be used. Even children and adults who don't require help with daytime breathing may require respiratory support at night, since respiratory failure during sleep can occur.

Braces or surgery may be necessary to treat scoliosis, dislocated hips, and foot deformities. Since individuals with central core disease can develop malignant hyperthermia during surgery, they should consult a **neurologist** or anesthesiologist prior to these or other surgeries.

Recovery and rehabilitation

Given the rarity of the congenital myopathies, the potential for rehabilitation in these disorders is largely unknown. Speech, physical, and occupational therapies may be recommended. Though intellect is typically normal, educational support through early intervention services and/or through an individualized education plan (IEP) may also be appropriate for some children. In severe cases, consideration may be given to placement in a residential care facility that can provide 24-hour care and support services.

The goal of rehabilitation for the congenital myopathies is to maintain or improve the patient's existing functions. Physical therapy may be recommended to improve mobility and muscle strength. For example, people with central core disease can benefit from **exercise**, under the direction of a physician. Speech therapy can help a person with a congenital myopathy to learn speech and/or ways to communicate. For example, a boy with X-linked myotubular myopathy who has a tracheostomy may need help learning how to communicate with sign language and, later, with writing boards. Occupational therapy can teach patients to use adaptive techniques and devices that may help compensate for muscle weakness. For example, someone with a severe form of nemaline myopathy may benefit from a walker, wheelchair or other device in order to get around.

Clinical trials

As of March 2004, one clinical trial was recruiting patients with congenital myopathy. A study designed to learn more about the natural history of inherited neurological disorders and the role of heredity in their development will be conducted in the United States. Updated information on this trial can be found at <http://www.clinicaltrials.gov> or by contacting the patient recruitment and public liaison office of the National Institute of Neurological Disorders and Stroke (NINDS) at 1-800-411-1222 or <prpl@mail.cc.nih.gov>.

Prognosis

The outlook for children with central core disease is generally positive. Although they begin life with some developmental delays, many improve as they get older and stay active throughout their lives. The outcome for patients with nemaline rod myopathy is quite variable. Depending upon disease severity, affected individuals can have normal life span, despite progressive muscle weakness, or they can die in infancy due to respiratory problems. Severe neonatal respiratory disease and the presence of arthrogryposis (limited joint movement due to contracted muscles and tendons) generally predict a poor outcome with death by age one. The prognosis for myotubular myopathy varies according to the presence and severity of respiratory disease and scoliosis. X-linked myotubular myopathy was once described as fatal in the first few months of life. Yet, it is now known that support of feeding (G-tube) and ventilation (tracheostomy) can significantly improve life expectancy and quality of life.

Special concerns

Malignant hyperthermia, a problem seen in some individuals with central core disease is a severe and potentially life-threatening complication of anesthesia. People with central core disease or a family history of the disease should consult their doctors about anesthesia risks. Also, wearing a medical alert bracelet may be advised.

Individuals with even mild cases of myotubular myopathy can experience potentially serious breathing problems such as **hypoxia** (lack of oxygen) during sleep. It is crucial that even patients with minimal disease severity be monitored for respiratory problems as they may require help with breathing at night.

Resources

BOOKS

Wallgren-Pettersson, Carina A., and Angus Clarke. "Congenital Myopathies." In *Principles and Practice of Medical Genetics.* 4th ed., edited by David Rimoin, MD, PhD, Michael Connor, Reed E. Pyeritz, MD, PhD, and Bruce Korf, MD, PhD, 4th ed. New York: Churchill Livingstone, 2002.

"Muscle Diseases." In *Textbook of Primary Care Medicine.* 3rd ed. edited by John Noble, MD, Harry Greene, II, MD, Wendy Levinson, MD, Geoffrey A. Modest, MD, Cynthia D. Mulrow, MD, Joseph Scherger, MD; and Mark J. Young, MD. St. Louis, MO: Mosby, 2000.

PERIODICALS

Bruno, C., and C. Minetti. "Congenital myopathies." *Current Neurol Neurosci Rep* 4 (January 2004): 68–73.

Jungbluth, H., C. A. Sewry, and F. Muntoni. "What's new in neuromuscular disorders? The congenital myopathies." *European Journal of Paediatric Neurology* 7 (2003): 23–30.

Prasad, A. N., and C. Prasad. "The floppy infant: contribution of genetic and metabolic disorders." *Brain Dev* 25 (October 2003): 457–76.

Quinllivan, R. M., C. R. Muller, M. Davis, N. G. Laing, G. A. Evans, J. Dwyer, J. Dove, A. P. Roberts, and C. A. Sewry. "Central core disease: clinical, pathological, and genetic features." *Archives of Disease in Childhood* 88 (December 2003): 68–1051–1055.

Sanoudou, D., and A. Beggs. "Clinical and genetic heterogeneity in nemaline myopathy—a disease of skeletal muscle thin filaments." *Trends in Molecular Medicine* 7 (August 2001): 362–368.

WEBSITES

Muscular Dystrophy Association (MDA). *Central Core Disease Page.* <http://www.mdausa.org/disease/ccd.html>.

Muscular Dystrophy Association (MDA). *Nemaline Myopathy Page.* <http://www.mdausa.org/disease/nm.html>.

Muscular Dystrophy Association (MDA). *Myotubular Myopathy Page.* <http://www.mdausa.org/disease/mm.html>.

National Institute of Neurological Disorders and Stroke (NINDS). *Congenital Myopathies Information Page.* <http://www.ninds.nih.gov/health_and_medical/disorders/myopathy_congenital.htm>.

ORGANIZATIONS

Muscular Dystrophy Association, 3300 East Sunrise Drive, Tucson, AZ 85718. (520) 529-2000 or (800) 572-1717; Fax: (520) 529-5300. mda@mdausa.org. <http://www.mdausa.org>.

Myotubular Myopathy Resource Group. 2602 Quaker Drive, Texas City, TX 77590. (409) 945-8569. info@mtmrg.org. <http://www.mtmrg.org>.

Nemaline Myopathy Foundation. P. O. Box 5937, Round Rock, TX 78683-5937. <http://www.davidmcd.btinternet.co.uk>.

Dawn J. Cardeiro, MS, CGC

Conjugate eye movements *see* **Visual disturbances; Traumatic brain injury**

Corpus callosotomy

Definition

Corpus callosotomy is a treatment for **epilepsy**, in which a group of fibers connecting the two sides of the brain, called the corpus callosum, is cut.

Purpose

Corpus callosotomy is used to treat epilepsy that is unresponsive to drug treatments. A person with epilepsy may be considered good candidate for one type of epilepsy surgery or another if he or she has **seizures** that are not adequately controlled by drug therapy, and has tried at least two (perhaps more, depending on the treatment center's guidelines) different anti-epileptic drugs.

The seizures of epilepsy are due to unregulated spreading of electrical activity from one part of the brain to other parts. In many people with epilepsy, this activity begins from a well-defined focal point, which can be identified by electrical testing. Surgical treatment of focal-origin seizures involves removal of the brain region containing the focal point, usually in a procedure called temporal lobectomy. In other people, no focal point is found, or there may be too many to remove individually. These patients are most likely to receive corpus callosotomy.

The purpose of a corpus callosotomy is to prevent spreading of seizure activity from one half of the brain to the other. The brain is divided into two halves, or hemispheres, that are connected by a thick bundle of nerve fibers, the corpus callosum. When these fibers are cut, a seizure that begins in one hemisphere is less likely to spread to the other. This can reduce the frequency of seizures significantly.

The initial surgery may cut the forward two-thirds of the corpus callosum, leaving the rest intact. If this does not provide sufficient seizure control, the remaining portion may be cut.

Corpus callosotomy is most often performed for children with "drop attacks," or atonic seizures, in which a sudden loss of muscle tone causes the child to fall to the floor. It is also performed in people with uncontrolled generalized tonic-clonic, or grand mal, seizures, or with massive jerking movements. Of the 20,000 to 70,000 people in the United States considered candidates for any type of epilepsy surgery, approximately 5,000 receive surgery per year. Between 1985 and 1990, more than 800 corpus callosotomies were performed, and the number has increased since then. Corpus callosotomy is performed by a special neurosurgical team, at a regional epilepsy treatment center.

Description

During corpus callosotomy, the patient is under general anesthesia, lying on the back. The head is fixed in place with blunt pins attached to a rigid structure. The head is shaved either before or during the procedure.

Incisions are made in the top of the skull to remove a flap of bone, exposing the brain. The outer covering is cut, and the two hemispheres are pulled slightly apart to expose the corpus callosum. The fibers of the corpus callosum are cut, taking care to avoid nearby arteries and ventricles (fluid-filled cavities in the brain).

Once the cut is made and any bleeding is controlled, the brain covering, bone, and scalp are closed and stitched.

Preparation

The candidate for any type of epilepsy surgery will have had a wide range of tests prior to surgery. These include **electroencephalography** (EEG), in which electrodes are placed on the scalp, on the brain surface, or within the brain to record electrical activity. EEG is used to attempt to locate the focal point(s) of the seizure activity.

Several neuroimaging procedures are used to obtain images of the brain. These may reveal structural abnormalities that the neurosurgeon must be aware of. These procedures may include **magnetic resonance imaging (MRI)**, x rays, computed tomography (**CT**) **scans**, or **positron emission tomography (PET)** imaging.

Neuropsychological tests may be done to provide a baseline against which the results of the surgery are measured. A Wada test may also be performed. In this test, a drug is injected into the artery leading to one half of the brain, putting it to sleep, allowing the **neurologist** to determine where language and other functions in the brain are localized, which may be useful for predicting the result of the surgery.

Aftercare

The patient remains in the hospital for about a week, possibly more depending on any complications that have occurred during surgery and on the health of the patient. There may be some discomfort afterwards. Tylenol with codeine may be prescribed for **pain**. Bending over should be avoided if possible, as it may lead to **headache** in the week or so after the procedure. Ice packs may be useful for pain and itchiness of the sutures on the head. Another several weeks of convalescence at home are required before the patient can resume normal activities. Heavy lifting or straining may continue to cause headaches or nausea, and should be avoided until the doctor approves. A diet rich in fiber can help avoid constipation, which may occur following surgery. Patients remain on anti-seizure medication at least for the short term, and may continue to require medication.

Risks

There is a slight risk of infection or hemorrhage from the surgery, usually less than 1%. Disconnection of the two hemispheres of the brain can cause some neuropsychological impairments such as decreased spontaneity of speech (it may be difficult to bring the right words into one's mind) and decreased use of the non-dominant hand. These problems usually improve over time. Complete cutting of the corpus callosotomy produces more long-lasting, but very subtle deficits in connecting words with images. These are usually not significant, or even noticed, by the patient.

Serious morbidity or mortality occurs in 1% or less of patients. Combined major and minor complication rates are approximately 20%.

Normal results

Patients typically experience a marked reduction in number and severity of seizures, with a small percentage of people becoming seizure free. Drop attacks may be eliminated completely in approximately 70% of patients. Other types of seizure are also reduced by 50% or more from corpus callosotomy surgery.

Resources

BOOKS

Devinsky, O. *A Guide to Understanding and Living with Epilepsy*. Philadelphia: EA Davis, 1994.

ORGANIZATIONS

Epilepsy Foundation. <www.epilepsyfoundation.org>.

Richard Robinson
Rosalyn Carson-DeWitt, MD

▌Corticobasal degeneration

Definition

Corticobasal degeneration (CBD) is a rare, progressive, neurodegenerative disease that causes **movement disorders** and **dementia**.

Description

CBD occurs when brain cells in two areas of the brain—the cortex and the basal ganglia—die off. The cause of this neurodegeneration is unknown. CBD is also called cortical basal degeneration and corticobasal ganglionic degeneration.

Demographics

It is not known exactly how many people have CBD. In the United States, the number is probably fewer than 10,000. Men and women are equally affected. Symptoms usually appear when a person is 50 or 60 years old.

Causes and symptoms

The ultimate cause of CBD is unknown. No genes have been found to be responsible, and no environmental or other risk factors have been identified. The brain areas affected are the cerebral cortex and the basal ganglia. The cerebral cortex is the center of mental activities such as planning, memory, language, and reasoning. The basal ganglia help control movements.

The symptoms of CBD may begin with either movement disorders or cognitive disorders. The movement disorders seen in CBD are similar to those in **Parkinson's disease** (PD), and CBD is often initially misdiagnosed as PD. In CBD, movements become slow and stiff, and may be accompanied by sustained abnormal postures (**dystonia**) or sudden violent jerks (**myoclonus**). Cognitive symptoms include memory impairment, loss of judgment, and difficulty planning or executing movements. Additional features may include impaired speech, and the "alien hand" phenomenon, in which the patient feels disconnected from, and not in control of, a hand or limb. Loss of sensation may also occur.

Diagnosis

Corticobasal degeneration is diagnosed with a neurological exam (testing of reflexes, coordination, sensation, etc.) and neuroimaging studies, including computed tomography (CT) scan and **magnetic resonance imaging (MRI)** to detect characteristic loss of brain tissue. **Neuropsychological testing** is also usually done to determine the kind and degree of cognitive impairment.

Treatment team

The treatment team includes a **neurologist, neuropsychologist**, speech/language pathologist, geriatric medicine specialist, and possibly a physical or occupational therapist.

Treatment

There are no treatments that can slow or reverse the course of CBD. Some symptoms can be lessened with drugs, although these are inconsistently effective and become less effective as time passes.

Key Terms

Basal ganglia   Brain structure at the base of the cerebral hemispheres involved in controlling movement.

Neurodegenerative   Relating to degeneration of nerve tissues.

Drugs used against PD are often prescribed, although they are rarely as effective in CBD. These drugs include levodopa and dopamine agonists, as well as **anticholinergics** such as trihexyphenidyl. Drugs used for Alzheimer's disease may also be tried for the cognitive symptoms.

A speech/language pathologist can help the patient with swallowing difficulties, although over time this problem will become worse and the patient may require the use of a feeding tube. The same specialist can advise about the use of assistive communication devices to improve communication as the ability to speak is lost.

Prognosis

Ability to move without a wheelchair is usually lost within five years of diagnosis. Within 10 years, swallowing difficulties often put the patient at risk for developing aspiration pneumonia, or lung infection from food in the airways. Death from pneumonia is common in CBD.

Resources

WEBSITES

WE MOVE. (April 19, 2004.) <http://www.wemove.org>.
National Institute of Neurological Disorders and Stroke (NINDS). *Corticobasal Degeneration Information Page.* (April 19, 2004). <http://www.ninds.nih.gov/health_and_medical/disorders/cortico_doc.htm>.

Richard Robinson

Cranial arteritis *see* **Temporal arteritis**

Craniosynostosis

Definition

Craniosynostosis is a defect in which one or more of the flexible and fibrous joints (cranial sutures) between the skull bones closes too soon; it occurs before birth or within a few months after birth. The skull cannot expand normally with growth of the brain, and so assumes an abnormal shape. Craniosynostosis can occur alone or as part of a syndrome of craniofacial defects.

Key Terms

Cranial sutures The fibrous joints (sutures) that hold together the five bones comprising the skull of a newborn.

Description

The skull of a newborn is composed of five bones that are held together by the fibrous sutures positioned at the front, top, sides, and back of the skull. By remaining open, the sutures allow the skull to normally expand in all directions as the brain is growing.

The premature closing of one or more of these cranial sutures stops the normal capacity of the skull to expand in early childhood. As not all of the cranial sutures will close, the skull expands in the areas that are still flexible. This results in an abnormally shaped skull or face. The forehead may be very pronounced and inclined forward. Viewed from above, the skull may be more rectangular in shape rather than oval.

Other forms of craniosynostosis include coronal craniosynostosis (affecting the coronal suture that crosses the top of the skull from temple to temple), metopic craniosynostosis (affecting the metopic suture of the forehead), sagittal craniosynostosis (affecting the sagittal suture that unites the two parietal bones), and lambdoidal craniosynostosis (affecting the lambdoid suture between the occipital and parietal bones of the skull).

Demographics

Craniosynostosis is a rare occurrence. The sagittal form of the disorder, in which the sagittal suture closes prematurely, is the most common form of craniosynostosis, occurring in three to five of every 1,000 babies, typically males. The frequencies of the various types of craniosynostosis are 50–60% sagittal, 20–30% coronal, 4–10% metopic, and 2–4% lambdoid.

Causes and symptoms

Craniosynostosis is usually caused by a genetic mutation. Mutations in several genes (designated TWIST, FGFR-1, FGFR-2, and FGFR-3) have been linked with craniosynostosis. In particular, the protein encoded for by TWIST is critical in the initiation and maintenance of the cranial suture process. As of 2004, the favored hypothesis is that the protein that normally functions to ensure that the formation of the cranial sutures occurs at the right time in development somehow goes awry and causes premature fusion of the bones of the brain.

Research published in 2003 in the *Annals of the Royal College of Surgeons of England* identified Saethre-Chotzen syndrome (a rare disorder characterized by an exaggerated forehead and drooping eyelids) as a genetic disorder that produces craniosynostosis.

Craniosynostosis can also be caused by maladies that affect the metabolism (rickets, vitamin D deficiency, overactive thyroid) and by bone marrow disorders. Furthermore, some cases have been associated with an abnormally small head (**microcephaly**) and the accumulation of cerebrospinal fluid in the brain (**hydrocephalus**).

Involvement of the different sutures produces different effects. Closure of the sagittal suture (located at the top of the skull and to the rear) produces an elongated head, prominent and protruding forehead, and narrow temples. Closure of the coronal suture (located on the side of the skull) produces a flattened forehead, higher-than-normal eye socket, abnormal nose, and a skull that slants from side to side. Closure of the metopic suture (which runs down the front-middle portion of the skull) results in a pointed-shaped forehead, triangular-shaped skull, closer-than-normal eyes, and a protruding rear portion of the skull. Finally, closure of the lambdoidal suture (located at the back of the skull) produces a mild flattening of the back of the head, forward-shifted ears, and the coronal symptoms.

Diagnosis

Diagnosis is made on the basis of a physical examination.

Treatment team

Treatment involves medical specialists (pediatric neurosurgeons, pediatric plastic surgeons, craniofacial surgeons) and specialized nurses.

Treatment

Surgery is the common treatment for craniosynostosis. The traditional surgeries involve the exposure of the skull, physical breakage of the fused suture region, and the restoration of the scalp. These surgeries all carry the risks associated with surgery in the brain region. Also, the surgeries produce much bleeding (sometimes a blood transfusion is necessary) and leave a large scar, and transient swelling and bruising can occur.

A new surgical technique called endoscopic strip craniectomy has been pioneered by two pediatric surgeons from the University of Missouri Health Care Center. This surgery is much less invasive, produces only a relatively small scar, and leaves little physical after effects

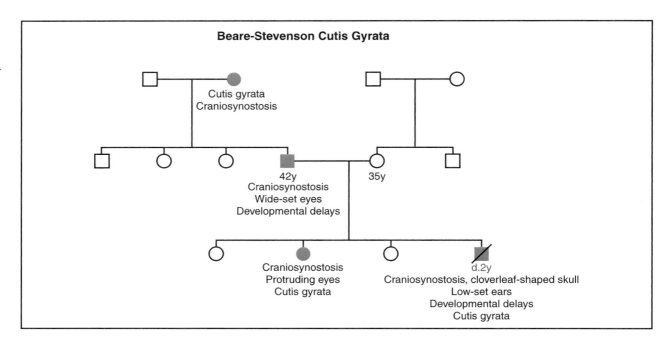

Beare-Stevenson Cutis Gyrata

Cutis gyrata
Craniosynostosis

42y
Craniosynostosis
Wide-set eyes
Developmental delays

35y

Craniosynostosis
Protruding eyes
Cutis gyrata

d.2y
Craniosynostosis, cloverleaf-shaped skull
Low-set ears
Developmental delays
Cutis gyrata

See Symbol Guide for Pedigree Charts. *(Gale Group.)*

such as swelling and bruising. In the procedure, an endoscope is used to remove the closed suture through incisions that are only several inches in length. In the more than 100 surgeries performed as of January 2001, most of the infants were in a condition satisfactory enough to leave the hospital the following day. Endoscopic strip craniectomy can only be done on infants under six months of age. After the surgery, the baby wears a protective helmet for several months, which molds the growing head into the correct shape.

Recovery and rehabilitation

Regardless of the type of surgery performed to correct the defects associated with craniosynostosis, the child will be restricted from vigorous activity or rough play while healing. The protective helmet is required for children after endoscopic strip craniectomy, while permanent plates inserted during other corrective surgeries eliminate the need for the helmet. Children who have had surgery to repair craniosynostosis will continue to need periodic examination by the surgeon until approximately age 18, when the skull has grown to its adult size and shape.

Clinical trials

The National Institute for Neurological Diseases and Stroke directly undertakes and funds a range of studies examining the mechanisms of early neurological development. However, there are no **clinical trials** scheduled to study craniosynostosis as of January 2004.

Prognosis

The outlook for a complete recovery for a child with craniosynostosis depends on whether just one suture is involved or whether multiple sutures have closed. Also, the presence of other abnormalities can lessen the confidence of a satisfactory outcome. Without surgical intervention, craniosynostosis can lead to increased brain pressure, delayed mental development, **mental retardation, seizures**, or blindness. After surgery is accomplished, the prognosis is excellent.

Resources

PERIODICALS

Johnson, D. "A Comprehensive Screen of Genes Implicated in Craniosynostosis." *Annals of the Royal College of Surgeons of England* (November 2003): 371–377.

OTHER

Sheth, R.D. "Craniosynostosis." *eMedicine.* January 22, 2004 (March 30, 2004). <http://www.emedicine.com/neuro/topic80.htm>.

National Institute of Neurological Disorders and Stroke. *Craniosynostosis Information Page.* January 22, 2004 (March 30, 2004). <http://www.ninds.nih.gov/health_and_medical/disorders/craniosytosis_doc.htm>.

University of Missouri Health Care. "Craniosynostosis: A New and Better Treatment." *MU Health.* January 19, 2004 (March 30, 2004). <http://www.muhealth.org/~neuromedicine/craniosynostosis.shtml>.

ORGANIZATIONS

March of Dimes Birth Defects Foundation. 1275 Mamaroneck Avenue, White Plains, NY 10605. (914) 428-7100 or

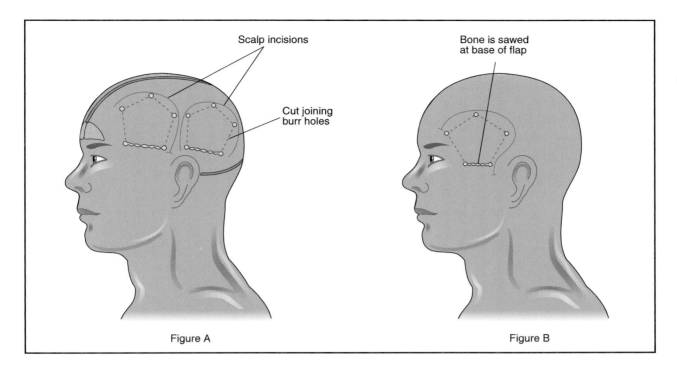

Scalp incisions

Cut joining
burr holes

Bone is sawed
at base of flap

Figure A

Figure B

In a craniotomy, the skin over a part of the skull is cut and pulled back. Small holes are drilled into the skull, and a special saw is used to cut the bone between the holes. The bone is removed, and a tumor or other defect is visualized and repaired. The bone is then replaced and the skin closed. *(Illustration by Electronic Illustrators Group.)*

(888) 663-4637; Fax: (914) 428-8203. askus@ marchofdimes.com. <http://www.marchofdimes.com>.

National Organization for Rare Disorders. 55 Kenosia Avenue, Danbury, CT 06813-1968. (203) 744-0100 or (800) 999-6673; Fax: (203) 798-2291. orphan@rarediseases.org. <http://www.rarediseases.org>.

World Craniofacial Foundation. 7777 Forest Lane, Suite C-621, Dallas, TX 75251-5838. (972) 566-6669 or (800) 533-3315; Fax: (972) 566-3850. worldcf@worldnet. att.net. <http://www.worldcf.org/cran_3c5.html>.

Brian Douglas Hoyle, PhD

Craniotomy

Definition

A craniotomy is a procedure to remove a lesion in the brain through an opening in the skull (cranium).

Purpose

A craniotomy is a type of brain surgery. It is the most commonly performed surgery for brain tumor removal. It also may be done to remove a blood clot (hematoma), to control hemorrhage from a weak, leaking blood vessel (cerebral aneurysm), to repair **arteriovenous malformations** (abnormal connections of blood vessels), to drain a brain abscess, to relieve pressure inside the skull, to perform a **biopsy**, or to inspect the brain.

Demographics

Because craniotomy is a procedure that is utilized for several conditions and diseases, statistical information for the procedure itself is not available. However, because craniotomy is most commonly performed to remove a brain tumor, statistics concerning this condition are given. Approximately 90% of primary brain cancers occur in adults, more commonly in males between 55 and 65 years of age. Tumors in children peak between the ages of 3 and 12. Brain tumors are presently the most common cancer in children (4 out of 100,000).

Description

There are two methods commonly utilized by surgeons to open the skull. Either an incision is made at the nape of the neck around the bone at the back (occipital bone) or a curving incision is made in front of the ear that arches above the eye. The incision penetrates as far as the thin membrane covering the skull bone. During the skin incision, the surgeon must seal off many small blood vessels because the scalp has a rich blood supply.

Key Terms

Abscess A localized collection of pus or infection that is walled off from the rest of the body.

Arteriogram An x-ray study of an artery that has been injected with a contrast dye.

Arteriovenous malformation Abnormal, direct connection between the arteries and veins. Arteriovenous malformations can range from very small to large.

Cerebral aneurysm An abnormal, localized bulge in a blood vessel that is usually caused by a congenital weakness in the wall of the vessel.

Cranium Skull; the bony framework that holds the brain.

Computed tomography (CT) An imaging technique that produces three-dimensional pictures of organs and structures inside the body using a 360° x-ray beam.

Edema An accumulation of watery fluid that causes swelling of the affected tissue.

Hematoma An accumulation of blood, often clotted, in a body tissue or organ, usually caused by a break or tear in a blood vessel.

Hemorrhage Very severe, massive bleeding that is difficult to control.

Magnetic resonance imaging (MRI) An imaging technique that uses magnetic fields and radio waves to create detailed images of internal body organs and structures, including the brain.

The scalp tissue is then folded back to expose the bone. Using a high-speed drill, the surgeon drills a pattern of holes through the cranium (skull) and uses a fine wire saw to connect the holes until a segment of bone (bone flap) can be removed. This gives the surgeon access to the inside of the skull and allows him to proceed with surgery inside the brain. After removal of the internal brain lesion or other procedure is completed, the bone is replaced and secured into position with soft wire. Membranes, muscle, and skin are sutured into position. If the lesion is an aneurysm, the affected artery is sealed at the leak. If there is a tumor, as much of it as possible is resected (removed). For arteriovenous malformations, the abnormality is clipped and the repair redirects the blood flow to normal vessels.

Diagnosis/Preparation

Since the lesion is in the brain, the surgeon uses imaging studies to definitively identify it. Neuroimaging is usually accomplished by the following:

• **Computed tomography** (**CT**) uses x rays and injection of an intravenous dye to visualize the lesion.

• **Magnetic resonance imaging** (**MRI**) uses magnetic fields and radio waves to visualize a lesion.

• An arteriogram is an x ray of blood vessels injected with a dye to visualize a tumor or cerebral aneurysm.

Before surgery the patient may be given medication to ease anxiety and to decrease the risk of **seizures**, swelling, and infection after surgery. Blood thinners (Coumadin, heparin, aspirin) and nonsteroidal anti-inflammatory drugs (ibuprofen, Motrin, Advil, Naprosyn,

Daypro) have been correlated with an increase in blood clot formation after surgery. These medications must be discontinued at least seven days before the surgery to reverse any blood thinning effects. Additionally, the surgeon will order routine or special laboratory tests as needed. The night before surgery the patient should not eat or drink after midnight. The patient's scalp is shaved in the operating room just before the surgery begins.

Aftercare

Craniotomy is a major surgical procedure performed under general anesthesia. Immediately after surgery, the patient's pupil reactions are tested, mental status is assessed after anesthesia, and movement of the limbs (arms/legs) is evaluated. Shortly after surgery, breathing exercises are started to clear the lungs. Typically after surgery patients are given medications to control **pain**, swelling, and seizures. Codeine may be prescribed to relieve **headache**. Special leg stockings are used to prevent blood clot formation after surgery. Patients can usually get out of bed in about a day after surgery and usually are hospitalized for five to fourteen days after surgery. The bandages on the skull are be removed and replaced regularly. The sutures closing the scalp are removed by the surgeon, but the soft wires used to reattach the portion of the skull that was removed are permanent and require no further attention. Patients should keep the scalp dry until the sutures are removed. If required (depending on area of brain involved) occupational therapists and physical therapist assess patients status postoperatively and help the patient improve strength, daily living skills and capabilities, and speech. Full recovery may take up to two months, since it is common for patients to feel fatigued for up to eight weeks after surgery.

Risks

The surgeon will discuss potential risks associated with the procedure. Neurosurgical procedures may result in bleeding, blood clots, retention of fluid causing swelling (edema), or unintended injury to normal nerve tissues. Some patients may develop infections. Damage to normal brain tissue may cause damage to an area and subsequent loss of brain function. Loss of function in specific areas can cause memory impairment. Some other examples of potential damage that may result from this procedure include deafness, double vision, numbness, paralysis, blindness, or loss of the sense of smell.

Normal results

Normal results depend on the cause for surgery and the patient's overall health status and age. If the operation was successful and uncomplicated recovery is quick, since there is a rich blood supply to the area. Recovery could take up to eight weeks, but patients are usually fully functioning in less time.

Morbidity and mortality rates

There is no information about the rates of diseases and death specifically related to craniotomy. The operation is performed as a neurosurgical intervention for several different diseases and conditions.

Resources

BOOKS

Connolly, E. Sanders, ed. *Fundamentals of Operative Techniques in Neurosurgery.* New York: Thieme Medical Publishers, 2002.

Greenberg, Mark S. *Handbook of Neurosurgery.* 5th ed. New York: Thieme Medical Publishers, 2000.

Miller, R. *Anesthesia.* 5th ed. Philadelphia, PA: Churchill Livingstone, 2000.

PERIODICALS

Gebel, J. M. and W. J. Powers. "Emergency Craniotomy for Intracerebral Hemorrhage: When Doesn't It Help and Does It Ever Help?" *Neurology* 58 (May 14, 2002): 1325-1326.

Mamminen, P. and T. K. Tan. "Postoperative Nausea and Vomiting After Craniotomy for Tumor Surgery: A Comparison Between Awake Craniotomy and General Anesthesia." *Journal of Clinical Anesthesia* 14 (June 2002): 279-283.

Osguthorpe, J. D. and S. Patel, eds. Skull Base Tumor Surgery. *Otolaryngologic Clinics of North America* 34 (December 2001).

Rabinstein, A. A., J. L. Atkinson, and E. F. M. Wijdicks. "Emergency Craniotomy in Patients Worsening Due to

WHO PERFORMS THE PROCEDURE AND WHERE IS IT PERFORMED?

The procedure is performed in a hospital with a **neurosurgery** department and an **intensive care unit**. The procedure is performed by a board certified neurosurgeon, who has completed two years of **general surgery** training and five years of neurosurgical training.

QUESTIONS TO ASK THE DOCTOR

- How is this procedure done?
- What kinds of tests and preparation are necessary before surgery?
- What risks are associated with the procedure?
- How often is normal brain tissue damaged during this type of surgery?
- What is the expected outcome of the surgery?
- What complications may result from this type of surgery?
- What is the recovery time?
- How many of these procedures have you done in the past year?

Expanded Cerebral Hematoma: To What Purpose?" *Neurology* 58 (May 14, 2002): 1367-1372.

ORGANIZATIONS

American Association of Neurological Surgeons. 5550 Meadowbrook Drive, Rolling Meadows, IL 60008. (888) 566-AANS (2267). Fax: (847) 378-0600. info@aans.org. <http://www.neurosurgery.org/aans/index.asp>.

Laith Farid Gulli, M.D., M.S.
Nicole Mallory, M.S., PA-C
Robert Ramirez, B.S.

Creutzfeldt-Jakob disease

Definition

Creutzfeldt-Jakob disease (CJD) is a rapidly progressive disease causing damage to the brain. It is one of a group of rare diseases that affects humans and animals, known as transmissible spongiform encephalopathies (TSE) and is believed to be caused by a prion, a newly identified type of disease-causing agent. Creutzfeldt-Jakob disease is characterized by **dementia** and walking difficulties. Death can occur up to two years after the first symptoms; however, most people die within seven months. There is no treatment or cure.

Description

Creutzfeldt-Jakob disease is a serious progressive degenerative disorder of the brain that was first described in the 1920s by two German researchers, and is characterized by sudden development of rapidly progressive neurological and neuromuscular symptoms. When symptoms begin, affected individuals may develop confusion, **depression**, behavioral changes, impaired vision, and/or impaired coordination. As the disease progresses, there may be rapidly progressive deterioration of thought processes and memory (dementia), resulting in confusion and disorientation, impairment of memory control, personality disintegration, agitation, and restlessness. Affected individuals also develop neuromuscular abnormalities such as muscle weakness and loss of muscle mass (wasting); irregular, rapid, shock-like muscle spasms (**myoclonus**); and/or relatively slow, involuntary, continual writhing movements, particularly in the arms and legs. Later stages of the disease may include further loss of physical and intellectual functions, a state of unconsciousness (coma), and increased susceptibility to repeated infections of the respiratory tract. In many affected individuals, life-threatening complications may develop less than a year after the disorder becomes apparent.

There are three main forms of CJD, each one with its distinctive basic features. The sporadic CJD, which accounts for approximately 85% of all cases worldwide and occurs by chance, is associated with the presence of a misshapen protein in the brain, known as a prion ("proteinaceous infectious particle"). Sporadic CJD cannot be caught from another person or animal, is not related to diet, nor can it be inherited. On the contrary, inherited (or familial) CJD accounts for 5–10% of all cases of CJD and is caused by a faulty gene called prion-related protein (PRPN) that is passed down from parents to their children in a dominant inheritance, which means patients will develop the disease if they inherit a defective gene from just one parent. Symptoms are similar to sporadic CJD, but they appear earlier and have a longer time course.

Unlike the previous two CJD forms, acquired CJD affects those people who have not inherited the condition by two other ways. The iatrogenic CJD occurs due to accidental infection after medical procedures such as human pituitary hormone injection or dura mater transplantation. The variant CJD (vCJD), a type of CJD that was first identified in 1996, is passed from cows with bovine spongiform **encephalopathy** (BSE, or "mad cow disease") to

---

Key Terms

Encephalopathy A disease or dysfunction of the brain.

Myoclonus Twitching muscular contractions.

Prion A protein particle lacking nucleic acid and thought to be the cause of certain infectious diseases of the central nervous system, such as Creutzfeldt-Jakob disease.

---

humans. The variant form affects mostly younger adults and has different clinical and pathological characteristics.

All forms of CJD can be present in a person for long periods (often more than 20 years) during which there are no symptoms. The duration of the illness before death varies from a matter of weeks (typical of sporadic CJD) to three to twelve months (typical of variant CJD). However, there have been exceptions in both types.

Demographics

CJD appears to affect males and females in equal numbers. It occurs worldwide with an incidence rate that has remained stable at approximately one case per million people, annually. It usually first appears in mid-life, beginning between ages 20 and 68, with the average age at onset of symptoms being around age 50. The onset of the iatrogenic form depends on the age of exposure.

Causes and symptoms

All forms of CJD are caused by the presence of a faulty protein in the brain, called prion. Prions occur in both a normal form, which is a harmless protein found in the body's cells, and in an infectious form, which causes disease. The harmless and infectious forms of the prion protein are nearly identical, but the infectious form takes a different folded shape. Sporadic CJD may develop because some of a person's normal prions spontaneously change into the infectious form of the protein and then alter the prions in other cells in a chain reaction by a mechanism that is not yet understood. Misfolded protein molecules then spread through the brain and stick together to form fibers and/or clumps called plaques that can be seen with powerful microscopes. These bundles of twisted protein disrupt brain cells and eventually leave large holes in the brain tissue, giving the brain a spongy appearance. Fibers and plaques may start to accumulate years before symptoms of CJD begin to appear. It is still unclear what role these abnormalities play in the disease or how they might affect symptoms.

About 5–10% of all CJD cases are inherited. These cases arise from a mutation, or change, in the gene PRPN that controls formation of the normal prion protein. While prions themselves do not contain genetic information and do not require genes to reproduce themselves, infectious prions can arise if a mutation occurs in the gene for the body's normal prions. If the prion gene is altered in a person's sperm or egg cells, the mutation can be transmitted to the person's offspring. Several different mutations in the prion gene have been identified. The particular mutation found in each family affects how frequently the disease appears and what symptoms are most noticeable. However, not all people with mutations in the prion gene develop CJD. This suggests that the mutations merely increase susceptibility to CJD and that other, still-unknown factors also play a role in the disease.

CJD does not cause any symptoms at first. The first symptoms to appear include slow thinking, difficulty concentrating, impaired judgment, memory loss, personality and behavioral changes, and difficulties with coordination and vision. These symptoms rapidly give way to increasing mental deficits leading to severe, progressive dementia (mental decline) associated with self-neglect, apathy or irritability, and prominent muscle spasms (myoclonus). **Seizures** commonly occur as the disease progresses. Symptoms continue to worsen until both mental and physical functions are lost; patients are completely bedridden, and eventually lapse into coma. Comatose patients may die as a result of infection associated with being immobile, such as pneumonia.

Diagnosis

There is currently no single diagnostic test for CJD. Indeed, the only definitive diagnosis can be assessed by a postmortem examination (autopsy) of the brain or examining a sample of brain tissue (brain **biopsy**). However, CJD should be considered in adults who experience a sudden onset of rapidly progressive dementia and neuromuscular symptoms such as myoclonus.

An electroencephalogram (EEG) and a **magnetic resonance imaging (MRI)** scan may be useful in determining abnormalities in the brain. People may be diagnosed as having "probable CJD." Although not definitive, all those who have been diagnosed as probable CJD in life, and who subsequently had an autopsy, were found to have been a CJD patient. Genetic testing can be carried out in people suspected of having the inherited form of CJD, in order to increase certainty of diagnosis. Such people usually report a family history of the disease.

Iatrogenic CJD is usually diagnosed on the basis of the affected person's medical history. Those at risk include people having received hormones derived from humans before 1992, or dura mater transplant grafts before 1985.

Treatment team

A **neurologist** or a psychiatrist is normally the primary consultant for CJD, and continual nursing care may be necessary as disease progresses. Physical therapist may also be required.

Treatment

As of 2004, no treatment has been shown to be effective against CJD. Treatments are available to alleviate some symptoms, such as morphine for muscle **pain**, and clonazepam (Rivotril) or sodium valproate (Epilim) for jerky movements. A wide range of drugs has been tested for their ability to slow the progress of the disease, but none has been shown to be useful.

At present, care consists of managing the specific problems faced by patients with CJD. Speech therapy and occupational therapy may help, and the support of district nurses and social services is often invaluable for people with CJD and their caregivers.

Recovery and rehabilitation

Because CJD is an incurable, fatal disease with a fast progression, recovery and rehabilitation are not possible. The emphasis in treatment is placed upon comfort and support of the affected individual and the caregivers.

Clinical trials

As of mid 2004, there are no ongoing **clinical trials** for CJD.

Prognosis

The outcome for a person with CJD is usually very poor. Complete dementia commonly occurs within six months or less after the appearance of the first symptoms, with the person becoming totally incapable of self-care. The disorder is fatal in a short time, usually within seven months, but a few people survive as long as one or two years after diagnosis. The cause of death is usually infection, heart failure, or respiratory failure.

Special concerns

Hospitals and health care providers take special precautions to minimize the risk of transferring prions from surgical equipment or donated tissues. Medical histories of potential cornea donors that indicate a familial history of possible Creutzfeldt-Jacob disease rule out the use of those corneas for transplantation. Additionally, regulations and records regarding livestock feed and transfer of livestock are maintained by the United States Department of Agriculture.

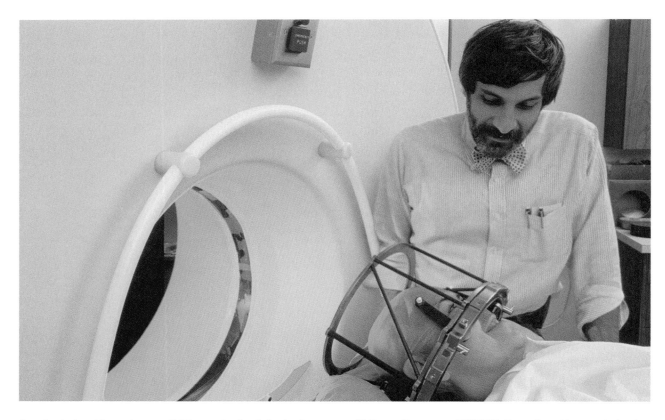

A patient about to undergo a CAT scan to check for brain cancer. *(© Roger Ressmeyer/CORBIS. Reproduced by permission.)*

Resources

BOOKS

Staff. *The Official Patient's Sourcebook on Creutzfeldt-Jakob Disease: A Revised and Updated Directory for the Internet Age.* San Diego: Icon Group International, 2003.

PERIODICALS

Mastaglia, F. L., M. J. Garllep, B. A. Phillips, and P. J. Zilko. "Inflammatory Myopathies: Clinical, Diagnostic and Therapeutic Aspects." *Muscle & Nerve* (April 2003): 407–425.

"U.S. to Expand Testing of Cattle for Disease." *New York Times* March 16, 2004: pA25.

OTHER

"New 'Mad Cow' Link to Humans and Livestock." *CNN.com.* August 29, 2000 (May 27, 2004). <http://edition.cnn.com/2000/HEALTH/08/29/britain.madcow/>.

NINDS Creutzfeldt-Jakob Disease Information Page. National Institute of Neurological Disorders and Stroke. April 20, 2004 (May 27, 2004). <http://www.ninds.nih.gov/health_and_medical/disorders/cjd.htm>.

ORGANIZATIONS

Creutzfeldt-Jakob (CJD) Foundation Inc. P.O. Box 5312, Akron, OH 44334. (330) 668-2474 or (800) 659-1991. crjakob@aol.com. <http://www.cjdfoundation.org>.

Marcos do Carmo Oyama
Iuri Drumond Louro, MD, PhD

CT scan

Definition

Computed tomography (also known as CT, CT scan, CAT, or computerized axial tomography) scans use x rays to produce precise cross-sectional images of anatomical structures.

Description

With the development of modern computers, the scans enhanced digital capabilities allowed the development of computed tomography imaging (derived from the Greek *tomos*, meaning "to slice"). The diagnostic potential of CT scans was first realized by English physician Godfrey Hounsfield.

CT scans differ from conventional x ray by collecting x rays that have passed through the body (those not absorbed by tissue) with an electronic detector mounted on a rotating frame rather than on film. The x-ray source and collector rotate around the patient as they emit and absorb x rays. CT technology then utilizes advanced computer-based mathematical algorithms to combine different readings or views of a patient into a coherent picture usable for diagnosis.

Key Terms

Computerized axial tomographic (CAT) scan A scanning method, also called CT scanning, that uses diagnostic x rays and a computer to give cross-sectional images at different angles of the brain and other parts of the body.

Radiologist A physician who specializes in imaging techniques such as x rays, CAT scans, MRI scans, and certain scans using radioactive isotopes.

X ray Electromagnetic radiation of very short wavelength, and very high energy.

CT scans increase the scope and safety of imaging procedures that allow physicians to view the arrangement and functioning of the body's internal structures. With particular regard to neurology, CT scans are used to determine the presence or absence of brain tumors. CT scans usually take about an hour and a half, including preparation time, with the actual examination of neural tissue in a brain scan taking 15–45 minutes.

CT scanners are now often combined with **positron emission tomography (PET)** scanners into one unit. PET-CT scanners have the ability to link the functional image created by a **PET** scan with the anatomical image produced by a CT scan. The combined scanning technique enhances a physician's ability to detect metabolic abnormalities (some no larger than 0.15 in [4 mm] in size) and to precisely map the location of the anomaly.

Increased accuracy reduces the number of unusable results and also results in less retesting.

The combined PET-CT scanners offer physicians the opportunity to differentiate, for example, between Alzheimer's disease and **multi-infarct dementia**. In addition, the enhanced images allow the differentiation of brain tumors from cerebral necrosis.

The physics

The physical basis of the CT scans lies in the fact that different tissues absorb x rays at different rates. The density and atomic number of the elements present are critical factors in determining whether a particular x ray is absorbed or passes through the body. The opacity of an image is related directly to the type of tissue or element. Dense bone appears white, while gaseous air in the lungs appears black.

CT scans are also used by some security agencies to examine packages and baggage.

CT scan procedures

CT scan allow the construction of detailed images and offer another, and in many cases, more affordable means of diagnosis without invasive surgical procedures. CT scans can also be used to guide the course of surgical procedures.

CT scans often utilize a medium or contrast enhancer, provided in the form of a drinkable liquid or via injection into the patient's bloodstream. Approximately 45 minutes before a patient is examined, the individual is given an intravenous injection of a radiopharmaceutical tracer. A brain scan and scan of the spinal cord can take less than 30 minutes.

Radiation exposure from a CT exam is roughly equal to a normal year's worth of exposure to natural background radiation—more than from a conventional x-ray examination, but less than that of other x-ray exams such as a skull x ray.

Because x rays are high energy rays that can damage critical cells in the developing embryo, women who suspect that they are pregnant should inform their doctor and the CT scan technologist prior to the exam. Nursing mothers are often advised to wait 24 hours after the injection of the contrast medium before resuming breast-feeding.

Because CT scans provide only axial cross-sections, an **MRI** test is often used to more carefully examine unusual or suspect findings.

Resources
WEBSITES

"Computed Tomography." *EcureME.* May 9, 2004 (May 27, 2004). <http://www.ecureme.com/emyhealth/data/Computed_Tomography.asp>.

The CT: Computed Tomography Test. University of Iowa Department of Neurology. May 9, 2004 (May 27, 2004). <http://www.vh.org/adult/patient/neurology/computedtomographytest/>.

Paul Arthur

Cumulative trauma disorders *see* **Repetitive motion disorders**

Cushing syndrome

Definition

Cushing syndrome was first described by an American neurosurgeon in the early twentieth century named Harvey Cushing. Cushing recognized a specific set of symptoms that collectively he identified as part of a syndrome. In this disease, prolonged exposure to abnormal levels of the hormone cortisol results in the collection of symptoms that Harvey Cushing described. Cushing Syndrome can also be associated with abnormal levels of another hormone, adrenocorticotropin (ACTH), and both ACTH and cortisol overproduction can often occur as part of other disorders.

Description

Cushing syndrome affects the body in many ways and can lead to severe medical complications if untreated. Effects of the disorder are manifested clinically, physically, and emotionally. Physically, patients develop an abnormal fat distribution that sometimes leads to feelings of insecurity or unattractiveness. Clinically, people with Cushing syndrome are often at risk for a variety of significant medical problems including diabetes, high blood pressure, hair loss (especially in women), and heart disease. Cushing syndrome is relatively rare. Severe **fatigue** can also develop and this has many ramifications in terms of complications related to daily living. Cushing syndrome is sometimes referred to as hypercortisolism.

Demographics

According to the National Institute of Diabetes & Digestive & Kidney Diseases (NIDDK), an estimated 10 to 15 individuals out of every million people will be affected each year with Cushing syndrome. These individuals are usually adults between the ages of twenty to fifty years old. Pituitary adenomas cause the majority of Cushing syndrome cases, and women that have these types of tumors are at a five-fold higher risk for developing the disease than men.

Causes and symptoms

The function of cortisol is to regulate blood pressure, act as an anti-inflammatory mediator, and to regulate insulin metabolism. Cortisol plays a role during the metabolic activities associated with fat, protein, and carbohydrate metabolism. High levels of cortisol can cause sodium and water retention. Therefore, overproduction of cortisol can have medically important health-related implications that affect muscle contractions, heartbeat, and blood cell function.

The adrenal glands are located on top of each kidney, and are responsible for releasing cortisol. The site of cortisol production is in the outer layer of the adrenal gland called the adrenal cortex. Release of cortisol is stimulated by ACTH, which is produced by another gland. This gland, called the pituitary gland, is juxtaposed to the base of the brain and serves as a type of control center for many other glands in the body. ACTH production occurs only when there is a low concentration of cortisol in the blood.

Therefore, cortisol production can be abnormal due to abnormalities in the function of the adrenal gland or the pituitary gland. It can also be overproduced by abnormal regulation of ACTH.

The role of cortisol in tumor formation

Cortisol overproduction can also be caused by many different types of tumors resulting in abnormalities in the function or regulation of the adrenal or pituitary glands. These tumors are usually not malignant and are found in the pituitary and adrenal glands. In the pituitary gland, a specific type of tumor called an adenoma can develop. Pituitary adenomas often can excessively overproduce ACTH in the absence of the normal stimulatory signals. People that develop Cushing syndrome are most likely to develop this disease due to these types of tumors. ACTH overproduction can also occur when the tumor is located outside of the pituitary gland; this condition is known as ectopic ACTH syndrome. These tumors, unlike pituitary adenomas, tend to be cancerous. Tumors can also develop in the adrenal gland and result in excessive cortisol production. Adrenal tumors can often result in malignancy, and patients with these tumors often quickly become symptomatic due to the high levels of cortisol produced.

Familial Cushing syndrome

Cushing syndrome can also develop in multiple individuals from the same family. This familial form is due to a genetically inherited susceptibility to developing specific endocrine tumors. The specific nature of the genetic components have not been clearly elucidated, except in cases of a rare genetic disease called Multiple Endocrine Neoplasia (MEN). MEN is caused by a genetic mutations in a specific gene involved in cell cycle regulation resulting in pituitary tumors that can lead to Cushing syndrome.

The symptoms associated with Cushing syndrome can be easily recognizable by an experienced physician. These clinical manifestations include physical characteristics that involve the face, neck, shoulders, and abdomen. Generally, most affected individuals develop obesity of the upper portion of their bodies. They often have thin arms and legs. The facial feature that characterizes Cushing syndrome is the typically developed round, moon-shaped face. An accumulation of fat pads are often observed on or below the base of the neck, on the patients back, between the patient's shoulders, as well as on the abdomen. Abdominal fat accumulation can be significant and can also be associated with vertical purplish striations (stretch marks). Stretch marks also can be observed on their thighs, arms, breasts, and buttocks. Affected children often suffer from obesity along with growth retardation.

Other clinical manifestations resulting from excessive cortisol production can be quite serious. **Myopathy**, or

Key Terms

Adrenocorticotropic hormone (ACTH) Also called adrenocorticotropin or corticotropin, this hormone is produced by the pituitary gland to stimulate the adrenal cortex to release various corticosteroid hormones.

Cortisol A steroid hormone secreted by the adrenal cortex that is important for maintenance of body fluids, electrolytes, and blood sugar levels. Also called hydrocortisone.

Pituitary gland The most important of the endocrine glands (glands that release hormones directly into the bloodstream), the pituitary is located at the base of the brain. Sometimes referred to as the "master gland," it regulates and controls the activities of other endocrine glands and many body processes including growth and reproductive function. Also called the hypophysis.

wasting away of the muscles often occurs. Due to the abnormal blood cell development that results from cortisol overproduction, the skin bruises more frequently and wounds do not heal as quickly. Skin tends to be fragile and thin. People with Cushing syndrome are susceptible to developing fractures, especially in the pelvic and spinal regions. Women are at a higher risk for developing osteoporosis or brittle bones. Men also frequently develop weak bones. For all affected individuals, difficulty with activities such as lifting objects or getting up from a sitting position can lead to **back pain** and fractures. Because cortisol is also important for regulating insulin, patients with Cushing syndrome are at risk for developing diabetes.

Diagnosis

The diagnosis of Cushing syndrome is based on the patient's family history and the results from several laboratory tests. The most definitive diagnostic laboratory test is to monitor cortisol production in the person's urine during a 24-hour collection period. A 50–100 microgram result represents the normal cutoff, with any higher value suggestive of Cushing syndrome.

When cortisol is found to be high, x rays are usually requested to identify pituitary or adrenal tumors. A dexamethasone suppression test is often requested with a positive finding on x ray and is used to distinguish between ACTH overproduction due to pituitary adenomas or other tumors. Dexamethasone is a synthetic hormone that, when used to help diagnose Cushing syndrome, is usually orally administered for four days at increasing

dosages, during which time the urine is collected. The effect on blood and urine cortisol concentrations can be determined and the different effects can distinguish these two types of ACTH-producing tumors. Radiological imaging such as **MRI** scans sometimes allow endocrinologists (physicians who specialize in hormone-related health concerns) to directly visualize the glands and determine their size and shape.

Treatment team

Several types of medical doctors are usually required for the diagnosis and treatment of Cushing syndrome. This includes an oncologist, a pathologist, or an endocrinologist. Although it is unlikely that a child would develop this disease, treatment would depend on whether the child has progressed through puberty. As Cushing syndrome in children can result in growth retardation, a pediatric endocrinologist would be the most likely specialist to monitor the child's development.

Treatment

Determining the appropriate treatment for individuals with Cushing syndrome relies on the accurate determination of the cause of excessive cortisol production. As there are a variety of causes, selecting the appropriate treatment depends on characterizing the disease based on the precipitating spectrum of clinical manifestations. For example, abnormal function of the pituitary gland or the adrenal cortex can be important indicators of causation. For this reason, it is important that affected individuals have a comprehensive clinical evaluation by an experienced physician. Tumors of the pituitary gland or the adrenal cortex can stimulate overproduction of ACTH or cortisol. Medical treatments with cortisone for unrelated conditions may also alter the amount of cortisol exposure and concentration circulating within the body.

In cases that involve pituitary tumors as the cause of Cushing syndrome, surgical removal represents a formidable treatment in cases where chemotherapy or **radiation** is ineffective. Transsphenoidal adenomectomy, a surgical procedure, is the most widely used treatment for pituitary adenomas that cause Cushing syndrome. This usually requires a specialized surgeon or treatment center, as it is a relatively rare and difficult procedure. The success rate is high and synthetic hormone replacement therapy, typically with prednisone, is only necessary for approximately one year. As an alternative, radiation therapy is also a possibility. There are also therapeutic agents that inhibit cortisol production that can be used.

Adrenal gland tumors are usually always surgically removed, whether they are benign or malignant. Adrenal gland removal typically does not affect endocrine function due to compensation from other glands in producing hormones. Hormone therapy is required with removal of both adrenal glands.

If the cause of Cushing syndrome is drug-induced, due to prolonged exposure to steroids called **glucocorticoids** that are used to treat other ailments, the physician will lower this dose as long as symptoms continue to be manifested.

Recovery and rehabilitation

Transsphenoidal adenomectomy performed by an experienced surgeon has a high success rate, with more than 80% of patients cured. In the event that the surgery is not successful or it provides only a temporary cure, it is often repeated with fairly favorable results. For radiation therapy, adding one of many drugs that suppresses cortisol production such as mitotane can enhance recovery time. These drugs have been considered to be effective when used alone in up to 40% of patients.

As scientists and clinicians better understand how cortisol and ACTH are produced and how disturbances in hormonal regulation affect the body, more treatment modalities will likely become available.

Clinical trials

The National Institutes of Health sponsors several scientists in clinical translational research in Cushing syndrome treatment, as well as the development of drugs leading to **clinical trials**. As of early 2004, there were at least eight ongoing clinical trials recruiting patients. These include long term post-operative follow ups, the evaluation of novel imaging techniques, understanding the role of stress and **depression** in Cushing syndrome, and other studies investigating adrenal and pituitary gland tumors. Further information on clinical trials can be found at the National Institutes of Health website on clinical trials, *ClinicalTrials.gov,* available at: <http://www.clinicaltrials.gov/ct/search?term=cushing+syndrome>.

Prognosis

The prognosis for individuals who receive treatment for Cushing syndrome is good with a high likelihood of being cured. However, in affected individuals that are not treated, the prognosis can be poor, with death eventually resulting from complications from hypertension, diabetes, or heart disease.

Resources

BOOKS

Icon Health Publications. *The Official Patient's Sourcebook on Cushing's Syndrome: A Revised and Updated Directory for the Internet Age.* San Diego: Icon Group, Int., 2002.

DeGroot, Leslie J., ed., et al. "Cushing's Syndrome." In *Endocrinology,* Vol. 2, pp. 1741–1769. Philadelphia: W. B. Saunders Company, 1995.

Wilson, Jean D., ed, et al. "Hyperfunction: Glucocorticoids: Hypercortisolism (Cushing's syndrome)," pp. 536–562. In *Williams Textbook of Endocrinology,* No. 8. Philadelphia: W. B. Saunders, 1992.

PERIODICALS

Boscaro, M., L. Barzon, F. Fallo, and N. Sonino. "Cushing Syndrome." *Lancet* 357, no. 9258 (March 10, 2001): 783–91.

OTHER

NINDS Cushing's Syndrome Information Page. National Institute of Neurological Disorders and Stroke. (January 20, 2004.) <http://www.ninds.nih.gov/health_and_medical/disorders/cushings_doc.htm>.

Cushing's Syndrome. National Institute of Diabetes & Digestive & Kidney Diseases. (January 20, 2004). <http://www.niddk.nih.gov/health/endo/pubs/cushings/cushings.htm>.

ORGANIZATIONS

Cushing's Support and Research Foundation, Inc. 65 East India Row 22B, Boston, MA 02110. (617) 723-3824 or (617) 723-3674. cushinfo@csrf.net. <http://csrf.net/>.

Pituitary Network Association. P.O. Box 1958, Thousand Oaks, CA 91358. (805) 499-9973; Fax: (805) 480-0633. pna@pituitary.org. <http://www.pituitary.org>.

Bryan Richard Cobb

Cytomegalic inclusion body disease

Definition

Cytomegalic inclusion body disease (CIBD) is a condition caused by infection with cytomegalovirus (CMV), a type of herpes virus. A hallmark of CIBD is the periodic reappearance of symptoms throughout life, as the virus cycles through periods of latency and active infection.

Description

CMV is one of the members of the herpes virus group, which includes herpes simplex types 1 and 2, and the viruses that cause chicken pox and infectious mononucleosis. The virus causes enlargement of cells of some organs and the development of inclusion bodies—bits of cellular material—in the cytoplasm or nucleus of these cells. A hallmark of the virus group is the ability to infect a host and then become dormant. CMV can remain dormant for years. Even in periods without symptoms, the

Key Terms

Cytomegalovirus A member of the herpes virus group found throughout all geographic locations and socioeconomic groups; virus usually remains dormant throughout life, reactivating when the body's immune system is severely debilitated.

Immunocompromised An abnormal condition in which the body's ability to fight infection is decreased, due to a disease process, certain medications, or a condition present at birth.

Inclusion body A small intracellular body found within the cytoplasm or nucleus of another cell, characteristic of disease.

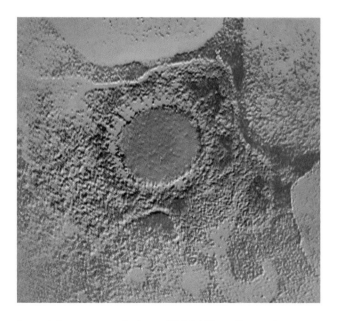

Part of the cytomegalovirus. *(CNRI / Photo Researchers, Inc.)*

virus can still be periodically shed from the body in fluids like tears, saliva, blood, semen, and breast milk. The virus can infect another person through close contact.

Many people with CMV can harbor the virus and display no symptoms. However, if the immune system is damaged or otherwise not functioning efficiently, the virus can reactivate from its dormancy. Cytomegalic inclusion body disease is also known as giant cell inclusion disease, cytomegalovirus infection, and salivary gland disease.

Demographics

The latent infection caused by CMV occurs virtually all over the world and is very common in any population. In the United States, up to 50–85% of people will be infected by the age of 40. CMV infection without symptoms is common in infants and young children. CMV infection is most widespread in economically debilitated regions, although people in developed countries are also susceptible.

Additionally, the virus can be readily transferred from a pregnant mother to the fetus. An infected pregnant woman may not display any symptoms. However, the fetus of a mother with CIBD is at risk for problems, including lung disease, bleeding, anemia, liver damage, or brain damage. CIBD is also a problem among those whose immune systems are not functioning properly or have not yet matured. This includes the unborn, people infected with the human immunodeficiency virus (HIV), and those whose immune systems have been deliberately disabled (i.e., organ transplant recipients).

Causes and symptoms

The cytomegalovirus is the cause of CIBD. When the infection occurs in healthy people after birth, symptoms can be minimal or even nonexistent. Some people experience mild symptoms similar to those of mononucleosis, including a prolonged fever, **fatigue**, mild hepatitis, and tender lymph nodes.

In a fetus, newborn, or a person with a compromised immune system, CIBD can be much more severe. With CIDB, people suffering from acquired immunodeficiency syndrome (**AIDS**) or people recovering from kidney and or other transplant surgeries can also develop inflammation of the retina of the eyes (retinitis) or encephalitis. Retinitis is more common, and in severe cases, blindness can result.

CIBD can cause death of a fetus or a premature birth. In infected newborns, CIBD can be apparent as a lung infection, excessive bleeding, anemia, liver damage, enlargement of the spleen, **seizures**, and inhibited brain development. The latter can result in hearing loss, developmental delays, and difficulty in coordination.

CMV-related polyradiculopathy also causes leg weakness, bowel dysfunction, and bladder dysfunction in end-stage AIDS patients suffering CMV infection.

Diagnosis

Diagnosis is based on the detection of the symptoms of CIBD. Because symptoms can be absent, diagnosis is often overlooked or difficult. If the virus is actively dividing, antibodies to the virus may be detectable by immunological tests of the blood such as the enzyme-linked immunosorbant assay (ELISA). As the antibodies persist for life, their detection is not a guarantee of an ongoing infection. The virus can also be isolated from urine and other body fluids.

One diagnostic feature associated with retinitis is the description of moving black spots in the eye. Although these "floaters" are common even in healthy individuals, they can also be the result of inflammation of the retina, and can alert a physician to the possibility of CIBD.

Treatment team

Treatment is usually maintained by the primary care physician for otherwise healthy patients. For those who are deliberately immunocompromised, newborns, and AIDS patients, a battery of specialists, including immunologists and specialists in infectious disease, can be involved in treatment and care.

Treatment

There is no cure for CIBD. Typically, good hygiene, including proper hand washing, is recommended to avoid transmission of the virus from person to person. **Antiviral drugs** such as ganciclovir and acyclovir can be administered, particularly to AIDS patients to reduce the amount of virus in the body. These drugs are taken throughout life. There are no vaccines for CIBD.

Recovery and rehabilitation

The CMV infection persists throughout life, therefore, rehabilitation efforts focus on supportive measures to combat CMV-caused complications, minimize the effect of symptoms, and minimize the possibility for transmission of the virus.

Clinical trials

As of February 2004, there are no specific CIBD **clinical trials** underway.

Prognosis

Most people who are infected with CMV display no symptoms and have no residual effects of the infection. However, in immunocompromised people, newborns, and unborn babies, the infection can cause serious illness or death.

Resources

BOOKS

Parker, J. N., and P. M. Parker. *The Official Patient's Sourcebook on Cytomegalic Inclusion Body Disease. A Revised and Updated Directory for the Internet Age.* San Diego: Icon Health Publications, 2003.

OTHER

Cytomegalic Inclusion Body Disease Information Page. National Institute of Neurological Disorders and Stroke. (May 20, 2004). <http://www.ninds.nih.gov/health_and_medical/disorders/cytomegalic.htm>.

Cytomegalovirus (CMV). New Mexico AIDS InfoNet. (May 20, 2004). <http://www.thebody.com/nmai/cmv.html>.

Cytomegaolavirus (CMV) Infection. Centers for Disease Control and Prevention. (May 20, 2004). <http://www.cdc.gov/ncidod/diseases/cmv.htm>.

ORGANIZATIONS

Centers for Disease Control and Prevention (CDC). 1600 Clifton Road, Atlanta, GA 30333. (404) 639-3311 or (800) 311-3435. <http://www.cdc.gov>.

National Institute of Allergy and Infectious Disease (NIAID). 31 Center Drive, Rm. 7A50, MSC 2520, Bethesda, MD 20892-2520. (301) 402-1663; Fax: (301) 402-0120. niadnews@niad.nih.gov. <http://www.ninds.nih.gov>.

National Institute for Neurological Diseases and Stroke (NINDS). 6001 Executive Boulevard, Bethesda, MD 20892. (301) 496-5751 or (800) 352-9424. <http://www.ninds.nih.gov>.

Brian Douglas Hoyle, PhD

Cytomegalovirus infection *see* **Cytomegalic inclusion body disease**

D

Dancing eyes-Dancing feet syndrome *see*
Opsoclonus myoclonus

Dandy-Walker syndrome

Definition

Dandy-Walker syndrome refers to a group of specific, congenital (present at birth) brain malformations, and is a common cause of **hydrocephalus** (increased fluid in the brain).

Description

Dandy-Walker syndrome is more often referred to as Dandy-Walker malformation (DWM) or Dandy-Walker complex. The condition is named for doctors Walter E. Dandy and Arthur E. Walker, who described the signs and symptoms of the condition in the early 1900s.

The brain contains four ventricles, which are inner, hollow portions filled with cerebrospinal fluid (CSF). The first and second (lateral) ventricles are inside the cerebral hemispheres, and the third and fourth ventricles are below them, closer to the brainstem. DWM consists of a specific group of brain malformations, including enlargement of the fourth ventricle, complete or partial agenesis (lack of development) of the cerebellar vermis (the middle portion of the **cerebellum**, which lies directly behind the cerebral hemispheres), and cyst formation and dilation of the posterior fossa (a small, hollow section between the lower cerebellum and skull).

A further defining characteristic of DMW is blockage or closure of the foramina (openings) of Magendie and Luschka, two channels at the base of the brain through which CSF normally flows. When these openings are obstructed, CSF produced in the ventricles has no outlet for normal circulation. This causes fluid pressure to build, and the ventricles to enlarge (always the fourth, and often the third and lateral ventricles).

Demographics

About one in 1,000 children is born with hydrocephalus. Of those, 10% have DWM as the underlying cause of their condition. DWM has not been shown to be more frequent in any particular ethnic group or race. About 85% of babies born with DWM have one or more other congenital malformations, or some type of recognizable syndrome. The 15% that have no other malformations may be said to have "isolated" DWM.

Causes and symptoms

The true cause of DWM is unknown. However, the components of the malformation seem to be related to a disruption in development of the middle portion of the lower part of the brain in the embryonic stage. This affects growth and development of the cerebellum, especially the vermis, and the brainstem such that the foramina of Magendie and Luschka are partially or completely closed.

Most cases of isolated DWM occur by chance (sporadic) and have very little risk of recurrence in siblings or children of the affected individual. In a few cases, DWM may be inherited as an autosomal recessive trait, which would imply a 25% risk for recurrence in siblings.

Some syndromes that may occur with DWM are chromosomal (abnormal number of chromosomes in every cell of the body—usually sporadic), while others are hereditary. The empiric recurrence risk for non-syndromic DWM with other anomalies is about 5% for siblings or children of the affected individual.

Outward physical signs of DWM may be a bulging occiput (lower rear portion of the skull) and an increased total head circumference. Symptoms of DWM are those caused by hydrocephalus (if present) and dysgenesis/agenesis of the cerebellar vermis. In infants, symptoms can include irritability, **seizures**, vomiting, abnormal breathing, nystagmus (jerky eye movements), and slow motor development. Older children and adults may have **headaches**, **ataxia** (difficulties with coordination), **visual disturbances**, and/or developmental delay/mental retardation.

Key Terms

Cerebellum The part of the brain involved in the coordination of movement, walking, and balance.

Cerebrospinal fluid The clear, normally colorless fluid that fills the brain cavities (ventricles), the subarachnoid space around the brain, and the spinal cord and acts as a shock absorber.

Hydrocephalus An abnormal accumulation of cerebrospinal fluid within the brain. This accumulation can be harmful by pressing on brain structures, and damaging them.

Ventricles The four fluid-filled chambers, or cavities, found in the two cerebral hemispheres of the brain, at the center of the brain, and between the brain stem and cerebellum, and linked by channels, or ducts, allowing cerebral fluid to circulate through them.

Ventriculoperitoneal shunt A tube equipped with a low-pressure valve, one end of which is inserted into a cerebral ventricle, the other end of which is routed into the peritoneum, or abdominal cavity.

Diagnosis

DWM may be diagnosed in pregnancy by ultrasound as early as 12–14 weeks after conception, although ultrasounds later in pregnancy are more sensitive. A level II ultrasound, a more detailed examination that can only be performed 18 weeks or later after conception, may be suggested to confirm the diagnosis of DWM and will look for the presence of other malformations. An amniocentesis, a procedure to analyze fetal chromosomes, is also usually offered.

After birth, DWM may be suspected because of physical or neurological signs, but it is only possible to establish the diagnosis of DWM by performing imaging studies of the brain through a computed tomography (CT) scan or **magnetic resonance imaging (MRI)**.

Treatment team

A neurosurgeon would perform any surgical procedures (such as shunts) needed to help relieve hydrocephalus or intracranial cysts. Depending on the severity of any neurological symptoms and the presence or absence of other congenital malformations, various specialists involved in the care of a child with DWM can include a neonatologist (specialist in the care of newborns), developmental pediatrician, geneticist, **neurologist**, specialized nursing care, and occupational/physical therapists (OT/PT).

Treatment

The primary treatment for DWM and associated hydrocephalus is the placement of a ventriculoperitoneal (VP) shunt. This is a procedure in which a neurosurgeon places one end of a small tube in a ventricle in the brain, and threads the other end under the skin down to the peritoneal (abdominal) cavity. The tube helps to direct excess CSF to the peritoneal cavity where it is reabsorbed by the body.

In some cases, the neurosurgeon may attempt a procedure called endoscopic fenestration. In this procedure a small, flexible viewing device, called an endoscope, is inserted into the brain and an opening is made between the third and fourth ventricles or in the foramina at the base of the brain. It is hoped that opening these passages will equalize CSF pressure throughout the **central nervous system**.

Other treatments include those for the symptoms of hydrocephalus and cerebellar agenesis, such as anti-seizure medications, and OT/PT for neuromuscular problems.

Recovery and rehabilitation

Some children recover completely after a shunt is placed, while others receive partial benefit. Shunting procedures are not always successful, and they carry a risk for serious infection. A child who retains neurologic deficits will likely require long-term care by a neurologist and OT/PT. Special accommodations for home care may also be needed.

Clinical trials

There are no **clinical trials** for Dandy-Walker syndrome.

Prognosis

Prognosis for DWM varies anywhere from excellent to fatal. The overall prognosis for DWM that occurs and is diagnosed as part of a known syndrome will depend on the possible prognoses for that particular syndrome, although the presence of DWM may have a negative impact. In other cases, DWM without other anomalies has a much better prognosis. As noted, prognosis is also critically dependent on the degree of hydrocephalus already present at birth or at the time of diagnosis.

Resources

BOOKS

Volpe, Joseph, J. *Neurology of the Newborn*, 4th edition. Philadelphia: W.B. Saunders Company, 2001.

PERIODICALS

Ecker, Jeffrey L., et al. "The Sonographic Diagnosis of Dandy-Walker and Dandy-Walker Variant: Associated Findings and Outcomes." *Prenatal Diagnosis* 20 (2000): 328–332.

Klein, O., et al. "Dandy-Walker Malformation: Prenatal Diagnosis and Prognosis." *Childs Nervous System* 19 (August 2003): 484–9.

Koble, Nicole, et al. "Dandy-Walker Malformation: Prenatal Diagnosis and Outcome." *Prenatal Diagnosis* 20 (2000): 318–327.

OTHER

NINDS Dandy-Walker Syndrome Information Page. The National Institute of Neurological Disorders and Stroke. April 2, 2003 (March 30, 2004). <http://www.ninds.nih.gov/health_and_medical/disorders/dandywalker.htm>.

ORGANIZATIONS

Dandy-Walker Syndrome Network. 5030 142nd Path W, Apple Valley, MN 55124. (952) 423-4008.

Hydrocephalus Association. 870 Market Street, Suite 705, San Francisco, CA 94102. (888) 598-3789; Fax: (415) 732-7044. <http://www.hydroassoc.org>.

Hydrocephalus Research Foundation. 1670 Green Oak Circle, Lawrenceville, GA 30243. (770) 995-9570; Fax: (770) 995-8982.

Hydrocephalus Support Group, Inc. PO Box 4236, Chesterfield, MO 63006-4236. (636) 532-8228; Fax: (314) 995-4108.

National Hydrocephalus Foundation. 12413 Centralia Road, Lakewood, CA 90715-1623. (888) 857-3434; Fax: (562) 924-6666. <http://nhfonline.org>.

Scott J. Polzin, MS, CGC

Dawson disease *see* **Subacute sclerosing parencephalitis**

de Morsier syndrome *see* **Septo-optic dysplasia**

Deafness *see* **Hearing disorders**

Decerebrate posturing *see* **Abnormal body posture**

Decorticate posturing *see* **Abnormal body posturing**

Deep brain stimulation

Definition

In deep brain stimulation (DBS), electrodes are implanted within the brain to deliver a continuous low electric current to the target area. The current is passed to the electrodes through a wire running under the scalp and skin to a battery-powered pulse generator implanted in the chest wall.

Purpose

DBS is used to treat **Parkinson's disease** (PD) and essential tremor (ET). It has also been used to treat **dystonia**, chronic **pain**, and several other conditions

The **movement disorders** of PD and ET are due to loss of regulation in complex circuits within the brain that control movement. While the cause of the two diseases differ, in both cases, certain parts of the brain become overactive. Surgical treatment can include destruction of part of the overactive portion, thus rebalancing the regulation within the circuit. It was discovered that the same effect could be obtained by electrically stimulating the same areas, which is presumed to shut down the cells without killing them.

DBS may be appropriate for patients with PD or ET whose symptoms are not adequately controlled by medications. In PD, this may occur after five to ten years of successful treatment. Continued disease progression leads to decreased effectiveness of the main treatment for PD, levodopa. Increasing doses are needed to control symptoms, and over time, this leads to development of unwanted movements, or dyskinesias. Successful DBS allows a reduction in levodopa, diminishing dyskinesias.

For PD, deep brain stimulation is performed on either the globus pallidus internus (GPi) or the subthalamic nucleus (STN). Treatment of essential tremor usually targets the thalamus. Each of these brain regions has two halves, which control movement on the opposite side of the body: right controls left, and left controls right. Unilateral (one-sided) DBS may be used if the symptoms are much more severe on one side. Bilateral DBS is used to treat symptoms on both sides.

Precautions

DBS is major brain surgery. Bleeding is a risk, and patients with bleeding disorders or who are taking blood thinning agents may require special management. DBS leaves metal electrodes implanted in the head, and patients are advised not to undergo diathermy (tissue heating) due to the risk of severe complications or death. Diathermy is used to treat chronic pain and other conditions. Special cautions are required for patients undergoing **MRI** after implantation.

Description

In DBS, a long thin electrode is planted deep within the brain, through a hole in the top of the skull. To make sure the electrode is planted in the proper location, a rigid "stereotactic frame" is attached to the patient's head before surgery. This device provides a three-dimensional coordinate system, used to locate the target tissue and to track the placing of the electrodes.

A single "burr hole" is made in the top of the skull for a unilateral procedure. Two holes are made for a bilateral procedure. This requires a topical anesthetic. General anesthesia is not used, for two reasons. First, the brain does not feel any pain. Second, the patient must be awake and responsive in order to respond to the neurosurgical team as they monitor the placement of the electrode. The target structures are close to several nerve tracts that carry information throughout the brain. Abnormalities in vision, speech, or other cognitive areas may indicate that the electrode is too close to one of these regions, and thus needs repositioning.

Other procedures may be used to ensure precise placement of the electrode, including electrical recording and injection of a contrast dye into the spinal fluid. The electrical recording can cause some minor odd sensations, but is harmless.

The electrode is connected by a wire to an implanted pulse generator. This wire is placed under the scalp and skin. A small incision is made in the area of the collarbone, and the pulse generator is placed there. This portion of the procedure is performed under general anesthesia.

Preparation

A variety of medical tests are needed before the day of surgery to properly locate the target (GPi, thalamus, or STN), and fit the frame. These may include CT scans, MRI, and injection of dyes into the spinal fluid or ventricles of the brain. The frame is attached to the head on the day of surgery, which may be somewhat painful, although the pain is lessened by local anesthetic. A mild sedative is given to ease anxiety.

Aftercare

Implantation of the electrodes, wire, and pulse generator is a lengthy procedure, and the patient will require a short hospital stay afterward to recovery from the surgery. Following this, the patient will meet several times with the **neurologist** to adjust the stimulator settings, in order to get maximum symptomatic improvement. The batteries in the pulse generator must be replaced every three to five years. This is done with a small incision as an outpatient procedure.

The patient's medications are adjusted after surgery. Most PD patients will need less levodopa after surgery, especially those who receive DBS of the STN.

Risks

Risks from DBS include the surgical risks or hemorrhage and infection, as well as the risks of general anesthesia. Patients who are cognitively impaired may become

more so after surgery. Electrodes can be placed too close to other brain regions, which can lead to visual defects, speech problems, and other complications. If these occur, they may be partially reduced by adjusting the stimulation settings. DBS leaves significant hardware in place under the skin, which can malfunction or break, requiring removal or replacement.

Normal results

Deep brain stimulation improves the movement symptoms of PD by 25–75%, depending on how carefully the electrodes are placed in the optimal target area, and how effectively the settings can be adjusted. These improvements are seen most while off levodopa; DBS does little to improve the best response to levodopa treatment. DBS does allow a reduction in levodopa dose, which usually reduces dyskinesias by 50% or more. This is especially true for DBS of the STN; DBS of the GPi may lead to a smaller reduction. Levodopa dose will likely be reduced, leading to a significant reduction in dyskinesias.

DBS in essential tremor may reduce tremor in the side opposite the electrode by up to 80%.

Resources

BOOKS

Jahanshahi, M., and C. D. Marsden. *Parkinson's Disease: A Self-Help Guide.* New York: Demos Medical Press, 2000.

WEBSITES

National Parkinson's Disease Foundation. (December 4, 2003). <www.npf.org>.

WE MOVE. (December 4, 2003). <www.wemove.org>.

ORGANIZATIONS

International Essential Tremor Foundation. P.O. Box 14005, Lenexa, Kansas 66285-4005. 913-341-3880 or 888-387-3667; Fax: 913-341-1296. staff@essentialtremor.org. <http://www.essentialtremor.org/>.

Richard Robinson

Delirium

Definition

Delirium is a transient, abrupt, usually reversible syndrome characterized by a disturbance that impairs consciousness, cognition (ability to think), and perception.

Description

The word delirium is derived from the Latin *delirare* which literally translates "to go out of the furrow." Delirium is typically an acute change in thinking with a disturbance in consciousness. Delirium is not a disease, but a syndrome that can occur as a result of many different underlying conditions. Typically, there is a broad range of accompanying symptoms. Delirium is also called acute confusional state. Delirium is a medical emergency and affects 10–30% of hospitalized patients with medical illness. It is a widespread condition that affects more than 50% of persons in certain high-risk population. Often the condition can be reversed, but delirium is associated with increased morbidity and mortality rates.

Demographics

Patients who develop delirium during hospitalization have a mortality rate of 22–76% and a high death rate months after discharge. Approximately 80% of patients develop delirium near death, and 40% of patients in the intensive care units have symptoms of delirium. The prevalence of postoperative delirium following general surgery is 5–10%, and 42% following orthopedic surgery. Delirium is very common in nursing homes. The exact incidence of delirium in emergency departments is unknown. Delirium is present in approximately 20% of medical patients at the time of hospital admission. The prevalence in hospitalized patients is approximately 10% on a general medical service, 8–12% on a psychiatric service, 35–80% on a geriatric unit, and 40% on a neurologic service. In the elderly and postoperative patients, delirium may result in long-term disability, increased complications, and prolonged hospital stay. Geriatric patients have the highest risk for developing delirium. The incidence is higher among young children, females, and Caucasians. Medications are the most common cause of delirium in the elderly, which accounts for 22–39% of cases. Medications are the most common reversible causes of delirium. Approximately 25% of hospitalized patients with cancer and 30–40% of patients with HIV (**AIDS**) infection develop delirium during hospitalizations.

Abnormal mechanisms causing delirium

There are three types of delirium based on the state of arousal. They include hyperactive delirium, hypoactive delirium, and mixed delirium. The hyperactive delirium is associated with drug intake such as alcohol withdrawal (or intoxication), amphetamine, phencyclidine (PCP), and lysergic acid diethylamide (LSD), a psychedelic compound. Hypoactive delirium is observed in patients with hypercapnia and hepatic **encephalopathy**. Patients who exhibit mixed delirium often exhibit nocturnal agitation, behavioral problems, and daytime sedation. The exact pathophysiological mechanisms that elicit delirium are not fully understood. Research that primarily studied subjects with alcohol withdrawal and hepatic encephalopathy indicated that delirium is caused by a reversible impairment of cerebral oxidative metabolism and multiple neurotransmitter abnormalities.

Key Terms

Central nervous system (CNS) Contains the brain and spinal cord.

Cerebral oxidative metabolism Using oxygen to generate energy by complex chemical reactions that occur in brain cells.

Dementia A disorder characterized by loss of intellectual abilities; impairments in judgment, abstract thinking, and memory; and personality changes.

Hepatic encephalopathy A change in mental state due to toxic substance buildup in the blood that is caused by liver failure.

Hypercapnia Excess carbon dioxide in the blood.

Hypoglycemia Low levels of glucose in the blood.

Interleukins Chemicals released in the body as a result of stress to the body.

Neurotransmitter abnormality

Acetylcholine is an excitatory chemical in the **central nervous system** (CNS). Anticholinergic medications, which disrupt release of acetylcholine, typically cause acute confusional states (delirium). Additionally, patients with diseases such as Alzheimer's disease with impaired cholinergic transmission and decreased acetylcholine are susceptible to delirium. Patients who develop postoperative delirium have an increase in serum anticholinergic activity.

Another neurotransmitter in the brain called dopamine causes delirium if there is an excess of dopaminergic activity. Dopaminergic and cholinergic activity in the brain exhibit a reciprocal relationship (i.e., a decrease in cholinergic activity leads to delirium, while an increase in dopaminergic activity leads to delirium). Studies have demonstrated that serotonin levels are increased in patients with septic delirium and encephalopathy. Serotoninergic agents, which are medications that may have unwanted side effects, leading to impaired serotonin release, can also cause delirium. Gama-aminobutyric acid (GABA) is an inhibitory neurochemical in the central nervous system. GABA is increased in patients with hepatic encephalopathy; this is probably caused by increases in ammonia levels.

Inflammatory mechanisms

Recent research indicates that there is a role for specific chemical mediators such as interleukin-1 (IL-1) and interleukin-6 (IL-6). These chemical mediators are released from cells after a broad range of infectious and toxic insults. Head trauma and ischemia, which are frequently associated with delirium, cause brain responses that are mediated by IL-1 and IL-6. Abnormal release can cause damage to nerve cells.

Structural mechanisms

Specific objective nerve pathways in the brain that induce delirium are unknown. Neuroimaging studies in patients with **traumatic brain injury** (TBI), **stroke**, and hepatic encephalopathy indicate that certain anatomical nerve pathways may contribute to a delirious state more than others. A specific pathway called the dorsal tegmental is also involved in delirium.

Summary of causes

In general, the causes of delirium fall within 11 categories: infectious, withdrawal, acute metabolic, trauma, CNS disease, hypoxic, deficiencies, environmental, acute vascular, toxins/drugs, and heavy metals. Examples of diseases or disorders in each category include:

- infectious: sepsis (infections that spread in blood and cause infections in the brain), encephalitis, meningitis, syphilis, CNS abscess

- withdrawal: as a result of drug withdrawal from alcohol or sedatives

- acute metabolic: acidosis, electrolyte disturbance, liver and kidney failure, other metabolic disturbances (glucose, Mg++, Ca++, conditions that affect the body's regulation of acid and electrolyte balance)

- trauma: head trauma, burns (delirium can occur secondary to traumatic events or severe burns)

- CNS disease such as stroke, bleeding in the brain, or seizures

- **hypoxia**: as a result of hypoxia (lack of oxygen), chronic obstructive lung disease (e.g., emphysema, bronchitis), or low blood pressure

- deficiencies of vitamins, especially B-complex vitamins

- environmental: severe changes in body temperature, either a decrease (hypothermia) or an increase (hyperthermia); hormonal imbalance (diabetes and thyroid problems)

- acute vascular: conditions affecting blood vessels in the brain, such as hemorrhage or blockage of a blood vessel from a clot

- toxins/drugs: chemical toxins such as street drugs, alcohol, pesticides, industrial poisons, carbon monoxide, cyanide, and solvents

- heavy metals: exposure to certain metals such as lead or mercury

Other common causes of delirium include hypoglycemia and hyperthermia.

Diagnostic criteria for delirium

The diagnosis of delirium is clinical, requiring physical examination and the analysis of symptoms because there is no single test that can successfully measure this condition. A careful history is essential to establish the diagnosis. Delirium is clinically characterized by an acutely transient alteration in mental status. Patients can have problems in orientation and short-term memory, difficulty sustaining attention, poor insight, and impaired judgment. In the hyperactive subtype of delirium, patients have an increased state of arousal, hypervigilance, and psychomotor abnormalities. Conversely, patients with the hypoactive subtype are typically withdrawn, less active, and sleepy. The mixed subtype category often presents with delirium as the primary symptom of an underlying illness. Mental status can be checked quickly and should include assessment of memory, attention, concentration, orientation, constructional tasks, spatial discrimination, writing, and arithmetic ability. Two of the most sensitive indicators for delirium are dysgraphia (impaired writing ability) and dysnomia (inability to name objects correctly).

Psychological deficit

The psychological diagnostic criteria for delirium include:

- change in cognition (i.e., disorientation, language disturbance, perceptual disturbance): this alteration cannot be accounted for by a preexisting, established, or evolving dementia

- disturbance of consciousness (i.e., reduced clarity of awareness of the environment) occurs with a reduction in ability to focus, maintain, or shift (change) attention

- the alterations develop over a short period (hours to days) and exhibit fluctuation during the day

- evidence exists from history, medical and/or laboratory findings, which indicates that the delirium is caused by a general medical condition, substance intoxication, substance withdrawal, medication use, or more than one cause (multiple etiologies)

Diagnostic instruments

There are several instruments that help establish the diagnosis of delirium. They include the Confusion Assessment Method (CAM), the Delirium Symptom Interview (DSI), and the Folstein Mini-Mental State Examination (MMSE). Delirium symptom severity can be assessed utilizing the Memorial Delirium Assessment Scale (MDAS) and the Delirium Rating Scale (DRS).

Lab studies

Glucose levels can help diagnose delirium causes by hypoglycemia or uncontrolled diabetes. A complete blood count with differential cell analysis can help to diagnose infection and anemia. Electrolyte analysis can diagnose high or low levels. Renal (kidney) and liver function test (LFTs) can diagnose liver and/or kidney failure. Other tests that can assist with identifying the underlying cause of delirium include urine analysis (urinary tract infections), urine/blood drug screen (to diagnose the presence of toxic substance), thyroid function tests (to diagnose an underfunctioning thyroid gland, a condition called hypothyroidism), and special tests to diagnose bacterial and viral causes of infection.

Neuroimaging studies such as computerized axial tomography (CAT) and **magnetic resonance imaging (MRI)** can be helpful to establish a diagnosis due to structural lesions or hemorrhage. Electroencephalogram (EEG), a special test that records brain activity in waves can be helpful to establish a diagnosis, especially in patients with hepatic encephalopathy (diffuse slow waves) and alcohol/sedative withdrawal (faster wave pattern).

Treatment

Clinicians must be vigilant to aggressively identify the underlying etiology of delirium, since the condition is a medical emergency. Symptomatic treatment for delirium may include the use of antipsychotic drugs. These medications help to control hallucinations, agitation, and help to improve the level of orientation and attention abilities (sensorium). Haloperidol (Haldol) is a highly researched medication and is often administered in the symptomatic management of delirium. The typical dose for patients with delirium of moderate severity is 1–2 mg twice daily and repeated every four hours as needed. Haldol can be administered orally, intravenously, or by intramuscular injection. Elderly patients should start with lower doses of Haldol, typically 0.25–1.0 mg twice daily and repeated every four hours as needed.

Environmental interventions

Treatment of delirium can be worsened by over stimulation or under stimulation in the environment. It is important to provide support and orientation to the patient. Additionally, providing the patients an environment with few distractions such as removing unnecessary objects in the room, use of clear language when talking to them, and avoidance of sensory extremes can be conducive to treatment planning.

Clinical trials

Information concerning **clinical trials** and research on delirium can be obtained from the National Institutes of Health (NIH). Research related to delirium is active at the Mayo Clinic Foundation, including research on Alzhiemer's disease, postoperative delirium in orthopedic surgical patients, and pharmacological treatment of **Parkinson's disease**.

Resources

BOOKS

Marx, John A., et al. (eds). *Rosen's Emergency Medicine: Concepts and Clinical Practice*, 5th ed. St. Louis: Mosby, Inc., 2002.

PERIODICALS

Chan, D., and N. Brennan. "Delirium: Making the Diagnosis, Improving the Prognosis." *Geriatrics* 54, no. 3 (March 1999).

Francis, J. "Three Millennia of Delirium Research: Moving Beyond Echoes of the Past." *Journal of the American Geriatrics Society* 47, no. 11 (1999).

Gleason, O. "Delirium." *American Family Physician* (March 2003).

Samuels, S., and M. M. Evers. "Delirium: Pragmatic Guidance for Managing a Common, Confounding, and Sometimes Lethal Condition." *Geriatrics* 57, no. 6 (June 2002).

WEBSITES

Delirium. (May 20, 2004) <http://omni.ac.uk>.

National Cancer Institute. (May 20, 2004) <http://www.cancer.gov>.

Association of Cancer Online Resources. (May 20, 2004) <http://www.acor.org>.

ORGANIZATIONS

National Institute of Neurological Disorders and Stroke (NINDS) Neurological Institute. P.O. Box 5801, Bethesda, MD 20824.

Laith Farid Gulli, MD
Nicole Mallory, MS, PA-C
Robert Ramirez, DO

Dementia with Lewy bodies *see* **Lewy body dementia**

Dementia, subcortical *see* **Binswanger disease, Dementia**

Dementia

Definition

The term dementia refers to symptoms, including changes in memory, personality, and behavior, that result from a change in the functioning of the brain. These declining changes are severe enough to impair the ability of a person to perform a function or to interact socially. This operating definition encompasses 70–80 different types of dementia. They include changes due to diseases (Alzheimer's and Creutzfeld-Jakob diseases), changes due to a heart attack or repeated blows to the head (as suffered by boxers), and damage due to long-term alcohol abuse.

Dementia is not the same thing as **delirium** or **mental retardation**. Delirium is typically a brief state of mental confusion often associated with hallucinations. Mental retardation is a condition that usually dates from childhood and is characterized by impaired intellectual ability; mentally retarded individuals typically have IQ (intelligence quotient) scores below 70 or 75.

Description

The absent-mindedness and confusion about familiar settings and tasks that are hallmarks of dementia used to be considered as part of a typical aging pattern in the elderly. Indeed, dementia historically has been called senility. Dementia is now recognized not to be a normal part of aging. The symptoms of dementia can result from different causes. Some of the changes to the brain that cause dementia are treatable and can be reversed, while other changes are irreversible.

Demographics

An estimated two million people in the United States alone have severe dementia. Up to five million more people in the United States have milder forms of cognitive impairment of the dementia type. The elderly are most prone to dementia, particularly those at risk for a **stroke**. The historical tendency of women to live longer than men has produced a higher prevalence of dementia in older women. However, women and men are equally prone to dementia. Over age 80, more than 20% of people have at least a mild form of dementia.

Causes and symptoms

Dementia is especially prominent in older people. The three main irreversible causes are Alzheimer's disease, dementia with Lewy bodies, and **multi-infarct dementia** (also called vascular dementia).

Degenerative forms of dementia are long lasting (chronic) and typically involve a progressive loss of brain cell function. In disorders like Alzheimer's and Creutzfeld-Jakob diseases, this can involve the presence of infectious agents that disturb the structure of proteins that are vital for cell function. Other forms of dementia are chemically based. For example, **Parkinson's disease** involves the progressive loss of the ability to produce the neurotransmitter dopamine. Interrupted transmission of nerve impulses causes the progressive physical and mental deterioration. Huntington's disease is an inherited form of dementia that occurs when neurons (brain cells) degenerate.

Key Terms

Amyloid plaques A waxy protein substance that forms clumps in brain tissues, leading to brain cell death as in Alzheimer disease.

Lewy bodies Spheres, found in the bodies of dying cells, that are considered to be a marker for Parkinson's disease.

Multi-infarct dementia Deterioration in mental function caused by numerous areas in the brain where narrowing of blood vessels has resulted in atherosclerotic plaque formation and damage to brain cells.

Alzheimer's disease is the most common cause of dementia. The progressive death of nerve cells in the brain is associated with the formation of clumps (amyloid plaques) and tangles of protein (neurofibrillary tangles) in the brain. The loss of brain cells with time is reflected in the symptoms; minor problems with memory become worse, and impairment in normal function can develop. Alzheimer's patients also have a lower level of a chemical that relays nerve impulses between nerve cells. As the brain damage progresses, other complications can ensue from the damage and these can prove fatal. Put another way, people die with Alzheimer's, not from it.

Dementia resulting from the abnormal formation of protein in the brain (Lewy bodies) is the second most common form of dementia in the elderly. It is unclear whether these structures are related to the brain abnormalities noted in Alzheimer's patients. Lewy body formation differs from Alzheimer's in that the speed of brain functions is affected more so than memory.

In multi-infarct dementia, blood clots can dislodge and impede the flow of blood in blood vessels in the brain. The restricted flow of blood can lead to death of brain cells and a stroke.

Dementias that are caused by the blockage of blood vessels are generally known as vascular dementia. This type of dementia can sometimes be reversed if the blood-vessel blockage can be alleviated. In contrast, the dementia associated with Alzheimer's disease is non-reversible.

Less common causes of dementia include Binwanger's disease (another vascular type of dementia), Parkinson's disease, Pick's disease, Huntington's disease, **Creutzfeldt-Jakob disease**, and acquired immunodeficiency syndrome (**AIDS**).

A study published in 2002 documented a link between elevated levels of an amino acid called homocysteine in the blood and the risk of developing dementia, likely vascular dementia. As homocysteine concentration can be modified by diet, the finding holds the potential that one risk factor for dementia may be controllable.

Symptoms of dementia include repeatedly asking the same question; loss of familiarity with surroundings; increasing difficulty in following directions; difficulty in keeping track of time, people, and locations; loss of memory; changes in personality or emotion; and neglect of personal care. Not everyone displays all symptoms. Indeed, symptoms vary based on the cause of the dementia. Also, symptoms can progress at different rates in different people.

Diagnosis

Diagnosis of dementia typically involves a medical examination, testing of mental responses (such as memory, problem solving, and counting), and knowledge of the patient's medical history (e.g., prescription and non-prescription drug use, nutrition, results of a physical examination, and medical history). Testing of the composition of the blood and urine can be helpful in ruling out specific causes such as thyroid disease or a deficiency in vitamin B_{12}. Some blood tests can help alert clinicians to the possibility of dementia. For example, persons infected with the human immunodeficiency virus (HIV) have distinct proteins in their blood that are often associated with the presence of dementia.

Visual examination of the brain can reveal structural abnormalities associated with dementia. Tests that are typically performed are computerized tomography (CT), **magnetic resonance imaging (MRI)**, and **positron emission tomography (PET)**. While accurate, such tests are not commonplace, and are rarely encountered outside of the research setting. Neuroimaging (**CT** or **MRI** scans) can be useful in excluding the possibility that dementia has resulted from an occlusion of a blood vessel, as in a stroke or due to the presence of a tumor.

Treatment team

Family physicians, medical specialists such as neurologists and psychiatrists, physical therapists, counselors, personal caregivers, and family members can all be part of the treatment team for someone afflicted with dementia.

Treatment

Drugs can help delay the progression of symptoms, particularly for Alzheimer's disease. The high blood pressure that is associated with multi-infarct dementia can also be controlled by drug therapy. Other stroke risk factors that can be treated include cholesterol level, diabetes, and

smoking. Medicines such as antidepressants, antipsychotics, and **anxiolytics** can also be used to treat behaviors associated with dementia, including insomnia, anxiety, **depression**, and nervousness.

Other treatments that do not involve drugs are the maintenance of a healthy diet, regular **exercise**, stimulating activities and social contacts, and making the home as safe as possible. Hobbies can help keep the mind occupied and stimulated. "Things-to-do" lists can be a helpful memory prompt for persons with early dementia. With more advanced disease, a facility specializing in Alzheimer's treatment often provides a stimulating modified environment along with meeting increasing medical and personal care needs.

Recovery and rehabilitation

Irreversible causes of dementia reduce or eliminate the chances of recovery and rehabilitation. Stimuli such as favorite family photographs and calendars provide clues to cognitive orientation, while devices such as walkers help maintain mobility for as long as possible.

Clinical trials

As of early 2004, there are 64 **clinical trials** for dementia study and treatment in the United States that are recruiting subjects. The trials range from improved strategies of care and telephone support to active interventions in the outcome of various forms of dementia. The bulk of the trials are concerned with Alzheimer's disease. Information about the trials can be found at the National Institutes of Health (NIH) sponsored clinical trials website.

Prognosis

For those with irreversible progressive dementia, the outlook often includes slow deterioration in mental and physical capacities. Eventually, help is often required when swallowing, walking, and even sitting become difficult. Aid can consist of preparing special diets that can be more easily consumed and making surroundings safe in case of falls. Lift assists in areas such as the bathroom can also be useful.

For those with dementia, the expected lifespan is often reduced from that of a healthy person. For example, in Alzheimer's disease, deterioration of areas of the brain that are vital for body functions can threaten survival.

Special concerns

Caring for an individual with dementia almost always challenges family resources. Licensed social service providers at hospitals and facilities for the elderly can provide information and referrals regarding support groups, mental health agencies, community resources, and personal care providers to assist families in caring for a person with dementia.

Resources

BOOKS

Bird, T. D. "Memory Loss and Dementia." In *Harrison's Principles of Internal Medicine*, 15th edition. Edited by A. S. Franci, E. Daunwald, and K. J. Isrelbacher. New York: McGraw Hill, 2001.

Castleman, Michael, et al. *There's Still a Person in There: The Complete Guide to Treating and Coping With Alzheimer's.* New York: Perigee Books, 2000.

Mace, Nancy L., and Peter V. Rabins. *The 36-Hour Day: A Family Guide to Caring for Persons with Alzheimer Disease, Related Dementing Illnesses, and Memory Loss in Later Life.* New York: Warner Books, 2001.

PERIODICALS

Sullivan, S. C., and K. C. Richards. "Special Section—Behavioral Symptoms of Dementia: Their Measurement and Intervention." *Aging and Mental Health* (February 2004): 143–152.

Seshadri, S., et al. "Plasma Homocysteine as a Risk Factor for Dementia and Alzheimer's Disease." *New England Journal of Medicine* (February 2002): 476–483.

OTHER

Mayo Clinic. *Dementia: It's Not Always Alzheimer's.* December 23, 2003 (March 30, 2004). <http://www.mayoclinic.com/invoke.cfm?id=AZ00003>.

National Institute on Aging. *Forgetfulness: It's Not Always What You Think.* December 23, 2003 (March 30, 2004). <http://www.niapublications.org/engagepages/forgetfulness.asp>.

ORGANIZATIONS

Alzheimer's Association. 919 Michigan Avenue, Suite 1100, Chicago, IL 60611-1676. (312) 335-8700 or (800) 272-3900; Fax: (312) 335-1110. info@alz.org. <http://www.alz.org>.

Alzheimer's Disease Education and Referral Center. P. O. Box 8250, Silver Spring, MD 20907-8250. (301) 495-3334 or (800) 438-4380. adear@alzheimers.org. <http://www.alzheimers.org>.

National Institute on Aging. 31 Center Drive, MSC 2292, Building 31, Room 5C27, Bethesda, MD 20892. (301) 496-1752 or (800) 222-2225. karpf@nia.nih.gov. <http://www.nia.nih.gov>.

National Institute for Neurological Disorders and Stroke. P. O. Box 5801, Bethesda, MD 20824. (301) 496-5761 or (800) 352-9424. <http://www.ninds.nih.gov>.

National Institute of Mental Health. 6001 Executive Boulevard, Room 8184, MSC 9663, Bethesda, MD 20892-9663. (301) 443-4513 or (866) 615-6464; Fax: (301) 443-4279. nimhinfo@nih.gov. <http://www.nimh.nih.gov>.

Brian Douglas Hoyle, PhD

Depression

Definition

When discussing depression as a symptom, a feeling of hopelessness is the most often described sensation. Depression is a common psychiatric disorder in the modern world and a growing cause of concern for health agencies worldwide due to the high social and economic costs involved. Symptoms of depression, like the disorder itself, vary in degree of severity, and contribute to mild to severe mood disturbances. Mood disturbances may range from a sudden transitory decrease in motivation and concentration to gloomy moods and irritation, or to severe, chronic prostration.

With treatment, more than 80% of people with depression respond favorably to medications, and the feeling of hopelessness subsides. With treatment, most people are able to resume their normal work and social activities.

Depression may occur at almost any stage of life, from childhood to middle or old age, as a result of a number of different factors that lead to chemical changes in the brain. Traumatic experiences, chronic stress, emotional loss, dysfunctional interpersonal relationships, social isolation, biological changes, aging, and inherited predisposition are common triggers for the symptoms of depression. Depression is classified according to the symptoms displayed and patterns of occurrence. Types of depression include major depressive disorder, bipolar depressive disorder, psychotic depressive disorder, postpartum depression, premenstrual dysphoric disorder, and seasonal disorder. Additional types of depression are included under the label of atypical depressive disorder. Many symptoms overlap among the types of depression, and not all people with depression experience all the symptoms associated with their particular type of the disorder.

Description

Symptoms of a depressive disorder include at least five of the following changes in the individual's previous characteristics: loss of motivation and inability to feel pleasure; deep chronic sadness or distress; changes in sleep patterns; lack of physical energy (apathy); feelings of hopelessness and worthlessness; difficulty with concentration; overeating or loss of appetite; withdrawal from interpersonal interactions or avoidance of others; death wishes, or belief in his/her own premature death. In children, the first signs of depression may be irritation and loss of concentration, apathy and distractibility during classes, and social withdrawal. Some adults initially complain of constant **fatigue**, even after long hours of sleep, digestive disorders, headaches, anxiety, recurrent memory lapses, and insomnia or excessive sleeping. An episode of major

Key Terms

Anorexia Loss of appetite.

Bipolar disorder A mood disorder characterized by periods of excitability (mania) alternating with periods of depression.

Dysthymia A chronic mood disorder characterized by mild depression.

Major depressive disorder A mood disorder characterized by overwhelming and persistent feelings of hopelessness, often accompanied by sleep disturbances, withdrawal from normal social and personal care activities, and an inability to concentrate.

Manic A period of excess mental activity, often accompanied by elevated mood and disorganized behavior.

Serotonin A type of neurotransmitter, a brain chemical that carries messages between brain cells. Low levels of serotonin in the brain are associated with feelings of depression.

depression may be preceded by a period of dysthymia, a mild but persistent low mood state, usually accompanied by diminished sexual drive, decreased affective response, and loss of interest in normal social activities and hobbies.

Most individuals with depression have difficulty in dealing with the challenges of daily life, and even minor obstacles or difficulties may trigger exaggerated emotional responses. Frustrating situations are frequently met with feelings of despair, dejection, resentment, and worthlessness, with people easily desisting from their goals. People with depression may try to avoid social situations and interpersonal interactions. Some people with depression overeat, while others show a sharp loss of appetite (anorexia). In some individuals, medical treatments for some other existing illness may also cause depression as an adverse reaction. For instance, antihypertensive drugs, steroids, muscle relaxants, anticancer drugs, and opioids, as well as extensive surgery such as a coronary bypass, may lead to depression. Cancer and other degenerative diseases, chronic painful conditions, metabolic diseases or hormonal changes during adolescence, or after childbirth, menopause, or old age may be potential triggers for depression. When the first onset of depression occurs after the age of 60, there is a greater possibility that the causative factor is a cerebrovascular (blood vessels in the brain) degeneration.

Molecular genetics research has recently shown that mutations in a gene coding for a protein that transports serotonin (a neurotransmitter) to neurons may determine how an individual will cope with stressful situations. A two-decade study involving 847 people of both sexes has shown that those who inherited two copies of the long version of the gene 5-HTT have a 17% risk of suffering a major depressive episode due to exposure to four or more identified stressful situations in their lives, whereas those with one long and one short version of the gene had the risk increased to 33%. The study has also shown that individuals with two short copies of the gene have a 43% probability of a major depressive episode when exposed to four or more stressful life events. The shorter version of the gene 5-HTT does not directly causes depression, but offers less protection against the harmful effects of traumatic or stressful situations to the brain. Studies of population genetics have also shown that about 50% of the world's Caucasian population carry one short and one long version of 5-HTT genes.

Depressive episodes may be associated with additional psychiatric disorders. Neurotic depression is often triggered by one or more adverse life events or traumatic experiences that have historically caused anxiety in the life of the person experiencing depression. For example, loss of social or economical status, chronic failure in living up to the expectations of parents, teachers, or bosses, death of a close relation, work-related competitive pressures, and other stressful situations such as accidents, urban violence, wars, and catastrophic events may lead to a depressive episode. Conversely, anxiety disorders such as panic syndrome, phobias, generalized anxiety, and post-traumatic stress disorder may trigger a major depressive crisis. Psychotic depressive disorders are likely to be associated with other psychiatric diseases or caused by them. Eating disorders such as bulimia, anorexia nervosa, and binge-eating disorder are generally accompanied by depression or may be caused by an existing depressive state. Neurodegenerative diseases such as Alzheimer's, Huntington's, and Parkinson's diseases frequently have depression among their symptoms.

Dysthymia is a mild but chronic depressed state, characterized by melancholic moods, low motivation, poor affective responsiveness, and a tendency for self isolation. A dysthymic state lasting two years or longer is a risk factor for the onset of a major depressive episode. However, many dysthymic individuals experience a chronic low mood state throughout their daily lives. Dysthymia is a frequent occurrence in individuals involved in chronic dysfunctional marriages or unsatisfying work conditions. Such chronic stressful situations alter the brain's neurochemistry, thus the opportunity arises for symptoms of depression to develop.

Psychotic depression is a particularly serious illness and possesses biological and cognitive (thought) components. Psychotic depression involves disturbances in

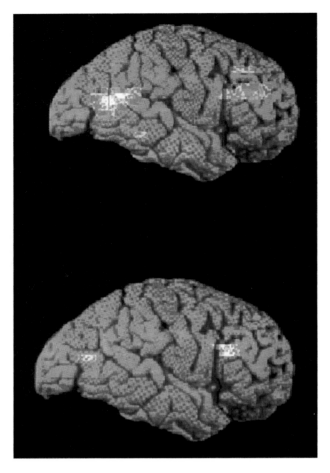

Colored positron emission tomography (PET) scans showing the brain of a depressed person (top) and the brain of a healthy person. (*© Photo Researchers. Reproduced by permission.*)

brain neurochemistry as a consequence of either a congenital (from birth) condition or due to prolonged exposure to stress or abuse during early childhood. Prolonged exposure to severe stress or abuse in the first decade of life induces both neurochemical and structural permanent changes in the developing brain with a direct impact on emotional aspects of personality. Normal patterns of perception and reaction give way to flawed mechanisms in order for a person to cope with chronic fear, abuse, and danger. Perception becomes fear-oriented and conditioned to constantly scan the environment for danger, with the flight-or-fight impulse underlying the individual's reactions. Delusions, misinterpretation of interpersonal signals, and a pervading feeling of worthlessness may impair the individual's ability to deal with even minor frustrations or obstacles, precipitating deep and prolonged episodes of depression, often with a high risk of suicide. Hallucinations may also occur, such as hearing voices or experiencing visions, as part of depression with psychosis.

A major depressive disorder (MDD) or clinical depression may consist of a single episode of severe depression requiring treatment or constitute the initial sign of a more complex disorder such as bipolar disorder. MDD may last for several months or even years if untreated and is associated with a high risk of suicide. In bipolar disorder, manic (hyper-excited and busy) periods alternate with deep depressive episodes, and are characterized by abnormal euphoria (an exaggerated feeling of happiness and well-being) and reckless behavior, followed by deep distress and prostration, often requiring hospitalization.

Major episodes of depression may last for one or more years if not treated, leading to a deep physical and emotional prostration. The person with major depression often moves very slowly and reports a sensation of heaviness in the arms and legs, with simple walking requiring an overwhelming effort. Personal hygiene is neglected and the person often desires to stay secluded or in bed for days or weeks. Suicidal thoughts may frequently occupy the mind or become recurrent patterns of thinking. Painful or unsettling memories are often recalled, and contribute to feelings of helplessness.

Atypical depression causes a cyclic behavior, alternating periods of severe and mild depressive states, punctuated by mood swings, hypersensitivity, oversleeping, overeating, with or without intermittent panic attacks. This depressive disorder is more common in women, with the onset usually occurring during adolescence.

Premenstrual dysphoric disorder (PDD) is not premenstrual stress. It is a more severe mood disorder that can cause deep depression or episodes of heightened irritation and aggressiveness, starting one or two weeks before menstruation and usually persisting during the entire period. Premenstrual dysphoric disorder is associated with abnormal changes in levels of hormones that affect brain neurochemistry.

Seasonal affective disorder (SAD) is caused by disturbances in the circadian cycle, a mechanism that controls conversion of serotonin into melatonin in the evening and mid-afternoon, and the conversion of melatonin into serotonin during daytime. Serotonin is the neurotransmitter responsible for sensations of satiety and emotional stability, which is converted at nighttime into melatonin, the hormone that regulates sleep and other functions. Some people are especially susceptible to the decreased exposure to daylight during long winter months and become depressed and irritable. Overeating and oversleeping during the winter season are common signs of seasonal affective disorder, along with irritation and depressed moods. However, as the amount of light increases during the spring and summer seasons, the symptoms disappear.

Postpartum depression is a severe and long-lasting depressive state also associated with abnormal changes in hormone levels affecting brain neurochemistry. If untreated, postpartum depression may last for months or even years, and is highly disruptive to family and maternal-child relations.

Without treatment, the risk of suicide as a consequence of depression should not be underestimated. Suicide accounts for approximately 15% of deaths among people with significant depression, and half of all suicide attempts in the United States are associated with depression. Persistent and recurrent depressive episodes are important contributors to other diseases alike such as myocardial infarction, hypertension, and other cardiovascular disorders.

Resources

BOOKS

Klein, Donald F., MD. *Understanding Depression: A Complete Guide to Its Diagnosis and Treatment.* New York: Oxford Press, 1995.

Solomon, Andrew. *The Noonday Demon: An Atlas of Depression.* New York: Scribners, 2002.

PERIODICALS

Manji, H. K., W. C. Drevets, and D. S. Charney. "The Cellular Neurobiology of Depression." *Nature Medicine* (May 2001) 7: 541–546.

Teicher, Martin H. "Wounds That Won't Heal—The Neurobiology of Child Abuse." *Scientific American* (March 2002): 68–75.

OTHER

National Institute of Mental Health. *Depression.* February 12, 2004 (March 31, 2004). <http://www.nimh.nih.gov/publicat/depression.cfm#ptdep1>.

ORGANIZATIONS

National Institute of Mental Health (NIMH). Office of Communications, 6001 Executive Boulevard, Room 8184, MSC 9663, Bethesda, MD 20892-9663. (301) 443-4513 or (800) 615-NIMH (6464); Fax: (301) 443-4279. nimhinfo@nih.gov. <http://www.nimh.nih.gov>.

Sandra Galeotti

Dermatomyositis

Definition

Dermatomyositis is one member of a group of diseases that are collectively called inflammatory myopathies. A **myopathy** is a disorder of a muscle. Hallmarks of dermatomyositis disease are a widespread rash and muscle weakness.

Description

Dermatomyositis is characterized by the onset of symptoms that can be severe, with rash and muscle weakness occurring over a large portion of the body. The term dermatomyositis stems from the root word "derm," referring to the skin, and the word "myositis," which means inflammation of muscles. Dermatomyositis, therefore, means an inflammation of the muscles and the skin. The disease was first described in 1887 in Germany.

Demographics

Both children and adults can be affected with dermatomyositis, but females are twice as likely to have the disorder as males. One-third of the cases occur in people over the age of 50. People of European ancestry have typically been more affected than people of African ancestry. As of 2004, however, the incidence of dermatomyositis is rising faster in African Americans than in whites. In the United States, the estimated prevalence of the disease is 5.5 cases per million people.

Causes and symptoms

The cause of dermatomyositis is a disruption in the functioning of the immune system, although the precise details of the malfunction are not yet known. While the basis of the disease may be due to a genetic mutation, conclusive evidence is lacking. Infection with certain viruses, or a bacterium called *Borrelia* (the cause of **Lyme disease**), has been suggested as possible triggers of the disease.

Dermatomyositis is often first apparent as a rash. The rash, which can be bluish-purple in color, reminiscent of bruising, typically occurs in patches on the face, neck, shoulders, upper portion of the chest, elbows, knuckles, knees, and back. Sometimes there can be accumulation of calcium as hard bumps underneath the skin in the region of the rash. The skin may break open and become very itchy, to the point of disturbing sleep.

The other principle symptom, which usually appears after the rash, but which can also be coincident with the rash, is muscle weakness. The muscles most often affected are those that are near the central part of the body, such as muscles of the chest and the upper arms and legs. As the disease progresses, muscles toward the outer parts of the arms and legs can weaken. As well, the affected muscles can become sore and painful to the touch.

The muscle weakness can make it hard for the affected person to get up from a sitting position, climb up stairs, lift even moderately heavy objects, and to reach up over their head. Swallowing can become difficult. People may also feel tired, lose weight, and develop a slight fever.

Except for the presence of rash, the symptoms of dermatomyositis are virtually the same as a related disease

Key Terms

Glucocorticoid medications A group of medications that produces effects of the body's own cortisone and cortisol. Glucocorticoids are commonly called steroids and, among other functions, work to reduce inflammation.

Myositis Inflammation of a muscle.

known as **polymyositis** (inflammation of many muscles). In about 40% of those with dermatomyositis, only the skin is affected. In these people, the disease can also be called amyopathic dermatomyositis (ADM), or DM sine myositis.

Diagnosis

Diagnosis is based on the presence of skin rash, muscle weakness, and higher than normal levels of some muscle enzymes (due to breakdown of muscle cells). A muscle **biopsy**, in which a sample of muscle is obtained, can reveal inflammation and the death of muscles cells associated with the weakening muscle.

Because of the presence of cancer in a significant proportion of elderly people who develop the disease, diagnosis is often accompanied by procedures like a chest x ray, mammogram in women, prostate examination in men, and sometimes a scan of the abdomen using the technique of computed tomography.

Treatment team

The treatment team for a case of dermatomyositis is typically made up of the family physician, **neurologist**, physical therapists, and family members or caregivers. Sometimes the team also includes a dermatologist (specialist in the structure, functions, and diseases of the skin) and a rheumatologist (specialist in conditions that cause swelling or **pain** in the muscles and joints).

Treatment

Treatment principally consists of therapy with glucocorticoid medications, which help quell an immune response that can exacerbate the rash. The steroid that is typically given is prednisone. In some people, this drug is not effective or tolerated well. Alternate drugs that can be given are azathioprine and methotrexate. An immune compound called immunoglobulin can also be given intravenously.

Recovery and rehabilitation

Physical therapy is often used to try to maintain or minimize the loss of muscle strength and function. As dermatomyositis is a chronic condition, emphasis is placed not on recovery, but on maintaining optimum muscle function.

Clinical trials

As of April 2004, there are seven **clinical trials** related to dermatomyositis or other related conditions recruiting participants in the United States. Some of the trials are evaluating new treatments such as novel drugs and irradiation. Other trials are trying to uncover how the disorder develops in children. Updated information about ongoing trials can be found at the National Institutes of Health website for clinical trials at <http://www.clinicaltrials.org>.

As well as the clinical trials, research is being undertaken to unravel the mechanisms of development of the disease, with a goal to prevent, treat, and ultimately, cure dermatomyositis.

Prognosis

The disease is seldom fatal, although muscle weakness can persist for life. Most cases of dermatomyositis do respond to therapy, which improves a person's outlook. However, the prognosis may not be as good if the disease is accompanied by heart or lung problems. In the latter cases, a person may become confined to a wheelchair. On rare occasions, heart or lung muscles weakened by dermatomyositis can cause death.

Special concerns

Approximately one-third of older people who develop dermatomyositis also have cancer. In some cases, the cancer may not yet be diagnosed. Therefore, a thorough physical examination of all body systems is important after receiving a diagnosis of dermatomyositis.

Resources

BOOKS

Parker J. N., and P. M. Parker. *The Official Parent's Sourcebook on Dermatomyositis: A Revised and Updated Directory for the Internet Age.* San Diego, Icon Group International, 2002.

PERIODICALS

Grogan, P. M., and J. S. Katz. "Inflammatory Myopathies." *Current Treatment Options in Neurology* (March 2004): 155–161.

OTHER

Callen, J. P. "Dermatomyositis." *eMedicine.* April 14, 2004 (May 27, 2004). <http://www.emedicine/com/derm/topic98.htm>.

"NINDS Dermatomyositis Information Page." *National Institute of Neurological Disorders and Stroke.* April 12, 2004 (May 27, 2004). <http://www.ninds.nih.gov/health_and_medical/disorders/dermato_doc.htm>.

ORGANIZATIONS

American Autoimmune Related Diseases Association. 22100 Gratiot Avenue, Eastpointe, MI 48201-2227. (586) 776-3900 or (800) 598-4668; Fax: (586) 776-3903. aarda@aol.com. <http://www.aarda.com>.

Myositis Association. 1233 20th Street, NW, Washington, DC 20036. (202) 887-0084 or (800) 821-7356; Fax: (202) 466-8940. tma@myositis.org. <http://www.myositis.org>.

National Institute for Neurological Diseases and Stroke (NINDS), 6001 Executive Boulevard, Bethesda, MD 20892. (301) 496-5751 or (800) 352-9424. <http://www.ninds.nih.gov>.

National Institute of Arthritis and Musculoskeletal and Skin Diseases (NIAMS). 31 Center Dr., Rm. 4C02 MSC 2350, Bethesda, MD 20892-2350. (301) 496-8190 or (877) 226-4267. NIAMSinfo@mail.nih.gov. <http://www.niams.nih.gov>.

National Organization for Rare Disorders. 55 Kenosia Avenue, Danbury, CT 06813-1968. (203) 744-0100 or (800) 999-6673; Fax: (203) 798-2291. orphan@rarediseases.org. <http://www.rarediseases.org>.

Brian Douglas Hoyle, PhD

Developmental dyspraxia *see* **Dyspraxia**

Devic syndrome

Definition

Devic Syndrome is a rare neurological disorder that affects both the protective sheet that lines the spinal cord and the optic nerve of the eye. People that have Devic syndrome lose the fatty covering of the spinal cord (myelin) and experience eye **pain** due to an exaggerated inflammatory response that occurs in the eye. The resulting spinal cord damage is known as **transverse myelitis** and the resulting eye inflammation is known as optic neuritis. Devic syndrome is a severe neurodegenerative disorder that can lead to blindness, paralysis, and incontinence (loss of bowel or bladder control).

Description

Devic syndrome is an autoimmune disorder that is considered by many scientists to be a form of **multiple sclerosis**, another neurodegenerative disease that affects the protective coating of the spinal cord called the myelin sheath. In Devic syndrome, the course of the disease is more rapid and severe. Symptoms typically observed in

---

Key Terms

Ataxia Loss of coordinated muscle movement caused by a disturbance of the nervous system.

Myelin sheath Insulating layer around some nerves that speeds the conduction of nerve signals.

Optic neuritis Inflammation of the optic nerve, often accompanied by vision loss.

Transverse myelitis A neurologic syndrome caused by inflammation of the spinal cord.

---

patients that have multiple sclerosis usually appear after symptoms associated with Devic syndrome, distinguishing the two neurodegenerative diseases. Devic syndrome is also known as Devic disease and neuromyelitis optica.

It is still controversial whether Devic syndrome is a variant of multiple sclerosis. It is considered by some scientists to be a variant of a disease caused by exposure to the varicella zoster virus that results in **acute disseminated encephalomyelitis** (ADEM).

Demographics

Devic syndrome can occur spontaneously, or in conjunction with multiple sclerosis or systemic **lupus** erythematosus. It affects males and females equally. Devic syndrome is a rare disorder, affecting less than an estimated five persons per million population per year.

Causes and symptoms

Devic syndrome is a chronic and degenerative disorder that usually affects both eyes. The eyes develop diminished sensitivity to bright lights, color vision impairment, and diminished light reflexes. Approximately two-thirds of persons with Devic syndrome experience complete visual loss. The symptoms begin with significant loss of vision that precedes muscle weakness, **ataxia** (coordination difficulties and unsteady gait, or manner of walking), and numbness. Inflammatory sites of attack are usually the optic nerve chiasma, optic tract, and spinal cord. Usually, the optic neuropathy (damage to the optic nerve) is accompanied by severe transverse myelitis, which involves an acute inflammation of the spinal cord. The optic neuropathy usually happens before the transverse myelitis occurs, but in approximately 20% of patients it occurs in the reverse order.

Persons with Devic syndrome can also experience urinary, gastrointestinal, and sexual dysfunction. This occurs due to degeneration of the nerves that exit the spinal cord and serve the body's trunk and limbs. Patients with Devic syndrome rarely experience clinical signs that involve defects beyond symptoms arising from the spinal cord and optic nerve. There are also characteristic brain **MRI** scan findings including swelling and signal changes that are typically observed, as well as increased protein content in the cerebral spinal fluid.

Diagnosis

Diagnosis is usually made by a **neurologist** and an ophthalmologist, by examining the eye and initiating several neurological exams including an MRI of the brain.

Treatment team

The neurologist and an ophthalmologist are the physicians that will be involved in making the diagnosis and providing follow-up treatment for persons with Devic syndrome. Patients that lose their eyesight will also require an occupational therapist that specializes in assisting individuals that become blind.

Treatment

There is no cure available for Devic syndrome. Treatment, therefore, is based solely on lessening the symptoms and providing comfort care for individuals that are in the more advanced stages of the disease. Steroidal anti-inflammatory medications such as corticosteroids might be helpful and are commonly prescribed for patients with this disorder. There is no defined standard of treatment for the disorder.

Recovery and rehabilitation

Recovery from attacks manifested by acute inflammation is often variable. Devic syndrome is a chronic disease, often progressive, and complete rehabilitation is usually not observed, as with many neurodegenerative diseases.

Clinical trials

Currently, the National Institute of Neurological Disorder and Stroke (NINDS) at the National Institutes of Health (NIH) are investigating how to repair damage to the **central nervous system** while restoring full strength to injured areas. As of mid-2004, there is currently a Phase III clinical trial to determine the effectiveness of plasma exchange in the treatment of acute severe attacks of inflammatory demyelinating disease in patients with degenerative neurological disorders who do not respond to intravenous steroid therapy. Although the study is no longer recruiting participants, anticipated results are not yet published.

Prognosis

The prognosis for individuals that have Devic syndrome is poor, as the disorder is eventually fatal for many patients. Isolated acute demyelinated encephalomyelitis (ADE) affects the optic nerve and the spinal cord in a similarly to Devic syndrome, but occurs after an infection or a common cold, and is distinct from Devic syndrome. ADE patients can fully recover, although many have associated permanent deficits, and in rare cases ADE can also be fatal.

Resources

BOOKS
Johnson, Richard T., et. al., "Transverse Myelitis" in *Current Therapy in Neurologic Disease,* 6th. ed. New York: Elsevier, 2002.

PERIODICALS
"Proposed diagnostic criteria and nosology of acute transverse myelitis," *Neurology* 59, no. 4 (August 27, 2002): 499–505.

OTHER
Lynn, Joann. "Transverse Myelitis: Symptoms, Causes and Diagnosis." *The Transverse Myelitis Association.* <http://www.myelitis.org/tm.htm> (May 1, 2004).
"NINDS Devic Syndrome Information Page." National Institute of Neurological Disorders and Stroke. <http://www.ninds.nih.gov/health_and_medical/disorders/devics.htm> (May 2, 2004).
Swallow, Charles T. "Optic neuritis." *eMedicine.* March 26, 2002. <http://www.emedicine.com/radio/topic488.htm> (May 1, 2004).

ORGANIZATIONS
Multiple Sclerosis Foundation. 6350 North Andrews Avenue, Ft. Lauderdale, FL 33309-2130. (954) 776-6805 or (888) MSFocus; Fax: (954) 351-0630. support@msfocus. org. <http://www.msfocus.org>.
National Eye Institute (NEI), National Institutes of Health, DHHS. 31 Center Drive, Rm. 6A32 MSC 2510, Bethesda, MD 20892-2510. (301) 496-5248 or (800) 869-2020. 2020@nei.nih.gov. <http://www.nei.nih.gov>.
Transverse Myelitis Association. 3548 Tahoma Place West, Tacoma, WA 98466. (253) 565-8156. ssiegel@myelitis.org. <http://www.myelitis.org>.

Bryan Richard Cobb, PhD

Dexamethasone *see* **Glucocorticoids**

Diabetic neuropathy disease

Definition

Diabetic neuropathy (DN) is a neurological disorder caused by consequences of a primary disease—diabetes mellitus. The diabetic neuropathy may be diffuse, affecting

Key Terms

Autoimmune Pertaining to an immune response by the body against its own tissues or types of cells.

Biopsy The surgical removal and microscopic examination of living tissue for diagnostic purposes or to follow the course of a disease. Most commonly the term refers to the collection and analysis of tissue from a suspected tumor to establish malignancy.

Carpal tunnel syndrome A condition caused by compression of the median nerve in the carpal tunnel of the hand, characterized by pain.

Diabetes mellitus The clinical name for common diabetes. It is a chronic disease characterized by the inability of the body to produce or respond properly to insulin, a hormone required by the body to convert glucose to energy.

Electromyography (EMG) A diagnostic test that records the electrical activity of muscles. In the test, small electrodes are placed on or in the skin; the pat-

terns of electrical activity are projected on a screen or over a loudspeaker. This procedure is used to test for muscle disorders, including muscular dystrophy.

Gastroparesis Nerve damage of the stomach that delays or stops stomach emptying, resulting in nausea, vomiting, bloating, discomfort, and weight loss.

Insulin A hormone or chemical produced by the pancreas that is needed by cells of the body in order to use glucose (sugar), a major source of energy for the human body.

Ketoacidosis Usually caused by uncontrolled type I diabetes, when the body isn't able to use glucose for energy. As an alternate source of energy, fat cells are broken down, producing ketones, toxic compounds that make the blood acidic. Symptoms of ketoacidosis include excessive thirst and urination, abdominal pain, vomiting, rapid breathing, extreme tiredness, and drowsiness.

multiple parts of the body, or focal, targeting a specific nerve or body part.

Description

Neurological damage is the result of chronically elevated blood sugar. Among all complications of diabetes, DN can be one of the most frustrating and debilitating conditions, because of the **pain**, discomfort, and disability it may cause, and because available treatments are limited and not always successful.

There are three main types of DN:

• Sensory neuropathy (or **peripheral neuropathy**, usually just referred to as neuropathy)—affects the nerves that carry sensation information to the brain, from various parts of the body, i.e.: how hot or cold something is, what the texture of something feels like, or the pain caused by a sharp object. This is the most common form of diabetic neuropathy.

• Autonomic neuropathy—affects the nerves that control involuntary activities of the body, such as the action of the stomach, intestine, bladder, and even the heart.

• Motor neuropathy—affects the nerves that carry signals from the brain to muscles, allowing all motions to occur, i.e. walking, moving the fingers, chewing. This form of neuropathy is very rare in diabetes.

The longer a person has diabetes, the more likely the development of one or more forms of neuropathy. Approximately 60–70% of patients with diabetes show signs of neuropathy, but only about five percent experience painful symptoms.

According to the categories described above, DN can lead to muscular weakness, loss of feeling or sensation, and loss of autonomic functions such as digestion, erection, bladder control, sweating, and so forth.

Demographics

In the United States, DN occurs in 10–20% of patients newly diagnosed with diabetes mellitus (DM), and its prevalence is up to 50% in elderly patients with DM. Most studies agree that the overall prevalence of symptomatic DN is approximately 30% of all patients with DM. The incidence of DN in the general population is approximately two percent.

Internationally, DN is found in 20–30% of individuals with type-2 diabetes. This number depends on the fiber type being tested and the sensitivity of the exam. Individuals with type-1 diabetes usually develop neuropathy after more than ten years of living with the disease.

It affects men and women equally, but neuropathic pain appears more frequently in females. Minority group members have more secondary complications, such as lower extremity amputations. These individuals tend to also have more hospitalizations due to neuropathic complications.

Causes and symptoms

Causes of diabetic neuropathy are likely to be different for different types of the disorder. Nerve damage is probably due to a combination of factors, such as:

• Metabolic factors: high blood glucose, long disease duration, low levels of insulin and abnormal blood fat levels

• Neurovascular factors, leading to blood vessel damage and consequent insufficient delivery of oxygen and nutrients to the nerves

• Autoimmune factors, causing nerve inflammation

• Mechanical nerve injury, such as carpal tunnel syndrome

• Inherited traits that increase susceptibility to nerve disease

• Lifestyle factors, such as smoking or alcohol use

Symptoms depend on the neuropathy type and affected nerves. Some people show no symptoms at all. Often, symptoms are minor at first, and because most nerve damage occurs over several years, mild cases may go unnoticed for a long time. Symptoms may include:

• Numbness, tingling, or pain in the toes, feet, legs, hands, arms, and fingers

• Wasting of feet or hands muscles

• Indigestion, nausea, or vomiting

• Diarrhea or constipation

• **Dizziness** or faintness due to a drop in postural blood pressure

• Problems with urination

• Erectile dysfunction (impotence) or vaginal dryness

• Weakness

In addition, weight loss and **depression** are not a direct consequence of the neuropathy but, nevertheless, often accompany it.

Diagnosis

Diabetic neuropathy is diagnosed on the basis of a clinical evaluation, analyzing the patient's history, symptoms and the physical exam. During the exam, the doctor may check blood pressure and heart rate, muscle strength, reflexes, and sensitivity to position, vibration, temperature, or a light touch.

The physician may also do other tests to help determine the type and extent of nerve damage:

• A comprehensive foot exam assesses skin, circulation, and sensation. Other tests include checking reflexes and assessing vibration perception.

• Nerve conduction studies check the transmission of an electrical current through a nerve. This test allows the doctor to assess the condition of all the nerves in the arms and legs.

• Electromyography (EMG) shows how well muscles respond to electrical signals transmitted by nearby nerves. This test is often done at the same time as nerve conduction studies.

• Quantitative sensory testing (QST) uses the response to stimuli, such as pressure, vibration, and temperature, to check for overt neuropathy. QST is increasingly used to recognize sensation loss and excessive irritability of nerves

• Heart rate variability shows how the heart responds to deep breathing and to changes in blood pressure and posture.

• Nerve or skin biopsies are used in research settings

Treatment team

Proper management of diabetic patients requires a skilled team including collaborating specialists. Depending on the qualifications of the patient's primary physician, other professionals are recruited as needed, such as an ophthalmologist, podiatrist, cardiologist, nutritionist, nurse educator, **neurologist**, vascular surgeon, endocrinologist, gastroenterologist and urologist. A nurse educator can ease the interface between otherwise independent specialists. Without such a team mentality, the diabetic patient is often set adrift, forced to cope with conflicting instructions and unneeded repetition of tests.

Treatment

The first step is to bring blood glucose levels down to the normal range to prevent further nerve damage. Blood glucose monitoring, meal planning, **exercise**, and oral drugs or insulin injections are needed to control blood glucose levels. Although, symptoms may get temporarily worse when blood sugar is first brought under control, over time, maintaining normal glucose levels helps lessen neuropathic symptoms. Importantly, good blood glucose control may also help prevent or delay the onset of further complications.

Additional treatments depend on the type of nerve problem in consideration, and are include:

• Foot care—Clean the feet daily, using warm water and a mild soap. Inspect the feet and toes every day for cuts, blisters, redness, swelling, calluses, or other problems.

Always wear shoes or slippers to protect feet from injuries, and prevent skin irritation by wearing thick, soft, seamless socks. Schedule regular visits with a podiatrist.

- Pain relief—To relieve pain, burning, tingling, or numbness, the physician may suggest aspirin, acetaminophen, or nonsteroidal anti-inflammatory drugs (NSAIDs) such as ibuprofen. People with renal disease should use NSAIDs only under a doctor's supervision. A topical cream called capsaicin is another option. Tricyclic antidepressant medications such as amitriptyline, imipramine, and nortriptyline, or anticonvulsant medications such as **carbamazepine** or **gabapentin** may relieve pain in some people. Codeine may be prescribed for a short time to relieve severe pain. Also, mexiletine, used to regulate heartbeat, has been effective in reducing pain in several **clinical trials**.

- Gastrointestinal problems—To relieve mild symptoms of stomach discomfort, doctors suggest eating small, frequent meals, avoiding fats, and eating less fiber. When symptoms are severe, the physician may prescribe erythromycin to speed digestion, metoclopramide for the same reason and to help relieve nausea, or other drugs to help regulate digestion or reduce stomach acid secretion.

- Urinary and sexual problems—To treat urinary tract infections, physicians can prescribe antibiotics and suggest drinking plenty of fluids. Several methods are available to treat erectile dysfunction caused by neuropathy, including taking oral drugs, using a mechanical vacuum device, or injecting a vasodilating drug into the penis before intercourse. In women, vaginal lubricants may be useful when neuropathy causes vaginal dryness.

Recovery and rehabilitation

Physical therapy may be a useful adjunct to other therapies, especially when muscular pain and weakness are a manifestation of the patient's neuropathy. The physical therapist can instruct the patient in a general exercise program to maintain his/her mobility and strength.

Occupational therapy may be necessary in cases where a person loses a limb due to secondary complications and needs functional training to regain his/her independence.

Clinical trials

There are numerous open clinical trials for diabetic neuropathy disease:

- Gene Therapy to Improve Wound Healing in Patients With Diabetes, at the National Institute of Arthritis and Musculoskeletal and Skin Diseases (NIAMS)

- Long-Term Treatment and Re-Treatment of Lower Extremity Diabetic Ulcers with Regranex or Placebo, sponsored by Johnson & Johnson Pharmaceutical Research and Development

- RhVEGF (Telbermin) for Induction of Healing of Chronic, Diabetic Foot Ulcers, sponsored by Genentech

- Study of Three Fixed Doses of EAA-090 in Adult Outpatients with Neuropathic Pain Associated with Diabetic Neuropathy, sponsored by Wyeth-Ayerst Research

- Treatment for Symptomatic Peripheral Neuropathy in Patients with Diabetes, LY333531 Treatment for Symptomatic Peripheral Neuropathy in Patients with Diabetes and Treatment of Peripheral Neuropathy in Patients with Diabetes, sponsored by Eli Lilly and Company

- VEGF for Diabetic Neuropathy, at the Caritas St. Elizabeth's Medical Center of Boston.

For updated information on clinical trials, visit the website www.clinicaltrials.org, sponsored by the United States government.

Prognosis

The mechanisms of diabetic neuropathy are poorly understood. At present, treatment alleviates pain and can control some associated symptoms, but the process is generally progressive.

Complications of diabetic neuropathy may include:

- Progression to cardiovascular autonomic neuropathy, a relatively rare occurrence which can eventually cause death

- Peripheral neuropathy that leads to foot ulcers and leg amputations

- Injuries associated with automonic neuropathy, including those from dizziness and falling

- gastric distress leading to nausea and vomiting, diarrhea and dehydration, which could impair the ability to regulate blood sugar.

Special concerns

Prevention of diabetic neuropathy can be achieved by establishing good control over blood sugar levels at the onset of diabetes. Even when symptoms of neuropathy are already present, maintaining normal blood sugar levels reduces pain significantly. Drugs such as some over-the-counter anti-inflamatories may aid in prevention, as well as deterrence, of neuropathy by keeping inflammation to a minimum.

Resources
BOOKS

Parker, James N., Phillip M. Parker. *The Official Patient's Sourcebook on Diabetic Neuropathy: A Revised and Updated Directory for the Internet Age.* Icon Group, International, 2002.

U.S. Dept of Health and Human Services. *Diabetic Neuropathies: The Nerve Damage of Diabetes.* NIDDK, National Diabetes Information Clearinghouse, 2002.

PERIODICALS

Podwall D., and C. Gooch. "Diabetic neuropathy: clinical features, etiology, and therapy." *Curr Neurol Neurosci Rep 4.* (January 2004): 55–61.

Hughes, R. A. C. "Peripheral neuropathy." *BMJ* 324 (February 2002): 466–469.

Vinik, A. I., R. Maser, B. Mitchell, and R. Freeman. "Diabetic Autonomic Neuropathy." *Diabetes Care* 26 (2003): 1553–1579.

OTHER

Diabetic Neuropathies: The Nerve Damage of Diabetes. National Institute of Diabetes and Digestive and Kidney Diseases. (January 4, 2004). <http://diabetes.niddk.nih.gov/>.

ORGANIZATIONS

American Diabetes Association (National Service Center). 1701 North Beauregard Street, Alexandria, VA 22311. (703) 549-6995 or (800) 232-3472 or (800) DIA-BETES. customerservice@diabetes.org. <http://www.diabetes.org>.

Centers for Disease Control and Prevention (National Center for Chronic Disease, Prevention and Health Promotion, Division of Diabetes Translation). Mail Stop K-10, 4770 Buford Highway, NE., Atlanta, GA 30341-3717. (301) 562-1050 or (800) CDC-DIAB (800-232-3422). diabetes@cdc.gov. <http://www.cdc.gov/diabetes>.

Juvenile Diabetes Research Foundation International. 120 Wall Street, 19th floor, New York, NY 10005. (212) 785-9500 or (800) 533-2873; Fax: (212) 785-9595. info@jdrf.org. <http://www.jdrf.org>.

National Diabetes Education Program. 1 Diabetes Way, Bethesda, MD 20892-3600. (800) 438-5383. <http://ndep.nih.gov>.

National Institute of Neurological Disorders and Stroke. P.O. Box 5801, Bethesda, MD 20824. (800) 352-9424. <http://www.ninds.nih.gov>.

Greiciane Gaburro Paneto
Francisco de Paula Careta
Iuri Drumond Louro

▌ Diadochokinetic rate

Definition

Diadochokinetic rate (DDK) refers to an assessment tool, used by speech-language pathologists (SLPs), that measures how quickly an individual can accurately produce a series of rapid, alternating sounds. These sounds, also called tokens, may be one syllable such as "puh," two or three syllables such as "puh-tuh" or "puh-tuh-kuh," or familiar words such as "pattycake" or "buttercup." Other names for DDK rate include maximum repetition rate and The Fletcher Time-by-Count Test of Diadochokinetic Syllable Rate, the latter of which is named for the clinician who published DKK rate data in 1972.

Purpose

Diadochokinetic rate is one means of assessing oral motor skills. DDK rate provides information about a person's ability to make rapid speech movements using different parts of his mouth. For example, the sounds "puh," "tuh," and "kuh" use the front (the lips), middle (the tip of the tongue), and back of the mouth (the soft palate), respectively. Evaluation of diadochokinetic rate usually occurs as part of an oral motor skills assessment. Other aspects of an oral motor skills assessment include examination of oral facial structures (lips, tongue, jaw, teeth, palate, and pharynx) and evaluation of velopharangeal function and breathing.

In general, DDK rates increase as children age and their motor systems mature. Some studies have shown reduced DDK rates in children and adults with speech impairments when compared to rates for individuals with typical speech. Examples of conditions that may be associated with a slower or more variable DDK rate include **ataxia**, **dysarthria**, childhood **apraxia** of speech, and **stuttering**.

Description

The task of measuring DDK rate usually occurs in a single session and takes as little as 15–20 minutes for the SLP to administer and score. Prior to administering the test, the speech-language pathologist will demonstrate the sound(s) to be repeated and allow the patient to complete several practice trials. A trial is defined by a predetermined amount of time or number of repetitions. Generally, the SLP will administer a series of tests, each of which requires the client to produce a different sound or combination of sounds.

To measure the DDK rate, a SLP will record how many times the individual repeats the sound or combination of sounds in a given period of time (usually five to 15 seconds). DDK rates are measured in terms of iterations per second (it/s) or in terms of the time required to produce a certain number of iterations of a mono-, bi-, or trisyllabic token. The rate will be calculated and compared to the published norms. The SLP may use specialized recording equipment and a computer software program to record and analyze DDK rate. The DDK rate is calculated by dividing the total number of iterations by the duration of the trial or by determining the time it took the client to make a set number of iterations. The results are scored and compared to the published normative values. For example, in

Key Terms

Ataxia Childhood apraxia of speech.

Dysarthria Stuttering.

the data published by Fletcher (1972), the norm for 20 repetitions of the syllable "puh" for a child at age 10 is 3.7 seconds.

Some clients, especially preschool age children, may have difficulty complying with the instructions or completing the DDK tasks. In such cases, real words such as "buttercup," or "pattycake" may be used to test diadochokinetic rate. Also, preliminary findings from research published by Yaruss and Logan in 2002 indicate that other means of assessing DDK productions in young children, namely, measurement of accuracy and fluency, may be more useful diagnostic tools than standard measures of DDK rate.

Resources

PERIODICALS

Fletcher, S. G. "Time-by-Count Measurement of Diadochokinetic Syllable Rate." *Journal of Speech and Hearing Research* 15 (Dec 1972): 763–70.

Yaruss, J. S., and K. Logan. "Evaluating Rate, Accuracy, and Fluency of Young Children's Diadochokinetic Productions: A Preliminary Investigation." *Journal of Fluency Disorders* 27 (2002): 65–86.

Williams, P., and J. Stackhouse. "Diadochokinetic Skills: Normal and Atypical Performance in Children Aged 3–5 Years." *International Journal of Language and Communication Disorders* 33 (Suppl 1998): 481–6.

WEBSITES

Apraxia Kids home page. (May 30, 2004). <http://www.apraxia-kids.org/index.html>.

ORGANIZATIONS

American Speech Language Hearing Association (ASHA). 10801 Rockville Pike, Rockville, MD 20852-3279. (301) 897-5700 or (800) 638-8255; Fax: (301) 571-0457. actioncenter@asha.org. <http://www.asha.org>.

Dawn J. Cardeiro, MS, CGC

Diazepam

Definition

Diazepam is an antianxiety medication that is also useful in the treatment of muscle spasms and some types of **seizures**. The drug belongs to the class of medications

Key Terms

Benzodiazepines A class of drugs with hypnotic, antianxiety, anticonvulsive, and muscle relaxant properties, used in the treatment of anxiety or sleeping disorders, to relax muscles, or to control seizures.

known as **benzodiazepines** that depress activity of the **central nervous system**.

Purpose

Diazepam, which is marketed under the brand names of Valium, Diastat, T-Quil, and Valrelease, is taken by millions of people to relieve feelings of anxiety. As well, the drug can lessen muscle spasms and can control some types of seizures. Diazepam is also used to therapeutically lessen the agitation caused during alcohol withdrawal by someone who is physically addicted to alcohol. Additionally, diazepam is used in the treatment of irritable bowel syndrome and to lessen the symptoms of panic attacks.

Description

Diazepam is supplied as a tablet, as a capsule that releases the active drug at a slower rate, or as a liquid. All three of these forms of the drug are taken orally. The time-release capsule should be swallowed whole. Diazepam should be stored at room temperature in a tightly closed container to avoid alteration in the compound due to excessive heat or moisture. Valium is also available in an injectable form.

Recommended dosage

Diazepam dosage is determined by a physician taking into account the nature of the problem, severity of the symptoms, and the person's response to the drug. Typical adult doses range from 2–10 mg taken two to four times a day. Children and elderly adults will typically receive 1–2 mg one to four times daily.

The dosage of diazepam typically prescribed by a physician is taken anywhere from one to four times each day, depending on the strength of the individual dose. This maintains the concentration of the drug at a therapeutic level, as diazepam is quickly absorbed from the gastrointestinal tract. Peak levels of the drug are reached within a couple of hours after administration, with levels dropping below therapeutic effectiveness within six to eight hours.

Diazepam can be taken with or without food. The liquid form can be mixed with other fluids or select foods such as applesauce.

Precautions

The recommended dosage should not be exceeded, nor should it continue to be taken after the prescribed time. Such abuse can lead to a dependence on the drug, or the establishment of tolerance. As the effectiveness of diazepam is related to its concentration, it is important to take the drug regularly. Doses should not be skipped as this could lead to a worsening of the symptoms.

Diazepam should not be taken with other central nervous system depressants such as narcotics, sleeping pills, or alcohol. The combinations could lower blood pressure and suppress breathing to the point of unconsciousness and death.

Persons taking diazepam should **exercise** extreme caution when driving or operating machinery. These activities should be avoided during periods of drowsiness associated with diazepam therapy.

Pregnant and breast-feeding woman should not take diazepam, nor should someone with **myasthenia gravis**. The drug should be used cautiously in those with **epilepsy**, as diazepam may trigger an epileptic seizure.

Side effects

Some people are allergic to diazepam. In this case, other drugs can be substituted. These include alprazolam (Xanax), chlordiazepoxide (Librium), and triazolam (Halcion).

Common side effects from diazepam include drowsiness, **dizziness**, blurred vision, **headache**, **fatigue**, muscle weakness, memory loss, skin rash, diarrhea, dry mouth, stomach upset, decreased sexual drive, and an altered appetite. Less common side effects include jaundice, decreased white blood cell count (leukopenia), insomnia, hallucinations, and irritability.

Interactions

Diazepam can interact with other prescription medicines, especially antihistamines, as well as cimetidine (Tagamet), disulfiram (Antabuse), and fluoxetine (Prozac). Additionally, interaction can occur with medications given for the relief of **depression**, **pain**, **Parkinson's disease**, asthma, and colds, and with muscle relaxants, oral contraceptives, sedatives and sleeping pills, tranquilizers, and even some vitamins. In general, the result of the interaction is to increase the drowsiness caused by diazepam.

Resources

BOOKS

Diazepam: A Medical Dictionary, Bibliography, and Annotated Research Guide to Internet References. San Diego: Icon Health International, 2004.

OTHER

"Diazepam." *Drugs.com.* May 5, 2004 (May 22, 2004.) <http://www.drugs.com/diazepam.html>.
"Diazepam." *Medline Plus.* National Library of Medicine. May 5, 2004 (May 22, 2004). <http://www.nlm.nih.gov/medlineplus/druginfo/medmaster/a682047.html>.

Brian Douglas Hoyle, PhD

Dichloralphenazone, Isometheptene, and Acetaminophen

Definition

Dichloralphenazone, isometheptene, and acetaminophen are a combination medicine indicated for the treatment of symptoms associated with vascular (tension) headaches and migraine. Dichloralphenazone is a general sedative that slows down **central nervous system** (CNS) function, causing relaxation and minor **pain** relief. Isometheptene causes narrowing of blood vessels, aiding the specific relief of **headache** pain. Acetaminophen is a general, mild pain reliever and fever reducer.

Purpose

Dichloralphenazone, isometheptene, and acetaminophen do not prevent the occurrence of regular tension headaches or migraines. Rather, they relieve symptoms, including headache, nausea, altered vision, and sensitivity to light and sound at their onset.

Description

In the United States, dichloralphenazone, isometheptene, and acetaminophen are sold under the names Amidrine, Duradrin, I.D.A , Iso-Acetazone, Isocom, Midchlor, Midrin, Migrapap, Migquin, Migratine, Migrazone, Migrend, Migrex, Mitride. The medications exert their therapeutic effects individually. Dichloralphenazone aids relaxation, isometheptene relieves the throbbing pain associated with headaches, and acetaminophen acts as a general pain reliever.

Recommended dosage

Dichloralphenazone, isometheptene, and acetaminophen are most commonly available together in capsule, tablet, or dissolving tablet form. They are prescribed by physicians in varying dosages.

Dichloralphenazone, isometheptene, and acetaminophen are not indicated for routine use or headache prevention. For the treatment of tension headaches and

Key Terms

Migraine Recurrent severe headaches generally accompanied by an aura (classic migraine), nausea, vomiting, and dizziness.

migraines, they should be taken at the onset of headache symptoms or at the first warning signs of migraine. The usual initial dose for adults is one to two capsules. Treatment including dichloralphenazone, isometheptene, and acetaminophen may be appropriate for some children, but only when advised by a physician. The maximum daily dose for anyone taking dichloralphenazone, isometheptene, and acetaminophen usually is not greater than six to eight capsules.

A double dose of dichloralphenazone, isometheptene, and acetaminophen should not be taken at one time. If one dose fails to relieve symptoms associated with tension headache or migraine, follow instructions provided by the prescribing physician for taking supplemental doses every few hours. Do not take dichloralphenazone, isometheptene, and acetaminophen for several days in a row, even if symptoms persist, unless instructed by a physician. Any persistent, severe headache should be evaluated by a physician, especially if accompanied by fever, **visual disturbances**, confusion, stiff neck, or numbness and weakness on one side of the body.

Precautions

Dichloralphenazone, isometheptene, and acetaminophen may cause drowsiness and sleepiness for several hours. Caution is necessary to determine if it is safe to drive a car or operate machinery.

It is necessary to consult a physician before taking dichloralphenazone, isometheptene, and acetaminophen with certain non-perscription medications. While taking dichloralphenazone, isometheptene, and acetaminophen, patients should avoid alcohol and CNS depressants (medicines that can make one drowsy or less alert, such as antihistimines, sleep medications, and some pain medications). They can exacerbate side effects such as drowsiness, nausea, and loss of coordination.

Avoid additional general pain relievers containing acetaminophen (such as Tylenol) while using a dichloralphenazone, isometheptene, and acetaminophen combination medicine.

Dichloralphenazone, isometheptene, and acetaminophen may not be suitable for persons with a history of asthma or other chronic lung diseases, liver disease, kidney disease, mental illness, high blood presure, **seizures**,

angina (chest pain), irregular heartbeats, or other heart problems. Persons who have had a **stroke** or are obese should avoid taking dichloralphenazone, isometheptene, and acetaminophen. Patients should notify their physician if they consume a large amount of alcohol, have a history of drug use, are nursing, pregnant, or plan to become pregnant.

The effect of dichloralphenazone, isometheptene, and acetaminophen during pregnancy has not been fully established, but research demonstrates that the medications are passed into breast milk. Patients who become pregnant while taking dichloralphenazone, isometheptene, and acetaminophen should contact their physician.

Side effects

Patients and their physicians should weigh the risks and benefits of dichloralphenazone, isometheptene, and acetaminophen before beginning treatment. Most patients tolerate combination medications with dichloralphenazone, isometheptene, and acetaminophen well, but may experience a variety of mild to moderate side effects. Some possible side effects, such as upset stomach and nausea mirror the symptoms associated with migraine. Common side effects that do not usually require medical attention include:

- diziness or unsteadiness
- sleepiness or drowsiness
- feeling of warmth or heaviness
- flushing
- tingling feeling
- excessive sweating
- diarrhea

Other, less common side effects of dichloralphenazone, isometheptene, and acetaminophen may be serious. The sudden onset of some severe side efects may indicate an allergic reaction. Contact the prescribing physician immediately if any of the following symptoms occur:

- pinpoint red spots on skin
- dark stools
- rash, lumps, or hives
- redness or swelling of the face, lips, or eyelids
- change in vision
- wheezing and difficulty breathing
- chest pain or tightness in the chest
- irregular heartbeat
- faintness or loss of consciousness
- sudden or severe stomach pain
- fever

Interactions

Dichloralphenazone, isometheptene, and acetaminophen receptor agonists may have negative interactions with antibiotics, antidepressants, anticoagulants, antihistimines, asthma medications, and monoamine oxidase inhibitors (MAOIs). Patients should not take dichloralphenazone, isometheptene, and acetaminophen for several weeks after stopping treatment with MAOIs.

Dichloralphenazone, isometheptene, and acetaminophen combination medications should not be used in conjunction with other migraine treatment medications unless otherwise directed by a physician.

Resources

BOOKS

Lang, Susan, and Lawrence Robbins. *Headache Help: A Complete Guide to Understanding Headaches and the Medications That Relieve Them.* Boston: Houghton Mifflin, 2000.

OTHER

"Isometheptene, Dichloralphenazone, and Acetaminophen." *Web MD.* (April 23, 2004). <http://my.webmd.com/hw/drug_data/d03459a1?bn=amidrine>.

"Isometheptene, Dichloralphenazone, and Acetaminophen (Systemic)." *Yahoo Drug Index.* (April 12, 2004). <http://health.yahoo.com/health/drug/202306/overview>.

ORGANIZATIONS

ACHE (American Council for Headache Education). 19 Mantua Road, Mt. Royal, NJ 08601. (856) 423-0258. <http://www.achenet.org>.

National Headache Foundation. 428 W. St. James Place, 2nd Floor, Chicago, IL 60614. (703) 739-9384 or (888) NHF-5552. <http://www.headaches.org>.

Migraine Awareness Group. 113 South Saint Asaph Street, Suite 300, Alexandria, VA 22314. (703) 739-9384. <http://www.migraines.org>.

Adrienne Wilmoth Lerner

Dichloralphenazone

Definition

Dichloralphenazone is a general sedative-hypnotic that slows **central nervous system** (CNS) function, causing relaxation and **pain** relief. It is primarily indicated as a component of a drug that is used in the treatment of tension (muscle contraction) and vascular (migraine) headaches. Additional uses for dichloralphenazone include sedation and pain relief, and treatment for symptoms associated with insomnia.

Purpose

The combination medication, including isometheptene, dichloralphenazone, and acetaminophen, is used to treat tension and vascular **headaches**. Although the combination does not prevent the occurrence of tension headaches or migraines, isometheptene, dichloralphenazone, and acetaminophen act to relieve pain at its onset. The combination also relieves some symptoms associated with migraine such as altered vision and sensitivity to light and sound.

Description

Dichloralphenazone is not indicated for routine use. The medication should be taken only at the onset of pain, tension headache symptoms, or at the first warning signs of migraine.

Recommended dosage

Dichloralphenazone is most commonly available in capsule form, and is prescribed by physicians in varying dosages. The usual dose for adults is one to two capsules. Under the supervision of a physician, treatment that includes dichloralphenazone may be appropriate for some children.

A double dose of dichloralphenazone should not be taken. If the first dose fails to relieve pain or symptoms associated with tension headache or migraine, the patient should follow instructions provided by the prescribing physician for taking supplemental doses every few hours. If pain persists for several days, this medication should not be taken without consulting the prescribing physician.

Precautions

Dichaloralphenazone may cause drowsiness and sleepiness for several hours. Extreme caution should be used when driving or operating machinery.

A physician should be consulted before taking any form of dichloralphenazone with certain non-prescription medications. Patients taking dichloralphenazone should avoid alcohol and CNS depressants, including medicines that can make one drowsy or less alert such as antihistimines, sleep medications, and some pain medications. These medicines can exacerbate the side effects of dichloraphenazone.

Dichloralphenazone may not be suitable for persons with a history of **seizures**, **stroke**, asthma or other chronic lung diseases, liver disease, kidney disease, mental illness, high blood pressure, angina (chest pain), irregular heartbeats, or other heart problems. Patients should notify their physician if they smoke, consume a large amount of alcohol, have a history of drug use, are nursing, pregnant, or

Key Terms

Migraine A recurring, severe vascular headache, often accompanied by stomach upset and visual sensitivity to light, thought to be caused by changes in blood flow and certain chemical changes in the brain.

Sedative Medications that quiet nervous system excitement, producing a relaxed state.

plan to become pregnant. The effect of dichloralphenazone during pregnancy has not been fully established. Patients who become pregnant while taking dichloralphenazone should contact their physician.

Side effects

Patients and their physicians should weigh the risks and benefits of dichloralphenazone before beginning treatment, as some forms of dichloralphenazone may be habit forming. Most patients tolerate combination medications with dichloralphenazone well. However, some people may experience a variety of mild to moderate side effects. A few possible side effects such as headache, upset stomach, and nausea mirror symptoms associated with tension headaches and migraine. Common side effects that do not usually require medical attention include:

- dizziness or unsteadiness
- sleepiness or drowsiness
- feeling of warmth or heaviness
- increased sweating
- flushing
- tingling feeling
- diarrhea

Other, less common side effects of dichloralphenazone could indicate a potentially serious condition. The sudden onset of some severe side effects may indicate an allergic reaction. If any of the following serious side effects occur, the prescribing physician should be contacted immediately:

- rash, lumps, or hives
- redness or swelling of the face, lips, or eyelids
- change in vision
- wheezing and difficulty breathing
- chest pain or tightness in the chest
- irregular heartbeat
- faintness or loss of consciousness

- sudden or severe stomach pain
- persistent fever

Interactions

Dichloralphenazone may have negative interactions with antibiotics, antidepressants, anticoagulants, anti-epileptic drugs (AEDs), **anticonvulsants**, antihistimines, asthma medications, and monoamine oxidase inhibitors (MAOIs). Patients should not take dichloralphenazone for several weeks after stopping treatment with MAOIs.

Dichloralphenazone should not be used in conjunction with other migraine treatment medications unless otherwise directed by a physician.

Resources

BOOKS

Lang, Susan. *Headache Help: A Complete Guide to Understanding Headaches and the Medications That Relieve Them—Fully Revised and Updated.* New York: Houghton Mifflin, 2000.

Robbins, Lawrence. *Management of Headache and Headache Medications.* New York: Springer Verlag, 2000.

OTHER

"Isometheptene, Dichloralphenazone, and Acetaminophen (Systemic)." *Medline Plus Drug Information.* National Library of Medicine. May 6, 2004 (May 22, 2004). <http://www.nlm.nih.gov/medlineplus/druginfo/uspdi/202306.html>.

ORGANIZATIONS

ACHE (American Council for Headache Education). 19 Mantua Road, Mt. Royal, NJ 08601. (856) 423-0258. <http://www.achenet.org>.

National Headache Foundation. 428 W. St. James Place, 2nd Floor, Chicago, IL 60614. (703) 739-9384 or (888) NHF-5552. <http://www.headaches.org>.

Migraine Awareness Group. 113 South Saint Asaph Street, Suite 300, Alexandria, VA 22314. (703) 739-9384. <http://www.migraines.org>.

Adrienne Wilmoth Lerner

Diencephalon

Definition

The diencephalon is a complex of structures within the brain, whose major divisions are the thalamus and hypothalamus. It functions as a relay system between sensory input neurons and other parts of the brain, as an interactive site for the central nervous and endocrine systems, and works in tandem with the limbic system.

Description

The diencephalon is composed of several structures, the whole about the size of an apricot, situated near the core center of the brain, just above the brainstem. It is made up of the medulla oblongata, pons, and midbrain, below the telencephalon, the most basal part of the cerebrum. The two major components of the diencephalon are the thalamus and the hypothalamus. Other important structures within the diencephalon complex are the epithalamus, subthalamus, third ventricle, mammillary bodies, posterior pituitary gland, and the pineal body. The diencephalon interconnects with a larger, surrounding array of structures called the limbic system, which is the seat of emotions and memory.

The diencephalon functions in the following ways:

• As a junction and relay system that receives and filters afferent (incoming) sensory information, then relays it on to other parts of the brain, mainly the cerebral cortex, but also to the **cerebellum** and brainstem.

• As an interactive site between the **central nervous system** and the endocrine system.

• As an interactive complementary to the limbic system.

The upper part of the diencephalon, making up about 80% of its mass, is the thalamus, a small pillow of neural gray matter divided into two egg-shaped lobes. The lobes' long axes run toward the front and back of the head, and are connected to each other by a small stalk, the intermediate mass. The two thalamic lobes are filled with numerous pairs of nuclei, which are concentrations of synapsing afferent, or incoming, and efferent, or outgoing, neurons. Numerous such nuclei are situated throughout the brain.

The thalamic nuclei are named and classified according to their positions within the thalamus (medial, lateral, central, etc.), by their neural connections, and by their functions. In terms of function, there are three types of thalamic nuclei: sensory, motor, and arousal.

Layered sheets of myelinated axons, the internal thalamic medullary laminae, run vertically through the lobes of the thalamus. These laminae are full of neurons that interconnect various thalamic nuclei. The edges of the internal lamina reach the surfaces of the lobes. They show as narrow, whitish, cable-like bands, running across either lobe from its posterior underside, across the top, and forward, bifurcating into two bands (two vertical layers) toward the front. The main lamina divide the lobes of the thalamus into portions containing the medial and lateral geniculate nuclei, while the anterior bifurcations enclose the anterior nuclei.

The thalamus, the basal ganglia, and the cerebellum, which is the main movement coordination center of the brain, are neurally linked to the cerebral motor cortex in reciprocal, or feedback, fashion. Together, they regulate and fine-tune motor functions. The basal ganglia, which are part of the telencephalon, are groupings of gray matter within the white matter of the cerebral hemispheres. The basal ganglia function directly with the cerebellum to modify and fine-tune body movements.

A small part of the diencephalon, the epithalamus, extends rearward from, and slightly higher than, the thalamus. It holds the habenular nuclei, the stria medullaris thalami nerve tracts, and the pineal body, or epiphysis. The habenular nuclei play a role in emotional responses to odors. They receive afferent nerves from the septum, a complex of structures within the telencephalon and limbic system, and from the lateral preoptic nuclei of the basal forebrain, which is the lowermost region of the cerebrum; the stria medullaris tracts and the basal ganglia are the conduits. The habenular nuclei send efferents to the interpeduncular nucleus of the midbrain via the habenulo-interpeduncular nerve tract.

The pea-sized, conically shaped pineal body, on a short stalk, projects rearward and downward from the epithalamus. The pineal is a gland-like organ whose functions are still only poorly understood. It is a functional, light-sensitive remnant of an ancient and much more complex system of visually oriented organs, the pineal complex. The pineal is neurally connected with the suprachiasmatic nuclei of the hypothalamus, which hold the circadian internal clock. This is located just above the optic chiasma, the point at which the optic nerves from both eyes cross. The human pineal secretes melatonin, a hormone that seems to have a calming effect on the nervous system. The pineal, in response to the level of daylight, may induce sleepiness by increasing the output of melatonin.

All sensory input, except the olfactory (smell), passes through the thalamus, where it is filtered, integrated, and passed on to proper sites in the brain, most of them within the cerebral cortex. The route is as follows:

• Impulses from the auditory organs synapse in the medial geniculate thalamic nuclei, where they are sent to the auditory centers of the cerebral cortex.

• Impulses from the eyes, via the optic nerves, synapse in the lateral geniculate thalamic nuclei, and are sent on to the calcarine cerebral cortex.

• Other sensory input synapses in the ventral posteromedial thalamic nuclei, which receive, process, and pass on somatosensory input from the head, while the ventral posterolateral thalamic nuclei do likewise with input from the rest of the body.

• The thalamic nuclei also receive input from subcortical sources and feedback from the cortical areas. These operate in tandem to filter and control input to the cortex.

Key Terms

Autonomic nervous system A complex of nerve tracts, nuclei and organs within the brain that maintain homeostasis, or the functioning of body systems at proper levels.

Hypothalamus The lowermost part of the diencephalon, containing several nuclei, nerve tracts, and the pituitary gland; it is the regulatory seat of the autonomic nervous system.

Limbic system A complex of nerve tracts and nuclei that function as the seat of memory and emotions, containing the fornix, hippocampus, amygdala, and the cingulate gyrus.

Thalamus A small mass of gray matter composing the upper structure of the diencephalon, divided into two lobes and filled with numerous thalamic.

The ventral anterior and ventral lateral thalamic nuclei, involved with motor function, receive sensory input relayed through the basal ganglia and through the superior cerebellar peduncle, the main neural tract connecting the cerebellum and the red nuclei. The ventral anterior and ventral lateral thalamic nuclei project to the premotor and motor cerebral cortex. In addition, the ventral anterior thalamic nuclei are the main relay nuclei between the thalamus and the limbic system, receiving the mammillothalamic nerve tract from the mammillary bodies in the hypothalamus and projecting to the cingulate gyrus.

The cingulate gyrus, which is not a part of the diencephalon, is the part of the cerebrum closest to the limbic system, and serves to neurally connect the thalamus and hippocampus. The cingulate gyrus associates memories and emotional responses with smells, sights, and **pain**, and allows movement of attention among objects or ideas.

The medial dorsal thalamic nuclei receive nerve tracts from the amygdala of the limbic system and send efferents to the prefrontal cerebral cortex (not part of the diencephalon), which has numerous feedback connections with the thalamus, amygdala, and other subcortical structures.

The anterior thalamic nuclei connect with the mammillary bodies of the hypothalamus, and through them, via a nerve tract, the fornix, with the hippocampus and the cingulate gyrus.

The centromedian thalamic nuclei regulate excitability levels within the cerebral cortex and thus play a major role in arousal and alertness. The centromedian thalamic nuclei receive motor-related input from the basal ganglia, cerebellum, and the reticular formation of the brainstem and midbrain, and send efferent nerves to the cerebral cortex. The reticular formation is a network of nerves running through the brainstem and hindbrain, and containing the reticular activating system, which plays a key role in inducing arousal and alertness in tune with the circadian rhythm (sleeping and waking cycles). The reticular thalamic nuclei, which receive neural input from the reticular formation, regulate general thalamic output in accordance with the circadian rhythm.

The dorsomedial thalamic nuclei are involved with emotional arousal and the expression of emotionally based behavior, as well as memory, foresight, and feelings of pleasure. These nuclei receive input from many sites and interconnect with the prefrontal cerebral cortex.

That part of the diencephalon immediately below the two lobes of the thalamus is the subthalamus. It contains several nerve tracts and the subthalamic nuclei. Small portions of the red nuclei and the substantia nigra of the midbrain reach into the subthalamus. The subthalamic nuclei are interconnected with the basal ganglia and are involved in controlling motor functions.

The hypothalamus is the lowermost structure of the diencephalon. The thalamus, epithalamus, and hypothalamus surround and define most of the third ventricle of the brain, which, like all the ventricles, is filled with cerebrospinal fluid. The third ventricle communicates with the lateral ventricles and, via the cerebral aqueduct, with the fourth ventricle.

The hypothalamus contains several nuclei, nerve tracts, and the pituitary gland. It is the regulatory seat of the autonomic nervous system, while the hypothalamus and the pituitary are the major sites in which the two regulatory systems of the body, the central nervous system and the endocrine system, interact. The hypothalamus regulates the production of pituitary hormones, influencing and being influenced by emotional states, physical appetites, autonomic functions, temperature control, and diurnal rhythms. It is thus the main control center for homeostasis, or keeping physiological maintenance systems functioning at optimal states.

Efferent nerves from the hypothalamus extend into the brainstem and the spinal cord, where they synapse with neurons of the autonomic nervous system, which regulates a number of involuntary functions, among them the rate of heartbeat, urine release, and peristalsis. The hypothalamus responds to sensations of temperature extremes, the posterior hypothalamus stimulating muscle shivering to deal with cold, via efferent neurons to motor neurons within the spinal cord, and the anterior hypothalamus producing sweating as a reaction to overheating.

The pair of globular mammillary bodies are partially embedded in the underside of the hypothalamus. They are involved in olfactory reflexes and emotional responses to odors. Also on the underside of the hypothalamus, and toward the front, is the optic chiasma, where the two optic nerve cables of the eyes cross.

From the floor of the hypothalamus, the posterior pituitary gland, or neurohypophysis, extends forward and downward at the end of a long peduncle or stalk, the infundibulum. Efferent hypothalamic nerves extend through the infundibulum to the posterior portion of the pituitary gland, others extend to the trigeminal and facial nerve nuclei, to help control the head muscles involved in swallowing.

The posterior pituitary is an extension of the hypothalamus, but the anterior part of the pituitary is glandular tissue with an embryonic origin separate from that of the posterior pituitary. During embryonic development, the anterior and posterior lobes of the pituitary eventually meet and fuse.

The hypothalamus plays a pivotal role in regulating the endocrine system via its control of the pituitary gland's production of several hormones, while the hypothalamus is influenced in turn by hormones in the bloodstream and by nerve input. A partial list of hormones secreted by the pituitary includes cortisol, prolactin, antidiuretic hormone (ADH), oxytocin, growth hormone (GH), thyroid stimulating hormone (TSH), adrenocorticotropic hormone (ACTH), lipotropins, beta-endorphins, melanocyte stimulating hormone, luteinizing hormone, and follicle stimulating hormone.

Hormones influence functions as diverse as metabolism, growth and maturation, reproduction, dealing with stress, urine production, ion balance, sexual development, and sexual function. The hypothalamus regulates physical appetites for food, water, and sex. Afferent fibers synapsing in the hypothalamus carry input from the internal organs, the taste receptors of the tongue, the limbic system, the nipples, and the external genitalia. The hypothalamus responds to and accords with emotional states, and thus plays a major role in affecting emotions and moods, among them sexual pleasure, tranquility, rage, and fear.

The hypothalamus contributes to the regulation of the circadian rhythm via an internal clock within the suprachiasmatic nuclei. This internal clock communicates with the reticular formation of the midbrain. The reticular formation contains the reticular activating system, which plays a key role in inducing arousal and alertness, in tandem with the circadian rhythm.

The diencephalon is interconnected with a surrounding complex of brain structures, the limbic system, which functions as the center of emotional states and responses, and of memory. Besides the various structures within the diencephalon, the limbic system includes the olfactory cortex, hippocampus, amygdala, cingulate gyrus, septal nuclei, the dorsomedial nuclei of the thalamus, and the anterior nuclear complex of the thalamus.

Memories of vividly emotional experiences are recorded and kept within easy reach of consciousness within the limbic system. Connections between, and functions of, the hypothalamus and limbic system are intimately intertwined. The ventral anterior thalamic nuclei are the main relay nuclei connecting the thalamus and the limbic system, receiving the mammillothalamic tract and projecting to the cingulate gyrus.

The olfactory sense is the only one whose neurons directly connect with a processing center within the limbic system and outside the thalamus. Within the hypothalamus, relayed olfactory impulses are used to regulate appetite and sexual behavior, and to regulate autonomic reactions initiated by odors. Since the limbic system processes memory and stores important memories, the direct connection of the olfactory neurons to the limbic system helps explain why odors serve as alarms (e.g., the odor of smoke) and can trigger strong emotional responses and vivid, detailed memories of events and emotional states.

The hippocampus, the main processor of memory, is a paired structure looping over the tops of the thalamic lobes and rearwards, curving downward and forward and ending at the paired, globular, cherry-sized amygdala, below and in front of the hypothalamus. The amygdala connect with the hippocampus, the septal nuclei, the prefrontal area of the cerebrum, and the medial dorsal nucleus of the thalamus. The amygdala also send nerves to the hypothalamus via the ventral amygdalofugal pathway.

The amygdala are centers for associating strong emotions, good or bad, with memories of the experiences that triggered those emotions. Fear responses and fear-charged memories are centered in the amygdala, which can retain vivid memories of traumatic experiences, and initiate the survival fight-or-flight response.

The hippocampus sends efferents, via a cable of nerves, the fornix, to the mammillary bodies within the hypothalamus. The mammillary bodies send efferents to the anterior nuclei of the thalamus via the mammillothalamic tract.

Resources

BOOKS

Ackerman, Diane. *An Alchemy of Mind: The Marvel and Mystery of the Brain.* New York: Scribner, 2004.

Mai, Juergen, Joseph Assheuer, and George Paxinos. *Atlas of the Human Brain.* Philadelphia: Academic Press, 1997; Deluxe Edition, 1998.

PERIODICALS

Scientific American Mind: The Brain, A Look Inside, special edition, vol. 14, no 1, 2004.

WEBSITES

Brain Structure and Function. University of Idaho. (May 20, 2004). <http://www.sci.uidaho.edu/med532/start.htm>.

DienCephalon. Geocities. (May 20, 2004.) <http://biology.about.com/gi/dynamic/offsite.htm?site=http://www.geocities.com/HotSprings/3468/11%2D02.html%23DienCephalon>.

The Human Brain: Chapter 5: The Cerebral Hemispheres. *Virtual Hospital.* (May 20, 2004). <http://www.vh.org/adult/provider/anatomy/BrainAnatomy/Ch5Text/Section08.html>.

The Hypothalamus and Pituitary Gland: Introduction and Index. Colorado State University. (May 20, 2004). <http://arbl.cvmbs.colostate.edu/hbooks/pathphys/endocrine/hypopit/index.html>.

The MIND Institute Mental Illness and Neuroscience Discovery. (May 20, 2004). <http://www.themindinstitute.org>.

Neuroanatomy and Neuropathology on the Internet. (May 20, 2004). <http://www.neuropat.dote.hu/anatomy.htm>.

Penn State Hershey Medical Center: FRED (Faculty Research Expertise Database). (May 20, 2004). <http://www.hmc.psu.edu/fred/>.

"A Primate Brain Information System." *Braininfo.* (May 20, 2004). <http://braininfo.rprc.washington.edu/mainmenu.html>.

The Washington University School of Medicine Neuroscience Tutorial. (May 20, 2004). <http://thalamus.wustl.edu/course/>.

ORGANIZATIONS

The MIND Institute: Mental Illness and Neuroscience Discovery. 801 University Boulevard SE Suite 200, Albuquerque, NM 87106. (505) 272-7578; Fax: (505) 272-7574. info@themindinstitute.org. <http://www.themindinstitute.org>.

Society for Behavioral Neuroendocrinology. 4327 Ridge Road, Palmyra, VA 22963. srl@virginia.edu. <http://www.sbne.org>.

Kevin Fitzgerald

Diet and nutrition

Definition

Adequate nutrition and a well-balanced diet in every phase of life are essential requirements for normal development and growth, health maintenance, and disease prevention, as well as for the recovery from illness or injury. The human organism is a dynamic system, constantly using stored energy to perform physiologic functions such as blood circulation, respiration, immune surveillance and defense against infections, synthesis of proteins, hormones, and **neurotransmitters** necessary for muscle activity, sensory perception, thought processing, digestion of food and elimination of body wastes, cell and tissue detoxification, and DNA repair. Food is the main source of the micronutrients the organism utilizes to perform these vital functions, thus keeping the many physiologic systems in a state of homeostasis, or dynamic functional balance.

Description

Micronutrients are substances the body extracts from food through digestion, the process of breaking down large and complex molecules of food into more simple and smaller ones. Micronutrients are then absorbed through the walls of the small intestine into the blood vessels to be distributed to and processed by different organs and tissues. Different classes of micronutrients are used for several different purposes. For instance, some micronutrients such as vitamins are essential for cellular protection against naturally occurring metabolic toxins formed as a byproduct of cellular activity, or against toxins derived from the environment, such as pollution, chemicals, solar **radiation**, or drugs. Micronutrients are divided in the following categories: amino acids, fatty acids, sugars or carbohydrates, vitamins, and minerals.

Amino acids are the building blocks of all types of proteins that constitute cells, organs, tissues, and muscles. Some proteins are mediators of signals between cells of different organs, regulating intracellular physiology and growth. Although approximately 300 amino acids are known in nature, the human body only utilizes about 20 of them. The body itself manufactures half of the amino acids required by humans to make proteins. However, 10 of these are called essential amino acids because humans depend on their presence in food, since the body cannot adequately manufacture them. Eight of the 10 essential amino acids must be present in the diet throughout life, whereas two are necessary during development and growth, or when tissue repair is needed.

Some amino acids are created in the brain and play an important role in the regulation of mood, cognitive function, attention, and sleep pattern. The synthesis of neurotransmitters, chemical messengers in the brain that regulate neural activity, is also dependent on adequate dietary intake of essential amino acids. Examples of neurotransmitters are acetylcholine, gamma-aminobutyric acid (GABA), dopamine, and serotonin. The main source of essential amino acids is animal protein such as fish, meat, milk, and eggs. Plants are also a source of amino acids, although none contain all of the essential amino acids. It is important, therefore, to combine different types of plants within the same meal, such as nuts, beans, grains, fruits, especially in vegetarian diets.

Enzymes are another important type of protein that regulates all metabolic events. Some enzymes are responsible for the detoxification of cells and tissues, and

Key Terms

Amino acid   An organic compound composed of both an amino group and an acidic carboxyl group. Amino acids are the basic building blocks of proteins. There are 20 types of amino acids (eight are "essential amino acids" that the body cannot make and must therefore be obtained from food).

Antioxidant   Any substance that reduces the damage caused by oxidation, such as the harm caused by free radicals.

Free radical   An unstable molecule that causes oxidative damage by stealing electrons from surrounding molecules, thereby disrupting activity in the body's cells.

Homeostasis   The balanced internal environment of the body and the automatic tendency of the body to maintain this internal "steady state." Also refers to the tendency of a family system to maintain internal stability and to resist change.

Neurotransmitter   A chemical messenger that transmits an impulse from one nerve cell to the next.

the activation of medications, while others are involved in the regulation of the cellular cycle during cell proliferation. Some enzymes are essential for the digestion of larger nutrients such as dietary proteins, carbohydrates, and fatty acids, and are known as digestive enzymes. Other groups of enzymes regulate the synthesis and degradation of other enzymes involved in the processing and transport of micronutrients.

Deficiency in digestive enzymes causes slow and incomplete digestion of larger nutrients, thus reducing the availability of micronutrients to the body and resulting in a nutritional deficit. Although the body manufactures some digestive enzymes, a diet rich in fruits and vegetables provides a reliable source for digestive enzymes. Papaya, pineapple, cucumber (eaten with the skin), tomatoes, and green leafy vegetables are especially good sources for digestive enzymes.

Another frequent cause of nutritional deficiency is malabsorption of nutrients in the intestinal tract due to parasite infestation, infections, or disruption of the normal intestinal microorganism balance by some medications. Normally, a mixed population of bacteria permanently lives in the intestinal mucosa, helping to break down some larger molecules such as complex carbohydrates. When

this balance is disrupted, even though the daily diet contains the correct amounts of all necessary nutrients, nutritional deficiencies may occur due to the inability of the intestinal tract to absorb molecules that are not broken down by the beneficial bacteria.

Fatty acids are the components of lipids or fats that may be combined with proteins and/or sugars to form a variety of functional and structural molecules such as cholesterol, hormones, and enzymes. Fatty acids are also an important source of body energy and are stored in the adipose tissue (i.e., fat cells). Lipoproteins (such as cholesterol) are present in the structure of cell membranes and in blood plasma, and have a variety of other functions. For example, cholesterol is a precursor of bile acid and of steroid hormones such as testosterone, progesterone, and estrogen. Myelin, the white substance that involves nerve fibers as a multi-layered sheath, is constituted of lipids and proteins, and is essential for normal neural signal transmission, and muscle control and coordination. Fatty acids are present in whole milk, butter, fish, seafood, lard, meat, vegetable oils, margarine, nuts, olives, corn, soybean, and grains.

Carbohydrates encompass a variety of sugar molecules that play a multitude of roles in body physiology and are also a structural component of the cell membrane. Carbohydrates supply and store energy, aid in intercellular communication, and regulate many metabolic events in the body. The digestive process transforms carbohydrates into glucose, the main source of energy used by cells. Glucose, a simple sugar, is a component of many proteins known as glycoproteins, and is also present in the molecular structure of DNA as pentose. The central and peripheral nervous systems demand a constant supply of glucose in the blood, as does the muscular system. The body stores glucose in the form of glycogen that can be promptly mobilized when the level of glucose in the blood falls. Glycogen is mainly stored in skeletal muscles and in the liver, but it is also present in small amounts in virtually every cell of the body. Carbohydrates are present in milk, fruits, potatoes, cereals, sugar, and honey. Whole grains, lettuce, and fruits also contain a type of fibrous carbohydrate humans cannot digest, known as cellulose. Nevertheless, cellulose helps digestion because these fibers stimulate movement of the intestinal tract, preventing constipation and removing pathogenic germs.

The body needs to protect its cells and DNA from the damage oxygen and free radicals can do. Free radicals are highly reactive substances that form when oxygen interacts with other molecules during digestion or other cellular processes. To combat this damage, the body uses a defense system of antioxidant molecules that react safely with the free radicals. Some antioxidant molecules are naturally occurring enzymes. Vitamins are another important source of antioxidants.

Vitamins neutralize free radicals and protect tissue integrity and function. They are also essential for a number of other cellular functions such as tissue renewal and healing, red blood cell production, body resistance to infections, brain and muscle activity, DNA replication during cell cycle, adequate regulation of several metabolic events, recovery from disease, and prevention of chronic disease. Vitamins are divided in two categories according to their solubility: water-soluble vitamins and fat-soluble vitamins.

Vitamin C (ascorbic acid) and B-complex vitamins (thiamine, niacin, riboflavin, biotin, folic acid, cobalamin, pyridoxine, and pantothenic acid) are water-soluble vitamins. Since kidneys easily eliminate water-soluble vitamins through the urine, they must be present in the daily diet because only trace amounts are stored in the organism. The main dietary sources of vitamin C are tomatoes, green leafy vegetables, and citrus fruits such as oranges, although other fruits and vegetables do contain smaller amounts of vitamin C. Raw meat and fish also contain vitamin C that is lost in the cooking process. Vitamin C protects cells against oxidation, helps collagen formation, and the transformation of cholesterol into bile acids. The detoxification properties of vitamin C help in the elimination of the toxins and free radicals that build up in the extracellular fluids and in cells during infections.

B-complex vitamins participate as co-factors in a vast number of enzyme activities and act as co-antioxidants as well. Some B vitamins are required for red blood cell formation, while others are required for regulation of plasma cholesterol levels, energy release in tissues, amino acid synthesis, embryo development, brain development and neuronal activity, bone marrow formation, and infection resistance. Additionally, some B vitamins promote myelin sheath formation around nerve fibers and neurons during brain development in the fetus and during child growth as well. The main dietary sources of B-complex vitamins are whole milk, chicken, pork, egg, seafood, meat, liver, corn, wheat and whole grains, green leaves, and legumes. As not all B vitamins are present in each of these foods, it is important to keep a well-balanced and varied diet. Strict vegetarians, especially vegans, need supplementation of some B vitamins such as biotin and cobalamin as animal products are eliminated as a dietary source.

The fat-soluble vitamins are vitamins A, D, E, and K. The precursors of these vitamins are present in food, and are transformed by the body into the active vitamin form. Dietary precursors of vitamin A are beta-carotene and other carotenes found in carrots, yellow fruits and seeds, as well as in dark green vegetables. Retinol, found in animal products such as meat, fish, egg yolk, whole milk, and butter, is vitamin A itself. Vitamin A is essential for normal fetal development, child growth, tissue repair,

healing, and renewal, vision, cell protection against free radicals, and reproduction. Beta-carotene shows several benefits of its own, independently of being converted into vitamin A by the body. Some scientific evidence shows that adequate levels of beta-carotene in the diet help to prevent chronic and degenerative diseases such as skin cancer, cardiac diseases, and cataracts. This vegetable precursor of vitamin A also has its own antioxidant activity, and enhances immune system function. Whereas excessive intake of retinol may cause liver and nerve cell toxicity, beta-carotene does not offer such a risk.

Vitamin D is, in fact, a group of molecules that function as hormones. The dietary precursor of vitamin D in plants is known as ergocalciferol. Animal products contain some preformed active molecules of vitamin D. However, the main source of vitamin D in the organism is in the form of an intermediate molecule of cholesterol that is converted into calcitriol in the skin through the action of solar radiation. Long winter months in the northern hemisphere or little exposure to sunlight sometimes lead to deficiency of vitamin D, thus requiring greater dietary intakes of animal products such as fatty fish and egg yolk. Calcitriol, one active form of vitamin D, regulates the synthesis of proteins responsible for calcium and phosphate absorption in the intestinal tract. Vitamin D also regulates the levels of calcium in blood plasma, and helps the mineralization of bones. This micronutrient is essential for normal skeletal development of infants and children, and to prevent osteoporosis in adults, especially women and elderly men.

Tocopherols are different forms of vitamin E, such as alpha and beta tocopherols, and are important antioxidants that protect cholesterol and fatty acids against peroxidation, the chemical process that transforms lipids into rancid fat. Peroxidation of circulating cholesterol causes progressive vascular obstruction, which may lead to heart attack or **stroke**. Vitamin E also protects fatty acids and lipids that are components of cell membrane structure, thus maintaining the cell's normal functionality. The best dietary sources of vitamin E are vegetable oils.

Vitamin K occurs as phylloquinone in plants, and as menaquinone in bacteria of the intestinal flora. It is essential for the right formation of clotting factors, the proteins responsible for normal blood coagulation. Dietary sources are spinach, cabbage, egg yolk, and liver, although the normal intestinal bacterial flora constitutes a regular source of the vitamin as well.

Discrete (trace) amounts of some minerals are also vital for cell metabolism, neural and muscle activity, bone development and maintenance, electro-chemical reactions, and transport of nutrients and metabolic waste through the cell membrane. The most important minerals are calcium, phosphorus, potassium, magnesium, sodium, and iron.

Calcium and phosphorus are required by a variety of body functions such as bone formation and maintenance, neural signal transmission or synapses, smooth muscle contraction, and skeletal muscle activity. They also regulate glandular and enzymatic activity. Major sources of these nutrients are milk and dairy products. Magnesium works together with calcium, regulating calcium transport into cells and to and from bones. Magnesium controls the levels of calcium transported to heart tissue, maintaining the heartbeat in a steady pace. Magnesium is also important in cells of the immune system such as lymphocytes, in skeletal muscles, and as a facilitator of oxygen delivery. Magnesium participates in the production of ATP (adenosine triphosphate), the source of energy utilized by cells.

Sodium and potassium regulate levels of fluids entering and leaving the cells, and moving between blood vessels and the lymphatic system, and are, therefore, important agents in the regulation of blood pressure. Iron is an essential component of red blood cells (hemoglobin), which transport oxygen to all tissues. Iron is stored in the plasma in proteins known as ferritin. Adequate plasma levels of ferritin are required for hematopoiesis, or blood formation. However, excess ferritin in plasma increases cholesterol peroxidation, leading to cardiovascular disease. Trace amounts of minerals are present in fruits and other vegetables, as well as in animal products such as seafood, fish, liver, milk, meat, eggs, and poultry.

Dieticians are the best advisors when a specific diet is important, such as during pregnancy, or in infancy and early childhood development, in order to prevent nutritional deficits. Physicians can refer patients to trusted dieticians. Elderly citizens and ill people also need professional nutritional guidance to meet deficiencies associated with the aging process or disease. The same is true for professional athletes and individuals working in strenuous physical and/or mental conditions. For the general population, the United States Department of Agriculture has designed the Food Guide Pyramid, illustrating the groups of foods and the daily-required variety of foods for optimum nutrition and health maintenance.

Resources

BOOKS

Champe, Pamela C., and Richard A. Harvey. *Biochemistry*, 2nd ed. Philadelphia: Lippincott Williams & Wilkins, 1994.

Halliwell, Barry and Okezie I. Aruoma, (eds.) *DNA and Free Radicals*, 1st ed. London: Ellis Horwood Ltd., 1993.

Mayhan, L. Kathleen, and Sylvia Escott-Stump. *Krause's Food, Nutrition and Diet Therapy*. Philadelphia: W.B.Saunders, 2003.

PERIODICALS

Ghani H., D. Stevens, J. Weiss, and R. Rosenbaum. "Vitamins and the Risk for Parkinson's Disease." *Neurology* (2002) 59: E8–E9.

OTHER

USDA Food and Nutrition Information Center. *Food Guide Pyramid*. January 15, 2004 (May 20, 2004.) <http://www.nal.usda.gov/fnic/Fpyr/pyramid.html>.

U.S. Department of Agriculture. *Nutrition.gov.* January 15, 2004 (May 20, 2004). <http://www.nutrition.gov/home/index.php3>.

ORGANIZATIONS

National Institute of Neurological Disorders and Stroke, P.O. Box 5801, Bethesda, MD 20824. (301) 496-5751 or (800) 352-9424. <http://www.ninds.nih.gov/search.htm>.

American Dietetic Association. 120 South Riverside Plaza, Suite 2000, Chicago, IL 60606-6995. (800) 877-1600. education@eatright.org. <http://www.eatright.org>.

Sandra Galeotti

Diffuse sclerosis *see* **Schilder's disease**

Diplopia *see* **Visual disturbances**

Disc herniation

Definition

Intervertebral discs are circular ring-like flat structures that function as cushions between two spinal vertebrae, allowing spinal flexibility and acting as shock absorbers. Each intervertebral disc contains a nucleus (center) surrounded by a sack of fibrocartilage (fibrous, connective tissue), rich in collagens (fibrous protein). A herniated disc occurs when the outer sack partially ruptures and the interior of the sack expands, pushing part of the disc into the spinal canal near to where the spinal cord and other nerve roots are located. This causes either chronic or acute **pain** in the back or in the neck, and movement restriction of the affected area due to pressure exerted on the spinal nerve roots. This condition is also known as a slipped disc, an intervertebral disc hernia, a herniated intervertebral disc, and a herniated nucleus pulposus.

Description

Intervertebral disc disease is among the most common causes of neck and **back pain**. Cervical disc herniations (in the neck region) are less common than lumbar (lower back) herniations. Lumbar disc herniations affect an estimated four out of five patients complaining of back pain. Several factors may contribute to a herniated disc, such as poor posture, work-related strain, traumatic injuries due to falls or blows in the back, improper weight lifting, obesity, and sport-related muscular strain. Disc herniation may also occur because of age-related degenerative processes that cause progressive loss of disc elasticity.

Key Terms

Collagen The main supportive protein of cartilage, connective tissue, tendon, skin, and bone.

Spinal cord The elongated nerve bundles that lie in the spinal canal and from which the spinal nerves emerge.

Other risk factors associated with disc hernias are lack of regular physical exercises, inadequate nutrition, smoking, and genetic factors.

Demographics

Herniated disc is a common problem, with approximately one in 32, or 8.4 million people in the United States affected each year.

Causes and symptoms

Degenerative disc disease, usually related to aging, is more common in the lumbar area, where much of the wear-and-tear of a lifetime of activity is exerted, resulting in chronic back pain. However, in the cervical area the disc degenerative process usually starts with a traumatic twisting of the disc space that leads to chronic inflammatory pain in the neck, and may result in arm pain and numbness. The degenerative process may also be associated with occupational repetitive movements such as those required in construction, farming, mining, and other professional activities where workers are required to handle heavy loads.

Herniated discs sometimes cause pain that is incapacitating, and the condition accounts for a major cause of work disability and health care expense in the United States. Lumbar disc hernias are commonly associated with **sciatica** (inflammation of the sciatic nerve in the lower back) due to disc protrusion or herniation that compresses the spinal nerve root radiating to the femoral or sciatic nerve. A sensation of sharp, painful electric-like shock is felt during acute sciatica both in the back and along the involved limb. Other symptoms are a burning pain in the back, numbness or tingling sensation in the related leg, and weakness in one or both legs.

Growing scientific evidence also points to genetic factors in disc herniation, especially in families with a history of predisposition to early-onset sciatica and disk herniation. The causation factor seems to be a mutation in one of the three genes (COL9A1, COL9A2, and COL9A3), which are related to the formation of collagen.

Diagnosis

A clinical record of chronic back pain and progressive leg pain points to the possibility of a degenerative disc disease in progression; and physical palpation (examination by touch) by the physician may reveal whether a nerve root is affected. The straight leg-raising test (raising the leg straight, with no bend at the knee, until pain is experienced in the thigh, buttocks, and calf) can also point to nerve root irritation in the lumbosacral area due to herniated disc. X ray of the affected spinal area is the standard test for confirmation of a herniated disc. When surgery is being considered, other imaging tests are performed, such as a **magnetic resonance imaging (MRI)** scan or computed tomography (**CT**) **scan,** for confirmation of the diagnosis.

Treatment team

The orthopedist is the medical specialist often first consulted, and many orthopedic clinics offer the services of physical therapists whose interventions will be prescribed by the physician. In more severe cases, the intervention of a **neurologist**, neurosurgeon, or an orthopedic surgeon, along with a pain specialist may be required.

Treatment

In most cases, conservative treatments such as over-the-counter painkillers, anti-inflammatory drugs, and muscle relaxants associated with a period of bed rest are enough to curb the acute phase. To prevent further acute pain, physical therapy and specific exercises may be recommended by the physician, along with the identification of poor postural habits and posture-correction exercises. However, in more severe cases where conservative treatment fails, further treatment may be necessary, such as injections with cortisone. Surgery is only a real necessity when a progressive loss of neurological function is experienced, leading, for instance, to bladder or bowel incontinence or limb paralysis. In cases of frequently recurrent acute pain, the person with a herniated disc chooses surgical intervention to decrease pain and improve quality of life.

Prognosis

The vast majority of people (more than 90%) treated for herniated disc experience improvement with pain and mobility. About 5% of people who have experienced a herniated disc will eventually have recurring pain, and another 5% will experience a herniated disc at another vertebral site.

Resources
BOOKS
De Beeck, Rik Op, and Hermans Veerle. *Research on Work-Related Low Back Disorders.* Brussels: Institute for

Occupational Safety and Health/European Agency for Safety and Health at Work, 2000.

PERIODICALS

Humphries, Craig D., and Jason C. Eck. "Clinical Evaluation and Treatment Options for Herniated Lumbar Disc." *American Family Physician* (1999): February 1, 575–587.

OTHER

Herniated Disc—Factsheet. American Association of Neurological Surgeons. January 4, 2004 (March 18, 2004). <http://www.neurosurgery.org/health/patient/answers.asp?DisorderID=37>.

ORGANIZATIONS

National Institute of Arthritis and Musculoskeletal and Skin Diseases (NIAMS). 1 AMS Circle, Bethesda, MD 20892-3675. (301) 495-4484 or (877) 22-NIAMS; Fax: (301) 718-6366. niamsinfo@mail.nih.gov. <http://www.niams.nih.gov/>.

Sandra Galeotti

Dizziness

Definition

Dizziness is a general term that describes sensations of imbalance and unsteadiness, such as vertigo, mild turning, imbalance, and near **fainting** or fainting. Feelings of dizziness stem from the vestibular system, which includes the brain and the parts of the inner ear that sense position and motion, coupled with sensory information from the eyes, skin, and muscle tension.

Description

Because dizziness is a general term for a variety of feelings of instability, it spans a large range of symptoms. These symptoms range from the most dramatic, vertigo, to the least severe, imbalance. Included in these feelings is fainting, which results in a loss of consciousness.

Vertigo is an acute feeling of violent rotation. People with vertigo often feel as if they are tilting or falling through space. Vertigo is most often caused by problems with the vestibular system of the inner ear. Symptoms can be brief, or may last for extended periods of time and may be accompanied by changes in pulse and blood pressure, perspiration, nausea, and a type of rapid eye movement called nystagmus.

Mild turning is a less violent type of vertigo. People with mild turning are still able to function in normal daily routines. However, a feeling of turning may continue for weeks. Mild turning is usually a symptom of inner ear dysfunction. It may also result from **transient ischemic attack**, or a lack of blood flow to the brain. People who have suffered from strokes may feel mild turning for periods of time. Mild turning may also be associated with **multiple sclerosis**, **AIDS**, or head trauma.

Imbalance is a feeling of instability or floating. It is associated with many general medical problems such as the flu or infection. Imbalance can also be associated with arthritis, especially in the neck, or another neurological problem.

Fainting is a sudden loss of consciousness and near fainting is a feeling of extreme light-headedness with a sinking or falling feeling. Vision usually becomes hazy or dimmed and the extremities become weak. Both fainting and near fainting are caused by lack of blood flow to the brain. Anything that causes a rapid drop in blood pressure, such as a heart attack or an insulin reaction in a diabetic, can result in fainting or near fainting. Panic attacks that cause a person to exhale a lot of carbon dioxide can cause fainting or near fainting.

Vestibular system

The vestibular system is the sensory system located in the inner ear that helps the body to maintain balance. Balance in the human body is coordinated by the brainstem, which, with speed and precision, collects information from other parts of the brain and sensory organs throughout the body. It is the brainstem that sends neurological instructions to the muscles and joints. The sensory organs that play critical roles relaying information to the brainstem include the skin, eyes, muscles and joints, and the vestibular system in the inner ear. Dizziness may result with dysfunction in any of these components or in the nerves that connect them.

Brain

The **cerebellum**, which is responsible for coordination and the cerebral cortex, provides neurological information to the brainstem. For example, the cerebellum is the organ that informs the body how to shift weight when going down a flight of stairs and how to balance on a bicycle. These processes are accomplished without conscious thinking.

In order to maintain balance, the brainstem depends on input from sensory organs including the eyes, muscles, joints, skin and ears. This information is relayed to the brainstem via the spinal cord. The combined neurological receptor system, which involves the brainstem, spinal cord, and sensory organs, is called the proprioceptive system. Proprioceptive dysfunction may result in dizziness, and people with problems with their proprioceptive system may fall often. Additionally, as people age, problems with proprioception become more common.

Key Terms

Auditory nerve   A bundle of nerve fibers that carries hearing information between the cochlea the brain.

Benign positional paroxysmal vertigo (BPPV)   A common cause of dizziness thought to be caused by debris that has collected within a part of the inner ear.

Brainstem   The part of the brain extending from the base to the spinal cord, responsible for controlling basic functions such as respiration and breathing.

Cerebral cortex   The surface gray matter of the cerebral hemispheres (cerebrum) of the brain, responsible for receiving sensory information, for conscious thought, and for movement.

Cerebellum   Area of the brain lying below and behind the cerebrum, responsible for maintaining balance, and coordinating and controlling voluntary muscle movement.

Mèniére's disease   An inner ear disorder that can affect both hearing and balance, and can cause vertigo, hearing loss, along with ringing and a sensation of fullness in the ear.

Otolith organs   Organs in the vestibular apparatus that sense horizontal and vertical movements of the head.

Semicircular canals   A set of three fluid-filled loops in the inner ear that are important to balance.

Vertigo   Extreme dizziness.

Vestibular system   The sensory system located in the inner ear that allows the body to maintain balance.

Sensory organs

Visual information is of particular importance to maintaining balance. The visual systems most involved are the optokinetic and pursuit systems. The optokinetic system is the motor impulse responsible for moving the eyes when the head moves, so that the field of vision remains clear. The pursuit system allows a person to focus on a moving object while the head remains stationary. Both of these systems feed information about the person's position relative to the surroundings to the brainstem. A specific type of eye movement called nystagmus, which is repetitive jerky movements of the eye, most often in the horizontal direction, may cause dizziness. Nystagmus may indicate that neurologic signals from the optokinetic or pursuit systems are not in agreement with the other balance information received by the brain.

Sensory information from muscles, joints, and skin plays a key role in balance. The muscles and joints of the human body are lined with sensory receptors that send neurological information about the position of the body to the brainstem. For example, receptors in the neck muscles tell the brain which way the head is turned. The skin, in particular the skin of the feet and buttocks, is covered with pressure sensors that relay information to the brain regarding what part of the body is touching the ground.

Peripheral vestibular system

The ear, particularly the inner ear, plays a critical role in maintaining balance. The inner ear contains two major parts: the cochlea, which is mostly used for hearing, and the vestibular apparatus, also known as the peripheral

vestibular system, which is important in balance. A set of channels connects the two parts of the ear and therefore any disease that affects hearing may also affect balance, and vice versa.

The peripheral vestibular system consists of a series of canals and chambers, all of which are made of membranes. This membrane system is filled with a fluid called endolymph. The peripheral vestibular system is further embedded in the temporal bone of the skull. In the space between the temporal bone and the membranes of the peripheral vestibular system resides a second fluid called perilymph. Endolymph and perilymph each have a different chemical makeup consisting of varying concentrations of water, potassium, sodium, and other salts. Endolymph flows out of the peripheral vestiubular system into an endolymphatic sac and then diffuses through a membrane into the cerebrospinal fluid that bathes the brain. Perilymph flows out of the peripheral vestibular system and directly into the cerebrospinal fluid. When the flow pressures or chemical compositions of the endolymph and perilymph change, feelings of dizziness can occur. These types of changes may be related to Mèniére's disease.

The vestibular apparatus is made up of two types of sensory organs: otolith organs and semicircular canals. The otolith organs sense the direction of gravity, while the semicircular canals sense rotation and movement of the head.

Two otolith organs in each ear are called the saccule and the utricle. The saccule is oriented in a vertical direction when a person is standing and, best senses vertical motion of the head. The utricle is nearly horizontal when a person is standing, so it best senses horizontal motion of the head. Each organ consists of calcium carbonate crystals embedded in a gel. Special hair-producing cells extend into the gel from below. As the head moves, gravity and inertia cause the crystals to bend the hairs, which are in contact with nerves. Information on the position and motion of the head is thus relayed to the brain. If the hairs or the crystals in the otolith organs are damaged, feelings of dizziness may result.

In each ear, there are also three semicircular canals that lie on planes that are perpendicular to each other. The canals are connected together by a main chamber called a vestibule. The canals and the vestibule are filled with endolymph fluid. Near its connection to the vestibule, one end of each of the canals widens into a region called the ampulla. One side of the ampulla is lined with specialized sensory cells. These cells have hairlike structures that extend into a gelatinous structure called a cupula. As the head moves in a given plane, the endolymph inside the semicircular canal in that plane remains stationary due to inertia. The cupula, however, moves because it is attached to the head. This puts pressure on the cupula, which in turn moves the hairlike structures. The bending of the hairlike structures stimulates nerves, alerting the brain that the head is moving in a particular plane. By integrating information from all three planes in which the semicircular canals lie, the brain reconstructs the three-dimensional movement of the head. If information from one of the semicircular canals does not agree with that of another, or if the information generated by semicircular canals in one ear does not agree with the information produced by the other ear, feelings of dizziness may result.

All of the signals from the peripheral vestibular system travel to the brain along the eighth cranial nerve, also called the vestibular nerve. Damage to this nerve, either through head trauma or the growth of tumors, can also cause feelings of dizziness. Neurological information from the semicircular canals seems be more important to the brain than information from the otolith structures. If the eighth cranial nerve on one side of the head is damaged, but the other side remains intact, the brain learns to compensate over time; however, the mechanics involved in this process are not well understood.

Demographics

Dizziness is an extremely common symptom occurring in people of all ages, ethnicities, and socioeconomic backgrounds. Balance disorders increase with age, and by age 75, dizziness is one of the most common reasons for visiting a doctor. In the general population, dizziness is the third most common reason that patients visit doctors. According to the National Institutes of Health (NIH), about 42% of the population of the United States will complain of dizziness at some point in their lives. In the United States, the cost of medical care for patients with symptoms of imbalance is estimated to be more than $1 billion per year.

Diseases associated with dizziness

Because it involves so many different parts of the body, the balance system may exhibit signs of dysfunction for a variety of reasons. Dizziness may be caused by problems with the **central nervous system**, the vestibular system, the sensory organs, including the eyes, muscles and joints, or more systemic disorders such as cardiovascular disease, bacterial and viral diseases, arthritis, blood disorders, medications, or psychological illnesses.

Central nervous system dysfunction

Any problem that affects the nerves leading to the brain from vestibular or sensory organs, the spinal cord, the cerebellum, the cerebral cortex, or the brainstem may result in dizziness. In particular, tumors that affect any of these organs are of concern. In addition, disorders that affect blood supply to the central nervous system, such as transient ischemic attacks, **stroke**, migraines, **epilepsy**, or multiple sclerosis, may result in feelings of dizziness.

BRAIN TUMORS Although rare, acoustic neuroma is a benign tumor growing on the vestibulo-cochlear nerves, which reach from the inner ear to the brain. It may press as well on blood vessels that flow between the peripheral vestibular system and the brain. Symptoms included ringing in one ear, imbalance, and hearing loss. Distortion of words often becomes increased as the tumor grows and disturbs the nerve. Treatment requires surgical removal of the tumor, which nearly always returns the sense of balance to normal, although some residual hearing loss may occur.

Other brain tumors may also cause feelings of dizziness. These include tumors that originate in the brain tissue, such as meningiomas (benign tumors) and gliomas (malignant tumors). Sometimes tumors from other parts of the body may metastasize in the brain and cause problems with balance.

CEREBRAL ATROPHY Age causes atrophy (deterioration) of brain cells that may result in slight feelings of imbalance. More severe forms of dizziness may result from other neurological disorders.

BLOOD SUPPLY DISORDERS If the blood flow and oxygenation to the cerebellum, cerebral cortex, or brainstem is not adequate, feelings of dizziness can result. Such symptoms can result from several types of disorders, including anemia, transient ischemic attacks (TIAs), and stroke.

TIAs are temporary loss of blood supply to the brain, often caused by arteriosclerosis (hardening of the arteries). In addition to a brief period of dizziness or vertigo, symptoms include a transient episode of numbness on one side of the body, and slurred speech and/or lack of coordination. If the loss of blood supply to the brain is due to a blockage in one of the arteries in the neck, surgery may correct the problem.

Strokes, or cerebrovascular accidents (CVA), occur in three major ways. A thrombotic stroke occurs when a fatty deposit forms a clot in an artery, blocking blood supply to the brain. An embolic stroke occurs when part of a clot from another part of the body breaks off and obstructs an artery leading to the brain. A hemorrhagic stroke occurs when blood vessels in the brain hemorrhage, leaving a blood clot in the brain.

PERIPHERAL VESTIBULAR SYSTEM DYSFUNCTION
When balance problems are brief or intermittent, the peripheral vestibular system is usually the cause. Many different problems may be at the root of vestibular disorder.

BENIGN PAROXYSMAL POSITIONAL VERTIGO (BPPV)
Benign paroxysmal positional vertigo occurs following an abrupt change in position of the head. Often, onset of vertigo occurs when patients roll from their back onto the side, and it usually subsides in less than a minute. BPPV can result from head trauma, degeneration of the peripheral vestibular system with age, infection of the respiratory tract, high blood pressure, or other cardiovascular diseases. Those who suffer from an infection of their vestibular system, causing severe vertigo that lasts up to several days, can develop BPPV any time within the next eight years. BPPV is also associated with migraine **headaches**.

Two theories on the cause of BPPV currently exist. One suggests that BPPV will occur when the calcium carbonate crystals in the otolith organs (the saccule and the utiricle) are displaced and become lodged in the cupula of the semicircular canals due to head trauma, infection, or degeneration of the inner ear canals. This displacement will stimulate the nerves from the semicircular canals when the head rotates in a particular position, indicating to the brain that the person is spinning. However, the rest of the sensory organs in the body report that the body is stationary. This conflicting information produces vertigo. The calcium carbonate crystals dissolve after a brief time, and the symptom is rectified. The second theory suggests that cellular debris accumulates into a mass that moves around the semicircular canals, exerting pressure on the cupula and causing vertigo. When the mass dissolves, the symptoms subside.

INNER EAR INFECTIONS
Inner ear infection, or vestibular neuronitis, occurs some time after a person has suffered from a viral infection. Onset includes a violent attack of vertigo, including nausea, vomiting, and the inability to stand or walk. Symptoms subside in several days, although feelings of unsteadiness may continue for a week or more. A swelling of the vestibular nerve following a viral infection causes vestibular neuronitis.

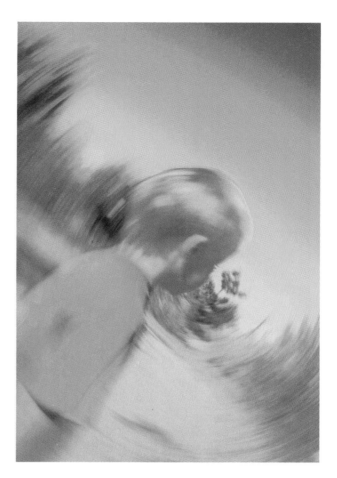

Photographic representation of vertigo. *(© 1993 J. S. Reid/Custom Medical Stock Photo. Reproduced by permission.)*

Sometimes the inflammation can recur over several years. A viral infection affecting the inner ear, but not the vestibular nerve, is called viral labyrinthitis. Labyrinthitis can cause hearing loss, but all other symptoms are similar to vestibular neuronitis.

Severe bacterial infections can also cause inflammation of the inner ear. These cases include risk of deafness, inflammation of the brain, and meningitis (inflammation of the membranes surrounding the brain and spinal cord). Otitis occurs when fluid accumulates in the middle ear, causing feelings of imbalance, mild turning, or vertigo. When the infection reaches the inner ear, the disease is called acute suppurative labyrinthitis. Treatment for any bacterial infection in the ear is critical to prevent long-term damage to hearing and balance organs.

PERILYMPH FISTULA
Perilymph fistulas are openings that occur between the middle ear and the inner ear. This allows a hole through which perilymph can flow, changing the pressure of perilymph flowing into the brain and causing dizziness. Fistulas often form as a result of head

trauma or abrupt changes in pressure. Symptoms may also include hearing loss, ringing in the ears, coordination problems, nystagmus, and headaches. Most fistulas heal with time; however, in severe cases, surgical procedures are used to close the hole, using a tissue graft.

MÈNIÉRE'S DISEASE In 1861, French physician Prosper Mèniére described Mèniére's disease as having four particular symptoms: vertigo lasting for an hour or more, but less than 24 hours; ringing or buzzing sounds in the ear; feeling of pressure or fullness in the ear; and some hearing loss. Some people are affected in both ears; others just one ear. Onset of Mèniére's may be related to stress, although not in all cases. Nystagmus is usually associated with the attacks.

Mèniére's disease is thought to be caused by an accumulation of endolymph within the canals of the inner ear, a condition called endolymphatic hydrops. This causes produces a swelling in the canals containing endolymph, which puts pressure on the parts of the canals containing perilymph. The result affects both hearing and balance. In severe cases, it is feared that the endolymphatic compartments may burst, disrupting both the chemical and pressure balances between the two fluids.

The cause of the accumulation of endolymph is unknown, although it can be related to trauma to the head, infection, degeneration of the inner ear, or some other regulatory mechanism. Syphilis is often associated with Mèniére's disease, as are allergies and leukemia. Some suggest that Mèniére's disease is an autoimmune dysfunction. There may be a genetic predisposition to Mèniére's disease.

Mèniére's disease is usually treated with meclizine (Antivert), antihistamines, and sedatives. Diuretics can be used to rid the body of excess endolymph. Salt-free diets can also help to prevent the accumulation of fluid in the ears.

Systemic disorders

Dizziness may be a symptom of a disorder that affects the whole body, or systems within the body. Dizziness may also be the result of systemic toxicity to substances such as medications and drugs.

POSTURAL HYPOTENSION The major symptom of postural hypotension, also called orthostasis, is low blood pressure. When a person stands up from a prone position, blood vessels in the legs and feet must constrict to force blood to the brain. When blood pressure is low, the blood vessels do not constrict quickly or with enough pressure and the result is a lag before blood reaches the brain, causing dizziness. Postural hypotension can be treated with an increase in fluid intake or with blood pressure medication.

HEART CONDITIONS A variety of heart conditions can cause feelings of dizziness. In particular, arrhythmia, a dysfunction of the heart characterized by an irregular heartbeat, decreases blood supply to the brain in such a way as to cause balance problems. In most cases, symptoms of dizziness associated with arrhythmia result from problems with heart valves, such as narrowing of the aorta and mitral valve prolapse.

INFECTIOUS DISEASES Influenza and flu-like diseases can cause dizziness, especially if accompanied by fever. The virus herpes zoster oticus causes painful blisters and **shingles**. If the virus attacks the facial nerve, it may result in vertigo. Several bacterial diseases can result in dizziness, including tuberculosis, syphilis, meningitis, or encephalitis. One of the major symptoms of **Lyme disease**, which is caused by infection of a microorganism resulting from a deer tick bite, is dizziness.

BLOOD DISORDERS A variety of diseases of the blood result in feelings of dizziness. These diseases include anemia, or a depletion of iron in the blood, sickle-cell anemia, leukemia, and polycythemia.

DRUGS AND OTHER SUBSTANCES A variety of substances ingested systemically to prevent disorders of diseases can result in feelings of dizziness. In particular, overdose of aspirin and other anti-inflammatory drugs can cause problems with balance. Antibiotics taken for extended periods of time are also known to cause dizziness. Streptomycin is known to damage the vestibular system, if taken in large doses. Medicines that are used to treat high blood pressure can lower blood pressure so much as to cause feelings of light-headedness. Quinine, which is taken to treat malaria, can cause dizziness, as can antihistamines used to prevent allergy attacks. Chemotherapy drugs are well known to have various side effects, including dizziness. Alcohol, caffeine, and nicotine are also known to cause dizziness, when taken in large doses.

Diagnosis

Because maintaining posture integrates so many different parts of the body, diagnosing the actual problem responsible for dizziness often requires a battery of tests. The cardiovascular system, the neurological system, and the vestibular system are all examined.

Blood pressure is one of the most important cardiovascular measurements made to determine the cause of imbalance. Usually the physician will measure blood pressure and heart rate with the patient lying down, and then again after the patient stands up. If blood pressure drops significantly and the heart rate increases more than five beats per minute, this signals the existence of postural

Dizziness

hypotension. Dizziness in people suffering from diabetes or on blood pressure medicine may be caused by postural hypotension.

Neurological tests

Because the central nervous system is integral to maintaining balance, neurological tests are often performed on patients with symptoms of dizziness. A test of mental status is often performed to ascertain that mental function is healthy. Physicians may test tendon reflexes to determine the status of peripheral and motor nerves, as well as spinal cord function. Nerves in different parts of the body may also be evaluated. In addition, physicians may test muscle strength and tone, coordination, and gait.

Neurologists may also perform a variety of computerized scans that determine if tumors or acoustic neuromas are present. These tests include **magnetic resonance imaging (MRI)**, computerized tomography (**CT**), and electroencephalogram (EEG).

Tests of the vestibular system

Most often performed by a otolaryngologist, the battery of tests performed to determine the health of the vestibular system include the Dix-Halpike test, electrostagmography, hearing tests, rotation tests, and posturography.

DIX-HALPIKE TEST The Dix-Halpike test, also called the Halpike test, is performed to determine if a patient suffers from benign paroxysmal positional vertigo (BPPV). The patient is seated and positioned so that his or her head hangs off the edge of the table when lying down. The patient's head is moved 45 degrees in one direction. The patient is then asked to lie down, without moving his or her head. The same procedure will be repeated on the other side. If feelings of vertigo result from this movement, BPPV is usually diagnosed.

ELECTRONYSTAGMOGRAPHY (ENG) Considered one of the most telling diagnostic tests to determine the cause of dizziness, electronystagmography consists of a series of evaluations that test the interactions between the vestibular organs and the eyes, also called the vestibulo-ocular reflex. Results from this test can inform the physician whether problems are caused by the vestibular system or by the central nervous system.

The most common diagnostic feature observed during ENG is nystagmus, an involuntary movement of the pupils that allows a person to maintain balance. In healthy persons, nystagmus consists of a slow movement in one direction in response to a change in the visual field and quick corrective movement in the other direction. In persons with disorders of the vestibular organs, nystagmus will produce quick movements in the horizontal direction. People with neurologic disorders will show signs of nystagmus in the vertical direction or even in a circular pattern.

In most of the ENG tests, electrodes taped to the patient's head record nystagmus as the patient is exposed to a variety of moving lights or patterns of stripes that stimulate the vestibular system. The patient may be asked to stand and lie in various positions for the tests. Also, included in the ENG is a caloric test in which warm water and cool water are circulated through the outer ear. This causes a slight expansion or contraction of the endolymph in the inner ear and simulates movement cues to the brain.

HEARING TESTS Because the cochlea and the vestibular organs are adjacent to one another, hearing dysfunction can often be related to problems with dizziness. Audiograms include tests for both hearing and interpreting sounds, and can determine whether or not problems exist in the middle ear, the inner ear, or the auditory nerve.

ROTATION TESTS Rotation tests evaluate the vestibulo-ocular reflex and provide important information when the dysfunction is common to both ears. Electrodes are usually taped to the face to monitor eye movement, and the patient is placed in a chair. The chair rotates at different speeds through different arcs of a circle. The audiologist may also ask the patient to focus on different objects as the chair is rotated.

POSTUROGRAPHY During posturography tests, a patient stands on a platform that measures how weight is distributed. During the test, the patient will close and open his or her eyes or look into a box with different visual stimuli. The platform is computer controlled so that it can gently tip forward or backward or from side to side. Posturography measures how much the patient sways or moves in response to the stimuli. This provides information on the function of the proprioceptive system, as well as the vestibular system.

Treatment

If symptoms of dizziness are found to be associated with systemic diseases such as diabetes, hypotension, or other infectious diseases, or with neurological disorders, treatment for the dizziness is usually successful.

In many patients, dizziness caused by vestibular dysfunction tends to dissipate with time and with little treatment. However, available and common treatments for vestibular problems include physical therapies, medications, and surgeries. In addition, low-salt diets, relaxation techniques, and psychological counseling may be used as treatment.

Exercises and therapy

The physical therapies to decrease dizziness fall into two major groups. Compensation therapies help train the patient's brain to rely on the sensory information it receives to maintain balance, and to ignore information from damaged organs. Exercises in a compensation program are designed to focus on the movements that cause dizziness so that the brain can adapt to these behaviors. In addition, exercises that teach the patient how to keep the eye movements separate from head movements and to practice balancing in various positions are used.

Specific exercises aimed at relieving benign paroxysmal positional vertigo (BPPV), called canalith repositioning procedures, have recently been developed. By turning the head to one side and moving from a sitting to lying position in a certain sequence, BPPV can be quickly relieved. The movements in the canalith repositioning procedures are intended to move calcium carbonate crystals from the semicircular canals back to the utricle. The success rate with these exercises can be up to 90%.

Medications

A variety of medications are used to treat vertigo. These include vestibular suppressants, which seem to work by decreasing the rate of firing of nerve cells. Common vestibular suppressants are meclizine (Antivert, Bonine, and Vetrol). Also prescribed are anti-nausea medications such as promethazane (Phenergan) and antihistamines (Benadryl, Dramamine). For dizziness brought on by anxiety attacks, anti-anxiety drugs such as **diazepam** (Valium) and lorazepam (Ativan) may be used. These drugs all have side effects and are seldom prescribed for long periods of time.

Surgery

Surgery is usually the last step in the treatment of dizziness, only used after therapy and medications have failed. One of the more common surgical procedures for treating vestibular disorders is patching perilymph fistulas, or tears, at the tops of the semicircular canals. Surgery may also be used to drain excess fluid from the endolymphatic canals to relieve endolymphatic hydrops. Cutting the vestibular nerve just before it joins with the auditory nerve to form the eighth cranial nerve can also be performed to alleviate severe problems with dizziness. Finally, the entire labyrinth can be destroyed in a procedure called a labyrinthectomy, although this is usually only performed when hearing has been completely lost as well.

Resources

BOOKS

Blakely, Brian W., and Mary-Ellen Siegel. *Feeling Dizzy: Understanding and Treating Dizziness, Vertigo, and Other Balance Disorders.* New York: Macmillan USA, 1997.

Olsen, Wayne, ed. *Mayo Clinic on Hearing: Strategies for Managing Hearing Loss, Dizziness, and Other Ear Problems.* Rochester, MN: Mayo Clinic Health Information, 2003.

OTHER

"Vestibular Disorders: An Overview." *The Vestibular Disorders Association.* November 3, 2003. (April 4, 2004). <http://www.vestibular.org/overview.html>.

"Equilibrium Pathologies." *Archives for Sensology and Neurootology in Science and Practice.* January 2004 (April 4, 2004). <http://www.vertigo-dizziness.com/english/equilibrium_pathologies.html>.

"Dizziness." *The Mayo Clinic.* October 10, 2002 (April 4, 2004). <http://www.mayoclinic.com/invoke.cfm?id=DS00435>.

"Dizziness and Motion Sickness." *The American Academy of Otolaryngology and Head and Neck Surgery.* January 30, 2004 (April 4, 2004). <http://www.entnet.org/healthinfo/balance/dizziness.cfm>.

"Balance, Dizziness and You." *National Institute on Deafness and other Communication Disorders.* November 20, 2003 (April 4, 2004). <http://www.nidcd.nih.gov/health/balance/baldizz.asp>.

ORGANIZATIONS

Vestibular Disorders Association. P.O. Box 4467, Portland, OR 97208. (503) 229-7705 or (800) 837-8428. <http://www.vestibular.org>.

Juli M. Berwald, PhD

Donepezil *see* **Cholinesterase inhibitors**

▌Dopamine receptor agonists

Definition

Dopamine receptor agonists are a class of drugs with similar actions to dopamine, a neurotransmitter that occurs naturally in the brain. A neurotransmitter is a chemical that allows the movement of information from one nerve cell (neuron) across the gap between the adjacent neuron. Dopaminergic receptors are protein complexes on the surface of certain neurons of the sympathetic autonomic nervous system that bind to dopamine.

Purpose

Dopamine stimulates the heart, increases the blood flow to the liver, spleen, kidneys, and other visceral organs, and controls muscle movements and motor coordination through an inhibitory action over stimuli response. Abnormal low levels of dopamine are associated with

tremors, muscular rigidity, low blood pressure, and low cardiac input. Therefore, dopamine and dopaminergic agonist drugs are administered to treat shock and congestive heart failure and to improve motor functions in patients with **Parkinson's disease** and other **movement disorders**. The balance between two neurotransmitter levels, acetylcholine and dopamine, is essential for motor and fine movement coordination. The balance is frequently found altered in movement disorders, due to a dopamine deficiency that results in excessive stimulation of skeletal muscles. In Parkinson's disease, either dopamine levels or the number of dopamine receptors are progressively decreased, resulting in tremors, slowness of movements, muscle rigidity, and poor posture and gait (manner of walking). Symptoms of Parkinson's disease are treated with anticholinergic drugs and/or dopamine receptor agonists. Dopaminergic agonist drugs such as levodopa (L-dopa) along with carbidopa, bromocriptine mesylate, cabergoline, pergolide mesylate, pramipexole, and ropinirole hydrochloride are prescribed to treat the symptoms of Parkinson's disease, either alone or in combinations.

Description

L-dopa (levodopa) is a precursor of dopamine, i.e., is converted into dopamine by the body. Levodopa thus increases dopamine levels in the motor areas of the **central nervous system** (CNS), especially in the initial stages of the disease. However, as the disease progresses, the drug loses its efficacy (effectiveness). When administered with carbidopa, levodopa's effects are enhanced because carbidopa increases L-dopa transport to the brain and decreases its gastrointestinal metabolism. Therefore, two beneficial effects are achieved: better results with lower doses of levodopa (4–5 times lower doses than in L-dopa therapy alone); and reduction or prevention of levodopa side effects, such as nausea, anorexia, vomiting, rapid heart rate, low blood pressure, mood changes, anxiety, and **depression**.

Bromocriptine mesylate is a derivative of ergotamine that inhibits the production of prolactin hormone by the pituitary gland. It is used in association with levodopa, in order to allow lower doses of the latter, especially in long-term therapy. Bromocriptine is also used to treat some menstrual disorders and infertility. This drug shows poor results in patients who do not respond to levodopa.

Pergolide mesylate has an action similar to that of bromocriptine, also inhibiting prolactin secretion. Also used in Parkinson's in association with L-dopa and carbidopa, pergolide is eliminated from the body through the kidneys. Cabergoline also inhibits prolactin secretion and is used to decrease abnormally high levels of this hormone, whether due to endocrine dysfunction or due to an

Key Terms

Dopamine A neurotransmitter in the brain involved in regulating nerve impulses associated with muscle movement, blood pressure, mood, and memory.

Dyskinesia Difficulty in moving, or a movement disorder.

Neurotransmitter A chemical that is released during a nerve impulse that transmits information from one nerve cell to another.

existing pituitary tumor. The drug is also prescribed to regulate the menstrual cycle in cases of polycystic ovaries, and to control symptoms in Parkinson's disease.

Pramipexole and ropinirole are dopaminergic agonists that show good results in controlling Parkinson's symptoms in patients still in the initial stages of the disease and not yet treated with L-dopa, thus postponing the need of levodopa administration to a later phase. They work as well in those patients with advanced Parkinson's symptoms already taking levodopa.

Precautions

Levodopa may worsen psychotic symptoms when administered to psychiatric patients and anti-psychotic drugs should not be taken with this medication. L-dopa is also contraindicated to patients with glaucoma, because it increases pressure within the eye. Patients with cardiac disorders must be carefully monitored during levodopa administration due to the risk of altered heart rhythms.

Bromocriptine is contraindicated (not advised) for children under 15 years old, in pregnancy, severe cardiac disease, and severely decreased kidney or liver function. Alcoholic beverages are contraindicated during bromocriptine use as well as the administration of diuretics or anti-psychotic drugs. Psychiatric disorders may worsen with the administration of this drug.

Pergolide is contraindicated in women who are breast-feeding or those with preexisting movement disorders or a psychotic condition. Patients with heart rhythm disturbances should be not take this medication.

Cabergoline is not indicated in cases of severe or uncontrolled hypertension (high blood pressure) or for women who are breast-feeding, and requires careful monitoring in patients with significant kidney or liver dysfunction. Pregnant women who are at risk for eclampsia should not take this medication as well.

Pramipexole and ropinirole are eliminated through the kidneys, and the simultaneous use of medications that decrease kidney function (such as cimetidine) requires medical monitoring. Patients with reduced kidney function also require careful follow up and dosage adjustments.

Side effects

Bromocriptine may cause gastrointestinal discomfort, constipation, abdominal cramps, **fatigue**, anxiety, urinary incontinence or retention, depression, insomnia, hypotension, anorexia (loss of appetite), and rapid heart rate.

Pergolide side effects include **dizziness** when rising, increased heart rate, hallucinations, mood and personality disorders, **ataxia** (loss of coordination), muscle rigidity, blurred vision, anorexia, diarrhea, depression, insomnia, **headache**, confusion, numbness, gastritis, fluid retention, and swelling of the hands, face, and feet.

Cabergoline side effects include gastrointestinal irritation, gases, abdominal **pain**, digestive difficulties, dry mouth, loss of appetite, depression, mood changes, anxiety, insomnia, depression, increased sex drive, low blood pressure, fatigue, body weight changes.

Both pramipexole and ropinirole may cause **hallucination** (especially in elderly patients), dizziness and low blood pressure when rising, nausea, and gastrointestinal discomfort such as nausea and constipation. Pramipexole may also cause general swelling, fever, anorexia, and difficulty swallowing, decreased sex drive, amnesia and mental confusion, as well as insomnia and vision abnormalities. Ropinirole sometimes causes dizziness and **fainting**, with or without a slow heart rate.

Interactions

Pyridoxine (vitamin B_6) interferes with the transport of levodopa to the central nervous system by increasing its metabolism in the gastrointestinal tract. Dopamine antagonists (i.e., inhibitors of dopamine), such as metoclopramide and phenothiazines interfere with levodopa and other dopaminergic agonists, thus decreasing its effectiveness. The simultaneous concomitant use of phenelzine and dopamine agonists may induce severe high blood pressure.

Resources

BOOKS

Champe, Pamela C., and Richard A. Harvey, eds. *Pharmacology,* 2nd ed. Philadelphia, PA: Lippincott Williams & Wilkins, 2000.

Weiner, William J., M.D. *Parkinson's Disease: A Complete Guide for Patients and Families.* Baltimore: Johns Hopkins University Press, 2001.

OTHER

"Dopamine Agonists." *WE MOVE.* <http://www.wemove.org/par/par_dopa.html> (April 23, 2004).

"Pergolide." *Medline Plus.* National Library of Medicine. <http://www.nlm.nih.gov/medlineplus/druginfo/medmaster/a601093.html> (April 23, 2004).

ORGANIZATIONS

National Parkinson Foundation. 1501 N.W. 9th Avenue, Bob Hope Research Center, Miami, Fl 33136-1494. (305) 243-6666 or (800) 327-4545; Fax: (305) 243-5595. mailbox@parkinson.org. <http://www.parkinson.org/>.

Sandra Galeotti

Dural sinuses *see* **Cerebral circulation**

Dysarthria

Definition

Dysarthria is a speech diagnostic term that can be used to classify various types of neuromuscular speech disturbances. Dysarthria results from notable degrees of one or more abnormalities involving speech musculature, including weakness, paralysis, incoordination, sensory deprivation, exaggerated reflex patterns, uncontrollable movement activities, and excess or reduced tone. Generally speaking, the dysarthrias are considered motor speech disorders because speaking difficulties are largely due to breakdowns in movement control of one or more muscle groups that compose the speech mechanism. The name of each dysarthria subtype is partially derived from the basic characteristics of the overlying movement disturbances. Notably, normal speech production involves the integration and coordination of five primary physiological subsystems: respiration (breath support); phonation (voice production); articulation (pronunciation of words); resonation (nasal versus oral voice quality); and prosody (rate, rhythm, and inflection patterns of speech).

Description

The pioneering works of Darley, Aronson, and Brown in 1975 led to the general model of dysarthria classification that continues to be used to date. These clinical researchers from the Mayo Clinic studied individuals with different neurological disorders for the primary purpose of identifying and describing in detail the various speech problems that they exhibited. These analyses helped to formulate predictable subtypes of speech abnormalities in individuals with specific kinds of neuropathologies. Besides the six primary forms of dysarthria identified, a seventh type has been added to the differential diagnostic scheme in the past decade. The seven dysarthria subtypes are spastic, unilateral upper motor neuron, ataxic, hypokinetic, hyperkinetic, flaccid, and mixed.

Demographics

There are no known figures regarding the overall incidence of the various dysarthrias in the general population. Moreover, because numerous possible neuropathological conditions can result in dysarthria, it is unproductive to speculate about either the specific or overall demographics of this multi-varied disorder.

Causes and symptoms

Spastic dysarthria

Spastic dysarthria is caused by damage to the primary voluntary motor pathways, which originate in the frontal lobes of the brain and descend to the brainstem and spinal cord. These central tracts constitute the pyramidal or upper motor neuron (UMN) system. Virtually all individuals with spastic dysarthria present with a broad spectrum of speech disturbances, including:

- abnormally excessive nasal speech quality

- imprecise articulation behaviors such as slurred sound productions and periods of speech unintelligibility

- slow-labored rate of speech

- strained or strangled voice quality

- limited vocal pitch and loudness range and control

- incoordinated, shallow, forced, uncontrolled, and overall disruptive speech breathing patterns

Individuals with spastic dysarthria often suffer from co-occurring weakness and paralysis of all four limbs. This occurs because the nerve tracts that supply movement control to these structures run in close parallel to those that regulate muscles of the speech mechanism, thereby making them equally susceptible to damage. The specific combination and severity of these features tend to vary from person to person based on the extent of associated UMN damage. In general, people with spastic dysarthria struggle with these speech difficulties because of widespread involvement of the tongue, lip, jaw, soft palate, voice box, and respiratory musculature. Problems with emotional breakdowns, such as unprovoked crying and laughing, also occur in many cases, due to uncontrolled releases of primitive reflexes and behaviors normally regulated, in part, by a mature and healthy UMN system. Finally, swallowing difficulties, known as dysphagia, are not uncommon in this population, because of underlying weakness and paralysis of the tongue and throat wall muscles.

The most common causes of spastic dysarthria include spastic **cerebral palsy**, **multiple sclerosis**, **amyotrophic lateral sclerosis** (ALS, or Lou Gehrig's disease), multiple strokes, and closed head injuries (particularly those that cause damage to the brainstem where the UMN tracts converge on the way to nerves that directly connect with the various muscles of the head, neck, limbs, and girdle).

Unilateral upper motor neuron (UMN) dysarthria

Unilateral UMN dysarthria is caused by damage to either the left or right UMN tract, anywhere along its course to the brainstem and spinal cord. The individual with this diagnosis generally presents with mild to moderate weakness and paralysis of the lower face, tongue, arm, and leg on the side of the body opposite the damaged UMN tract. The hemiplegia may necessitate use of a cane or wheelchair, and the facial and tongue musculature disturbances usually only result in mild speech production and swallowing difficulties because the unimpaired opposite half of the lips and tongue often compensate well for this unilateral problem.

Speech breathing and inflection patterns, voice characteristics, and nasal resonance features are not typically abnormal in the individual with unilateral UMN dysarthria. However, it is not uncommon for this person to suffer from a significant language processing disorder (i.e., **aphasia**) and/or **apraxia** in which the brain damage also involves areas of the cortex that normally regulate motor programming and language formulation abilities.

The most common causes of this dysarthria subtype are cerebral vascular accidents (i.e., strokes) and mild-to-moderate head injuries.

Ataxic dysarthria

Ataxic dysarthria is caused by damage to the **cerebellum** or its connections to the cerebral cortex or brainstem. This component of the **central nervous system** is chiefly responsible for regulating the force, timing, rhythm, speed, and overall coordination of all bodily movements. When the cerebellum is damaged the affected person may exhibit drunk-like motor patterns, characterized by a wide-based and reeling gait and slurred articulation patterns with intermittently explosive voice pitch and loudness outbursts. During purposeful movement efforts, this individual often suffers from intention **tremors**, which cause under- or overshooting of the intended target.

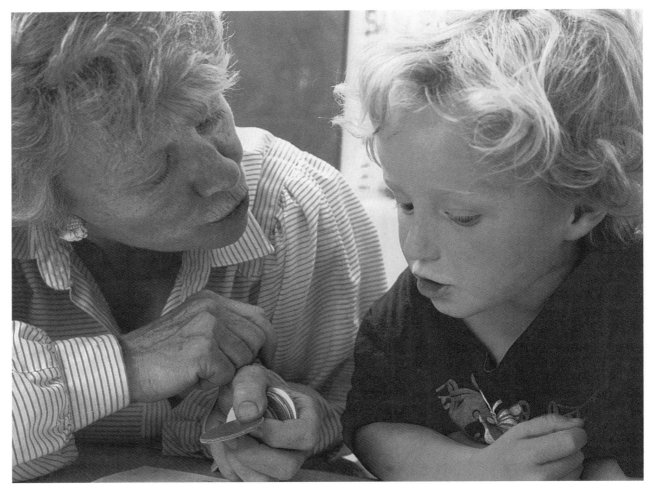

A speech therapist helps a young boy sound out words. *(© Photo Researchers. Reproduced by permission.)*

However, this shaking phenomenon tends to disappear at rest. Swallowing is not usually disturbed.

The most common causes of **ataxia** include cerebral palsy, multiple sclerosis, and closed head injuries.

Hypokinetic dysarthria

Hypokinetic dysarthria is caused by damage to the upper brainstem in a region that is richly composed of darkly pigmented (nigra) nerve cells. These neurons contain the neurochemical agent dopamine, which helps regulate muscle tone and smooth and complete bodily movements. When various speech muscles are involved, numerous communication deficits occur, including imprecise articulation of sounds, harsh-hoarse voice quality, and abnormal bursts of speech that sound like the individual is tripping over his or her tongue. These common dysarthric features are the result of widespread rigidity (i.e., stiffness and limited range of motion [hypokinesia]),

tremors, and incoordination of the tongue, lip, jaw, and voice box musculature.

Because the most common cause of hypokinetic dysarthria is **Parkinson's disease**, patients with these types of speech problems also exhibit numerous trunk and limb disturbances such as rest tremors of the hands, stooped posture, shuffling gait, and mask-like facial expressions due to involvement of associated body musculature. Swallowing difficulties may co-occur.

Hyperkinetic dysarthria

Hyperkinetic dysarthria is generally caused by damage to nerve pathways and centers within the depths of the brain (subcortex) known as the basal ganglia. These integrated central nervous system components form complex feedback loops between one another and the cerebral cortex. The basal ganglia are largely responsible for helping to maintain posture, muscle tone, bodily adjustments, and overall stability during gross voluntary movement patterns. Damage to these structures and their circuitry generally produces two different types of symptoms, depending upon the site(s) of injury: increased muscle tone and very slow movement, known as rigidity, as seen in patients with Parkinson's disease, or involuntary, excessive, and uncontrollable quick-jerky, slow-twisting, or trembling limb and speech musculature behaviors.

Patients with Huntington's disease and tic disorders frequently exhibit the quick and jerky forms of movement abnormalities. The slow, writhing, and twisting **movement disorders** are usually observed in patients with histories of **dystonia**, athetosis, torticolis, and **dyskinesia**. In fact, spasmodic dysphonia, characterized by strained-strangled or abnormally breathy vocal quality and episodes of periodic arrests of voice, is a form of hyperkinetic dysarthria in that dystonia involves the vocal cords. Tremors are common in patients with essential (organic) tremor disorders. In general, when tongue, lip, and jaw muscles are afflicted by such breakdowns, the articulation of speech sounds is inconsistent and imprecise, voice is hoarse-harsh in quality, the rhythm of speech is flat and irregular, and breathing patterns are sudden, forced, and shallow. All of these disturbances contribute in total to variable, but often-marked degrees of speech unintelligibility in these clinical populations.

Whereas in most cases the underlying cause of muscle hyperactivity is associated with one of the above listed disease-specific entities, occasionally severe head injuries and deep brain tumors can result in any of these types of movement control disorders. Swallowing difficulties can be a significant problem for these types of patients.

Flaccid dysarthria

Flaccid dysarthria is caused by damage to nerves that emerge from the brainstem (cranial) or spinal cord and travel directly to muscles that are involved in speech production. These nerves are generically referred to as lower motor neurons. Cranial nerves V, VII, X, and XII are of great importance because they supply the chief muscles of speech production, namely, the jaw, lips, voice box and palate, and tongue, respectively. The cervical spinal nerves innervate the diaphragm, and the thoracic spinal nerves stimulate the chest and abdominal wall muscles, all of which are involved in speech breathing activities. The types of neuromuscular problems that arise as a result of injuries to these nerves depend upon which and how many nerves are disturbed. In general, the types of abnormal muscle signs occurring in patients with damage to lower motor neurons include paralysis, weakness, reduced speed of movement, depressed tactile feedback, limited reflex behaviors, and atrophy or shrinkage of muscle tissue.

Analyses of the electrical activity of involved muscles using needle electrodes frequently reveal disturbed firing patterns or twitch-like behaviors known as fasciculations. In a structure like the tongue, which is not covered with thick overlying skin, fasciculations can sometimes be evident by shining a flashlight on the surface at rest. This pathologic feature is an important differential diagnostic sign of damage to the cranial nerve XII. Patients with limited lower motor neuron damage usually exhibit less severe flaccid dysarthria than those with more widespread damage. Additionally, the actual nerves that are damaged dictate the specific types of speech difficulties that may occur. For example, if a focal lesion involves only the cranial nerve VII, as in **Bell's palsy**, only the lip musculature will be weakened. The result in this case usually produces minimal dysarthria. However, damage to multiple cranial nerves, as often occurs in certain degenerative conditions like Lou Gehrig's disease, will likely cause severe speech difficulties. The most common speech signs observed in patients with flaccid dysarthria, regardless of the cause or severity, include articulation imprecision, hypernasal voice, hoarse and breathy vocal quality, and slow-labored speech rate.

Brain stem strokes, tumors on the brain stem or along the course of the cranial or spinal nerves, **muscular dystrophy**, and general injuries to these nerves as a result of head trauma or surgical complications are among the most frequent causes of flaccid dysarthria. If spinal nerves that supply the limbs are also damaged, as may be the case in some of these clinical populations, co-occurring paralysis of these structures is likely to complicate the rehabilitation program. Swallowing problems may occur in some cases, depending upon which and how many cranial nerves are involved.

Mixed dysarthria

Mixed dysarthria is caused by simultaneous damage to two or more primary motor components of the nervous system, such as the combined upper and lower motor neuron lesions that typically occur in Lou Gehrig's disease, or the co-occurring degeneration of the upper motor neuron and cerebellum pathways seen in patients with multiple sclerosis. In the first example, the patient usually suffers from mixed spastic-flaccid dysarthria. In the second case, the MS patient often presents with mixed spastic-ataxic dysarthria. The exact mixture of neurological damage governs the characteristic speech (and overall body) musculature difficulties.

It is not uncommon for severe head injuries to cause multi-focal nervous system lesions and nonspecific mixed dysarthrias. Many such patients also struggle with limb and trunk motor problems, as well as coexisting swallowing, cognitive, language, perceptual, and psychosocial deficits that worsen their underlying motor speech problems and complicate the rehabilitation course. The mixture may be of two or more of the previously described single-entity dysarthrias.

Diagnosis

In addition to clinical examinations, many dysarthric patients will need to submit to various laboratory studies for a thorough appraisal of the possible underlying causes, areas of brain damage, and overall prospects for improvement with appropriate treatment. Such testing might include:

- computed tomography (**CT**) or **magnetic resonance imaging (MRI)** scans of the head, neck, and/or chest

- skull x rays

- arteriography (imaging of arterial flow dynamics)

- spinal tap for cerebral spinal fluid analysis

- electroencephalography (EEG)

- electromyography (EMG)

- videoendosocopy of the vocal cords and soft palate

- pulmonary function studies

- videofluoroscopic examinations of swallowing proficiency

- speech aerodynamic and acoustic analyses

These diagnostic tests require the cooperation of many different clinical practitioners from various fields of study.

Familiarity with the variable speech subsystem abnormalities exhibited by dysarthric patients is indispensable to differential diagnosis. Additionally, because dysarthria is only a speech diagnostic term, and the underlying cause is some form of neurological problem, a medical examination, usually performed by a clinical **neurologist**, is critical both to the overall diagnosis in any given case and for effective treatment recommendations. Family members and friends can, however, facilitate this process by cursory investigations of the speech difficulties prior to visiting with diagnosticians for formal testing. This preparatory process may involve having the patient perform several physiologic tasks, as well as noting any generalized walking, balance, and limb coordination difficulties exhibited by the affected individual. If the possible cause is understood from the outset, it may help pinpoint the speech diagnosis. The individual can be engaged in general conversation to judge overall speech intelligibility. The listener can listen for signs of poor pronunciation of sounds, excessively nasal voice, hoarseness or strained vocal quality, breath support difficulties, and limited pitch and loudness inflection patterns. Any one or more of these problems may be evident in the speech profiles of individuals with different forms of dysarthria.

Treatment team

The rehabilitation team for an individual with dysarthria often varies, depending on the severity and cause of the dysarthria and the extent of associated limb and trunk musculature disabilities and co-occurring language, cognitive, and psychosocial deficits. In general, those individuals with multi-system breakdowns require a more complex array of team constituents than those who have more focal or mild problems. Most teams consist of the clinical neurologist, speech-language pathologist, physical therapist, occupational therapist, **neuropsychologist**, nurse practitioner, and social worker. In school-age patients, teachers and guidance counselors will also play very important roles in the treatment program. Naturally, the role of the speech pathologist is usually most critical in the communication treatment plan for dysarthric patients.

Treatment

Physical and occupational therapists focus on improving limb and trunk coordination, balance, and range of motion, particularly in relation to daily living functions such as walking, self-dressing, and feeding. Neuropsychologists often facilitate memory strategies, perceptual processes, and overall organizational skills required in various work-related settings and daily social circumstances. The administration of certain medications, daily health care and personal hygiene needs, and general tracheostomy care and feeding-tube monitoring may be indicated.

The speech pathologist must design specific speech musculature exercises to improve the strength, tone, range of motion, coordination, and speed of integrated tongue, lip, jaw, and vocal musculature contractions. These general objectives are often achieved following a hierarchy of exercises that may require two or more sessions of therapy per week. In some cases, when oral speech skills fail to improve with both speech and non-speech exercises, use of an alternative or augmentative communication system is required, such as computerized speech synthesizers and/or form or picture boards. These tools are most useful for those patients who possess at least some control of an upper limb to activate a keyboard or point to a picture. In very severely affected patients, a head pointer may be devised so that head movements meet these objectives.

Prognosis

The prognosis for speech improvement in any individual with dysarthria usually depends on the severity of the problem and the underlying cause. If the speech difficulties are mild to moderate, and the cause has been treated successfully through proper medical avenues and is non-progressive, the prognosis for notable improvements with good speech therapy is often very good. However, in the case of severe dysarthria, with a medically uncontrollable or progressively deteriorating etiology, the prognosis for significant gains, even with the best therapeutic programs possible, is almost always very guarded.

Special concerns

Depending on the cause and the severity of the dysarthria, and any coexisting motor, language, cognitive, intellectual, and psychosocial deficits, the affected individual may require many different methods of care. Formal nursing or group home settings are sometimes necessary for those individuals who are not self-sufficient or who lack home care assistance and supervision. Special education classes may be required in those cases with associated learning disabilities. Structural modifications of a wheelchair to facilitate upright head posturing and abdominal support during speech breathing efforts may be helpful for some patients, and construction of ramps in the home may also be necessary to accommodate wheelchair mobility requirements. Arrangements for use of a bell or light switch activator may be indispensable to certain patients who cannot verbally, or otherwise, get the attention of caregivers.

Resources

BOOKS

Darley, F. L., A. E. Aronson, and J. R. Brown. *Motor Speech Disorders*. Philadelphia: W. B. Saunders, Company, 1975.

Duffy, J. R. *Motor Speech Disorders: Substrates, Differential Diagnosis, and Management*. St. Louis: Mosby, 1995.

Dworkin, J. P. *Motor Speech Disorders: A Treatment Guide*. St. Louis: Mosby, 1991.

Dworkin, J. P., and R. A. Cullata. *Dworkin-Culatta Oral Mechanism Examination and Treatment System*. Farmington Hills, MI: Edgewood Press, 1996.

Robin, D. A., K. M. Yorkston, and D. R. Beukelman. *Disorders of Motor Speech*. Baltimore, MD: Paul H. Brookes Publishing, 1996.

Vogel, D., and M. P. Cannito. *Treating Disordered Speech Motor Control (2nd Ed)*. Austin, TX: Pro-Ed, 2001.

Yorkston, K., D. R. Beukelman, E. Strand, and K. Bell. *Management of Motor Speech Disorders in Children*. Austin, TX: Pro-Ed, 1999.

ORGANIZATIONS

Department of Otolaryngology, Head and Neck Surgery, Wayne State University, 5E-UHC, Detroit, MI 48331. (313) 745-8648. aa1544@wayne.edu.

James Paul Dworkin, PhD

Dysautonomia *see* **Autonomic dysfunction**

Dysesthesias

Definition

The word dysesthesias is derived from the Greek "dys," which means "bad," and "aesthesis," which means "sensation." Thus, dysesthesias are "bad sensations" and the word refers to **pain** or uncomfortable sensations, often described as burning, tingling, or numbness.

Description

Dysesthesias is a symptom of pain or abnormal sensation(s) that typically cause hyperesthesia, paresthesiae, or peripheral sensory neuropathy. Dysesthesias can be due to lesions (an abnormal change) in sensory nerves and sensory pathways in the **central nervous system** (CNS, consisting of the brain and the spinal cord). The pain or abnormal sensations in dysesthesias is often described as painful feelings of tingling, burning, or numbness. Dysesthesias can simply be described as a burning pain that is worse where touch sensation is poorest.

Dysesthesias can also be caused by lesions in peripheral nerves (the **peripheral nervous system**, or PNS, which consists of nerves that are outside the brain or spinal cord). Peripheral nerves travel to muscles and organs providing a nerve supply. Dysesthesias due to a lesion in the PNS usually occurs below the level of the lesion. There is a broad spectrum of diseases, disorders, and medications that cause dysesthesias. There are two broad categories of dysesthesias called paresthesiae and peripheral sensory neuropathy. Some of the common causes of dysesthesias within these categories will be considered.

Paresthesias

Paresthesias (abnormal neurological sensations that include numbness, tingling, burning, prickling, and increased sensitivity, or hyperesthesia) can include several conditions such as **carpal tunnel syndrome**, **thoracic outlet syndrome**, **multiple sclerosis**, strokes (cerebrovascular accidents), **Guillain-Barré syndrome**, **transverse myelitis**, and compartment syndrome/Volkmann's contracture.

Carpal tunnel syndrome

Carpal tunnel syndrome is caused by entrapment of the median nerve at the wrist. There is limited available space for the median nerve. There is a disease process (i.e. osteoarthritis) that entraps the nerve. Symptoms include paresthesiae of the first three fingers usually present overnight and typically relieved by shaking or elevating the hands. Symptoms progress to sensory loss and weakness of muscles. Treatment usually includes overnight splinting, diuretics (to reduce swelling), or surgery.

Thoracic outlet syndrome

Thoracic outlet syndrome is a condition caused by compression of nerves (and blood vessels) located between the armpit and the base of the neck. The neurologic symptoms associated with thoracic outlet syndrome include dysesthesias (numbness and tingling), weakness, and fatigability. The damage occurs in nerves leaving the spinal cord located behind the neck. Symptoms worsen with arm elevation above the level of the shoulder. Approximately 50% of persons affected report a history of a single traumatic event (i.e., motor vehicle accident) that caused a neck injury.

Multiple sclerosis/transverse myelitis

Multiple Sclerosis is an inflammatory process that involves white matter. There is focal neurologic deficit which can progress. The condition can go in remission but other attacks usually occur causing neurologic deficits. Transverse myelitis (usually associated with an inflammatory process) can cause **back pain**, leg weakness, and sensory disturbance. Transverse myelitis can occur after viral infections or may even occur as a feature of multiple sclerosis.

Stroke (cerebrovascular accident)

There are two major arteries implicated with **stroke**. These include the carotid arteries (in the neck and travels into the brain) and the basilar artery (an artery located in the base of the skull). The dysesthesias associated with carotid artery stroke consists of tingling and numbness on one side of the body. Stroke associated with the basilar artery can cause dysesthesias (tingling or numbness) in the cheeks, mouth, or gums.

Guillain-Barré syndrome

Guillain-Barré syndrome (also called acute inflammatory demyelinating polyneuropathy) is an immune mediated disorder that follows some infectious process (such as infectious mononucleosis, herpes viruses, cytomegalovirus, and mycoplasma), and is the most frequent caused of acute flaccid paralysis throughout the world. Initial symptoms consist of "pins-and-needles sensations" in the feet, lower back pain, and weakness (which develop within hours or days). Weakness is prominent in the legs. Progression of symptoms can occur abruptly and patients may have serious involvement of nerves responsible for respiration and swallowing, which may be life-threatening. The condition is serious and could cause rapid deterioration. Patients usually require hospitalization and treatment with high doses of human immunoglobulin and plasmapheresis (exchange of patient's plasma for the protein called albumin).

Key Terms

HIV Human immunodeficiency virus, which causes AIDS.

Lacinating pain Piercing, stabbing, or darting pain.

Lymphocytic meningitis Benign infection of brain coverings that protect the brain.

Radiculoneuritis Inflammation of a spinal nerve.

Rodenticide Chemical that kills rodents.

Compartment syndrome/Volkmann contracture

Compartment syndrome refers to any condition that causes a decrease in compartment size or increased compartment pressure. Compartment syndromes can be caused by crush injuries, internal bleeding, fractures, snake bites, burns, and excessive **exercise**. If a compartment (or area) is injured (i.e., a crushing injury to hand), the trauma will decrease the normal area of the hand (due to bleeding). This results in an increase in compartmental pressure which could impair blood flow to the area, causing irreversible tissue ischemia (tissue death). Compartment syndrome can occur from injuries to the upper extremity which can affect the forearm and hand since these areas have naturally occurring compartments made by anatomical structures such as muscle. Excessive swelling due to traumatic injury can cause nerves and blood vessels to be compartmentalized (in a sense, crushed against) muscle from abnormal swelling or internal bleeding. If left untreated the dead muscle and nerve tissue is replaced with fibrous tissue causing a Volkmann ischemic contracture (contractures of fingers or in severe cases the forearm). In severe cases there is a loss of nerve tissue. Damage shows signs in 30 minutes and measurable functional loss after 12 to 24 hours.

Peripheral neuropathy

Peripheral neuropathies are conditions that cause injury to nerves that supply sensation to the legs and arms. This category of dysesthesias can include conditions such as amyloidosis, **Charcot-Marie-Tooth** syndrome, diabetes, leprosy, syphilis, and **Lyme disease**.

Amyloid neuropathies/hereditary neuropathies

There are several types of amyloid neuropathies, and they are all associated with diseases that deposit a protein (amyloid) in nerves and even other tissues (like blood vessels). Sensory nerves are damaged causing dysesthesias.

These disorders are inherited, occur in midlife, and represent the most relevant inherited neurologic diseases. These include Charcot-Marie-Tooth disease and amyloid neuropathies. Charcot-Marie-Tooth disease refers to inherited disease that causes nerve degeneration usually in the second to fourth decades of life. Patients exhibit impairment of sensory function, and the nerves of the toes and feet are affected (can lead to foot drop.)

Diabetes (metabolic neuropathy)

The most frequent neuropathy world wide is diabetes. **Peripheral neuropathy** can be detected in approximately 70% of long-term diabetics. The cause of nerve involvement is unclear, but it is thought that a faulty mechanism (deleterious to nerve cells) is related to high blood glucose levels. The symptoms are insidious and typically include dysesthesias evoked by regular activity (i.e., bothersome tingling of toes under bed sheets). The pain can be throbbing or it may be a continuous burning type of dysesthesias. Additionally, person may describe abrupt, quick "lightning" pains which may affect the feet and legs.

Leprous neuropathy

Leprosy is an infectious disease transmitted by a bacterium called *Mycobacterium leprae.* The World Health Organization (WHO) estimates that there are 2.5 million persons affected by leprosy. The organism proliferates in coolest regions of skin (i.e., ears, face, fingers), causing a selective loss of pain sensation (dysesthesias) in cold areas of skin.

Neurosyphilis

Neurosyphilis refers to a disease caused by untreated syphilis infection that invades the central nervous system years after initial infection. In the United States the number of cases of neurosyphilis has risen from 10,000 in 1956 to over 50,000 in 1990. Approximately 28% of patients have **ataxia**, 23% have stroke, and 10% of affected persons describe "lightning" pains. Additionally 10% have headaches and 36% have cranial neuropathy. Treatment attempts include antimicrobial therapy.

Lyme disease (Boreliosis)

Lyme disease is an infection transmitted by an arthropod (a tick which harbors the infectious bacterium called *Borrelia burdorferi*). The bacteria can be transmitted to a human by the bite of infected deer ticks, and in 2002 caused 23,000 infections in the United States. After the initial symptoms ("bulls-eye" rash, fever, **fatigue**, muscle aches, and joint aches), early disease can cause neurologic

symptoms such as lymphocytic meningitis, cranial neuropathy (especially facial nerve palsy), and radiculoneuritis. Patients may also have musculoskeletal pain that includes muscle pain (myalgia) and joint aches (arthralgia). Late symptoms include **encephalopathy**, sleep disturbances, fatigue, and personality changes.

Other causes of dysesthesias
Toxic neuropathies

Toxic neuropathies can occur due to medications (used to treat illnesses), metal exposures, substance abuse, and exposure to industrial poisons/chemicals. For drug (medications) or chemical exposure induced neuropathies the cause (mechanism of damage) is usually obscure. Medications that can cause neuropathies include (but are not limited to) antivirals, chloramphenicol (antibiotic), cisplatin (anticancer), ethambutol (antitubercolosis), hydralazine (antihypertensive), isoniazid (antitubercolosis), metronidazole (antifungal), phenytoin (antiepileptic), pyridoxine (vitamin B-6), gold therapy, and vincristine/vinblastin (anticancer) therapy. Metals that can cause neuropathies include arsenic, lead, mercury, and thallium (a metal in rodenticides such as Gizmo mouse killer). Heavy metals such as lead found in lead-based paint in the automobile industry and manufacture of storage batteries and printing can cause neuropathies. Lead neuropathy can occur due to drinking bootleg whiskey distilled in lead pipes, or hand mixing of lead-based paints by artists. Occupational exposure in farming to arsenic-containing sprays, pesticides, and weed killers can cause arsenic neuropathy. Accidental ingestion of arsenic-containing rodenticides can cause arsenic neuropathy.

Chemical abuse with alcohol or by glue or nitrous oxide inhalation can cause neuropathies. Severe peripheral neuropathies can result from exposure to household and industrial chemicals.

Thallium neuropathy

Thallium neuropathy can occur in manufacturers of optic glass, industrial diamonds, and prisms. Thallium is also used as an additive in internal combustion engines. Accidental ingestion of thallium and subsequent neuropathy also occurs with rodent killer substances (rodenticides).

HIV infection

Before development of **AIDS**, persons with HIV infection can develop chronic inflammatory peripheral neuropathy. However, the most prevalent neuropathy associated with HIV infection is sensory neuropathy of AIDS, which causes pain on the soles of the feet and discomfort when walking. The pain is intense and affected persons may have motor impairment. The condition is caused by degeneration of sensory nerve fibers.

Shingles

Another condition called herpes zoster or **shingles** (caused by the varicella zoster virus which causes chicken pox) can cause a latent nerve neuropathy with localized cutaneous eruptions during periods of reactivation. There are over 500,000 cases of shingles estimated to occur annually in the United States. The abnormal skin sensations are localized and range from itching to tingling to severe pain. Treatment typically includes antiviral medications. Pain can persist for months or even years.

Bell's palsy

The cause of **Bell's palsy** is unclear. It is thought to be due to an infectious process, possibly viral, that involves a nerve in the face called the facial nerve. Pain is often sudden and patients often describe a "numbing of the face" sensation.

Biological toxins

The ingestion of a certain fish (ciguatera) and some shellfish can be the cause of acute peripheral neuropathy (paresthesia). The typical causes among ciguatera include red snapper and barracuda from waters in the West Indies, Florida and Hawaii. Shellfish, clams scallops and mussels from the waters of Alaska, New England and the west coast are also causative biologic toxins. The neuropathy is followed after a few hours from the initial symptoms of nausea and vomiting. Paresthesiae occurs around the face and spreads to limbs. The problem can quickly progress to respiratory paralysis (paralysis of the muscles responsible for respiration) which could be a life-threatening condition.

Vitamin Deficiency

Neuropathy can result due to vitamin deficiencies such as vitamin B-12, vitamin B-1 and vitamin E. Vitamin B-12 deficiency can cause dysesthesias (sensation of "pins-and-needles" and numbness) in the feet and hands. Usually patients are diagnosed since they have a blood disorder called macrocytic megaloblastic anemia. Patients who have a bowel problem called malabsorption may loose ingested fat substances in the feces undigested, causing a loss of essential vitamins and nutrients. Fat containing molecules like vitamin E may be lost causing a neuropathy with symptoms similar to vitamin B-12 deficiency. Vitamin B-1 deficiency can likely occur due to alcoholism. The neuropathy is mostly sensory and patients describe a painful hypersensitivity of the feet. In advanced cases there may be weakness in the limbs or even paralysis leading to wrist drop or **foot drop**.

Nerve root compression

Radiculopathy, commonly caused by disk herniation (nerve root compression) is generally accompanied by muscle weakness, sensory loss and absent tendon reflexes. Herpes zoster radiculopathy is a lesion in the nerve root characterized by a burning pain and skin eruptions in dermatomal distribution. The inflammatory reaction precipitates stimulation of nerves producing a burning pain that precedes and often accompanies the skin eruptions.

General Concepts of pain management: Acute vs. chronic pain

There are several key concepts for pain management. Pain is best treated early and a vigilant search for the cause is imperative. Pain scales should be utilized in order to gauge progression of pain (i.e. getting worse or better). Unrelieved pain is implicated with negative physiological and psychological conditions. For acute pain an opioid (morphine) is a suitable agent to control moderate to severe pain. Acute pain is usually a symptom of injury or illness and serves a biological purpose (i.e. to provoke treatment of the injury). Additionally, acute pain causes anxiety, has identifiable pathology (disease) and is present less than six months. In cases of chronic pain, the dysesthesias is the problem itself and serves no biological function. Chronic pain syndromes with dysesthesias are often implicated with **depression** due to chronicity (long-term illness). Chronic pain may or may not have identifiable pathology and is present for more than six months.

Management of Pain

The first step to management of patients with neuropathic pain is to gain a good explanation of the cause and origin of the pain. Tricyclic antidepressants have an important role for the treatment of neuropathic pain (especially the "burning pain" associated with diabetes). These medications seem to be effective in several "pain" syndromes. Tricyclics tend to help with "burning" type pains, lacinating pains and cutaneous hyperalgesia. Tricyclics have an analgesic effect, thought to be mediated by alterations in brain chemistry (two specific **neurotransmitters** called serotonin and norepinephrine). **Anticonvulsants** (antiepileptic medications) can help reduce lacinating pain. Topical local aesthetic preparations (i.e. EMLA cream, eutectic mixture of local anesthetics) can penetrate skin and temporarily relieve neuropathic pain. The use of long term opioid treatment is unclear and should be reserved to selective cases. The use of capsaicin (the active substance extracted from hot pepper, can relieve pain (if placed on skin) in approximately 33% of patients with painful post-herpetic neuralgia and diabetic neuropathy.

Resources

BOOKS

Canale, S. Terry. *Campbell's Operative Orthopedics,* 10th ed. St. Louis: Mosby, Inc., 2003.

DeLee, Jesse, G., and David Drez. *Delee and Drez's Orthopedic Sports Medicine,* 2nd ed. Philadelphia: Saunders, 2003.

Goetz, Christopher G., et al., eds. *Textbook of Clinical Neurology,* 1st ed. Philadelphia: W. B. Saunders Company, 1999.

Goldman, Lee, et al. *Cecil's Textbook of Medicine,* 21st ed. Philadelphia: W. B. Saunders Company, 2000.

Marx, John A., et al., eds. *Rosen's Emergency Medicine: Concepts and Clinical Practice.* 5th ed. St. Louis: Mosby, Inc., 2002.

Noble, John, et al., eds. *Textbook of Primary Care Medicine.* 3rd ed. St. Louis: Mosby, Inc., 2001.

PERIODICALS

Pascuzzi, Robert, M. "Peripheral neuropathies in clinical practice." *Medical Clinics of North America* 87, no. 3 (May 2003).

WEBSITES

National Institute of Neurological Disorders. <http://www.ninds.nih.gov>.

ORGANIZATIONS

NIH Neurological Institute. PO Box 5801, Bethesda, MD 20824. 301-496-5751 or 1-800-352-9424. <http://www.ninds.nih.gov>.

Laith Farid Gulli, M.D.
Nicole Mallory, M.S., PA-C
Alfredo Mori, M.B., B.S.

Dysgeusia

Definition

Dysgeusia is a disorder of the sense of taste.

Description

Any condition that affects the ability to taste is referred to as dysgeusia. While dysgeusia is often used to describe any change in the sense of taste, more specific terms include ageusia (complete loss of the sensation of taste); hypogeusia (decreased sense of taste); parageusia (bad taste in the mouth); and dysgeusia (distorted sense of taste, such as a metallic taste in the mouth). A wide variety of conditions can cause a deficit in the sense of taste, including any conditions that interfere with the functioning of the taste buds (the nerve cells on the tongue that process information about taste), conditions that interrupt the taste signal that is sent to the brain, or conditions that interfere with the normal brain processing of those signals. Processes that affect the functioning of the lingual nerve or the glossopharyngeal nerve may impair the sense of taste. Furthermore, the sense of taste is frequently dulled or impaired due to dysfunction of the sense of smell.

Causes and symptoms

There are a wide variety of conditions that can cause dysgeusia, including:

• smoking
• respiratory infections (colds, sinus infections, throat infection, or pharyngitis)
• strep throat
• inflammation of the tongue (glossitis)
• gingivitis
• influenza
• dry mouth (due to medications or disorders such as Sjogren's syndrome or salivary gland disorders or infections)
• vitamin deficiencies (such as B-12 and zinc)
• Cushing's disorder
• cancer
• diabetes
• hypothyroidism
• liver or kidney failure
• head injuries
• brain tumors or other tumors that destroy or injure areas of the nose, mouth, throat, or brain responsible for taste
• nasal polyps
• **Bell's palsy**
• **multiple sclerosis**

In addition, normal aging usually includes a decrement in the sense of taste as the numbers of taste buds decrease over time. A large number of medications can affect the sense of taste; antibiotics and cancer chemotherapeutic agents are common culprits. Examples of drugs that are known to cause dysgeusia include lithium, penicillamine, procarbazine, rifampin, vinblastine, vincristine, captopril, griseofulvin, and thyroid medications. **Radiation** therapy may cause dysgeusia.

Symptoms of dysgeusia include decreased acuity of the sense of taste or the distorted perception of an odd taste. Complete loss of taste sensation is relatively rare.

Diagnosis

Diagnosis can be made by having an individual taste and smell a variety of test substances. **CT** or **MRI** imaging may reveal the disorder underlying the development of dysgeusia.

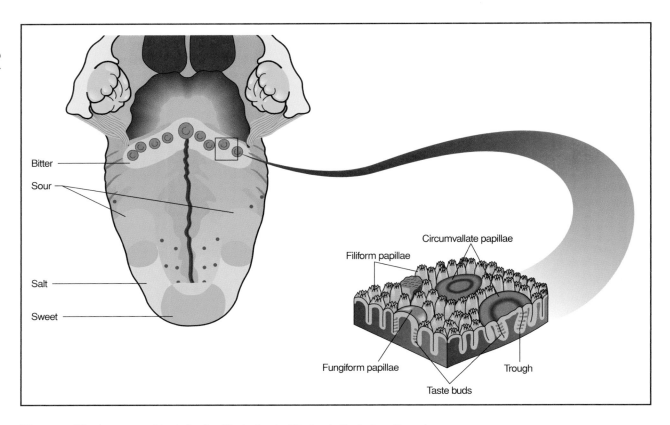

Bitter

Sour

Salt

Sweet

Filiform papillae

Circumvallate papillae

Fungiform papillae

Taste buds

Trough

Diagram of the tongue and taste buds. *(Illustration by Electronic Illustrators Group.)*

Treatment team

Dysgeusia may be treated by a **neurologist** or by the physician who is treating the underlying condition responsible for the disorder (such as an otorhinolaryngologist for various ear, nose, or throat conditions, such as nasal polyps).

Treatment

Some types of dysgeusia resolve on their own, particularly dysgeusia that occurs due to an infection. When the infection clears, the dysgeusia usually abates and the sense of taste returns. When smokers stop smoking, their sense of taste may improve over time. Stopping some medications may also lead to an improved sense of taste. Individuals who suffer from dry mouth (xerostomia) may benefit from artificial saliva. Individuals with nasal polyps may note improved sense of taste after polyp removal.

Prognosis

Dysgeusia secondary to infection or reversible conditions like Bell's palsy may improve partially or completely with resolution of the infection or condition; dysgeusia due to medication use or smoking may also improve partially or

completely when the individual stops using the medication or discontinues smoking. However, dysgeusia due to more permanent damage to the neurological apparatus responsible for taste or smell (such as head injury, multiple sclerosis, radiation treatments, or diabetes) may never improve.

Special concerns

Individuals with severely compromised taste or smell may inadvertently eat spoiled foods, leading to food-borne illness. Furthermore, without a good sense of smell or taste, there is an increased risk that an individual will not be able to protect him- or herself from exposure to other toxins, pollution, or smoke. Individuals with an impaired sense of taste may over-salt or over-sugar their food, in an attempt to compensate. They may not take in a reasonably balanced, nutritious diet with sufficient calories, because eating may become unenjoyable.

Resources
BOOKS

Pryse-Phillips, William, T. Jock Murray, and James Boyd. "Toxic Damage to the nervous system." In *Noble: Textbook of Primary Care Medicine*, edited by John Noble, et al. St. Louis: W. B. Saunders Company, 2001.

PERIODICALS

Bromley, Steven M. "Smell and Taste Disorders: A Primary Care Approach." *American Family Physician* (January 2000).

Ritchie, C. S. "Oral health, taste, and olfaction." *Clin Geriatr Med* 18, no. 4 (November 2002): 709–717

Rosalyn Carson-DeWitt, MD

Dyskinesia

Definition

Dyskinesias are a group of disorders characterized by involuntary movements of muscles.

Description

Dyskinesias are excessive abnormal movements that are involuntary. There are several different types of dyskinesias, and each has different clinical symptoms, causes, and treatments. Adults and children with certain chronic brain disorders often exhibit symptoms of dyskinesia. Movement can occur in the head, arms, legs, hand, feet, lips, or tongue. The dyskinesias can be categorized as **chorea**, **dystonia**, **myoclonus**, tremor, and paroxysmal tardive (late-onset type). Other forms of dyskinesia include athetosis, ballism, akathisia, tics, stereotypy, and restless legs. Dyskinesias can also be called hyperkinesia syndromes.

Chorea

Choreas are abnormal movements that are irregular, involuntary, nonrhymical, abrupt, rapid, and nonsustained jerking, which continuously flow from one body part to another. Movements are isolated, brief, and infrequent. Chorea can cause inability to maintain a sustained contraction, which causes affected persons to drop objects. Persons with chorea have an irregular dance-like gait. The cause of chorea is not completely understood.

Dystonia

Dystonia that occurs at rest may persist as the kinetic (clonic) form. Dystonias can be either focal or generalized. Focal dystonias are involuntary movements in a single body part, which commonly includes **blepharospasm** (upper facial), spasmodic torticollis (cervical), and writer's cramp. Dystonia affecting two or more body regions is called segmental dystonia. Generalized dystonia typically affects the trunk, one or both legs, and another body part. Other types of dystonias include Merge's syndrome (spasms of the jaw muscles when opening and closing of

the mouth). Spasmodic dystonias can cause speech impairment due to spasms of laryngeal (throat) muscles. The intensity of muscular movements in patients with dystonia can fluctuate, and symptoms worsen during **fatigue**, stress, activity, and change in posture. In some cases, the bizarre symptoms of dystonia can be mistaken for psychological illness. Dystonias can be inherited or acquired due to another primary cause. Inherited diseases that exhibit dystonia are rare and include dopa-responsive dystonia, idiopathic tension dystonia, and x-linked dystonia-Parkinsonism (found among Ashkenazi Jews).

Myoclonus

Myoclonus refers to muscular contractions (positive myoclonus) that are brief, sudden, and severe, and shock-like movements or inhibitions (negative myoclonus). Myoclonus could be generalized or isolated. The movements consist of rhythmical irregular jerks or oscillatory jerks that occur abruptly and then fade. The abnormal jerks are associated with environmental stimuli such as light, sound, movement, and visual threat. The condition can be misdiagnosed for **epilepsy**. Myoclonus usually occurs at rest, but can also appear when the affected body part is subjected to voluntary activity, which is referred to as action myoclonus. Action myoclonus is more disabling than rest myoclonus.

Tremor

Tremors are rhythmic oscillatory movements that are regular, but may vary in rate, location, amplitude, and constancy, and depend on type and severity of the tremor.

Key Terms

Ataxia Failure of muscular coordination due to muscle disorder.

Chronic Over a long period of time.

Flexion (flex) To move a limb toward the body.

Kinetic Word taken from the Greek (kinesis): motion.

Neuroleptic Negative effects of thinking and behavior, creating a state of apathy and lack of initiative.

Retrocollis Muscular spasms that affect the neck muscles located in the back.

Torticollis Contracted neck muscle, causing twisting of the neck in an abnormal position.

Unilateral On one side.

Tremors can occur with action, at rest, and with holding a position or posture. The tremor can be so rapid it is often described as a "flicker of light." Subtypes of tremors include tremors at rest, essential tremor, which is a postural tremor at either rest or activity and may be inherited, or tremor with movement (intention "kinetic" tremor). Resting tremors are usually slow, occur during an activity, and disappear when action is initiated (e.g., **Parkinson's disease**). Essential tremor is usually benign, but can cause disability due to impairment of handwriting and limitations of activities related to daily living. Essential tremor may be inherited.

Paroxysmal dyskinesias

Paroxysmal dyskinesia is a group of disorders that includes paroxysmal kinesigenic dyskinesia, episodic **ataxia**, paroxysmal hypnogenic dyskinesia, paroxysmal exertion-induced dyskinesia, and paroxysmal non-kinesigenic dyskinesia. The paroxysmal dyskinesias are a hyperkinetic disorder characterized by intermittent involuntary movements consisting of symptoms from other **movement disorders** such as chorea, athetosis, dystonia, and ballismus. Episodes of paroxysmal dyskinesias can last from a few seconds to several days. Episodic ataxias are characterized by intermittent episodes of ataxia that can last seconds to hours. Paroxysmal dyskinesias may be triggered by prolonged exertion, sleep, stress, alcohol, coffee, tea, fatigue, sudden voluntary movement, heat, or cold.

Athetosis

Athetosis is a disorder characterized by movements that are continuous, slow, and writhing. The movements are commonly appendicular and frequently involve muscles in the face, neck, and tongue. The condition may occur at rest or when executing voluntary movement. The speed of movements in affected persons can sometimes increase and symptoms are similar to those of chorea (called choreoathetosis). Athetosis movements can blend with those of dystonia, if the muscular contractions are sustained and cause abnormal posturing.

Ballism

Ballismus are large choreic movements that are fast and usually affect the limbs. Affected individuals exhibit flinging and flailing movements. Commonly, ballismus affects one side of the body (unilateral), producing a condition called hemiballismus.

Akathisia

Akathisia refers to complex movements such as tics, compulsions, and mannerisms that are stereotypic and usually relieved when executing a motor act. Typically,

when sitting, the akathitic persons may exhibit movements that include symptoms such as crossing and uncrossing the legs, squirming, pacing, stroking the scalp, or rocking the body. Patients may have burning sensations on the specific affected body part, and they may vocalize a continual moaning and groaning.

Tics

Tics can be divided into two disorders: motor tics (abnormal movements) and/or vocal tics (abnormal sounds). Children can present with a chronic disorder of both motor and vocal tics (Gilles de la **Tourette syndrome**). Movements of simple tics may be very similar to a choreic or myoclonic jerk (abrupt, single, sudden, isolated). Complex tics are movements that are distinctly coordinated patterns of sequential movements, but they may not be identical from occurrence to occurrence and they can occur in different body areas. Tics are rapid movements and, if contractions are sustained in affected body parts, they resemble dystonic movements.

One of the major clinical signs that help distinguish tics from other dyskinesias is the presence of involuntary ocular (eye) movement in persons affected with tics. The ocular manifestations of tics can include a brief jerk of the eyes or a sustained eye deviation. Two other dyskinesias, myoclonus and dystonia, can present with involuntary ocular manifestations.

With vocal tics, affected persons can exhibit grunts, throat-clearing sounds, or even the utterance of obscenities (coprolalia). Phonic tics (involving nasal and vocal muscles) can be divided into simple phonic tics such as throat-clearing or sniffing or complex phonic tics that include bark-like noises and verbalizations.

Stereotypies

Sterotypies are movements that are frequent and may last for minutes. These movements are repetitive and identical (continuous stereotypy.) The bizarre movements associated with **mental retardation**, **autism**, and **schizophrenia** are stereotypies. Continuous stereotypy is characteristic of another type of dyskinesia called tardive dyskinesia, which results from treatment with neuroleptic and antipsychotic medications.

Tardive dyskinesia

Tardive (late-onset) dyskinesia refers to a group of movement disorders that are characterized by hyperkinetic involuntary movements, consisting of mixed manifestations of orofacial dyskinesia, chorea, tics, and/or athetosis. Abnormal movement can affect muscles in the lips, face, trunk, tongue, and extremities, which can interfere with eating and dexterity. The most characteristic symptom of tardive dyskinesia is orofacial dyskinesia, which usually starts with slow, mild tongue movements followed by exaggerated movements of lips and tongue. Affected individuals can have symptoms that may progress to chewing movements, blinking, bulging cheeks, grimacing, arching eyebrows, and blepharospasms.

Tardive dyskinesias are commonly seen in patients taking certain medications such as neuroleptics and antipsychotic medication that are prescribed for schizophrenia, schizoaffective disorder, or bipolar disorder. Other types of tardive dyskinesias include tardive akathisia, tardive dystonia, tardive myoclonus, tardive Tourettism, tardive tremor, and blepharospasm. Approximately 50% of patients taking dopamine receptor blocker medication will develop a form of tardive dyskinesia.

Tardive akathisia refers tapping, squirming, and marching movements that are repetitive. Movements associated with tardive dystonia can include a fixed posturing of face and neck, trunk, and extremities. Persons affected with tardive myoclonus, which is a rare disorder, exhibit brief jerky movements of muscles in the face, neck, trunk, arms, and legs. Symptoms of tardive Tourettism usually begins in persons older than 21 years of age and include frequent, multiple tics that are both vocal and motor. This disorder should not be confused with Tourette syndrome, which commonly presents by seven years of age.

Tardive tremors often present as involuntary rhythmical, wave-like, and persistent movements of the head, neck, limbs, or voice. Tardive tremors are present both at rest and during voluntary movement.

Early myoclonic encephalopathy

Early myoclonic **encephalopathy** is a rare disorder, in which the incidence is approximately one in 40,000 children. It is characterized by brief and abrupt myoclonic jerks (common occurrence in 90% of patients) and **seizures**. The onset of symptoms usually occurs within the first three years of life. Treatment and management depends on the underlying cause of seizures. Typically, patients receive antiepileptic medications, and improvement of symptoms is usually associated with a good prognosis. If symptoms do not improve with antiepileptic medication(s), the prognosis is not favorable.

Resources

BOOKS

Goetz, Christopher G., et al. (eds). *Textbook of Clinical Neurology.* 1st ed. Philadelphia: W.B. Saunders Company, 1999.

Goldman, Lee, et al. *Cecil's Textbook of Medicine.* 21st ed. Philadelphia: W.B. Saunders Company, 2000.

Noble, John, et al, (eds). *Textbook of Primary Care Medicine.* 3rd ed. St. Louis: Mosby, Inc., 2001.

PERIODICALS

Brasic, James R. "Tardive Dyskinesia." *eMedicine Series* (December 2003).

Jankovic, J., and M. Demirkiran. "Paroxysmal Dyskinesias: An Update." *Annals Medical Science* 10 (2001).

Jenner, Peter. "Avoidance of Dyskinesia: Preclinical Evidence for Continuous Dopaminergic Stimulation." *Neurology* 62:1 (January 2004).

WEBSITES

Gardos, G., and J. O. Cole. *The Treatment of Tardive Dyskinesias.* (May 20, 2004). <http://www.acnp.org/g4/GN401000145/CH142.html>.

ORGANIZATIONS

American College of Neuropsychopharmacology. 320 Centre Building 2014 Broadway, Nashville, TN 37203. (615) 322-2075; Fax: (615) 343-0662. acnp@acnp.org.

Laith Farid Gulli, MD
Nicole Mallory, MS, PA-C

Dyslexia

Definition

Dyslexia is an unexpected impairment in reading and spelling despite a normal intellect.

Description

Dyslexia was first described by Hinshelwood in 1896. Orton originally hypothesized that dyslexia results from a dysfunction in visual memory and visual perception due to a delayment in maturation. Most dyslexics also display poor writing ability. Dyslexia is a classical primary reading disorder and should be differentiated from secondary disorders such as **mental retardation**, educational or environmental deprivation, or physical/organic diseases. The disorder results as a combination of genetic and environmental causes, which can induce variations in the behavioral, cognitive, and physiological measures related to reading disability. Dyslexia was previously called congenital word blindness. Dyslexia is a reading disorder, not caused by lowered motivation, inadequate learning opportunity or any overt neurological disability. Reading is a complex process which involves multiple systems to process the information cognitively and physiologically. In simple terms reading typically begins with a visual sensation stimuli and processing the text via the visual pathway in the brain (from the retina in the eye, the impulse goes in the brain to the lateral geniculate nuclei and primary visual cortex, the occipital lobe, located in the back of the head, which functions to process and integrate incoming visual information). Input information from vision is probably integrated with other neuronal systems that include language-specific rules, learned information and symbolic images into components of language thinking related to reading. Reading-related thinking is correlated with high activity in the left-hemisphere cortical regions, and language processing centers in the brain. Additionally, learning to read is also related to the learning process, which is mediated by the **cerebellum** and on relay feedback mechanisms between related areas of the brain.

Deficits in reading may stem from disruptions of simple sensory impairments to more complex problems involving thinking related to language. There are several subtypes of dyslexias and they can be categorized as either central or peripheral dyslexias (of which there are two, attentional dyslexia and neglect dyslexia), which result from impairment to brain processes that are capable of converting letters on the page into visual word forms. There are two types of peripheral dyslexias called attentional dyslexia, and neglect dyslexia. The attentional dyslexia subtype is a rare disorder of attention control, typically correlated with damage to the left parietal lobe (located on the sides of the head). The attentional dyslexia causes an impairment of reading words in sentences, since the defect causes many words to be visible at the same time. Neglect dyslexia is usually due to brain damage, and causes an impairment of reading because the affected person misidentifies letters in certain spatial regions of either a word or a group of words. The defect for neglect dyslexia subtype is associated with the right parietal lobe. Neglect dyslexia can be further divided into left neglect dyslexia and right neglect dyslexia. In the left neglect dyslexia subtype, the affected person experiences difficulty reading initial letters of the word, which may cause a letter(s) to be substituted, omitted or added. The right neglect dyslexia subtype causes a patient to have letter errors at the end of the word.

Letter-by-letter reading (LBL, pure alexia, or pure word blindness) is another form of peripheral dyslexia causing patients to have very slow reading performance with large effects on word length and response time. There is damage to the prestriate cortex of the occipital cortex and most patients also have a dense right visual field deficit. The damage impairs the word-form system in an abnormal way so that written words seem as random letter strings.

Central dyslexias are typically caused by disruption to neuronal processes correlated with sound analysis and meaning of written words. There are two major subtypes of central dyslexias which either impair semantic reading or nonsemantic reading. Semantic reading dyslexia is also referred to as deep and phonologic dyslexia. Semantic reading is due to extensive damage to the left hemisphere which results in a deficit whereby patients can only assemble the pronunciation of a word by first assessing its

Key Terms

Attention deficit/hyperactivity disorder (ADHD) A disorder associated with behavioral control, due to difficulty processing neural stimuli.

Dizygotic twins Twins that share the same environment during development in the uterus but are not identical.

Lateral geniculate nuclei A structure that receives and processes impulses from the optic nerve, and sends these impulses further into the brain for more processing of information.

Monozygotic twins Twins that are genetically identical and are always of the same gender.

Occipital lobe The back part of the brain that functions as a visual interpretation center.

Parietal lobe Part of the cerebral hemisphere, located on both sides of the brain.

Phoneme The smallest meaningful segment of language (e.g., the word "cat" has 3 phonemes, "kuh," "aah," and "tuh").

Retina Area of the eye that helps process visual information to send impulses to the brain.

Temporal lobe A lobe of the brain that contains auditory and receptive (stimuli) areas.

Visual field A field of vision that is visible without eye movement.

meaning. Affected individuals also make visual errors when reading. Nonsemantic reading, due to damage of the left temporal lobe causes patients to have difficulty reading exception words (i.e. shove), but can read correctly words that are common and similar (i.e. love).

Demographics

It is thought that dyslexia is the most common neurobehavioral disorder affecting children. The prevalence (existing cases) ranges from 5-10% of school-aged children (school and clinic identified) in the United States. However, these rates may be significantly more (up to 17.5%) in unselected populations. Research indicates that dyslexia is a chronic and persistent disorder. Evidence concerning gender predilection remains controversial. Dyslexia may also co-occur with another disorder called attention deficit/hyperactivity disorder (ADHD, 40% comorbidity). Dyslexia affects approximately 80% of children identified as manifesting a learning disorder.

Causes and symptoms

Persons affected with dyslexia have dysfunction developing an awareness of spoken and written words and segmenting smaller units of sound that are essential in an alphabetic language like English. Patients lose the ability to link and map printed symbols (letters) to sound.

Dyslexia runs in families. Studies demonstrate concordance rates of 68% for monozygotic twins and 37% for dizygote twins (Colorado Twin Study of Reading Disability). However, the genetic transmission is not simple and does not follow classical knowledge of trait heritability. Findings suggest that several genetic factors determine reading ability and the interactions of some or all factors determine the ultimate ability to read.

Evidence from neurobiological research utilizing high resolution imaging techniques, and brain measurement studies indicate differences in left temporo-parieto-occipital brain regions in dyslexic patients when compared to nonimpaired readers. Furthermore, evidence using functional brain imaging techniques in adult and children with dyslexia demonstrates a failure of normal left hemisphere posterior brain systems during reading with increased brain activation in frontal regions. This data indicates that impairment of posterior reading systems results in a disruption of the smoothly functioning and integrated reading system seen in nonimpaired persons. The impairment of posterior reading systems causes dyslexic persons to shift to ancillary neuronal systems to compensate for the deficit. It is the impairment in the posterior reading systems that prevents the development of skilled reading. Postmortem studies (confirmed in live subjects using **MRI** imaging) indicate a lack of symmetry in language-associated regions in the brain. The abnormal symmetry is associated with the common linguistic deficits that are characteristic of dyslexia.

The specific signs of dyslexia in both adults and school-aged children are similar. Patients exhibit inaccurate and labored decoding, word recognition, and text reading. They also exhibit difficulties in spelling and remain slow readers. Typical early symptoms can include difficulty playing rhyming games and problems with learning numbers and letters. Children often avoid reading independently and are unusually happy at the opportunity for parents to read to them.

Diagnosis

All cases and ages are diagnosed clinically by a combination of careful medical history, observation and psychological testing. There is no one test that is sufficient to render a definitive diagnosis. Rather, the diagnosis is made based on the results of all the clinical data attained.

Dyslexia can be distinguished from other **learning disorders** by identifying the phonologic deficit. Family history and collateral data obtained from school and test results are essential. Tests to determine attention, memory, intelligence and math and language skills may be administered to establish the diagnosis.

Treatment team

The treatment team can consist of a **neurologist**, a pediatrician, and special education instructors. A clinical psychologist can perform psychological assessments (psychometric testing) to help establish the diagnosis. School and/or college counselors also comprise part of an effective and integrated treatment team.

Treatment

The management for dyslexic patients is lifelong. Early identification and intervention (remediation) of reading deficits involves specialist education. Intervention programs must systematically and explicitly teach phonics ensuring a clear understanding of how letters are linked to sounds (phonemes) and spelling. Typically individualized teaching is recommended to provide a balanced remedial program providing systematic instruction on phonemic awareness, phonics, vocabulary fluency and comprehension strategies. A well-integrated treatment program also includes opportunities for writing, reading, and discussing literature. A well-executed treatment program considers each component of the reading process to improve phonemic awareness and the ability to manipulate speech sounds.

Treatment for older persons (high school, college, and graduate school) is accommodation rather than remediation. College students require extra time with examination and reading/writing assignments. Other accommodations include recorded books, tape recorders in the classroom, tutorial services, alternatives to multiple choice questions and computer availability with spelling checkers.

Recovery and rehabilitation

Rehabilitation for dyslexics is a lifelong process. Early intervention in younger patients consists of a highly structured, integrated, systematic and explicit treatment program. A balanced treatment program should include the meaning and phonetic approaches to reading to ultimately improve language development (since dyslexia is a language-based disorder.) The program should allow for personalized instruction. Older persons require accommodation in college and at work versus remediation.

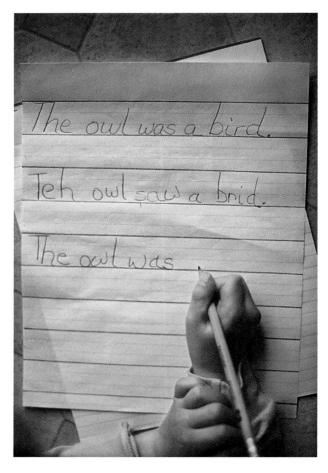

A child with dyslexia, writing words incorrectly. *(Photograph by Robert Huffman. Field Mark Publications. Reproduced by permission.)*

Clinical trials

There are two current clinical research trials entitled: Comprehensive Program to Improve Reading and Writing Skills in At-Risk and Dyslexic Children; and Using MRI to Evaluate Instructional Programs for Children with Developmental Dyslexia. Information can be obtained from http://www.ClinicalTrails.com.

Prognosis

Dyslexia is a lifelong disorder, but improvement is possible. Multiple learning disabilities can be expected, since the brain connections for reading, spelling, listening, speaking, and writing are part of the linguistic system. The prognosis can ultimately depend on associated comorbidities (other disorders associated with the primary disorder), early detection and intervention, and an intensive and comprehensive treatment plan.

Special concerns

Early recognition, intervention, and family members are important. Remediation programs must be delivered by highly-trained specialists, and treatment should be individualized.

Resources
BOOKS
Behrman, Richard, E., et al., eds. *Nelson Textbook of Pediatrics.* 17th ed. Philadelphia: Saunders, 2004.

PERIODICALS
Brow, W. E., A. L. Reiss, and S. Eliez. "Preliminary evidence of widespread morphological variations of the brain in dyslexia." *Neurology* 56, no. 6 (March 2001).

Bub, Danial. "Alexia and related reading disorders." *Neurological clinics* 21, no. 2 (May 2003).

Francks, C., and L. Macphie. "The genetic basis of dyslexia." *The Lancet Neurology* 1, no. 8 (December 2002).

Olitsky, Scott E. "Reading disorders in children." *Pediatric Clinics of North America* 50, no. 1 (February 2003).

Wood, F., and E. L. Grigorenko. "Emerging Issues in the Genetics of Dyslexia: A Methodological Preview." *Journal of Learning Disabilities* 34, no. 6 (November-December 2001).

WEBSITES
Dyslexia. <http://www.dyslexia.com>.

The International Dyslexia Association. <http://www.interdys.org>.

ORGANIZATIONS
The National Center for Learning Disabilities. 381 Park Avenue South, Suite 1401, New York, NY 10016. (212) 545-7510 or 888-575-7373; Fax: (212) 545-9665. <http://www.ncld.org>.

The International Dyslexia Association. 8600 LaSalle Road, Baltimore, MD 21286-2044. 410-296-0232 or 800-ABCD123; Fax: 410-321-5069. <http://www.interdys.org>.

Laith Farid Gulli, MD
Nicole Mallory, MS, PA-C
Robert Ramirez, DO

Dysphagia *see* **Swallowing disorders**

Dyspraxia
Definition

Dyspraxia is a neurological disorder of motor coordination usually apparent in childhood that manifests as difficulty in thinking out, planning out, and executing planned movements or tasks. The term dyspraxia derives from the Greek word *praxis*, meaning "movement process."

Description

The earliest description of a syndrome of clumsiness, termed "congenital maladroitness," dates back to the turn of the twentieth century. Since that time, numerous names have been given to this syndrome of impaired coordination, including dyspraxia, developmental dyspraxia, developmental coordination disorder, clumsy child syndrome, and sensory integration disorder. Some sources ascribe different meanings to these terms, while others use them interchangeably. Researchers commonly use the term developmental coordination disorder (DCD); DCD is classified by the *Diagnostic and Statistical Manual of Mental Disorders*, Fourth Edition, Text Revision (DSM-IV-TR) as a motor skills disorder.

Dyspraxia is a variable condition; it manifests in different ways at different ages. It may impair physical, intellectual, emotional, social, language, and/or sensory development. Dyspraxia is often subdivided into two types: developmental dyspraxia, also known as developmental coordination disorder, and verbal dyspraxia, also known as developmental **apraxia** of speech. Symptoms of the dyspraxia typically appear in childhood, anywhere from infancy to adolescence, and can persist into adult years. Other disorders such as **dyslexia**, learning disabilities, and attention deficit disorder often co-occur in children with dyspraxia.

Demographics

Estimates of the prevalence of developmental coordination disorder are approximately 6% in children aged 5–11. Some reports indicate a higher prevalence in the 10–20% range. Males are four times more likely than females to have dyspraxia. In some cases, the disorder may be familial.

Causes and symptoms

Developmental dyspraxia is apparent from birth or early in life. As of 2004, the underlying cause or causes for dyspraxia remain largely unknown. It is thought that any number of factors such as illness or trauma may adversely affect normal brain development, resulting in dyspraxia. Genes may also play a role in the development of dyspraxia. It is known that dyspraxia can be acquired (acquired dyspraxia) due to brain damage suffered as a result of **stroke**, an accident, or other trauma.

Symptoms of dyspraxia vary and may include some or all of the following problems:

• poor balance and coordination

• vision problems

• perceptual problems

• poor spatial awareness

• poor posture

• poor short-term memory

• difficulty planning motor tasks

• difficulty with reading, writing, and speech

• emotional and behavioral problems

• poor social skills

The symptoms of dyspraxia depend somewhat on the age of the child. Young children will have delayed motor milestones such as crawling, walking, and jumping. Older children may present with academic problems such as difficulty with reading and writing or with playing ball games.

Developmental verbal dyspraxia (DVD), a type of dyspraxia, can manifest as early as infancy with feeding problems. Children with DVD may display delays in expressive language, difficulty in producing speech, reduced intelligibility of speech, and inconsistent production of familiar words.

Diagnosis

The diagnosis of dyspraxia is based on observation of a patient's symptoms and on results of standardized tests. Findings from a neurological or neurodevelopmental evaluation may also be used to confirm a suspected diagnosis. The process of making a diagnosis of dyspraxia can be complex for a number of reasons. Dyspraxia may affect many different body functions, it can occur as a part of another syndrome, and symptoms of dyspraxia overlap with similar disorders such as dyslexia.

Diagnostic criteria

Various health professionals and organizations define the term dyspraxia differently. The Dyspraxia Foundation (England) describes it as "an impairment or immaturity of the organization of movement," and further adds that it may be associated with problems in language, perception, and thought. Other advocacy groups such as the Dyspraxia Association of Ireland and the Dyspraxia Foundation of New Zealand, Inc. offer slightly different definitions. The American Psychiatric Association lists four criteria in the DSM-IV-TR for the diagnosis of developmental coordination disorder:

• marked impairment in the development of motor coordination

• the impaired coordination significantly interferes with academic achievement or activities of daily living

- the coordination difficulties are not due to a general medical problem such as **cerebral palsy** or **muscular dystrophy** and do not meet the criteria for pervasive developmental disorder
- if **mental retardation** (MR) is present, the motor coordination problems exceed those typically associated with the MR

Treatment team

Treatment for individuals with dyspraxia is highly individualized because the manifestations vary from patient to patient. The treatment team for a child with dyspraxia may include a pediatric **neurologist**, a physical therapist, an occupational therapist, and a speech therapist, in addition to a family doctor or pediatrician. In some cases, the treatment team may also include a psychologist, a developmental optometrist, and specialists in early intervention or special education.

Treatment

Currently there is no cure for dyspraxia. Treatment mainly consists of rehabilitation through physical, occupational, and speech therapies. Other interventions such as special education, psychological therapy, or orthoptic exercises may be recommended on a case-by-case basis. The purpose of treatment for dyspraxia is to help the child to think out, plan out, and execute the actions necessary to try out new tasks or familiar tasks in novel ways.

Recovery and rehabilitation

There are specific therapies for dyspraxia. In physical therapy, a physical therapist may evaluate some or all of the following skill areas in order to formulate a plan of treatment with the patient's physician:

- muscle tone
- control of shoulders and pelvis
- active trunk extension and flexion (posture)
- hand-eye coordination (throwing a ball)
- foot-eye coordination (kicking a ball)
- midline crossing (writing)
- directional awareness (ability to move in different directions)
- spatial awareness (judge distances and direction)
- integration (moving both sides of the body simultaneously)
- knowledge of two sides/dominance of one side (knowing right from left)
- short-term memory

- motor planning (ability to plan movements needed to move from one position to another)
- self organization (dressing, eating, etc.)
- eye tracking

Physical therapy generally consists of activities and exercises designed to improve the specific skill weakness. For example, activities such as climbing, going through tunnels, and moving in and out of cones may assist a child who has poor spatial awareness. The physical therapist may also recommend that the child practice the treatment activities or exercises at home.

In occupational therapy, an occupational therapist may use standardized tests to evaluate the child's sensory integration skills. A therapeutic technique known as sensory integration may be recommended. Sensory integration techniques help a child to sort, store, and integrate information obtained by the senses so that it may be used for learning.

In speech therapy, a speech therapist may assist the child with areas such as muscle control, planning language, and forming concepts and strategies in order to communicate. The therapist may use language tests to assess language comprehension and production in order to develop a plan of treatment

Clinical trials

As of 2004, there was one clinical trial recruiting patients with a form of dyspraxia known as verbal dyspraxia. The aim of the study, entitled "Central Mechanisms in Speech Motor Control Studied with H2150 **PET**," is to use radioactive water (H2150) and **positron emission tomography (PET)** scan to measure blood flow to different areas of the brain in order to better understand the mechanisms involved in speech motor control. Information on this trial can be found at <http://www.clinicaltrials.gov> (see study number 92-DC-0178) or by contacting the National Institute on Deafness and Other Communication Disorders (NIDCD) patient recruitment and public liaison office at (800) 411-1010.

Prognosis

The prognosis for dyspraxia varies. Some children "outgrow" their condition, whereas others continue to have difficulties into adulthood. Though early diagnosis and prompt treatment may improve the outcome for a given patient, the precise factors that influence prognosis are not well understood. For example, it remains unclear how factors such as a child's specific deficits and the underlying cause for the disorder influence rehabilitation potential. Also, the prognosis for dyspraxia is situational; it depends on the age of the patient and the demands of a given setting or environment.

Special concerns

A child with a diagnosis of dyspraxia or developmental coordination disorder may be eligible to have an individual education plan (IEP). An IEP provides a framework from which administrators, teachers, and parents can meet the educational needs of a child with dyspraxia. Depending upon severity of symptoms and the presence of other problems such as learning difficulties, children may be best served by special education classes or by a private educational setting.

Resources

BOOKS

American Psychiatric Association. *Diagnostic and Statistical Manual of Mental Disorders*, 4th edition, text revision. Washington, DC: American Psychiatric Association, 2000.

Macintyre, C. *Dyspraxia 5–11: A Practical Guide.* London: David Fulton Publishers, 2001.

Portwood, M. *Understanding Developmental Dyspraxia: A Textbook for Students and Professionals.* London: David Fulton Publishers, 2000.

PERIODICALS

Cousins, M., and M. M. Smyth. "Developmental Coordination Impairments in Adulthood." *Hum Mov Sci* 22 (November 2003): 433–59.

Flory, S. "Identifying, Assessing and Helping Dyspraxic Children." *Dyslexia* 6 (July–September 2000): 205–8.

McCormick, M. "Dyslexia and Developmental Verbal Dyspraxia." *Dyslexia* 6 (July–September 2000): 210–4.

Payton, P., and M. Winfield. "Interventions for Pupils with Dyspraxic Difficulties." *Dyslexia* 6 (July–September 2000): 208–10.

WEBSITES

Apraxia Kids Home Page. (May 30, 2004). <http://www.apraxia-kids.org/index.html>.

The Dyspraxia Support Group of New Zealand Home Page. (May 30, 2004). <http://www.dyspraxia.org.nz/>.

Developmental Dyspraxia Information Page. The National Institute of Neurological Disorders and Stroke (NINDS). (May 30, 2004). <http://www.ninds.nih.gov/health_and_medical/disorders/dyspraxia.htm>.

ORGANIZATIONS

American Speech Language Hearing Association (ASHA). 10801 Rockville Pike, Rockville, MD 20852-3279. (301) 897-5700 or (800) 638-8255; Fax: (301) 571-0457. actioncenter@asha.org. <http://www.asha.org>.

The Dyspraxia Foundation. 8 West Alley, Hitchin, Hertfordshire SG5 1EG, United Kingdom. +44 (0) 14 6245 5016 or +44 (0) 14 6245 4986; Fax: +44 (0) 14 6245 5052. dyspraxia@dyspraxiafoundation.org.uk. <http://www.dyspraxiafoundation.org.uk/>.

The Dyspraxia Support Group of New Zealand, Inc. The Dyspraxia Centre, P.O. Box 20292, Bishopdale, Christchurch, New Zealand. +64 3 359 7072; Fax: +64 3 359 7074. praxisnz@xtra.co.nz. <http://www.dyspraxia.org.nz/>

Dawn J. Cardeiro, MS, CGC

Dyssynergia cerebellaris myoclonica *see* Ramsey-Hunt syndrome type II

Dystonia

Definition

Dystonia is a disabling movement disorder characterized by sustained contraction of muscles leading to twisting distorted postures. Dystonia may affect various parts of the body and has multiple causes, making classification and diagnosis challenging. The etiology behind the various forms of dystonia is unknown, although abnormal functioning of the cerebral cortex and basal ganglia and other pathways involved in movement are presumed. Clinical and basic science research on humans and primates, and identification of multiple genes causing dystonia have improved the understanding and treatment of this debilitating disorder.

Description

Dystonia as a term was first coined by Oppenheim in 1911 in reference to a childhood-onset syndrome he termed dystonia musculorum deformans. This entity, known as idiopathic torsion dystonia today, was noted to run in families, and although presumably inherited, was only recently proven to be of genetic cause. There is a wide range of variability in the manifestation of clinical symptoms of dystonia. Due to its various causes, dystonia is seen as a syndrome rather than a disease.

Dystonia can be classified by age of onset, cause, or by distribution of the body parts affected. Dystonia localized to a single body part such as the hand or neck is referred to as focal. Among body parts affected in focal dystonia, the eyelids, mouth, muscles controlling the voice, neck, hand, or arm may be affected. Dystonia localized to two contiguous body parts is referred to as segmental. Dystonia affecting body parts that are not next to each other is referred to as multifocal. Dystonia affecting one segment and another body part is classified as generalized. It may also affect only one half of the body and be called hemidystonia. Dystonia with a known environmental cause is referred to as secondary. The cause of primary or idiopathic dystonias is unknown or genetic.

The course and severity of dystonic symptoms may change over the duration of the illness. Symptoms may initially involve one body part and then spread to other body parts. The likelihood of spread often depends on the age and site of onset of symptoms. Early onset dystonia may start in a limb but tends to become generalized. Adult onset dystonia may start in the neck or face muscles and tends not to spread. Dystonia may first occur only with voluntary movements, but in time, occur at rest as well.

Demographics

Dystonia follows **Parkinson's disease** and essential tremor as the most frequent movement disorder. Prevalence is estimated as 3.4 per 100,000 for generalized forms and 29.5 per 100,000 for focal dystonia. Early onset dystonia may be more frequent in patients of Jewish ancestry, especially from Eastern Europe or Ashkenazi background.

Causes and symptoms
Causes

The exact cause of dystonia is unknown. Ongoing research on dystonia is directed at examining the abnormal brain activity in different parts of the brain such as the basal ganglia and cerebral cortex. The basal ganglia are a collection of nerve cells that are part of the brain pathways important for regulating aspects of normal movement. Abnormalities in the processing of information in these pathways are thought to underlie the various **movement disorders** such as Parkinson's disease, Huntington's disease, tremor, and dystonia. There is evidence for abnormalities in the spinal cord and peripheral nerves as well, suggesting that dystonia may involve abnormalities at multiple levels of the nervous system. Patients with dystonia may have abnormal touch perception and sensation, and theories propose that there may be defects in the preparation of movement as well as the translation of sensation to movement. Dystonia can be classified by cause into primary and secondary forms. Primary or idiopathic dystonia is presumed to be of genetic or unknown cause, whereas secondary dystonias are due to an attributable cause.

Primary dystonia

Primary or idiopathic dystonias have no identifiable etiology and are presumed to be genetic in cause. There are currently at least 13 different genetic dystonia syndromes, although only a few genes have actually been isolated. The only identified gene for primary dystonia is DYT1 on chromosome 9. DYT1 dystonia tends to occur in childhood and starts in a limb only to generalize. The appearance of the dystonia may differ in individuals with the same genetic abnormality, suggesting that there are environmental factors involved as well. Primary genetic dystonias may appear in multiple family members, but most are due to new mutations in genes and referred to as sporadic. Primary dystonias tend to develop gradually over the course of months to years.

Secondary dystonia

Secondary dystonia can be caused by a structural abnormality of the brain such as a **stroke** or infection, drugs or various toxins or metabolic abnormalities. These tend to occur over the course of days to weeks due to the nature of an inciting insult. Dystonia may occur after birth trauma and may be delayed in onset for up to a decade or later. Some may occur as part of a larger disease process affecting other parts of the body such as Wilson's disease, a defect of metabolism of copper that causes abnormal liver function and movement problems such as dystonia or tremor. Usually an abnormality will be found on brain imaging studies such as **MRI** or **CT scan**. Patients taking medications for psychiatric diseases such as **schizophrenia** or psychosis may develop dystonia as a drug reaction. Dystonia may be feigned as part of a psychiatric disorder and is then known as psychogenic.

Other dystonias

Dystonia may also be associated with other neurologic disorders. These are classified as dystonia-plus syndromes. Dystonia may be associated with Parkinson's disease or **myoclonus**, another movement disorder which consists of muscle jerking. Dystonia may be part of a larger syndrome of neurodegenerative disorders, a group of diseases which are caused by degeneration of nerve cells in certain portions of the brain. Such disorders include Huntington's disease and Parkinson's disease.

Symptoms

The symptoms of dystonia depend on the body part affected. Dystonia localized to the face may involve repetitive blinking, tongue protrusion, or jaw clenching. Blinking can become so severe that the patient can not see due to inability to open the eyes. Dystonia affecting the neck may lead to sustained flexion, extension, or twisting postures of the neck known as torticollis. Some dystonias are task-specific and only arise during the performance of certain tasks such as writing, typing, or playing instruments. The progression of these symptoms can lead to severe disability and inability to perform daily work. Generalized dystonia, the most severe form, can present as twisting movements of the head, trunk, and arms, completely disabling the affected individual. Dystonia can often be associated with a tremor in the affected body part.

All forms of dystonia impair normal movement and daily function to some degree. Dystonia can be worsened by stress and anxiety, whereas it may be relieved with relaxation and sleep. Symptoms may be improved by touching various parts of the body in a phenomenon called a "sensory trick."

Diagnosis

The diagnosis of dystonia is clinical and is usually made by a **neurologist** who may have expertise with movement disorders. Investigation of dystonia will usually involve a physical examination and medical history taken by the neurologist to look for secondary causes such as drug exposure or stroke or other family members affected, suggesting a genetic cause. An MRI of the brain may be performed to look for a structural abnormality causing the symptoms. Laboratory testing may reveal abnormalities of copper metabolism associated with Wilson's disease. Genetic testing for the DYT1 gene is not performed unless the dystonia is early in onset or there is a family history of similar symptoms.

Treatment team

Treatment for dystonia involves the interaction between a neurologist, psychiatrists, and physical and occupational therapists. Treatment may involve a neurosurgeon for symptoms that do not respond to medical management. Dystonia of childhood onset is treated by a pediatric neurologist cooperating with pediatricians and pediatric therapists.

Treatment

Treatment for dystonia is usually directed towards management of the symptoms and depends on the type of dystonia. Dystonia that is associated or caused by known etiologies such as drugs, Wilson's disease, or dopa-responsive dystonia may be improved by treating the underlying disease with resolution of symptoms. The various treatments available may be grouped into oral medications, **botulinum toxin** injections, and surgical modalities.

Medications

Various oral medications are available for the symptomatic treatment of dystonia. Among these are various medications that affect different neurochemical systems thought to be important in causing dystonia. Some patients with symptoms of early onset may have dystonia that responds dramatically to levodopa. **Anticholinergics**, dopamine depleting agents, **benzodiazepines**, baclofen, or atypical antipsychotics may be tried as well.

Botox

Chemical denervation using botulinum toxin has been used for many movement disorders including dystonia. Botulinum toxin blocks the transmission of nerve impulses to the muscle and paralyzes the overactive muscles involved. Focal forms of dystonia are more amenable to treatment due to the ease of localizing injectable muscles and less extensive involvement. Botox may be used in generalized dystonia to facilitate improvement in select muscles needed for daily function such as the arms and legs.

Surgical treatment

Selective destruction or high frequency stimulation of nerve centers involved in causing dystonia has been useful in treating selected patients with disabling symptoms. Patients with generalized dystonia or hemidystonia may benefit due to the widespread nature of symptoms, limiting the efficacy of medications and botox injections. Surgical lesioning of nerve cells in the globus pallidus or stimulation of cells in the globus pallidus or subthalamic nucleus have been shown to be effective in treating the symptoms of dystonia. The long-term benefit of surgical therapies on symptoms of dystonia has yet to be validated.

Recovery and rehabilitation

Symptoms of dystonia may fluctuate over the course of years. The course of disease in any given individual can not be predicted. Some may improve spontaneously, whereas others may progress and spread to involve other body parts. Physical therapists may aid in the treatment of symptoms of dystonia. Treatment is focused on maintaining or improving the patient's ability to walk. Occupational therapy may be helpful in improving hand use.

Clinical trials

Several **clinical trials** are currently in effect for treatment of dystonia. The National Institutes of Health (NIH) and National Institutes of Neurological Diseases and Stroke (NINDS) are recruiting patients for trials examining the effect of different medications, botulinum toxin treatment, and surgical treatment for patients with dystonia. Studies are also ongoing to study the effect of electrical stimulation of the brain and nerves with magnetic fields to treat dystonia. Updated information on clinical trials can be found at the National Institutes of Health clinical trials website at www.clinicaltrials.org.

Prognosis

The prognosis for dystonia depends on the distribution and the cause. The initial site of symptoms may predict the prognosis. Patients with symptoms that start in the leg have a higher likelihood (90%) of progression to involve other body parts and become generalized. Patients with symptoms starting in the neck and later in onset have a much lower likelihood of spread. Most focal dystonias respond to medications or botulinum toxin. Refractory and generalized dystonia may require surgical management. Most patients have a normal life expectancy although with continued disabling symptoms.

Special concerns
Educational and social needs

Dystonia in many cases is a chronic illness and due to the physical limitations and often disfiguring symptoms, may lead to feelings of **depression** or anxiety. These feelings may require treatment by a psychiatrist if severe enough. It is important for patients with dystonia to continue to be involved in community activities and social events.

Resources

BOOKS
Bradley, Walter G., Robert Daroff, Gerald Fenichel, and C. David Marsden. *Neurology in Clinical Practice.* Newton, MA: Butterworth-Heinemann, 2000.

Rowland, Lewis, ed. *Merritt's Textbook of Neurology.* Philadelphia, PA: Lippincott Williams & Wilkins, 2000.

PERIODICALS
Klein, C., and L. J. Ozelius. "Dystonia: clinical features, genetics, and treatment." *Current Opinion in Neurology* 15 (2002): 491–497.

Langlois, M., F. Richer, and S. Chouinard. "New Perspectives on Dystonia." *Canadian Journal of Neurological Sciences* 30, Suppl. 1 (2003): S34–S44.

Volkmann, J., and R. Benecke. "Deep Brain Stimulation for Dystonia: Patient Selection and Evaluation." *Movement Disorders* 17 (2002): S112–S115.

WEBSITES
NINDS Dystonias Information Page. National Institutes of Neurological Disorders and Stroke (NINDS). July 1, 2001. (June 7, 2004). <http://www.ninds.nih.gov/health_and_medical/disorders/the_dystonias.htm>

ORGANIZATIONS
Dystonia Medical Research Foundation. 1 East Wacker Drive, Suite 2430, Chicago, IL 60601-1905. (312) 755-0198; Fax: (312) 803-0138. dystonia@dystonia-foundation.org/ <http://www.dystonia-foundation.org>.

Worldwide Education & Awareness for Movement Disorders (WE MOVE). 204 West 84th Street, New York, NY 10024. (212) 875-8312 or (800) 437-6682; Fax: (212) 875-8389. wemove@wemove.org. <http://www.wemove.org>.

Peter T. Lin, MD

E

Edrophonium *see* **Cholinergic stimulants**

Electric personal assistive mobility devices

Definition

Electric personal assistive mobility devices are power-assisted devices for mobility such as wheelchairs, scooters, and more recent innovations such as the Segway™ Human Transporter. These devices make everyday life easier for someone who is partially or completely immobile.

Description

Currently there are approximately 160,000 people who use electric powered wheelchair and scooters in the United States alone. Of these, some 100,000 utilize wheelchairs and 60,000 use powered scooters. As baby boomers become senior citizens and mobility becomes more of a concern for this large population, the market for these aids is expected to increase. Industry estimates show the powered assistive device market as growing by about 7% each year through 2007. By 2007, sales of manual- and electric-powered wheelchairs and powered scooters is estimated to be $2.7 billion in the United States.

Wheelchairs

Electric wheelchairs appeared in the 1950s. Then, the less sophisticated mechanics of the chair produced a rougher and more jarring ride. Today's models are better described as electronic chairs rather than electric chairs. Electronic circuitry allows for a control of speed and a precise control of direction. Many of today's sophisticated powered wheelchairs conform to two basic styles. The first is called the traditional style and consists of a power source mounted behind or underneath the seat of the wheelchair. As the name implies, the traditional unit looks very much like a manual wheelchair.

The second design is known as a platform chair. In this design, the seating area, which can often be raised or lowered, sits on top of the power source. There are several groups of powered wheelchairs, based on the intended use. Wheelchairs designed strictly for indoor use have a smaller area between the wheels, allowing them to negotiate the tighter turns and more confined spaces of the indoor world. Other designs allow the electric wheelchair to be used both indoors and outdoors, on sidewalks, driveways, and hard, even surfaces. Finally, some electric wheelchairs are able to negotiate more rugged terrain such as uneven, stony surfaces.

Wheelchairs meant for indoor and indoor/outdoor use conserve weight by reducing the size of the rechargeable batteries that deliver the power to the device. Outdoor models deliver more power, more speed, and can operate for a longer period of time, at the cost of a heavier wheelchair. Electric wheelchairs can also be classified according to the location of the wheels that drive the device. Rear-wheel, mid-wheel, and front-wheel drive models are available. In a rear-wheel chair, the big wheels that drive the unit are positioned behind the rider's center of gravity. This is the traditional chair design.

In the mid-wheel design, the large wheels are positioned directly under the rider's center of gravity. This offers a shorter turning radius, which can be useful in tight places. However, sudden stops can cause the chair to rock or pitch forward. Finally, the front-wheel drive chair has the large wheels in front of the rider's center of gravity. This allows for a tight turning radius and even to climb over obstacles such as curbs.

For people who are immobile, some wheelchairs are capable of adjusting the person's position. Some chairs can recline and/or can tilt people back while they are still in the sitting position. Changes of position relieve pressure and can help lessen the development of skin irritation.

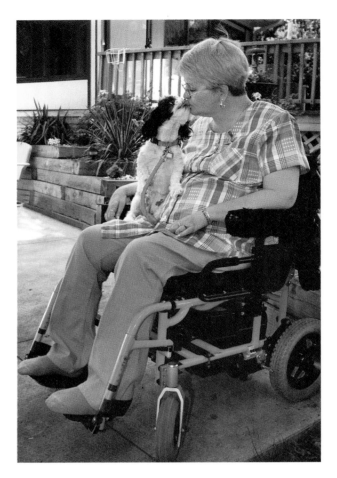

Roslyn Cappiello, a quadriplegic and president of the Omaha chapter of Mothers Against Drunk Driving. *(AP/Wide World Photos. Reproduced by permission.)*

Changing position can also help some people breathe more easily.

Some powered wheelchairs are also capable of raising or lowering a person. This can make life easier by allowing the person to retrieve fallen objects and to reach higher-placed objects. Some wheelchairs can even raise the person to a standing position. This increases the range of tasks a person can accomplish. A wheelchair-bound person can wash dishes, clean windows, work at a counter, and put dishes away in a cupboard, as a few examples, thus reducing the need to modify a home.

The controls to electric-powered wheelchairs vary depending on the mobility of the user. For those with arm function, a joystick can be used to propel the chair forwards or backwards, and to steer. Those who are paralyzed are able to perform these functions using a sip-and-puff setup via a straw. Some manufacturers even make voice-activated and -responsive wheelchairs.

This ability of fully paralyzed people to independently operate a wheelchair offers great potential in reducing the barriers that have prevented wheelchair users from participating fully in society.

Innovations in electric-powered wheelchairs

Construction materials used in wheelchair frames have reduced the weight of the chairs. Aluminum, stainless steel, and steel tubes are some of several materials that produce strength without excess weight.

In 1993, a new powered wheelchair marketed as the Hoveround was launched. It has features of both a wheelchair and a scooter. The most unique features are the round base and single rear wheel, which allow the chair to be turned in a full circle on the spot. A relatively recent innovation is known as the pushrim-activated power-assisted wheelchair (PAPAW). This design uses motors and an electric battery to supply forward thrust or braking capabilities that complement similar manual actions of the user. A PAPAW is best suited to a user who can manually operate a wheelchair, but not very efficiently due to **pain**, insufficient arm strength, heart and/or lung trouble, or inability to maintain effective posture.

User demand is driving new designs for mobility devices that do not look like wheelchairs. Indeed, newer designs for wheelchairs are more similar to scooters than to the traditional design of the wheelchair. The impetus for this new design has been people's desire for more independence and mobility, to the point of being able to mount curbs and travel over rough ground.

The Independence 3000 IBOT Transporter (IBOT) can change the way it moves in response to varying terrain. The two pairs of large rear wheels can operate at different height, allowing for actions like the mounting of curbs. In fact, the front pair of wheels can ride up the rear set, enabling the two pairs of wheels to balance vertically on each other.

Scooters

Scooters are designed for people who are able to walk, but have difficulty walking significant distances. Examples include people with milder forms of **cerebral palsy**, **multiple sclerosis**, postpolio syndrome, and those who have had a **stroke** or who suffer from arthritis. Scooters are not designed for those who are absolutely immobile. Scooters consist of a seat mounted on a movable platform. The rider uses handle bars to maintain balance and to steer, although some scooters use electronics that control the steering instead of the operator. The seats are typically removable to allow the scooter to be easily transported in car, truck, or other vehicle.

Scooters represent a hybrid between a manual and electric wheelchair. They appeal to those who do not have the physical capability to power a manual wheelchair, but who do not need the electronic controls and various seating configurations that can be selected in some electric wheelchairs. For users who have the upper arm and body strength necessary to use one and also to hold themselves in a sitting position for a prolonged time, a scooter can represent a more economical alternative to a powered wheelchair.

The basic setup of a scooter is known as the base unit. This consists of a frame made of steel or aluminum attached to a platform. Some units also have a windscreen as part of the unit. The seat post can be a permanent part of the frame, or may be detachable for easy transport.

Scooters can be front-wheel drive or rear-wheel drive. The scooters with rear-wheel drive, which has a larger motor and a longer distance between the front and rear wheels, typically supply more power and so are useful for tasks like climbing hilly terrain. Front-wheel drive scooters have a smaller motor and so are more maneuverable in tight places such as indoor use. They can also be used outside on flat, paved surfaces. The choice of scooter depends on the user's needs. Three- and four-wheeled scooters are also available. These provide more stability for users whose balance is faulty.

Other personal transport devices

For many years, golf cart-style vehicles have provided transportation for elderly people. In retirement communities, carts can be an everyday part of the landscape, being used even on the roads of gated communities. As the population ages and decreased physical mobility affects more people, the popularity of electric carts may well grow.

The Segway™ Human Transporter was introduced in the 1990s. It offers increased mobility for those with disabilities, but could also aid some persons who are unable to walk long distances. The machine operates on a principle called dynamic stabilization. Essentially, this means that the machine works in a manner similar to people's sense of balance. When people standing on the machine shift their center of gravity forward, the machine moves forward. Shifting the center of gravity backward stops the machine. There is no accelerator or brake.

While more of a curiosity than practical means of transport as of 2004, the transporter is an example of how increased mobility is possible in environments such as sidewalks and factories.

Resources

BOOKS

Iezzoni, Lisa. *When Walking Fails: Mobility Problems of Adults with Chronic Conditions.* Berkeley: University of California Press, 2003.

Karp, Gary. *Life on Wheels: For the Active Wheelchair User.* Sebastopol, CA: Patient-Centered Guides, 1999.

OTHER

Cooper, R. A., and R. Cooper. "Trends and Issues in Wheeled Mobility Technologies." *Center for Inclusive Design and Environmental Access.* April 10, 2004 (June 2, 2004). <http://www.ap.buffaloa.edu/idea/space%20w...s/WEB%20-%20Trends_Iss_WC%20(Cooper).htm>.

ORGANIZATIONS

Center for Inclusive Design and Environmental Access. School of Architecture and Design, University of Buffalo, Buffalo, NY 14214-3087. (716) 829-3485; Fax: (716) 829-3861. idea@ap.buffalo.edu. <http://www.ap.buffalo.edu/idea>.

Department of Rehabilitation Science and Technology. 420 Forbes Tower, University of Pittsburgh, Pittsburgh, PA 15260. (412) 383-6556; Fax: (412) 383-6597. shrsadm+@pitt.edu. <http://www.shrs.pitt.edu>.

Worldwide Education & Awareness for Movement Disorders (WE MOVE). 204 West 84th Street, New York, NY 10024. (212) 875-8312 or (800) 437-MOV2 (6682); Fax: (212) 875-8389. Wemove@wemove.org. <http://www.wemove.org>.

Brian Douglas Hoyle, PhD

Electroencephalography

Definition

Electroencephalography, or EEG, is a neurological test that involves attaching electrodes to the head of a person to measure and record electrical activity in the brain over time.

Purpose

The EEG, also known as a brain wave test, is a key tool in the diagnosis and management of **epilepsy** and other seizure disorders. It is also used to assist in the diagnosis of brain damage and diseases such as strokes, tumors, encephalitis, **mental retardation**, and sleep disorders. The results of the test can distinguish psychiatric conditions such as **schizophrenia**, paranoia, and **depression** from degenerative mental disorders such as Alzheimer's and Parkinson's diseases. An EEG may also be used to monitor brain activity during surgery to assess the effects of anesthesia. Additionally, it is used to determine brain status and brain death.

Precautions

There are few adverse conditions associated with an EEG test. Persons with seizure disorders may experience **seizures** during the test in reaction to flashing lights or by deep breathing.

Description

Before an EEG begins, a nurse or technologist attaches approximately 16–21 electrodes to a person's scalp using an electrically conductive, washable paste. The electrodes are placed on the head in a standard pattern based on head circumference measurements. Depending on the purpose for the EEG, implantable, or invasive, electrodes are occasionally used. Implantable electrodes include sphenoidal electrodes, which are fine wires inserted under the zygomatic arch, or cheekbone. Depth electrodes, or subdural strip electrodes, are surgically implanted into the brain and are used to localize a seizure focus in preparation for epilepsy surgery. Once in place, even implantable electrodes do not cause **pain**. The electrodes are used to measure the electrical activity in various regions of the brain over the course of the test period.

For the test, a person lies on a bed, padded table, or comfortable chair and is asked to relax and remain still while measurements are being taken. An EEG usually takes no more than one hour, although long-term monitoring is often used for diagnosis of seizure disorders. During the test procedure, a person may be asked to breathe slowly or quickly. Visual stimuli such as flashing lights or a patterned board may be used to stimulate certain types of brain activity. Throughout the procedure, the electroencephalography unit makes a continuous graphic record of the person's brain activity, or brain waves, on a long strip of recording paper or computer screen. This graphic record is called an electroencephalogram. If the display is computerized, the test may be called a digital EEG, or dEEG.

The sleep EEG uses the same equipment and procedures as a regular EEG. Persons undergoing a sleep EEG are encouraged to fall asleep completely rather than just relax. They are typically provided a bed and a quiet room conducive to sleep. A sleep EEG lasts up to three hours, or up to eight or nine hours if it is a night's sleep.

In an ambulatory EEG, individuals are hooked up to a portable cassette recorder. They then go about normal activities and take normal rest and sleep for a period of up to 24 hours. During this period, individuals and their family members record any symptoms or abnormal behaviors, which can later be correlated with the EEG to see if they represent seizures.

An extension of the EEG technique, called quantitative EEG (qEEG), involves manipulating the EEG signals with a computer using the fast Fourier transform algorithm. The result is then best displayed using a colored gray scale transposed onto a schematic map of the head to form a topographic image. The brain map produced in this technique is a vivid illustration of electrical activity of the brain. This technique also has the ability to compare the similarity of the signals between different electrodes, a measurement known as spectral coherence. Studies have

shown the value of this measurement in diagnosis of Alzheimer's disease and mild closed-head injuries. The technique can also identify areas of the brain having abnormally slow activity when the data are both mapped and compared to known normal values. The result is then known as a statistical or significance probability map (SPM). This allows differentiation between early **dementia** (increased slowing) or otherwise uncomplicated depression (no slowing).

Preparation

An EEG is generally performed as one test in a series of neurological evaluations. Rarely does the EEG form the sole basis for a particular diagnosis.

Full instructions should be given to individuals receiving an EEG when they schedule their test. Typically, individuals taking medications that affect the **central nervous system**, such as **anticonvulsants**, stimulants, or antidepressants, are told to discontinue their prescription for a short time prior to the test (usually one or two days). However, such requests should be cleared with the treating physician. EEG test candidates may be asked to avoid food and beverages that contain caffeine, a central nervous system stimulant. They may also be asked to arrive for the test with clean hair that is free of spray or other styling products to make attachment of the electrodes easier.

Individuals undergoing a sleep EEG may be asked to remain awake the night before their test. They may be given a sedative prior to the test to induce sleep.

Key Terms

Encephalitis Inflammation of the brain.

Fast Fourier transfer A digital processing of the recorded signal resulting in a decomposition of its frequency components.

Ictal EEG An EEG done to determine the type of seizure characteristic of a person's disorder. During this EEG, seizure medicine may be discontinued in an attempt to induce as seizure during the testing period.

Sphenoidal electrodes Fine wire electrodes that are implanted under the cheek bones, used to measure temporal seizures.

Subdural electrodes Strip electrodes that are placed under dura mater (the outermost, toughest, and most fibrous of the three membranes [meninges] covering the brain and spinal cord). They are used to locate foci of epileptic seizures prior to epilepsy surgery.

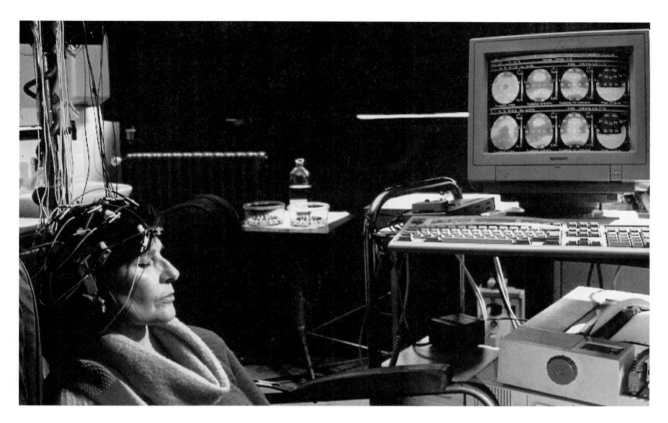

Woman undergoing an electroencephalogram (EEG). *(Photograph by Catherine Pouedras. Science Photo Library, National Audubon Society Collection/Photo Researchers, Inc. Reproduced by permission.)*

Aftercare

If an individual has suspended regular medication for the test, the EEG nurse or technician should advise as to when to begin taking it again.

Risks

Being off certain medications for one to two days may trigger seizures. Certain procedures used during EEG may trigger seizures in persons with epilepsy. Those procedures include flashing lights and deep breathing. If the EEG is being used as a diagnostic tool for epilepsy (i.e., to determine the type of seizures an individual is experiencing), this may be a desired effect, although the person needs to be monitored closely so that the seizure can be aborted if necessary. This type of test is known as an ictal EEG.

Normal results

In reading and interpreting brain wave patterns, a **neurologist** or other physician will evaluate the type of brain waves and the symmetry, location, and consistency of brain wave patterns. Brain wave response to certain stimuli presented during the EEG test (such as flashing lights or noise) will also be evaluated.

The four basic types of brain waves are alpha, beta, theta, and delta, with the type distinguished by frequency. Alpha waves fall between 8 and 13 Hertz (Hz), beta are above 13 Hz, theta between 4 and 7 Hz, and delta are less than 4 Hz. Alpha waves are usually the dominant rhythm seen in the posterior region of the brain in older children and adults, when they are awake and relaxed. Beta waves are normal in sleep, particularly for infants and young children. Theta waves are normally found during drowsiness and sleep and are normal in wakefulness in children, while delta waves are the most prominent feature of the sleeping EEG. Spikes and sharp waves are generally abnormal; however, they are common in the EEG of normal newborns.

Different types of brain waves are seen as abnormal only in the context of the location of the waves, a person's age, and one's state of consciousness. In general, disease typically increases slow activity such as theta or delta waves, but decreases fast activity such as alpha and beta waves.

Not all decreases in wave activity are abnormal. The normal alpha waves seen in the posterior region of the brain are suppressed merely if a person is tense. Sometimes the addition of a wave is abnormal. For example, alpha rhythms seen in a newborn can signify seizure activity. Finally, the area where the rhythm is seen can be telling. The alpha coma is characterized by alpha rhythms produced diffusely, or, in other words, by all regions of the brain.

Some abnormal beta rhythms include frontal beta waves that are induced by sedative drugs. Marked asymmetry in beta rhythms suggests a structural lesion on the side lacking the beta waves. Beta waves are also commonly measured over skull lesions such as fractures or burr holes, in an activity known as a breach rhythm.

Usually seen only during sleep in adults, the presence of theta waves in the temporal region of awake, older adults has been tentatively correlated with vascular disease. Another rhythm normal in sleep, delta rhythms, may be recorded in a wakeful state over localized regions of cerebral damage. Intermittent delta rhythms are also an indication of damage of the relays between the deep gray matter and the cortex of the brain. In adults, this intermittent activity is found in the frontal region, whereas in children it is in the occipital region.

The EEG readings of persons with epilepsy or other seizure disorders display bursts, or spikes, of electrical activity. In focal epilepsy, spikes are restricted to one hemisphere of the brain. If spikes are generalized to both hemispheres of the brain, multifocal epilepsy may be present. The EEG can be used to localize the region of the brain where the abnormal electrical activity is occurring. This is most easily accomplished using a recording method, or montage, called an average reference montage. With this type of recording, the signal from each electrode is compared to the average signal from all the electrodes. The negative amplitude (an upward movement) of the spike is observed for the different channels, or inputs, from the various electrodes. The negative deflection will be greatest as recorded by the electrode that is closest in location to the origin of the abnormal activity. The spike will be present but of reduced amplitude as the electrodes move farther away from the site producing the spike. Electrodes distant from the site will not record the spike occurrence.

A final variety of abnormal result is the presence of slower-than-normal wave activity, which can either be a slow background rhythm or slow waves superimposed on a normal background. A posterior dominant rhythm of 7 Hz or less in an adult is abnormal and consistent with **encephalopathy** (brain disease). In contrast, localized theta or delta rhythms found in conjunction with normal background rhythms suggest a structural lesion.

Resources
BOOKS
Chin, W. C., and T. C. Head. *Essentials of Clinical Neurophysiology*, 3rd edition. London: Butterworth-Heinemann, 2002.

Daube, J. R. *Clinical Neurophysiology*, 2nd edition. New York: Oxford University Press, 2002.

Ebersole, J. S., and T. A. Pedley. *Current Practice of Clinical Electroencephalography*, 3rd Edition. Philadelphia: Lippincott Williams & Wilkins, 2002.

Rowan, A. J., and E. Tolunsky. *Primer of EEG*. London: Butterworth-Heinemann, 2003.

PERIODICALS
De Clercq, W., P. Lemmerling, S. Van Huffel, and W. Van Paesschen. "Anticipation of Epileptic Seizures from Standard EEG Recordings." *Lancet* 361, no. 9361 (2003): 971–972.

Harden, C. L., F. T. Burgut, and A. M. Kanner. "The Diagnostic Significance of Video-EEG Monitoring Findings on Pseudoseizure Patients Differs between Neurologists and Psychiatrists." *Epilepsia* 44, no. 3 (2003): 453–456.

Stepien, R. A. "Testing for Non-linearity in EEG Signal of Healthy Subjects." *Acta Experimental Neurobiology* 62, no. 4 (2002): 277–281.

Vanhatalo, S., M. D. Holmes, P. Tallgren, J. Voipio, K. Kaila, and J. W. Miller. "Very Slow EEG Responses Lateralize Temporal Lobe Seizures: An Evaluation of Non-invasive DC-EEG." *Neurology* 60, no. 7 (2003): 1098–1104.

ORGANIZATIONS
American Association of Electrodiagnostic Medicine. 421 First Avenue SW, Suite 300 East, Rochester, MN 55902. (507) 288-0100; Fax: (507) 288-1225. aaem@aaem.net. <http://www.aaem.net/>.

American Board of Registration of EEG and EP Technologists. PO Box 891663, Longwood, FL 32791. (407) 788-6308. <http://www.abret.org/index.htm>.

American Society of Electroneurodiagnostic Technologists Inc., 204 W. 7th Carroll, IA 51401. (712) 792-2978. <http://www.aset.org/>.

Epilepsy Foundation. 4351 Garden City Drive, Landover, MD 20785-7223. (800) 332-1000 or (301) 459-3700. <http://www.efa.org>.

Joint Review Committee on Electroneurodiagnostic Technology. 3350 South 198th Rd., Goodson, MO 65659-9110. (417) 253-5810. <http://www.caahep.org>.

OTHER
Electroencephalography. Hofstra University. April 27, 2003 (February 18, 2004). <http://people.hofstra.edu/faculty/sina_y_rabbany/>.

Bergey, Gregory K., and Piotr J. Franaszczuk. "Epileptic Seizures Are Characterized by Changing Signal Complexity." April 17, 2003 (February 18, 2004). <http://erl.neuro.jhmi.edu/pfranasz/CN00/cn00.pdf>.

Rutherford, Kim, M.D. "EEG (Electroencephalography)." *Kid's Health For Parents*. June 2001 (February 18, 2004). <http://kidshealth.org/parent/system/medical/eeg.html>.

Epilepsy Information: Electroencephalography. National Society for Epilepsy. September 2002 (February 18,

2004). <http://www.epilepsynse.org.uk/pages/info/leaflets/eeg.cfm>.

L. Fleming Fallon, Jr., MD, DrPH

Electromyography

Definition

Electromyography (EMG) is an electrical recording of muscle activity that aids in the diagnosis of neuromuscular disease, which affects muscle and peripheral nerves.

Purpose

Muscles are stimulated by signals from nerve cells called motor neurons. This stimulation causes electrical activity in the muscle, which in turn causes contraction. A needle electrode inserted into the muscle and connected to a recording device detects this electrical activity. Together, the electrode and recorder are called an electromyography machine. EMG can determine whether a particular muscle is responding appropriately to stimulation, and whether a muscle remains inactive when not stimulated.

EMG is performed most often to help diagnose different diseases causing weakness. Although EMG is a test of the motor system, it may help identify abnormalities of nerves or spinal nerve roots that may be associated with **pain** or numbness. Other symptoms for which EMG may be useful include atrophy, stiffness, fasciculation (muscle twitching), cramp, deformity, and **spasticity**. EMG results can help determine whether symptoms are due to a muscle disease or a neurological disorder, and, when combined with clinical findings, usually allow a confident diagnosis.

EMG can help diagnose many muscle and nerve disorders, including:

- muscular dystrophy
- congenital myopathies
- mitochondrial myopathies
- metabolic myopathies
- myotonias
- peripheral neuropathies
- radiculopathies
- nerve lesions
- amyotrophic lateral sclerosis
- polio
- spinal muscular atrophy
- Guillain-Barré syndrome
- ataxias
- myasthenias
- inflammatory myopathies

Precautions

No special precautions are needed for this test. Persons with a history of bleeding disorder should consult with their treating physician before the test. If a muscle **biopsy** is planned as part of the diagnostic workup, EMG should not be performed at the same site, as it may affect the microscopic appearance of the muscle. Also, persons on blood thinners should relay this information to the physician performing the EMG.

Description

During an EMG test, a fine needle is inserted into the muscle to be tested. This may cause some discomfort, similar to that of an injection. Recordings are made while the muscle is at rest, and then during the contraction. The person performing the test may move the limb being tested, and direct the patient to move it with various levels of force. The needle may be repositioned in the same muscle for further recording. Other muscles may be tested as well. A typical session lasts from 30–60 minutes, with individual muscles usually studied for a period of two to five minutes.

A slightly different test, the "nerve conduction velocity test," is often performed at the same time with the same equipment. In this test, stimulating and recording electrodes are used and small electrical shocks are applied to measure the ability of the nerve to conduct electrical signals. This test may cause mild tingling and discomfort similar to a mild shock from static electricity. Evoked potentials may also be performed for additional diagnostic information. Nerve conduction velocity and evoked potential testing are especially helpful when pain or sensory complaints are more problematic than weakness.

Preparation

No special preparation is needed. The doctor supervising and interpreting the test should be given information about the symptoms, medical conditions, suspected diagnosis, neuroimaging studies, and other test results.

Aftercare

Minor pain and bleeding may continue for several hours after the test. The muscle may be tender for a day or two.

Risks

There are no significant risks to this test, other than those associated with any needle insertion (pain, bleeding, bruising, or infection).

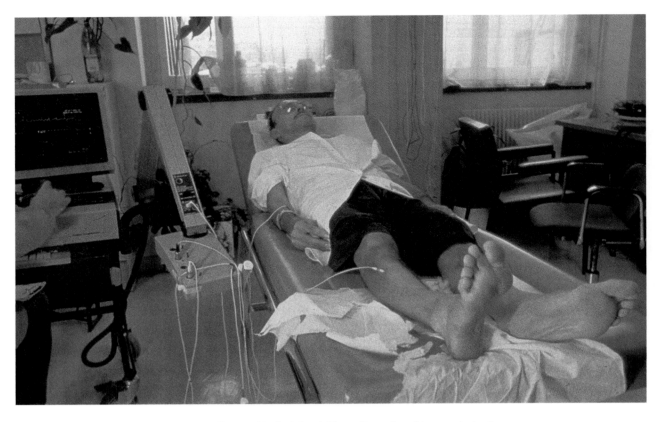

Patient undergoing electromyography. *(Custom Medical Stock Photo. Reproduced by permission.)*

Key Terms

Motor neurons Nerve cells that transmit signals from the brain or spinal cord to the muscles.

Motor unit action potentials Spikes of electrical activity recorded during an EMG that reflect the number of motor units (motor neurons and the muscle fibers they transmit signals to) activated when the patient voluntarily contracts a muscle.

Normal results

There should be some brief EMG activity during needle insertion. This activity may be increased in diseases of the nerve and decreased in long-standing muscle disorders in which muscle tissue is replaced by fibrous tissue or fat. Muscle tissue normally shows no EMG activity when at rest or when moved passively by the examiner. When the patient actively contracts the muscle, spikes (motor unit action potentials) should appear on the recording screen, reflecting the electrical activity within. As the muscle is

contracted more forcefully, more groups of muscle fibers are recruited or activated, causing more EMG activity.

The interpretation of EMG results is not a simple matter, requiring analysis of the onset, duration, amplitude, and other characteristics of the spike patterns.

Electrical activity at rest is abnormal; the particular pattern of firing may indicate denervation (for example, a nerve lesion, **radiculopathy**, or lower motor neuron degeneration), myotonia, or **inflammatory myopathy**.

Decreases in the amplitude and duration of spikes are associated with muscle diseases, which also show faster recruitment of other muscle fibers to compensate for weakness. Increases in the amplitude and duration of the spikes are typical of nerve diseases in which some degree of reinnervation (repair by new nerve connections to muscle) has occurred. Recruitment is reduced in nerve disorders.

Resources
BOOKS
Basmajian, J., and C. DeLuca. *Muscles Alive: Their Function Revealed by Electromyography*, 5th ed. Baltimore: Williams & Wilkins, 1985.

Richard Robinson

Empty sella syndrome

Definition

Empty sella syndrome is the appearance, by radiograph (x ray) of the skull, that the sella turcica, which normally contains the pituitary gland, is empty.

Description

Sella turcica is Latin for "Turkish saddle," which roughly describes the U–shaped appearance of this bony pocket when seen by x ray. It is a concavity in the middle of the sphenoid bone measuring about $1.5 \times 1.0 \times 0.5$ cm. The sphenoid bone forms a portion of the base of the skull just behind the eyes, at about the midpoint and just below the cerebral hemispheres.

The pituitary gland has a bulbous shape, extending on a stalk below the hypothalamus. The pituitary normally completely fills the sella turcica. The subarachnoid space, filled with cerebrospinal fluid (CSF), surrounds the pituitary stalk. The dura mater (see **Meninges**) normally extends away from the bony upper portion of the sella turcica forming a barrier between the subarachnoid space and the pituitary gland below. This barrier formed by the dura mater surrounding the top of the pituitary gland is known as the diaphragma sella.

In most cases when an empty sella is seen by x ray, the sella turcica is not truly empty. In fact, CSF has entered the space normally occupied by the pituitary and has compressed the gland against the wall of the sella. A truly empty sella, i.e., missing pituitary gland, is rare.

Demographics

The true incidence of empty sella syndrome in the population is not known. However, statistics collected from autopsies have shown that an empty sella is found as an incidental finding in anywhere from 5% to 25% of cases. These do not include cases in which the pituitary gland was surgically removed or irradiated.

Most cases of empty sella syndrome are seen in middle–aged, obese women, who often have hypertension. Children with empty sella syndrome are more often symptomatic, which most often manifests as growth hormone deficiency. About half of children with growth hormone deficiency are found to have an empty sella, but only 2% of children with normal pituitary function have the finding.

Causes and symptoms

Primary empty sella syndrome is thought to be congenital (present at birth) in most cases, and is caused by a failure or opening of the diaphragma sella. This may be an accidental occurrence, with no known triggering or causative factors. In some cases the sella turcica may grow larger than normal.

Secondary empty sella (acquired) may be caused by a medical procedure, such as surgery or **radiation** for a pituitary tumor. Disease or trauma may also reduce the size of the pituitary, or eliminate it completely. Abnormally low production of one or more pituitary hormones is known as hypopituitarism. A specific type of acquired empty sella syndrome associated with hypopituitarism, known as Sheehan's syndrome, is caused by infarction (loss of blood supply) of the pituitary brought on by shock or hemorrhage after labor and delivery. In cases of acquired empty sella, the condition is a byproduct of some other process.

Probably less than 10% of individuals with primary empty sella syndrome have some symptoms of hypopituitarism. Symptoms related to secondary empty sella syndrome would be those of the underlying cause, except in the case of empty sella syndrome due to trauma.

Hypopituitarism can result in one or more of the following:

• Hypothyroidism. Decreased production of the thyroid gland, which can result in diminished metabolism, intolerance of cold temperatures, **fatigue**, mental and physical sluggishness, constipation, muscle aches, dry skin, and dry hair.

• Hypogonadism. Decreased production of sex hormones, which can result in loss of pubic hair, decreased sex drive, impotence in men, and amenorrhea (absence of menstrual cycle) in women.

Key Terms

Cerebrospinal fluid The clear, normally colorless fluid that fills the brain cavities (ventricles), the subarachnoid space around the brain, and the spinal cord and acts as a shock absorber.

Hypopituitarism A condition characterized by underactivity of the pituitary gland.

Pituitary gland The most important of the endocrine glands (glands that release hormones directly into the bloodstream), the pituitary is located at the base of the brain. Sometimes referred to as the "master gland," it regulates and controls the activities of other endocrine glands and many body processes including growth and reproductive function. Also called the hypophysis.

- Hypoadrenalism. Decreased production of the adrenal gland, which can result in low blood pressure and hypoglycemia (low blood sugar).

Diagnosis

Other than those cases detected directly at autopsy (usually incidentally), empty sella syndrome is always diagnosed by some type of imaging study of the brain (x ray, **CT scan**, or **MRI**). Again, in many of these cases the empty sella is detected as a coincidental finding on an imaging study ordered for some other reason. Only occasionally is the diagnosis made because empty sella syndrome was suspected from some type of endocrinological abnormality suggesting hypopituitarism.

Treatment

Treatment of symptomatic empty sella syndrome would typically involve replacement therapy for any deficient hormones. For instance, hypothyroidism would require treatment with synthetic thyroid hormone, hypoadrenalism could be treated with steroids (cortisol), and hypogonadism might require sex hormone replacement therapy. Treatment of endocrinological dysfunction can be especially difficult because of the complicated way in which the many hormones of the body interact with and affect each other. In addition, all treatments for empty sella syndrome would be symptomatic treatments; there is no method to restore the pituitary gland to its normal size.

Prognosis

In most cases in which hypopituitarism accompanies empty sella syndrome, treatment for the symptoms would be lifelong. In all cases in which disease or medical intervention has reduced or eliminated the pituitary gland, there is no method of completely restoring normal pituitary function. Replacement therapies are effective when well-managed. However, even someone with optimum therapy is unlikely to feel completely "well," in relation to normal pituitary function, all of the time.

Special concerns

Symptoms of empty sella syndrome may be subtle, and may mimic other conditions. Since an accurate diagnosis of empty sella syndrome requires imaging studies of the brain, there is a risk that the condition could be misdiagnosed, or go undiagnosed.

Resources

BOOKS

DeMyer, William. *Neuroanatomy*, 2nd ed. Baltimore: Williams & Wilkins, 1998. pp. 312-316.

Gilroy, John. *Basic Neurology*, 3rd ed. New York: McGraw-Hill, 2000. pp. 521-523.

Reinhardt, Shelley, et al, eds. *Basic & Clinical Endocrinology*, 6th ed. Philadelphia: McGraw Hill, 2001. pp. 128-129.

Wilson, Jean D., et al, eds. *Williams Textbook of Endocrinology*, 9th ed. Philadelphia: W.B. Saunders Company, 1998..

OTHER

Empty Sella Syndrome Information Page. The National Institute of Neurological Disorders and Stroke. (September 10, 2003). http://www.ninds.nih.gov/health_and_medical/disorders/emptysella.htm.

Scott J. Polzin, MS, CGC

Encephalitis and meningitis

Definition

Encephalitis is an acute inflammatory process that affects brain tissue and is almost always accompanied by inflammation of the adjacent **meninges** (tissues lining the brain). There are many types of encephalitis, most of which are caused by viral infections.

Meningitis is an inflammation of the membranes (meninges) that surround the brain and spinal cord. Meningitis may be caused by many different viruses and bacteria, or by diseases that can cause inflammation of tissues of the body without infection (such as systemic **lupus** erythematosus). Viral meningitis is sometimes called aseptic meningitis to indicate it is not the result of a bacterial infection.

Description

Encephalitis can be divided into two forms, primary and secondary encephalitis, according to the two methods by which the viruses infect the brain. Primary encephalitis occurs when a virus directly invades the brain and spinal cord. Primary encephalitis can happen to people at any time of the year (sporadic encephalitis), or can be part of an outbreak (epidemic encephalitis). Secondary, or post-infectious encephalitis occurs when a virus first infects another organ and secondarily enters the brain.

Meningitis is an inflammation of the membranes that surround the brain and spinal cord, and may be caused by many different viruses and bacteria, or by non-infectious inflammatory diseases. Encephalitis is a distinct disease from meningitis, although, clinically, the two often share signs and symptoms of inflammation of the meninges.

Demographics

Determining the true incidence of encephalitis in the United States is difficult because reporting policies are neither standardized nor rigorously enforced. Several thousand cases of viral encephalitis are reported yearly. HSE (herpes simplex encephalitis), the most common cause of sporadic encephalitis in other western countries, is still relatively rare in the United States, with an overall incidence of two cases per one million persons per year.

Arboviruses (viruses transmitted to humans by blood-sucking insects such as mosquitoes and ticks) are the most common causes of episodic encephalitis. These statistics may be misleading because most people bitten by arbovirus-infected insects do not develop clinical disease, and only 10% of those develop overt encephalitis. Among less common causes of viral encephalitis, varicella-zoster encephalitis (a complication of the condition commonly known as **shingles**) has an incidence of one in 2000 infected people.

Internationally, Japanese virus encephalitis (JE), occurring principally in Japan, Southeast Asia, China, and India, is the most common viral encephalitis outside the United States.

In 1995, there were 5755 cases of bacterial meningitis reported in United States. This is a dramatic decrease from the 12,920 cases reported in 1986, probably due to the decrease in *Haemophilus influenzae* meningitis since the introduction of the Hib vaccine. The occurrences by infectious agents in 1995 are as follows:

• *Streptococcus pneumoniae*: 1.1 per 100,000 persons

• *Neisseria meningitides*: 0.6 per100,000 persons

• *Streptococcus*: 0.3 per 100,000 persons

• *Listeria monocytogenes*: 0.2 per 100,000 persons

• *Haemophilus influenzae*: 0.2 per 100,000 persons

The incidence of meningitis in newborns has shown no significant change in the last 25 years. Viral meningitis is the most common form of aseptic meningitis and, since the introduction of the mumps vaccine, is caused by enteroviruses in up to 85% of cases. The incidence of encephalitis is more difficult to estimate because of difficulty in establishing the diagnosis. One report estimates an incidence of one in 500–1,000 infants and in the first six months of life.

Causes and symptoms

Causes

The causes of encephalitis are usually infectious, but may also be due to some noninfectious causes. Three broad categories of viruses—herpes viruses, viruses responsible for childhood infections, and arboviruses

Key Terms

Arboviruses Viruses harbored by arthropods (mosquitoes and ticks) and transferred to humans by their bite. Arboviruses are one cause of encephalitis.

Electroencephalogram A procedure that uses electrodes on the scalp to record electrical activity of the brain. Used for detection of epilepsy, coma, and brain death.

Encephalitis Inflammation of the brain.

Meningitis Inflammation of the meninges, the membranes that surround the brain and spinal cord.

Pathogen A disease-causing organism.

Seizure A convulsion, or uncontrolled discharge of nerve cells that may spread to other cells throughout the brain.

(viruses harbored by mosquitoes and ticks, and transferred through their bite)—typically trigger encephalitis.

ENCEPHALITIS AND HERPES VIRUSES Some herpes viruses that cause common infections may also cause encephalitis. These include:

• Herpes simplex virus. There are two types of herpes simplex virus (HSV) infections. HSV type 1 (HSV-1) causes cold sores or fever blisters around the mouth. HSV type 2 (HSV-2) causes genital herpes. HSV is the most common cause of sporadic encephalitis, with HSV-1 being the more common culprit. When untreated, the mortality rate from herpes simplex encephalitis is between 60–80%. That number drops to 15–20% with treatment.

• Varicella-zoster virus. This virus is responsible for chicken pox and shingles. It can cause encephalitis in adults and children, but the cases tend to be mild.

• Epstein-Barr virus. This herpes virus causes infectious mononucleosis. If encephalitis develops, it's usually mild, but more severe forms can result in death in up to 8% of cases.

ARBOVIRUSES The mosquito season varies according to geographic location. Arbovirus transmission, therefore, also varies according to season, the cycle of viral transmission, and local climatic conditions. Six encephalitis disease groups caused by arboviruses are monitored by the United States Centers for Disease Control (CDC) and include:

• St. Louis encephalitis

• West Nile encephalitis

- Powassan encephalitis
- Eastern equine encephalitis
- Western equine encephalitis
- California serogroup viral encephalitis, which includes infections with the following viruses: La Crosse, Jamestown Canyon, snowshoe hare, trivittatus, Keystone, and California encephalitis viruses.

OTHER CAUSES OF ENCEPHALITIS Bacterial pathogens (disease-causing organisms), such as rickettsial disease, mycoplasma, and cat scratch disease, are rare, but often involve inflammation of the meninges. Encephalitis can be due to parasites and fungi. Insects, such as mosquitoes in the eastern and southeastern United States can also spread encephalitis.

CAUSES OF MENINGITIS Viral meningitis is the most common infection of the **Central Nervous System** (CNS). It most frequently occurs in children younger than one year of age. Enteroviruses (viruses that causes infections of the gastrointestinal tract) are the most common causative agent and are a frequent cause of febrile illnesses in children. Other viral pathogens include paramyxoviruses, herpes, influenza, rubella, and adenovirus. Meningitis may occur in up to half of children younger than three months with enteroviral infections. Enteroviral infections can occur any time during the year, but are normally associated with outbreaks in the summer and fall. Viral infections cause an inflammatory response, but to a lesser degree than bacterial infections. Damage from viral meningitis may be due to an associated encephalitis and increased intracranial pressure.

Bacterial meningitis is fairly uncommon, but can be extremely serious. There are two main types of bacterial meningitis, which cause most of the reported bacterial cases: meningococcal and pneumococcal. *Haempohilus influenzae* type b (Hib), which was recently a major cause of bacterial meningitis, has now been almost eliminated by the vaccination of infants. The most common causative organisms in the first month of life are *Escherichia coli* and group B streptococci. *Listeria monocytogenes* infection also occurs in patients in this age range and accounts for 5–10% of cases. In people older than two months, *S. pneumoniae* and *N. meningitides* currently cause the majority of the cases of bacterial meningitis. *H. influenzae* may still occur, especially in children who have not received the Hib vaccine.

Symptoms

Symptoms of encephalitis include sudden fever, **headache**, vomiting, heightened sensitivity to light, stiff neck and back, confusion and impaired judgment, drowsiness, weak muscles, a clumsy and unsteady gait (manner of walking), bulging in the soft spots (fontanels) of the skull in infants, and irritability. More severe or late symptoms include loss of consciousness, **seizures**, muscle weakness, or sudden severe **dementia**.

Symptoms of meningitis, which may appear suddenly, often include high fever, severe and persistent headache, stiff neck, nausea, and vomiting. Changes in behavior such as confusion, sleepiness, and difficulty waking up are extremely important symptoms and may require emergency treatment.

In infants, symptoms of meningitis may include high-pitched cry, moaning cry, whimpering, dislike of being handled, fretfulness, arching of the back, neck retraction, blank, staring expression, difficulty in waking, lethargia, fever, cold hands and feet, refusing to feed or vomiting, pale, blotchy skin color. In adults, symptoms of meningitis may include vomiting, headache, drowsiness, seizures, high temperature, joint **pain**, stiff neck, and aversion to light.

Arboviral infections may be asymptomatic or may result in illnesses of variable severity. Arboviral meningitis is characterized by fever, headache, and stiff neck. Arboviral encephalitis is characterized by fever, headache, and altered mental status that ranges from confusion to coma. Signs of brain dysfunction such as numbness or paralysis, cranial nerve palsies, visual or hearing deficits, abnormal reflexes, and generalized seizures may also be present.

Diagnosis

Encephalitis or meningitis is suspected by a physician when the symptoms described above are present. The physician diagnoses encephalitis or meningitis after a careful examination and testing. The examination includes special maneuvers to detect signs of inflammation of the membranes that surround the brain and spinal cord (meninges). Tests that are used in the evaluation of individuals suspected of having encephalitis or meningitis include blood counts, blood cultures, coagulation studies, bacterial antigen studies of urine and serum, brain scanning, and spinal fluid analysis.

The most common method of diagnosing encephalitis and meningitis is to analyze the cerebrospinal fluid surrounding the brain and spinal cord. A needle inserted into lower spine extracts a sample of fluid for laboratory analysis, which may reveal the presence of an infection or an increased white blood cell count, a signal that the immune system is fighting an infection. The cerebrospinal fluid may also be slightly bloody if small hemorrhages have occurred. Diagnosis of herpes simplex encephalitis can be difficult, but advances using sensitive DNA methods have allowed detection of the virus in spinal fluid.

Electroencephalography (EEG) measures the waves of electrical activity produced by the brain. It is often used

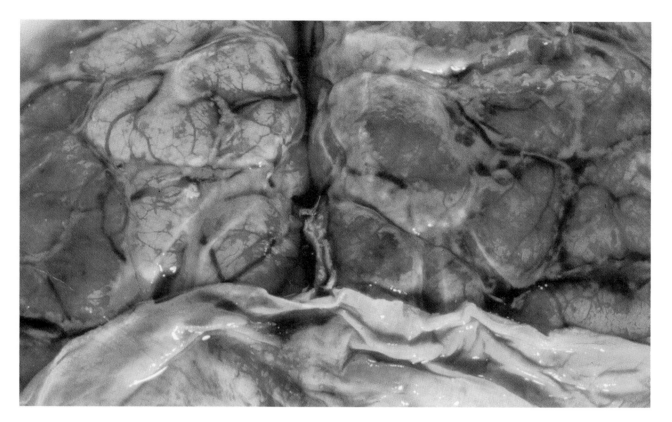

Occipital lobes of brain with acute meningitis. Dura mater has been reflected from surface of brain, revealing intensely discolored red (hyperemic) arachnoid mater and subarachnoid pus (white-gray purulent material). The patient, a three-and-a-half-year-old boy, was well except for an upper respiratory infection with cough one day prior to death. *(Joseph R. Siebert. photograph. © Custom Medical Stock Photo. Reproduced by permission.)*

to diagnose and manage seizure disorders. A number of small electrodes are attached to the scalp. The patient remains still during the test and at times may be asked to breathe deeply and steadily for several minutes or to stare at a patterned board. At times, a light may be flashed into eyes. These actions are meant to stimulate the brain. The electrodes pick up the electrical impulses from brain and send them to the EEG machine, which records the brain waves on a moving sheet of paper. An abnormal EEG result may suggest some of diseases, but a normal result does not rule them out.

Brain imaging, using computed tomography (CT) or **magnetic resonance imaging (MRI)** may reveal swelling of brain. These techniques may reveal another condition with signs and symptoms that are similar to encephalitis, such as a concussion.

Rarely, if diagnosis of herpes simplex encephalitis isn't possible using DNA methods or by CT or MRI scans, a physician may take a small sample of the brain tissue, or **biopsy**, for analysis to determine if the virus is present. Physicians usually attempt treatment with antiviral medications before suggesting brain biopsy.

Blood testing can confirm the presence of West Nile virus in the body by drawing a sample of blood for laboratory analysis. When infected with West Nile virus, an analysis of blood sample may show a rising level of an antibody against the virus, a positive DNA test for the virus or a positive virus culture.

Treatment team

The treatment team may include a pediatrician or a general practitioner, an infectious disease specialist and/or a critical care specialist, a neurosurgeon, a **neurologist** or a neonatologist. Others professionals may give support during hospitalization for intravenous antibiotics or other specific procedures.

Treatment

Treatment for meningitis depends on the cause and on the symptoms. Antiviral medications may be used if a virus is involved. Antibiotics are prescribed for bacterial infections. If the causative organism is unknown, antibiotic regimes can be based on the child's age. In infants

Causes of Encephalitis	How Spread
Enteroviruses	Contact with body fluids
Herpes simplex virus	Person to person contact
HIV (human immunodeficiency virus)	When an infected person's blood or body fluids are introduced into the bloodstream of a healthy person
Arboviruses	Bites from mosquitoes that pick up the virus from infected birds, chipmunks, squirrels, or other animals
Animal-borne illnesses	Bites from infected animals such as cats, dogs, and bats

(Illustration created by Frank Forney.)

aged 30 days or younger, ampicillin is usually prescribed along with an aminoglycoside or a cephalosporin (cefotaxime) medication. In children aged 30–60 days, ampicillin and a cephalosporin (ceftriaxone or cefotaxime) can also be used. However, since *S. pneumoniae* occasionally occurs in this age range, vancomycin should be part of treatment instead of ampicillin. In older children, cephalosporin or ampicillin plus chloramphenicol can be used. Often, rifampicin is given (in meningococcal bacterial meningitis cases) as a preventative measure to roommates, close family members, or others who may have come in contact with an infected person.

In addition, anticonvulsant medications may be used if there are seizures. Corticosteroids may be needed to reduce brain swelling and inflammation. Dexamethasone is usually indicated for children with suspected meningitis who are older than six weeks and is recommended for treatment of infants and children with *H. influenzae* meningitis. Sedatives may be needed for irritability or restlessness and over-the-counter medications may be used for fever and headache.

Until a bacterial cause of CNS inflammation is excluded, the treatment should include parenteral (given by injection) antibiotics. Treatment with a third-generation cephalosporin antibiotic, such as cefotaxime sodium

(Claforan) or ceftriaxone sodium (Rocephin), is usually recommended. Vancomycin (Lyphocin, Vancocin, Vancoled) should be added in geographic areas where strains of *S. pneumoniae* resistant to penicillin and cephalosporins have been reported.

Encephalitis can be difficult to treat because the viruses that cause the disease generally don't respond to many medications. The exceptions are herpes simplex virus and varicella-zoster virus, which respond to the antiviral drug acyclovir, and is usually administered intravenously in the hospital for at least ten days.

Treatment is available for many symptoms of encephalitis. Patients with headache should rest in a quiet, dark environment and take analgesics. Narcotic therapy may be needed for pain relief; however, medication induced changes in level of consciousness should be avoided. Anticonvulsant medication and anti-inflammatory drugs to reduce swelling and pressure within the skull are usually prescribed. Otherwise, treatment mainly consists of rest and a healthy diet including plenty of liquids.

Recovery and rehabilitation

As opposed to many untreatable neurological conditions, encephalitis and meningitis are diseases that, given the adequate treatment described above, often resolve with complete recovery. It is very important that the disease's cause is promptly identified and treated before any complication is irreversibly established. Physical and speech therapy are often helpful when neurological deficits remain, as are occupational therapists and audiologists.

Clinical trials

The National Institute of Allergy and Infectious Diseases (NIAID) and the National Institute of Neurological Disorders and Stroke (NINDS) support and conduct research on encephalitis and meningitis. Much of this research is aimed at learning more about the cause(s), prevention, and treatment of these disorders. Ongoing **clinical trials** as of early 2004 include:

- Valacyclovir for long-term therapy of Herpes simplex encephalitis; IVIG—West Nile encephalitis: Safety and Efficacy; Structure of the Herpes Simplex Virus Receptor; sponsored by National Institute of Allergy and Infectious Diseases

- Natural History of **West Nile Virus Infection**; Omr-IgG-am™ for Treating Patients with or at High Risk for West Nile Virus Disease; sponsored by Warren G. Magnuson Clinical Center

- Intrathecal Gemcitibine to Treat Neoplastic Meningitis; Intrathecal Gemcitabine in Treating Patients with Cancer and Neoplastic Meningitis; sponsored by Baylor College of Medicine

Updated information on clinical trials can be found at the National Institutes of Health clinical trials website at www.clinicaltrials.org.

Prognosis

The prognosis for encephalitis varies. Some cases are mild, short and relatively benign and patients have full recovery. Other cases are severe, and permanent impairment or death is possible. The acute phase of encephalitis may last for one to two weeks, with gradual or sudden resolution of fever and neurological symptoms. Neurological symptoms may require many months before full recovery. Prognosis for people with viral meningitis is usually good.

With early diagnosis and prompt treatment, most patients recover from meningitis. However, in some cases, the disease progresses so rapidly that death occurs during the first 48 hours, despite early treatment. Permanent neurological impairments including memory, speech, vision, hearing, muscle control, and sensation difficulties can occur in people who survive severe cases of meningitis and encephalitis.

The prognosis for appropriately treated meningitis has improved, but there is still a 5% mortality rate and significant morbidity (lasting impairment). The prognosis

varies with the age of the person, clinical condition, and infecting organism.

Special concerns

A person's exposure to mosquitoes and other insects that harbor arboviruses can be reduced by taking precautions when in a mosquito-prone area. Insect repellents containing DEET provide effective temporary protection form mosquito bites. Long sleeves and pants should be worn when outside during the evening hours of peak mosquito activity. When camping outside, intact mosquito netting over sleeping areas reduces the risk of mosquito bites. Communities also employ large-scale spraying of pesticides to reduce the population of mosquitoes, and encourage citizens to eliminate all standing water sources, such as in bird baths, flower pots, and tires stored outside to eliminate possible breeding grounds for mosquitoes.

Although large epidemics of meningococcal meningitis do not occur in the United States, some countries experience large, periodic outbreaks. Overseas travelers should check to see if meningococcal vaccine is recommended for their destination. Travelers should receive the vaccine at least one week before departure, if possible. A vaccine to prevent meningitis due to *S. pneumoniae* (also called pneumococcal meningitis) can also prevent other forms of infection due to *S. pneumoniae*. The pneumococcal vaccine is not effective in children under two years of age, but it is recommended for all individuals over 65 years of age and younger people with certain chronic medical conditions.

Resources

BOOKS

Kandel, Eric R. *Principles of Neural Science.* New York: McGraw-Hill/Appleton & Lange, 2000.

Kolb, Bryan, and Ian Q. Whishaw. *Introduction to Brain and Behavior.* New York: W. H. Freeman & Co, 2001.

Roos, Karen L. *Meningitis: 100 Maxims.* London: Edward Arnold, 1996.

PERIODICALS

Chandesris, M. O., et al. "A case of Influenza virus encephalitis in south of France." *Rev Med Interne* 25 (2004): 78–82.

Kurt-Jones, E. A., et al. "Herpes simplex virus 1 interaction with Toll-like receptor 2 contributes to lethal encephalitis." *Proc Natl Acad Sci USA* (2004): 1315–1320.

OTHER

Information on Arboviral Encephalitides. Centers for Disease Control and Prevention. (April 10, 2004). <http://www.cdc.gov/ncidod/dvbid/arbor/arbdet.htm>

NINDS Encephalitis and Meningitis Information Page. National Institutes of Neurological Disorders and Stroke. (April 10, 2004). <http://www.ninds.nih.gov/health_and_medical/disorders/encmenin_doc.htm>

Top 20 Meningitis FAQs. Meningitis Foundation of America. (April 10, 2004). <http://www.musa.org/faqs.htm>

ORGANIZATIONS

Meningitis Foundation of America, Inc. 7155 Shadeland Station Suite 190, Indianapolis, Indiana 46256-3922. (317) 595-6383 or (800) 668-1129; Fax: (317) 595-6370. support@musa.org. <http://www.musa.org/>.

National Institute of Allergy and Infectious Diseases (NIAID). 31 Center Drive, Rm. 7A50 MSC 2520, Bethesda, Maryland 20892-2520. (301) 496-5717. <http://www.niaid.nih.gov/>.

Centers for Disease Control and Prevention (CDC), Division of Vector-Borne Infectious Diseases. P.O. Box 2087, Fort Collins, Colorado 80522. (800) 311-3435. dvbid@cdc.gov. <http://www.cdc.gov/ncidod/dvbid/index.htm>.

Bruno Marcos Verbeno
Iuri Drumond Louro, M.D., Ph.D.

Encephalitis lethargica

Definition

Encephalitis lethargica is an inflammation of the brain caused by two trypanosomes (microscopic protozoan parasites). The illness, which can be fatal, is transmitted from one infected person to another by the tsetse fly. While it can occur globally, encephalitis lethargica is especially prevalent in Africa.

Description

Encephalitis lethargica is a vector-borne disease, meaning it is transmitted to a susceptible person by a living creature. The tsetse fly lives in moist vegetation near lakes and rivers and in grassy areas. People living near these regions are most susceptible the bite of a tsetse fly infected with the trypasosomes that cause encephalitis lethargica. The disease is also known as African trypanosomiasis, sleeping sickness, sleepy sickness, and von Economo's disease. Another form of the trypanosome-borne disease that occurs in North, Central, and South America is called Chagas disease.

Other subspecies of the trypanosome parasite can infect animals such as cattle, who can also harbor the trypanosomes that are infectious to humans.

Demographics

The form of encephalitis lethargica known as African trypanosomiasis occurs only in the sub-Saharan area of Africa. Tsetse flies are endemic in this region. However, for as yet unknown reasons, there are regions where tsetse flies are found, but the disease is absent. There have been several epidemics in Africa in the nineteenth and twentieth centuries. From 1896–1906, Uganda and the Congo basin were affected. A more wide-ranging epidemic occurred in 1920. Finally, an epidemic that began in 1970 is still occurring.

The latest epidemic is a result of the relaxed surveillance for the disease that happened with the near-eradication of the disease in the 1960s. As of 2004, the disease is a threat to more than 60 million people in 36 sub-Saharan African countries. In 1999, nearly 45,000 cases were reported, according to the World Health Organization (WHO). These cases represent individuals who were able to seek treatment and receive a definitive diagnosis at local health care centers. The actual number of cases was likely much higher, with estimates ranging from 300,000–500,000 cases actually occurring. In Africa, the disease occurs primarily in rural areas, where health care is least available. Poverty and encephalitis lethargica are associated with one another.

Causes and symptoms

The disease is caused by *Trypanosoma brucei gambiense* and *Trypanosoma brucei rhodesiense*. The first species is found in central and West Africa. The infection is chronic; it persists for months or years with no display of symptoms. When they do emerge, the disease is at an advanced stage and the symptoms are more severe. *T. brucei rhodesiense* is found primarily in southern and eastern Africa. It causes an infection whose symptoms appear quickly (acute infection). This disease is more severe. Fortunately, the rapid appearance of symptoms offers more of a chance for quick detection.

Both trypanosomes are transferred to the tsetse fly when the fly obtains a blood meal from an infected person. The trypanosomes then multiply in the blood of the fly, and can be transferred to a susceptible person on whom the fly subsequently feeds.

The early symptoms of the disease include fever, severe **headache**, joint **pain**, and swelling of the lymph nodes. These symptoms can disappear and reoccur. Later, symptoms of what is called the neurological phase emerge and often include the characteristic symptoms of the disease: extreme weakness, paralysis of eye muscles, sleepiness, disruption of the sleep cycle, and a lapse into a deep and fatal coma. Transmission of the trypanosomes across the placenta from a pregnant woman to the fetus can occur. Typically this causes spontaneous abortion or death of the fetus.

Diagnosis

The most useful diagnostic sign is swollen cervical glands. This indicates the presence of the parasite. Populations can be screened for clinical signs of the disease (the

Key Terms

Encephalitis Inflammation of the brain, usually caused by a virus. The inflammation may interfere with normal brain function and may cause seizures, sleepiness, confusion, personality changes, weakness in one or more parts of the body, and even coma.

Parasite An organism that lives and feeds in or on another organism (the host) and does nothing to benefit the host.

Vector-borne disease A disease that is delivered from one host to another by a vector or carrier organism.

early phase symptoms) and the use of tests that detect antibodies to the parasite in the blood. An early diagnostic sign of the bite of the tsetse fly is the appearance of a painful red sore (chancre) at the site of the bite.

A type of diagnosis called phase diagnosis can be used to help determine the level of advancement of the disease. Cerebro-spinal fluid is obtained by the technique of lumbar puncture and analyzed. Phase diagnosis requires medical and laboratory staff, and is typically done in a clinic. The long period, symptom-free period of a Trypanosoma brucei gambiense infection can complicate and delay diagnosis.

Treatment team

Physicians and nurses are the primary team involved in treating encephalitis lethargica. Additionally, public health workers in Africa and other areas affected with the tsetse fly receive help from health agencies throughout the world, who provide aid and strategies to reduce populations of the fly, educate local peoples to bite prevention methods, and treat affected individuals. Warring factions, with resulting political instability and hunger in the Sub-Saharan region of Africa have led to difficulty in controlling the spread of the tsetse fly and the disease.

Treatment

The choice of treatment depends on whether the disease is detected earlier or later in the infection. Early-stage infections can be treated using two drugs; suramine and pentamidine. An agreement between the World Health Organization and the drug's manufacturer (Aventis) has guaranteed continued production of the compounds.

Treatment of the later, neurological symptoms requires a drug that can cross the blood-brain barrier to reach the parasite. Currently only one drug (melarsoprol) is commercially available. The drug causes harsh side effects and itself has a fatal complication rate approaching 10%. As well, resistance of the trypanosomes to the drug is increasing. A second drug (eflornithine) exists, but is not commercially available. It is active only against *Trypanosoma brucei gambiense*. There is no vaccine for the disease.

Recovery and rehabilitation

Recovery from the early stage of the disease can be complete. Recovery from the neurological stage is typically incomplete, with varying degrees of impaired brain function often resulting. Once the person reaches the stage of coma, the disease is invariably fatal.

Clinical trials

As of early 2004, there were no **clinical trials** in progress for the study of encephalitis lethargica. Rather, efforts to increase screening of susceptible populations and to increase the supply of drugs is the identified priority for scientists working with the disease.

Prognosis

If treated early, a person with encephalitis lethargica can be cured. If not treated early, the prognosis is much less favorable due to resulting brain damage. Encephalitis lethargica is fatal if untreated.

Resources

BOOKS

Dumas, Michel, et. al. *Progress in Human African Trypanosomiasis, Sleeping Sickness.* New York: Springer Verlag, 1999.

Ramen, Fred. *Sleeping Sickness and Other Parasitic Tropical Diseases (Epidemics).* New York: Rosen Publishing Group, 2002.

OTHER

African Trypanosomiasis or Sleeping Sickness. World Health Organization. (January 27 2004). <http://www.who.int/int-fs/en/fact259.html>

East African Trypanosomiasis. Centers for Disease Control and Prevention. (January 27 2004). <http://www.cdc.gov/ncidod/dpd/parasites/...osomisasis/factsht_ea_trypanosomiasis.htm>

ORGANIZATIONS

Centers for Disease Control and Prevention (CDC). 1600 Clifton Road, Atlanta, GA 30333. (404) 639-3311 or (800) 311-3435. <http://www.cdc.gov>.

World Health Organization (WHO). Avenue Appia 20, 1211 Geneva, Geneva, Switzerland. +41 22 791 21 11; Fax: +41 22 791-3111. info@who.int. <http://www.who.int>.

Brian Douglas Hoyle, PhD

Encephaloceles

Definition

Encephaloceles refers to defects in the development of a fetal structure called the neural tube. The tube fails to close completely during development of the fetus, resulting in portions of the brain and its surrounding membranes that protrude from the skull in sac-like formations. Often, normal brain function is impaired and children with encephaloceles experience delays in development.

Description

In normal fetal development, the neural tube forms by the closure of the neural structure. When this does not occur in the case of an encephalocele, the result is a groove. The groove can form down the middle region of the upper part of the skull, or between the forehead and the nose, or down the back of the skull. The incomplete closure also creates areas where the brain and its overlaying membrane can bulge outward in sac-like protrusions. The larger deformities, in particular those that occur at the back of the skull, are readily evident and are recognized very soon after birth. These deformities are also associated with abnormal structure and functioning of the brain. Some encephaloceles are less evident, even to the point of being undetectable at birth. Defects in the region of the forehead and nose are examples.

Demographics

Encephaloceles occur rarely. At a rate of one per 5,000–10,000 live births, an encephalocele is less common than **spina bifida**, another neural tube defect. Geographical differences occur with respect to the type of encephalocele. Malformation of the back portion of the head is more common in Europe and North America, whereas involvement of the front portion of the head occurs more frequently in Southeast Asia, Malaysia, and Russia.

Causes and symptoms

The exact cause of encephaloceles is not yet known. The disorder is passed on from generation to generation, and is more prevalent in families where there is a history

Key Terms

Cerebrospinal fluid A clear fluid that is produced in the ventricles of the brain and circulates around and within the brain and spinal cord.

Neural tube defect A birth defect caused by abnormal closure or development of the neural tube, the embryonic structure that gives rise to the central nervous system.

Teratogen A substance that has been demonstrated to cause physical defects in the developing human embryo.

of spina bifida. It is clear that one or more genetic abnormalities lie at the heart of the condition. However, fetal development is an extremely complex process, with interactions between various genes, and influence of the external environment determining which genes are activated at which time. Thus, pinning down the crucial genes whose expression or changed activity produces abnormal neural tube formation is a difficult task.

Research using animal models has shown that teratogens, compounds like x rays, trypan blue, and arsenic, which can damage the developing fetus, cause encephaloceles in the animals. Whether exposure of a human fetus to such agents contributes to encephalocele formation in humans is not known.

Most often, the symptoms of encephaloceles are not difficult to recognize. These include the excessive build-up of cerebrospinal fluid in the brain (a condition called **hydrocephalus**), paralyzed arms and legs (spastic quadriplegia), an abnormally small head (**microcephaly**), difficulty in tasks like walking and reaching because of a lack of coordination (**ataxia**), delayed or impaired mental and physical development (although intelligence is not always affected), problems with vision, and **seizures**.

If the bulging portion contains only cerebrospinal fluid and the overlaying membrane, the malady can also be called a cranial meningocele or a meningocele. If brain tissue is also present, the malady can also be referred to as an encephalomeningocele.

Diagnosis

Diagnosis is based at the discovery of the physical abnormalities at birth or sometime later, and on the failure to attain the various physical and mental developmental milestones that are a normal part of early life.

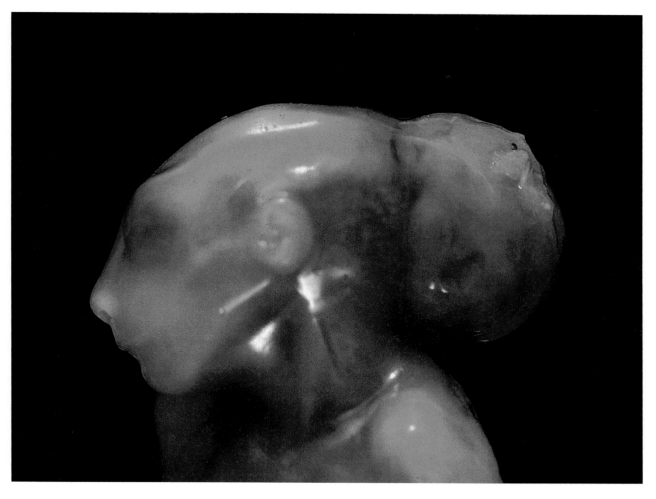

Encephalocele, a brain formation growing outside the skull, on a 16-week-old fetus. *(© Siebert/Custom Medical Stock Photo. Reproduced by permission.)*

Treatment team

Medical treatment involves family physicians, neurosurgeons, and nurses. Special education professionals, physical therapists, and caregivers are also an important part of the treatment team, as an affected person may require assistance in everyday activities throughout life.

Treatment

Treatment typically involves surgery. The surgery is usually accomplished soon after birth, and re-positions the bulging brain back into the skull, removes any of the sac-like protrusions, and corrects the skull deformities. Often, shunts are placed during surgery to drain excess cerebrospinal fluid from the brain. While delicate, the operation typically relieves the pressure that would otherwise impede normal brain development. Other treatment involves dealing with specific symptoms and producing as comfortable and satisfying everyday life as is possible.

Recovery and rehabilitation

Prospects for recovery are difficult to predict prior to surgery. Nonetheless, if surgery is successful, and other developmental difficulties have not occurred, an individual can develop normally. Where neurological and developmental damage has occurred, the focus shifts from recovery to maximizing mental and physical abilities.

Clinical trials

As of April 2004, no clinical trails for specific study of encephaloceles were being conducted. However, research is underway to more clearly define the mechanisms of brain development, and several **clinical trials** related to neural tube defects are recruiting participants. Updated information can be found at the National Institutes of Health clinical trials website at: http://clinicaltrials.gov.

Prognosis

As for recovery and rehabilitation, the prognosis is varies and cannot be predicted beforehand. In general, when the bulging material consists of mainly cerebrospinal fluid, a complete recovery can occur 60–80% of the time. However, the presence of brain tissue in the protruding material can reduce the chances of a complete recovery considerably.

Special concerns

Folic acid, a B vitamin, has been shown to help prevent neural tube defects when taken before and in early pregnancy. The March of Dimes organization and the United States Public Health Service recommend that all women who may become pregnant take a multi-vitamin that contains 400 micrograms of folic acid every day.

Resources

BOOKS

McComb, G. G., ed. *Neural Tube Defects.* American Association of Neurological Surgeons, 1998.

PERIODICALS

"Beaumont surgeons correct rare defect for Caribbean boy." *Health Week* (July 1, 2002): 17.

OTHER

NINDS Encephaloceles Information Page. National Institute of Neurological Disorders and Stroke. (April 7, 2004). <http://www.ninds.nih.gov/health_and_medical/disorders/encephaloceles.htm>

Prevention of Neural Tube Defects. The Arc. (April 10, 2004). <http://www.thearc.org/faqs/folicqa.html>

ORGANIZATIONS

Birth Defect Research for Children. 930 Woodcock Road, Suite 225. Orlando, FL 22808. (407) 895-0802 or (800) 313-2232; Fax: (407) 895-0824.

March of Dimes Birth Defects Foundation. 1275 Mamaroneck Avenue, White Plains, NY 10605. (914) 428-7100 or (888) 663-4637; Fax: (914) 428-8203. askus@marchofdimes.com. <http://www.marchofdimes.com>.

National Institute for Neurological Diseases and Stroke (NINDS). 6001 Executive Boulevard, Bethesda, MD, 20892. (301) 496-5751 or (800) 352-9424. <http://www.ninds.nih.gov>.

National Organization for Rare Disorders. 55 Kenosia Avenue, Danbury, CT 06813-1968. (203) 744-0100 or (800) 999-6673; Fax: (203) 798-2291. orphan@rarediseases.org. <http://www.rarediseases.org>.

Brian Douglas Hoyle, PhD

Encephalopathy

Definition

Encephalopathy is a condition characterized by altered brain function and structure. It is caused by diffuse brain disease.

Description

Encephalopathy may be caused by advanced and severe disease states, infections, or as a result of taking certain medications. The three main causes of encephalopathy are liver disease, kidney disease, and lack of oxygen in the brain. The associated symptoms can include subtle personality changes, inability to concentrate, lethargy, progressive loss of memory and thinking abilities, progressive loss of consciousness, and abnormal involuntary movements. Symptoms vary with the severity and type of encephalopathy.

Encephalopathy may vary in severity from only subtle changes in mental state to a more advanced state that can lead to deep coma. Cerebral edema is a common manifestation of severe encephalopathy, which causes an increase in intracranial pressure. The major related causes of death include sepsis, circulatory collapse, and brain failure related to a syndrome encompassing cerebral edema, damaged blood-brain-barrier, increased intracranial pressure, brainstem herniation, and/or neurotoxins leaking into the brain and killing brain cells. Additionally, patients with severe encephalopathy usually develop intracranial hypertension, which can produce cerebral ischemia injury and cerebral herniation.

Demographics

There is no statistical information available for encephalopathy per se. Encephalopathy can occur at any age and there seems to be no gender or racial predilection, because encephalopathy is a manifestation of a primary illness.

Causes and symptoms

Causes

There is a wide variety of conditions that cause encephalopathy. Encephalopathy can be caused by infections (bacteria, viruses, or prions); lack of oxygen to the brain; liver failure; kidney failure; alcohol/drug overdose; prolonged exposure to toxic chemical (solvents, paints, industrial chemicals, drugs, **radiation**); metabolic diseases; brain tumor; increased intracranial pressure; and poor nutrition.

HYPOXIC ENCEPHALOPATHY Hypoxic encephalopathy refers to a lack of oxygen to the entire brain, which

Key Terms

Cerebral herniation Movement of the brain against the skull.

Cerebral ischemia Lack of oxygen to the brain, which may result in tissue death.

Encephalogram Machine that detects brain activity by measuring electrical activity in the brain.

Intracranial hypertension Increase in pressure in the brain.

typically results in brain damage. Cerebral **hypoxia** can be caused by drowning, low blood pressure, birth injuries, cardiac arrest, strangulation, asphyxiation caused by smoke inhalation, severe hemorrhage, carbon monoxide poisoning, high altitudes, choking, tracheal compression, complications of anesthesia, paralysis of respiratory muscles, and respiratory failure.

Cardiac arrest is the most common condition that causes cerebral hypoxia. When the heart stops pumping, oxygen-rich blood cannot be delivered to vital organs such as the brain. Hypoxia to the brain causes irreversible brain damage after two minutes.

HEPATIC ENCEPHALOPATHY Hepatic encephalopathy refers to a condition of brain and nervous system damage caused by liver (hepatic) failure. Diseases that damage the liver causing impairment of the detoxification and functional capabilities of the liver can cause hepatic encephalopathy. Examples of disorders that decrease liver function are hepatitis or cirrhosis. Impairment in the detoxification capabilities of the liver causes accumulation of toxic chemicals in the blood such as ammonia, in addition to many other impurities that all collectively cause damage to the nervous system.

KIDNEY FAILURE The main function for the kidneys is to eliminate excess fluid and waste material from the blood. When the kidneys lose the ability to filter the blood, dangerous levels of waste products accumulate in the body. Chronic renal failure can be caused by diabetes, analgesic nephropathy (due to long-term use of aspirin or nonsteroidal anti-inflammatory drugs), kidney diseases (polycystic kidney disease, pyelonephritis, and glomerulonephritis), renal artery stenosis (a narrowing of the artery that supplies blood to the kidneys), and lead poisoning.

SEVERE INFECTIONS Severe infections, especially those that affect the brain, can cause encephalopathy. Infections that specifically target the brain are encephalitis, which is inflammation of the brain, typically caused by a

virus, or meningitis, which is inflammation of the tissue that surrounds and protects the brain.

CHRONIC ALCOHOL USE Long-term use of alcohol not only causes destruction of brain cells but can cause cirrhosis of the liver or hepatitis, which results in the destruction of liver cells. Chronic alcoholism leads to progressive destruction of liver cells, which can cause end-stage liver failure. A subtype of hepatitis infection called hepatitis C typically causes progressive destruction to liver cells.

UREMIC ENCEPHALOPATHY Uremia describes the final stage of progressive renal insufficiency, which culminates in end-stage kidney failure with neurologic involvement. This is called uremic encephalopathy. The cause is unknown and no single metabolite or toxin is responsible for symptoms, but rather it is an accumulation of several chemicals/toxins in the blood that causes symptoms of encephalopathy.

Symptoms

The hallmark of encephalopathy is altered mental state. In mild cases, hypoxia can cause an altered mental state, which includes symptoms such as motor incoordination, poor judgment, and inattentiveness. Mild cases have no lasting effects. Patients who have severe hypoxia or anoxia (total lack of oxygen delivery, usually from cardiac arrest) lose consciousness within seconds. Other symptoms of encephalopathy include lethargy, nystagmus (rapid, involuntary eye movement), tremor, **dementia**, **seizures**, **myoclonus** (involuntary twitching of a muscle or group of muscles), muscle weakness and atrophy, and loss of ability to speak or swallow. An early and characteristic feature of hepatic encephalopathy is called constitutional **apraxia**, which is inability to reproduce simple designs such as a star. Patients with liver failure may exhibit a symptom called asterixis, an involuntary jerking tremor of the hands.

Diagnosis

The diagnosis of encephalopathy depends on the presence of acute or chronic liver disease; altered mental state such as confusion, stupor, or coma; symptoms of **central nervous system** damage; and abnormal wave patterns on an encephalogram. Diagnostic tests that may be utilized to establish the diagnosis include, but are not to limited to: complete blood count; liver function tests; ammonia and glucose levels; lactate levels (often elevated due to impaired tissue perfusion and because of decreased clearance by the liver); arterial blood gases (may reveal hypoxemia); kidney function tests; blood cultures (to detect infectious agents); virology testing (for hepatitis); neuroimaging studies; and ultrasound studies.

Treatment team

The causes of encephalopathies are broad. Additionally, the symptoms are also broad, ranging from mild changes of consciousness to coma or death. Therefore, the treatment team can consist of a broad spectrum of specialists that can include, but is not limited to, an internist, oncologist, pulmonologist, critical care physician, radiologist, hepatologist (specialist in liver diseases), and surgeon. The disorder can also occur in the pediatric ages or even at birth. In these critical situations, specialists in pediatric critical care, a neonatologist, and a perinatologist (specialist in maternal-fetal health) would be involved.

Treatment

Hypoxia or anoxic encephalopathy is an emergency, and immediate measures are necessary to prevent further damage to the brain and to restore breathing and circulation. It is necessary to treat hepatic encephalopathy early to prevent long-term damage. Specific treatment for hepatic encephalopathy is aimed at eliminating toxic substances and/or treatment of the primary illness that caused encephalopathy. Elimination of toxins such as ammonia can be accomplished by decreasing absorption of protein from the gut. By giving the patient a compound called lactulose, absorption of ammonia can be decreased. Persons with hepatic encephalopathy should not consume protein, and constipation should be avoided. Uremic encephalopathy caused by chronic renal failure is treated with transplantation or dialysis.

Recovery and rehabilitation

Recovery is an emergency for all patients with severe hypoxia or anoxia. Vital functions such as breathing, cardiac function, and delivery of oxygen-rich blood to the brain should be restored within two to five minutes. If anoxia persists for more than two minutes, there will be permanent and severe damage to the brain.

Clinical trials

There are four active government-sponsored **clinical trials** that are recruiting patients. There is a phase III clinical trial concerning birth asphyxia (hypoxic-ischemic encephalopathy) in infants up to six hours old. A phase II clinical trial is investigating the neuroimaging findings associated with persistent encephalopathy caused by the tick-transmitted infection called Lyme's disease (persistent Lyme encephalopathy). A third study is investigating a genetic form of familial dementia that causes encephaolpathy due to neurodegeneration of brain tissue. A fourth study investigates a disorder called neuronal ceroid lipofuscinosis (NCLS), which is a common heritable form of encephaopathy that occurs in one of 12,500 children. Detailed information about each of these studies can be obtained online from the website <http://www.clinicaltrials.gov>.

Prognosis

The outcome for patients who present with symptoms of encephalopathy depends on the cause. If the cause can be corrected in time, the outcome can be favorable. However, if encephalopathy is a manifestation of more advanced chronic disease, or if it is part of a rapidly fulminating disorder, the outcome can be poor and death may ensue due to the primary cause.

Special concerns

Persons who present with encephalopathy have advanced disease or the beginning of an advanced disease process. Vigilance on the part of the primary care provider is necessary to take all precautions to prevent this process.

Resources

BOOKS

Goetz, Christopher G., et al. (eds). *Textbook of Clinical Neurology*, 1st ed. Philadelphia: W.B. Saunders Company, 1999.

Goldman, Lee, et al. *Cecil's Textbook of Medicine*, 21st ed. Philadelphia: WB. Saunders Company, 2000.

Noble, John, et al. (eds). *Textbook of Primary Care Medicine*, 3rd ed. St. Louis: Mosby, Inc., 2001.

Rakel, Robert A. *Textbook of Family Practice*, 6th ed. Philadelphia: WB Saunders Company, 2002.

Rosen, Peter. *Emergency Medicine: Concepts and Clinical Practice*, 4th ed. St Louis: Mosby Year Book, Inc., 1998.

PERIODICALS

"Encephalopathy." *eMedicine Series* (July 2001).

Saas, David A. "Fulminant Hepatic Failure." *Gastroenterology Clinics* 32:4 (December 2003).

WEBSITES

NINDS Encephalopathy Information Page. National Institute of Neurological Disorders and Stroke. (May 20, 2004). <http://www.ninds.nih.gov/health_and_medical/disorders/encephalopathy.htm>.

ORGANIZATIONS

National Institute of Neurological Disorders and Stroke NIH Neurological Institute. P.O. Box 5801, Bethesda, MD 20824. (301) 496-5751 or (800) 352-9424. <http://www.ninds.nih.gov>.

Laith Farid Gulli, MD
Alfredo Mori, MB, BS

Encephalotrigeminal angiomatosis *see*
Sturge-Weber syndrome

Endovascular embolization

Definition

Endovascular embolization is a procedure that utilizes chemical agents or metallic coils to stop bleeding and treat **aneurysms** or brain tumors.

Purpose

The purpose is either to cut off blood supply or to fill a sac (also creating a thrombus). Endovascular embolization is a procedure used to treat hemorrhage, cranial tumors, or aneurysms. The procedure can be life saving. Bleeding can be stopped in cases of trauma, epistaxis (nosebleed), coughing up blood from the lungs (hemoptysis), gastrointestinal bleeding, hemorrhage to solid organs, and postcesarean, postoperative, or postpartum bleeding in the abdomen or pelvis. Additionally, endovascular embolization is used to cut off the blood supply to cranial tumors which eventually causes tumor cell destruction and tumor mass shrinkage from lack of oxygen and nourishment. The procedure can also be utilized for packing an aneurysm with coils, to prevent rupture and possible death from intracranial hemorrhage.

Precautions

Embolization is an indication for treatment of many clinical entities. The procedure is performed under general anesthesia and elective cases require pre-procedural evaluation with an anesthesiologist. The procedure requires a brief inpatient stay for one to two days. Dietary restrictions and medical work-up are usually indicated before elective surgery (i.e., cranial tumors). If an aneurysm or tumor cannot be safely embolized, the procedure is terminated. For bleeding, the procedure may likely be an emergency.

Description

Embolization is a useful procedure in a broad spectrum of clinical disorders. Typically embolization for any reason begins with a diagnostic **angiography** procedure to identify the source of the problem. The diagnostic angiography is usually performed in an artery. A catheter is usually inserted into the groin artery and dye is injected into the system. The catheter is wiggled through to the desired location using a television monitor. The target area may be a region where there is bleeding or it may be an aneurysm or cranial tumor. Once at the target area, chemicals or metal coils (for an aneurysm) are introduced by a microcatheter. In the case of an aneurysm, soft metal coils are placed with a microcatheter in the aneurysm until it is packed with about five to six coils. Filling the aneurysm will prevent blood flow into the aneurysm sac, since the sac is filled with coils and a thrombus after the procedure. Endovascular embolization can help to stop bleeding or re-bleeding for patients who are hemorrhaging. For cranial tumors the goal is to inject emboli in blood vessels that nourish brain tumors. This causes destruction of the tumor mass due to lack of blood supply. For any reason, when a blood vessel requires embolization, coils are the instrument of choice.

Preparation

Routine blood tests are done one to two days before an elective embolization. For scheduled procedures the patient should not eat or drink liquids after midnight the night before the procedure. The procedure is usually performed in a neuroangiography unit. A nurse will shave the patient's groin area since the catheter is inserted in the groin artery (also called the femoral artery). Emergency preparation may be initiated for persons who are actively bleeding.

Aftercare

After elective embolization, patients are taken to a neurosurgical intensive care unit or a step-down unit for close monitoring and recovery. It is necessary to lie flat for eight hours after the procedure to allow the groin area (where the catheter was inserted) to heal. Usually the next day the patient will be transferred to a regular ward room and discharged to home the following day.

Risks

The risk of embolization is low. Possible complications include weakness in an arm or leg, dysesthesia, speech or visual deficits, and **stroke**.

Normal results

Normal results depend on the indications for the procedure. For bleeding the desired goal is rapid cessation of bleeding source. Aneurysm will likely develop saccular occlusion (occlusion of the aneurysm sac), reducing the risk of rupture and fatal intracranial hemorrhage. The desired effect for an intracranial tumor is obliteration of tumor vasculature, which eventually causes destruction of the tumor mass, secondary to oxygen deprivation.

Resources

BOOKS

Grainger, Ronald G., and David Allison. *Grainger & Allison's Diagnostic Radiology: A Textbook of Medical Imaging,* 4th Ed. Churchill Livingstone, Inc.

WEBSITES

Arteriovenous Malformations. The Mayfield Clinic. <http://mayfieldclinic.com/PE/PE-AVM.HTM>.

Endovascular Embolization of Cranial Tumors. University of North Carolina at Chapel Hill. <http://www.cs.unc.edu/Research/intel/brain.html>.

Endovascular Embolization Treatment of Aneurysms. The University of Toronto. <http://nrainavm.uhnres.utoronto.ca/malformations/content/treat_embo_aneurysm.htm>.

ORGANIZATIONS

International Radiosurgery Support Association. PO Box 5186, Harrisburg, PA 17110. (717) 260-9808; Fax: (717) 260-9809. getinfo@irsa.org. <http://www.irsa.org>.

Laith Farid Gulli, MD
Robert Ramirez, DO

Epidural hematoma

Definition

An epidural hematoma is a pocket of blood that forms immediately outside the dura mater. The dura mater is the fibrous outermost sheath or membrane that encloses the brain and spinal cord. Epidural means outside the dura, and hematoma means mass of blood.

Description

Epidural hematomas usually form when a violent blow breaks a blood vessel in the space outside the dura mater, whether in the skull or in the spinal column. In the skull, the vessel most often responsible for epidural hematoma is the middle meningeal artery.

Blood from the broken vessel forms a pressurized pocket of blood, like a large, internal blood blister. The growing hematoma pushes against the rigid bone of the skull or spinal column and thus exerts pressure on the dura mater, which in turn pushes on the brain or spinal cord. This pressure may stretch and tear blood vessels or even force the brain to herniate (i.e., partially squeeze out) through the foramen magnum, the hole in the bottom of the skull through which the spinal cord enters, or through the tentorium cerebelli, the part of the dura mater that covers the **cerebellum** and supports the occipital lobes from below. Herniation of the brain is likely to be fatal.

Epidural hematomas are less common than subdural hematomas, which are the most common mechanism of fatal brain damage in head trauma. They are also distinguished from intracranial hematomas, volumes of blood that collect inside the brain rather than at its surface.

Demographics

Traumatic brain injuries such as those that can result in cranial epidural hematoma are common. About 500,000 patients are admitted to hospitals in the United States annually with head injuries that cause brain damage, and some 75,000–90,000 of these patients die. Motor vehicle accidents are the most common cause of closed-head injuries, accounting for 50–70% of such injuries. Falls are the second most common cause of closed head trauma. Alcohol is a contributing factor in about 40% of severe head injuries. Sports such as football can result in traumatic head injury, but do so relatively rarely. Three-quarters of patients with **traumatic brain injury** are male, and the risk of traumatic brain injury declines steadily with age.

Epidural hematoma occurs in about 1% of all patients with severe head injuries. The fraction of comatose head-injury patients with **subdural hematoma** is greater, but still only about 10%.

Causes and symptoms

Intracranial subdural hematoma

The most common cause of cranial epidural hematoma is head trauma, which is some kind of blow to the head. Epidural hematomas are most commonly found in the temporal or temporoparietal region, i.e., along the sides of the brain. Patients often lose consciousness due to the original head trauma, regain consciousness and undergo a period of clear-mindedness, then deteriorate neurologically.

Spinal epidural hematoma

Trauma is a common cause of spinal epidural hematoma. Non-trauma causes include anticoagulant therapy, hemophilia, liver disease, aspirin use, systemic **lupus** erythematosus, and, rarely, lumbar puncture. In 40–50% of cases of spinal epidural hematoma, no precipitating trauma or other cause is observed; these cases are considered spontaneous.

Spinal epidural hematoma causes compression of the spinal cord. Symptoms vary with the amount and location of this pressure. **Back pain** may be slight or absent. The patient may have loss of feeling (anesthesia) or less-than-normal feeling (hypoesthesia) in the legs, arm, or trunk. There may be weakening of the legs and loss of deep tendon reflexes. There may be bowel and bladder dysfunction

Key Terms

Dura mater The tough, fibrous outermost layer of the three meninges that surround the brain and spinal cord.

Hematoma A bruise or collection of blood within soft tissue that results in swelling.

(e.g., incontinence or inability to control the bladder or bowels).

Diagnosis

Neurologic assessment is the first step in determining the severity of a head injury. The patient's speech, eye-opening, and muscular responses are evaluated, along with the orientation (if conscious) to place, time, and commands to open eyes or the like. If the patient is unconscious, examination of the pupillary light reflex is important. An epidural or other hematoma increases intracranial pressure, which quickly has an effect on the third cranial nerve, which contains, among other nerve fibers, those that control constriction of the pupil. Pressure that blocks this nerve leads to fixed dilation of the pupil. Fixed pupil dilation in one or both eyes is a strong indicator that the patient may have an intracranial hematoma. To distinguish between epidural, subdural, and intracranial hematoma, computerized tomography (**CT**) or **magnetic resonance imaging (MRI)** is probably necessary. Surgeons determine if swelling on one side of the brain has shifted the midline of the brain. If a shift of more than 0.2 in (5 mm) is found, an emergency **craniotomy** (opening of the skull) may be performed.

Patients with spinal epidural hematoma may experience sudden onset of back or neck **pain** at the site of the bleed. Coughing or any other maneuver that increases pressure inside the torso may worsen the pain transiently. In children, the bleeding is more likely to be in the cervical (neck) region than in the thoracic (middle back) region.

When making the diagnosis of spinal epidural hematoma, physicians must decide whether the symptoms of spinal compression are being caused by a hematoma or by a tumor. CT or MRI are definitive in distinguishing between compression of the spinal cord caused by tumor or hematoma.

Treatment team

Treatment for hematoma is primarily surgical. A **neurologist** and a neurosurgeon will be essential members of the treatment team, as will nursing staff, in the operating room and out of it, who are specially trained in head trauma care.

Treatment

Emergency care for spinal trauma consists of immobilizing the patient and administering high-dose corticosteroids. However, the highest priority for any intracranial or spinal hematoma is relief of the pressure by surgical drainage of the hematoma.

Recovery and rehabilitation

Epidural hematoma can result in permanent paralysis or other neurological deficits. If spinal cord compression due to hematoma is alleviated within 6–12 hours, permanent symptoms may be avoided. Prevention of brain damage depends more on preventing the brain from being deformed by the pressure of the hematoma than on relieving that pressure. Rehabilitation needs will depend on how much permanent damage, if any, has been caused.

Clinical trials

As of 2004, no **clinical trials** were being conducted for epidural hematoma patients in the United States.

Resources

PERIODICALS

Marsh, Cherly. "Surgical Management of Patients with Severe Head Injuries." *AORN Journal* May 1, 1996.

Sung, Helen Minjung. "How to Diagnose and Treat Acute, Nontraumatic Spinal Cord Lesions." *The Journal of Critical Illness* April 1, 2000.

Trask, Todd. "Management of Head Trauma (Critical Care Review)." *Chest* August 1, 2002.

OTHER

Epidural Hematoma Patient/Family Resources. April 26, 2004 (May 30, 2004). <http://cchs-dl.slis.ua.edu/patientinfo/orthopedics/head/epidural-hematoma.htm>.

NINDS Traumatic Brain Injury Information Page. National Institute of Neurological Disorders and Stroke. April 26, 2004 (May 30, 2004). <http://www.ninds.nih.gov/health_and_medical/disorders/tbi_doc.htm>.

Larry Gilman

Epilepsy

Definition

The words "epilepsy" and "epileptic" are of Greek origin and have the same root as the verb "epilambanein," which means "to seize" or "to attack." Therefore, epilepsy means seizure, while epileptic means seized. In the modern understanding of epilepsy, it should not be considered a disease. Rather, it is a symptom indicating a medical condition in the brain that causes a potential for recurrent **seizures**. The condition of epilepsy has many causes and the kinds of seizures that occur can vary widely.

Description

The word epilepsy is actually a descriptive term. It takes into account an individual's risk of recurrent seizures. However, when people are suffering from meningitis and have a seizure, they would not be considered to have epilepsy unless they had a seizure after the meningitis resolved. In this case, these individuals have a risk for recurrent seizures and, hence, epilepsy. If an individual over time does not have any seizures off medications, then it could be said that epilepsy has resolved or gone into remission.

For thousands of years, epilepsy was looked upon differently than most other medical problems. Because of this, epilepsy has been fraught with social stigmas, even up to today. The ancient Greeks knew about the condition that led to a sudden attack upon the unfortunate. Although Hippocrates, in roughly 400 B.C., referred to epilepsy as the sacred disease, he did so to emphasize the general public's superstitious view of the condition. Of course, it certainly was not an affliction sent from a deity, nor was it even a demon. Nevertheless, seizures, which manifest in unusual behaviors, mystified observers who considered this illness, from all others, as coming from another world.

The current understanding of epilepsy is a recent development. Previously, it was not even believed that the brain had electrical properties. It was not until the last few centuries that the brain was considered the seat of the mind; it was the heart or the lungs that were commonly regarded as the organ of thought. Physicians struggled with what to even call a seizure. In general, any behavior that resulted in a loss of consciousness or convulsions was labeled a seizure. It is likely that episodes of **fainting** were erroneously called seizures.

Finally, in 1873, an adequate definition for the term seizure finally came into existence. The famous English **neurologist** John Hughlings Jackson explained epilepsy as "a sudden, excessive, and rapid discharge of gray matter of some part of the brain" that would correspond to the patient's experience.

Demographics

More than 2.5 million Americans suffer from epilepsy, and more than another 50 million worldwide. Epilepsy is more common than **Parkinson's disease**, **multiple sclerosis**, **cerebral palsy**, and **muscular dystrophy**

Key Terms

Automatisms Movements during a seizure that are semi-purposeful but involuntary.

Gelastic seizures Seizures manifesting with brief involuntary laughter.

Gray matter The portion of the brain that contains neurons, as opposed to white matter, which contains nerve tracts.

Spike wave discharge Characteristic abnormal wave pattern in the electroencephalogram that is a hallmark of an area that has the potential of generating a seizure.

---

all combined. The risk of experiencing one seizure in the course of a lifetime, from any cause, is close to 10%. However, there is an approximately 1% chance of developing epilepsy in the general population before the age of 20. The risk increases to 3% by age 75. Of course, depending on the age group being studied, the cause of epilepsy will vary. The incidence of epilepsy is relatively constant among different ethnic groups and similar between genders. However, there may be variation in incidence in underdeveloped countries due to access to care and endemic illness that can cause seizures, such as neurocystercercosis in Latin American countries.

Causes and symptoms

Epilepsy has many causes that, in part, have an affect on the clinical presentation of symptoms. In order for epilepsy to occur, there must be an underlying physical problem in the brain. The problem can be so mild that an individual is perfectly normal other than seizures. The brain has roughly 50–100 billion neurons. Each neuron can have up to 10,000 contacts with neighboring neurons. Hence, trillions of connections exist. However, only a very small area of dysfunctional brain tissue is necessary to create a persistent generator of seizures and, hence, epilepsy. The following are potential causes of epilepsy:

- genetic and/or hereditary
- perinatal neurological insults
- trauma with brain injury
- **stroke**
- brain tumors
- infections such as meningitis and encephalitis
- multiple sclerosis
- ideopathic (unknown or genetic)

Any of the above conditions have the potential for causing the brain or a portion of it to be dysfunctional and produce recurrent seizures. Regardless of the exact cause, epilepsy is a paroxysmal (sudden) condition. It involves the synchronous discharging of a population of neurons. This is an abnormal event that, depending on the location in the brain, will correspond to the particular symptoms of a seizure. The International League Against Epilepsy (ILAE) issued a classification of types of seizures. The list gives the kind of seizures that can occur. Individual seizure types are based on the clinical behavior (semiology) and electrophysiological characteristics as seen on an electroencephalogram (EEG). Generalized seizures included in the list are:

- tonic-clonic seizures (includes variations beginning with a clonic or myoclonic phase)
- clonic seizures, including without tonic features and with tonic features
- typical absence seizures
- atypical absence seizures
- myoclonic absence seizures
- tonic seizures
- spasms
- myoclonic seizures
- eyelid myoclonia, including without absences and with absences
- myoclonic atonic seizures
- negative **myoclonus**
- atonic seizures
- reflex seizures in generalized epilepsy syndromes

Focal seizures included in the ILAE list are:

- focal sensory seizures with elementary sensory symptoms (e.g., occipital and parietal lobe seizures) and experiential sensory symptoms (e.g., temporo-parieto-occipital junction seizures)
- focal motor seizures with elementary clonic motor signs, asymmetrical tonic motor seizures (e.g., supplementary motor seizures), typical (temporal lobe) automatisms (e.g., mesial temporal lobe seizures), hyperkinetic automatisms, focal negative myoclonus, and inhibitory motor seizures
- gelastic seizures
- hemiclonic seizures
- secondarily generalized seizures
- reflex seizures in focal epilepsy syndromes

In 1989, the International League Against Epilepsy also issued the following classification of epilepsies and epileptic syndromes:

- benign familial neonatal seizures
- early myoclonic encephalopathy

- Ohtahara syndrome
- migrating partial seizures of infancy (syndrome in development)
- West syndrome
- benign myoclonic epilepsy in infancy
- benign familial and non-familial infantile seizures
- Dravet's syndrome
- HH syndrome
- myoclonic status in nonprogressive encephalopathies (syndrome in development)
- benign childhood epilepsy with centrotemporal spikes
- early onset benign childhood occipital epilepsy (Panayiotopoulos type)
- late-onset childhood occipital epilepsy (Gastaut type)
- epilepsy with myoclonic absences
- epilepsy with myoclonic-astatic seizures
- **Lennox-Gastaut syndrome**
- Landau-Kleffner syndrome (LKS)
- epilepsy with continuous spike-and-waves during slow-wave sleep (other than LKS)
- childhood absence epilepsy
- progressive myoclonus epilepsies
- idiopathic generalized epilepsies with variable phenotypes include juvenile absence epilepsy, juvenile myoclonic epilepsy, and epilepsy with generalized tonic-clonic seizures only
- reflex epilepsies
- idiopathic photosensitive occipital lobe epilepsy
- other visual sensitive epilepsies
- primary reading epilepsy
- startle epilepsy
- autosomal dominant nocturnal frontal lobe epilepsy
- familial temporal lobe epilepsies
- generalized epilepsies with **febrile seizures** plus (syndrome in development)
- familial focal epilepsy with variable foci (syndrome in development)
- symptomatic focal epilepsies
- limbic epilepsies
- mesial **temporal lobe epilepsy** with hippocampal sclerosis
- mesial temporal lobe epilepsy defined by specific etiologies
- neocortical epilepsies
- Rasmussen syndrome

Classifying epilepsy can help in the evaluation and management of patients with seizure disorders. The combination of seizure type(s), etiology (cause), age of onset,

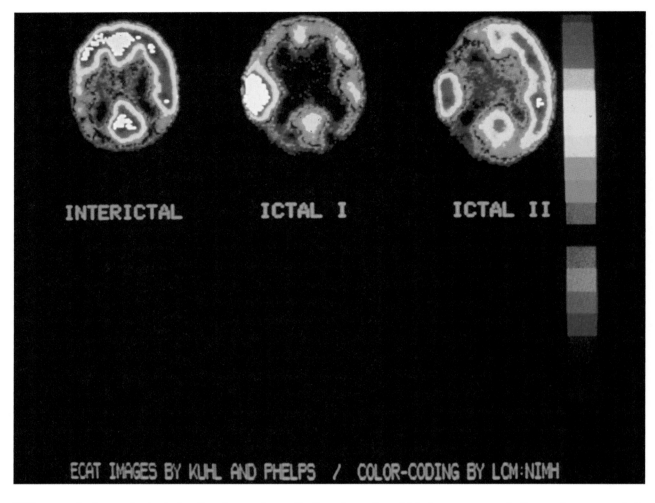

INTERICTAL   ICTAL I   ICTAL II

ECAT IMAGES BY KUHL AND PHELPS / COLOR-CODING BY LCM:NIMH

PET scans of a human brain during the stages of an epileptic seizure; the middle image represents the most severe period of the seizure. *(© Photo Researchers, Inc. Reproduced by permission.)*

family history, and other medical or neurological conditions can be used to identify an epilepsy syndrome. Classification helps clinicians and researchers understand the broader picture of seizure disorders. On a practical level, syndrome identification can help in planning the management of patients. Syndrome classification schemes are revised periodically as individual components of particular categories are better understood.

The term idiopathic refers to a cause that is suspected to be, if not genetic, then unknown. Cryptogenic is a term that suggests that an underlying cause is suspected, but not yet fully understood. Symptomatic is a term that is applied to epilepsies that are a result of understood underlying pathologies.

The management and prognosis vary considerably among these differing syndromes. Epilepsies that have a genetic basis can be inherited or occur spontaneously. A

detailed family history can often identify other family members who have had seizures. However, because seizures are common, it is possible to have more than one family member with epilepsy, though the etiologies may not be related. To say that a particular type of epilepsy is genetic does not mean that it is necessarily transmitted by heredity. Often, disorders can have a genetic cause, but be spontaneously occurring in only one member of a family. In this case, there may simply be a random mutation in that particular person's genes.

There are several mechanisms in which epilepsies can be inherited. So-called simple Mendelian inheritance occurs with benign familial neonatal convulsions and autosomal dominant nocturnal frontal lobe epilepsy. On the other hand, complex inheritance mechanisms can involve more than one gene, or a gene mutation in combination with environmental or acquired factors such as juvenile myoclonic epilepsy. As the genetics of the epilepsies become better understood, the classification scheme will evolve.

With epilepsy, symptoms vary considerably depending on the type. The common link among the epilepsies is, of course, seizures. The different epilepsies can sometimes be associated with more than one seizure type. This is the case with Lennox-Gastaut syndrome.

Diagnosis

Arriving at a diagnosis of epilepsy is relatively straightforward: when people suffer two or more seizures, they would be considered to have epilepsy. However, diagnosing the specific epilepsy syndrome is much more complex. The first step in the evaluation process is to obtain a very detailed history of the illness, not only from the patient but from the family as well. Since seizures can impair consciousness, the patient may not be able to recall the specifics of the attacks. In these cases, family or friends that have witnessed the episodes can fill in the gaps about the particulars of the seizure. The description of the behaviors during a seizure can go a long way to categorizing the type of seizure and help with the overall diagnosis. Moreover, in the initial visit with the physician, the entire history of the patient is obtained. In a child, this would include birth history, complications, if any, maternal history, and developmental milestones. At any age, so-called co-morbidities (other medical problems) are considered. Medications that have been taken or currently being prescribed are documented.

A complete physical examination is performed, especially a neurological exam. Because seizures are an episodic disorder, abnormal neurological findings may not be present. Frequently, people with epilepsy have a normal exam. However, in some, there can be abnormal findings that can provide clues to the underlying cause of epilepsy. For example, if someone has had a stroke that subsequently caused seizures, then the neurological exam can be expected to reveal a focal neurological deficit such as weakness or language difficulties. In some children with seizures, there can be a variety of associated neurologic abnormalities such as **mental retardation** and cerebral palsy that are themselves non-specific but indicate that the brain has suffered, at some point in development, an injury or malformation. Also, subtle findings on examination can lead to a diagnosis such as in **tuberous sclerosis**. This is an autosomal dominantly inherited disorder associated with **infantile spasms** in 25% of cases. On examination, patients have so-called ash-leaf spots and adenoma sebaceum on the skin. There can also be a variety of systemic abnormalities that involve the kidneys, retina, heart, and gums, depending on severity.

In the course of evaluating epilepsy, a number of tests are typically ordered. Usually, magnetic resonance image (**MRI**) of the brain is obtained. This is a scan that can help in finding many known causes of epilepsy such as tumors, strokes, trauma, and congenital malformations. However, while MRI can reveal incredible details of the brain, it cannot visualize the presence of abnormalities in the microscopic neuronal environment. Another test that is routinely ordered is an electroencephalogram (EEG). Unlike the MRI scan, this can be considered a functional test of the brain. The EEG measures the electrical activity of the brain. Some seizure disorders or epilepsies have a characteristic EEG with particular abnormalities that can help in diagnosis. Other tests that are frequently ordered are various blood tests that are also ordered in many medical conditions. These blood tests help to screen for abnormalities that can be a factor in the cause of seizures. Occasionally, genetic testing is performed in those instances where a known genetic cause is suspected and can be tested. A major concern in the course of an evaluation of epilepsy is to identify the presence of life-threatening causes such as brain tumors, infections, and cerebrovascular disease. Also, an accurate diagnosis can expedite the most effective treatment plan.

The symptoms of epilepsy are dependent in part on the particular seizures that occur and other medical problems that may be associated. Seizures, themselves, can take on a variety of features. A simple sustained twitching of an extremity could be a focal seizure. If a seizure arises in the occipital lobes of the brains, then a visual experience can occur. Aura is a term often used to describe symptoms that a person may feel prior to the loss of consciousness of a seizure. However, auras are, themselves, small focal seizures that have not spread in the brain to involve consciousness. Smells, well-formed hallucinations, tingling sensations, or nausea have each occurred in auras. The particular sensation can be a clue as to the location in the brain where a seizure starts. Focal seizures can then spread to involve other areas of the brain and lead to an alteration of consciousness, and possibly convulsions. In certain epilepsy syndromes such as Lennox-Gastaut, there can be more than one type of seizure experienced, such as atonic, atypical absence, and tonic-axial seizures.

Treatment

One challenge in predicting the course of epilepsy is that for any type, there can be a variable response to treatment. Sometimes, seizures may play a rather small role in the manifestation of a medical condition. For example, a severe head injury could result in seizures that readily respond to medication, but severe neurological impairments and disabilities may still be present. On the other hand, a different head injury may result in relatively mild neurological problems, but there may be seizures that are severe and be resistant to medications.

Whatever the case, the ultimate goals when treating epilepsy are to:

• strive for complete freedom from seizures

• have little to no side effects from medications

• be able to follow an easy regimen so that compliance with treatment can be maintained

Up to 60% of patients with epilepsy can be expected to achieve control of seizures with medication(s). However, in the remaining 40%, epilepsy appears to be resistant, to varying degrees, to medications. In these cases, the epilepsy is termed medically intractable.

Generally, the choice of medication is somewhat trial and error. There are, however, a number of considerations that guide the choice of treatment. Each medication has a particular side effect profile and mechanism of action. Some medications seem to be particularly effective for certain epilepsy syndromes. For example, juvenile myoclonic epilepsy responds well to valproic acid. On the other hand, ethosuxamide is primarily used for absence seizures.

As with any medication, individuals can have very different experiences with same drug. Consequently, it is difficult to predict the efficacy of treatment in the beginning. A key concept of treatment is to first strive for monotherapy (or single drug therapy). This simplifies treatment and minimizes the chance of side effects. Sometimes, however, two or more drugs may be necessary to achieve satisfactory control of seizures. As with any treatment, potential side effects can be worse than the disease itself. Moreover, there is little point in controlling seizures if severe side effects limit quality of life. If a seizure disorder is characterized by mild, focal, or brief symptoms that do not interfere with day-to-day life, then aggressive treatments may not be justified. Epilepsy medications do not cure epilepsy; the medications can only control the frequency and severity of seizures. A list of the most commonly used medications in the management of epilepsy includes:

• phenobarbital

• phenytoin (Dilantin, Phenytek)

• clonazepam (Klonipin)

• ethosuxamide (Zarontin)

• carbamazepine (Tegretol, Carbatrol)

• divalproex sodium (Depakote, Depakene)

• felbamate (Felbatol)

• gabapentin (Neurontin)

• lamotrigine (Lamictal)

• topiramate (Topamax)

• tiagabine (Gabatril)

• zonisamide (Zonegran)

• oxcarbazepine (Trileptal)

• leviteracetam (Keppra)

It has been found that the initial, thoughtfully chosen medication can be expected to make almost 50% of patients seizure free for extended periods of time. If the initial drug fails, another well-chosen drug may make an additional 14% of people seizure free. If that drug fails, then the likelihood of rendering someone with epilepsy seizure free is poor. This does not mean that trying more medications or combinations of them may not be successful, but rather, these statistics give the neurologist and the patient an understanding of the realities of epilepsy treatment. In cases where medications do not fully control epilepsy, it is recommended that a more extensive evaluation at a comprehensive epilepsy center be conducted where an epileptologist (a specialist in epilepsy) will more thoroughly assess the particular aspects of the seizures. When medications are clearly ineffective, the other types of therapy that can be considered are the ketogenic diet, brain surgery, and vagal nerve stimulation.

Ketogenic diet

The ketogenic diet is based on high-fat, low-carbohydrate, and low-protein meals. The ketogenic diet is named because of the production of ketones by the breakdown of fatty acids. The most common version of the diet involves long-chain triglycerides. These are present in whole cream, butter, and fatty meats.

The ketogenic diet is administered with the support of a nutritionist with experience in this treatment modality. It is mostly used in children with medically intractable epilepsy and whose diet can be controlled. The ketogenic diet can be considered a pharmacologic treatment. As such, there are potential side effects that limit its tolerance. This includes hair thinning, lethargy, weight loss, kidney stones, and possibly cardiac problems. Sugar-free vitamin and mineral supplementation is necessary. The diet may not be appropriate for certain individuals, particularly in children, who may have certain metabolic diseases.

Overall, the diet has been very helpful in the control of seizures in many patients. Roughly 50% of patients can hope to achieve complete control of seizures, 25% of the patients see improvements, and another 25% are non-responders. There are some patients who have an improvement in behavior. If the diet is well tolerated with good results, then it can be maintained for up to two years, followed by a careful gradual transition to regular meals.

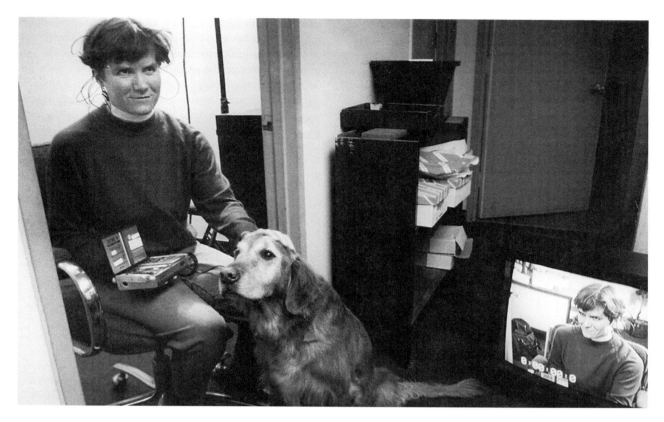

Elizabeth Rudy, who suffers from epilepsy, sits hooked up to brain wave monitor. Her left hand strokes her seizure-predicting dog, Ribbon. *(A/P Wide World Photos. Reproduced by permission.)*

Epilepsy surgery

Epilepsy surgery is an option in the attempt to either cure or significantly reduce the severity of medically resistant cases. It is thought that up to 100,000 patients in the United States could be potential candidates for a surgical treatment. However, only about 5,000 cases are performed throughout the United States annually. This is likely due to several factors, including the belief that any brain surgery is a last resort, the lack of awareness or understanding of the benefits of surgery, and the false hope that some medication will come along that will be effective.

There are several kinds of surgery that are available depending on the nature of the seizure disorder. A list of operations that are utilized regularly for epilepsy include:

• lobectomy

• lesionectomy

• corpus collosotomy

• multiple subpial transection

• hemispherectomy

The type of surgery that is performed depends on the nature of the individual seizure disorder. If a seizure can be localized to a particular area in the brain, then this abnormal region can potentially be surgically removed. Epileptic brain tissue is abnormal and its removal can provide a chance of a cure. Generally, surgery should be a consideration when the risk and benefits of it outweigh the long-term risks of uncontrolled epilepsy.

The approach taken in any brain surgery for epilepsy is highly individualized and great care is taken to avoid injury to essential brain tissue. The most common epilepsy surgery performed is the temporal lobectomy. Brain tumors are frequently associated with seizures. In many cases, surgery to remove the tumor is planned so that regions that may be causing seizures are removed as well. However, in many cases, epilepsy surgery cannot be done.

Vagus nerve stimulation

Another non-medicinal approach to treating epilepsy is a novel method that became available in July 1997. The Food and Drug Administration (FDA) approved the use of the vagal nerve stimulator (VNS) as add-on therapy in patients who experience seizures of partial onset. The VNS is designed to intermittently deliver small electrical stimulations to a nerve in the neck called the vagus nerve.

There are two vagal nerves, one on each side of the neck near the carotid arteries, making a pair of cranial nerves (there are 12 different paired cranial nerves). The vagus nerve carries information from the brain to many parts of the thoracic and abdominal organs. The nerve also carries information from these same organs back to the brain. VNS takes advantage of this fact and, by intermittent stimulation, there is an effect on many brain areas that can be involved in seizures.

About 50% of patients experience at least 50% reduction in the frequency of their seizures. The responses to VNS range from complete control of seizures (less than 10% of patients) to no noticeable improvement. The device is not a substitute for epilepsy surgery and should be considered only after there is an evaluation for epilepsy surgery. The implantation of the device requires relatively minor surgery with two incisions, one in the neck and the other in the left upper chest area.

The battery in the device lasts up to eight to ten years, after which the device can be replaced. Side effects of VNS therapy include voice hoarseness that typically does not impair communication. Like any surgery, there is an initial risk of infection, bleeding, and **pain**. Recovery takes a few weeks. Individuals can return to their usual activities once the incisions have healed.

Clinical trials

The National Institute of Neurological Disorders and Stroke list a number of **clinical trials**. There are also a number of studies being conducted at a more basic science stage evaluating the role of the following in seizures and epilepsy: **neurotransmitters**, non-neuronal cells, and genetic factors. Treatment strategies including **deep brain stimulation** and intracranial early seizure detection devices are being studied at different stages.

Prognosis

The prognosis of epilepsy varies widely depending on the cause, severity, and patient's age. Even individuals with a similar diagnosis may have different experiences with treatment. For example, in benign epilepsy of childhood with centrotemporal spikes (also called benign rolandic epilepsy), the prognosis is excellent with nearly all children experiencing remission by their teens. With childhood absence epilepsy, the prognosis is variable. In this case, the absence seizures become less frequent with time, but almost half of patients may eventually develop generalized tonic-clonic seizures. Overall, the seizures are responsive to an appropriate anticonvulsant. On the other hand, the seizures in Lennox-Gastaut syndrome are very difficult to control. In this case, however, the ketogenic diet can help. In seizures that begin in adulthood, one can expect that medications will control seizures in up to 60–70% of cases. However, in some of the more than 30% of medically intractable cases, epilepsy surgery can improve or even cure the problem.

Overall, most patients have a good chance of controlling seizures with the available options of treatment. The goal of treatment is complete cessation of seizures since a mere reduction in seizure frequency and/or severity may continue to limit patients' quality of life: they may not be able to drive, sustain employment, or be productive in school.

Resources

BOOKS

Browne, T. R., and G. L. Holmes. *Handbook of Epilepsy*, 2nd edition. Philadelphia: Lippincott Williams & Wilkins. 2000.

Devinski, O. *A Guide to Understanding and Living with Epilepsy*. Philadelphia: F.A. Davis Company. 1994.

Engel, J., Jr., and T. A. Pedley. *Epilepsy: A Comprehensive Textbook*. Philadelphia: Lippincott-Raven. 1998.

Freeman, M. J., et al. *The Ketogenic Diet: A Treatment for Epilepsy*, 3rd Edition. New York: Demos Medical Publishing, 2000.

Hauser, W. A., and D. Hesdorffer. *Epilepsy: Frequency, Causes, and Consequences*. New York: Demos Medical Publishing, 1990.

Pellock, J. M., W. E. Dodson, and B. F. D. Bourgeois. *Pediatric Epilepsy Diagnosis and Therapy*, 2nd Edition. New York: Demos Medical Publishing, 2001.

Santilli, N. *Managing Seizure Disorders: A Handbook for Health Care Professionals*. Philadelphia: Lippincott-Raven. 1996.

Schachter, S. C., and D. Schmidt. *Vagus Nerve Stimulation*, 2nd Edition. Oxford, England: Martin Dunitz, 2003.

Wyllie, E. *The Treatment of Epilepsy: Principles and Practice*, 3rd Edition. Philadelphia: Lippincott Williams & Wilkins, 2001.

PERIODICALS

Kwan, P., and M. J. Brodie. "Early Identification of Refractory Epilepsy." *New England Journal of Medicine* no. 342 (2000): 314–319.

ORGANIZATIONS

American Epilepsy Society. 342 North Main Street, West Hartford, CT 06117-2507. 860.586.7505. <www.aesnet.org>.

Epilepsy Foundation of America. 4351 Garden City Drive, Landover, MD 20785-7223. (800) 332-1000. <www.epilepsyfoundation.org>.

International League Against Epilepsy. Avenue Marcel Thiry 204, B-1200, Brussels, Belgium. + 32 (0) 2 774 9547; Fax: + 32 (0) 2 774 9690. <www.epilepsy.org>.

Roy Sucholeiki, MD

Erb's palsy *see* **Brachial plexus injuries**

Erb-Duchenne and Dejerine-Klumpke palsies *see* **Brachial plexus injuries**

Exercise

Definition

Exercise is physical activity that is undertaken in order to improve one's health. Physicians, physical therapists, and researchers have found that exercise plays an important role in the maintenance of brain, nerve, and muscle function in the human body. New research suggests that exercise may delay mental deterioration with age and disease, and perhaps even promote neurogenesis (nerve cell growth).

Description

Health care professionals recommend regular exercise because it increases energy, contributes to overall health, improves sleep, increases life expectancy, and enhances lifestyle. In terms of specific medical disorders, exercise has been shown to prevent or delay the onset of coronary artery disease, bone loss and osteoporosis, some types of cancer, and **stroke**.

Generally, exercise is categorized into the following four types:

- Aerobic exercise focuses on strengthening the heart, lungs, and circulatory system. Its major goal is to increase the heart rate and breathing rate. Examples of aerobic exercise include jogging, bicycling, swimming, and racket sports.

- Strength training focuses on strengthening muscles and joints. It also improves balance and increases metabolism. Weightlifting is the most common form of strength training.

- Balance exercises are used to improve stability. They stimulate the vestibular system, which includes muscles, joints, sensory organs, the inner ear, and the brain.

- Stretching exercises improve flexibility, which helps prevent injury during other forms of exercises and may decrease chronic pain. Stretching exercises include yoga, tai chi, and basic stretches.

All four types of exercises have been found to be important to maintaining brain, nerve, and muscle health.

Exercise and the brain

Exercise is particularly beneficial to the health of the brain. It has long been known that exercise causes the endocrine system to release serotonin and dopamine, hormones in the brain that produce feelings of euphoria and peacefulness. These hormones often allow people who exercise to think more clearly and perform mental tasks more easily. Exercise has also been successfully used as a treatment for **depression**, used in lieu of prescription antidepressants.

A 2003 study on mice suggests that new brain cells can grow as a result of exercise. This neurogenesis, previously thought not to occur in adult mammals, is concentrated in the hippocampus, the part of the brain responsible for learning and spatial memory. In addition, the study found that the mice subjected to an exercise regimen had stronger synapses than the mice that were sedentary. Other research shows that nerve growth factors, called neurotropins, are stimulated by exercise. Finally, exercise increases blood flow to the brain, as well as collateral circulation, enhancing mental function and nerve cell stimulation.

Exercise and aging

Aging naturally affects a variety of processes in the human body. Exercise has many positive benefits that prevent or slow the age-related deterioration of brain, nerve, and muscle functions.

In 2001, a study reported by the Mayo Clinic showed that regular exercise in older people slowed rates of mental deterioration, including Alzheimer's disease and **dementia**. On tests of mental acuity, older people who exercised regularly performed just as well as younger people who did not exercise. Another study found that regular walking greatly slowed rates of mental decline in older women.

Between the ages of 30 and 90, natural aging processes result in the loss of 15–25% of the brain tissue. In particular, losses are significant in the parts of the brain consisting of gray matter, which is associated with learning and memory. The February 2003 issue of *Journal of Gerontology: Medical Sciences* reported that this natural degradation of gray matter in older people was significantly decreased in people who exercised regularly compared to those who did not exercise. In the study, fitness levels were determined by treadmill-walking tests and tissue degradation was measured using **magnetic resonance imaging (MRI)**.

Balance is often affected as people age. Balance depends on input from the eyes, ears, and other sensory organs, all of which are affected by age. In addition, muscle strength and tone are required for balance. The natural aging process includes contraction of muscle tissue, and sedentary lifestyles only exacerbate the weakening of muscles. Joints supported by strong muscles are more stable than joints that are supported by weak muscles. Strength training, in particular, has the potential to counteract loss of muscle strength.

Physical therapy and the brain, nerves, and muscles

Therapeutic exercises have been designed to enhance a variety of aspects of physical fitness in patients suffering from diseases and dysfunctions. Goals of physical therapy include improving circulation, coordination, balance, and respiratory capacity. Exercises may be geared toward mobilizing joints and releasing contracted muscles and tendons.

Patients suffering from neurological disorders can be treated with a variety of physical therapies. For example, motor neuron damage or partial peripheral nerve damage may respond to a specific type of physical therapy called proprioceptive neuromuscular facilitation (PNF). PNF focuses on exercises that build muscle strength by applying resistance to muscle contraction. Patients who have experienced cerebrovascular accidents may undergo PNF combined with training for muscle strength, balance, and coordination. **Multiple sclerosis** is treated with PNF along with physical fitness training. Physical therapies for Parkinson disease focus on general physical fitness training, along with stretching exercises.

Resources

BOOKS

Putnam, Stephen C. *Nature's Ritalin for the Marathon Mind.* Hinesburg, VT: Upper Access Book Publishers, 2001.

Ratey, John. *A User's Guide to the Brain: Perception, Attention, and the Four Theaters of the Brain.* Vancouver, WA: Vintage Books, 2002.

OTHER

Effects on Neurologic Diseases and Mental Decline. Health and Age. (March 18, 2004). <http://www.healthandage.com/Home/gm=0!gc=2!gid6=2908>.

Frankenfield, Gay. "Exercise May Improve Learning and Memory." *WebMD* January 4, 2004 (March 18, 2004). <http://my.webmd.com/content/article/17/1676_50120.htm?lastselectedguid={5FE84E90-BC77-4056-A91C-9531713CA348}.

Lawrence, Star. "Train Your Brain with Exercise." *WebMD* July 28, 2003 (March 18, 2004). <http://my.webmd.com/content/article/67/79909.htm?lastselectedguid={5FE84E90-BC77-4056-A91C-9531713CA348}>.

Warner, Jennifer. "Exercise Saves Brain Cells." *WebMD* January 29, 2003 (March 18, 2004). <http://my.webmd.com/content/article/60/66925.htm?lastselectedguid={5FE84E90-BC77-4056-A91C-9531713CA348}>.

ORGANIZATIONS

Centers for Disease Control and Prevention, National Center for Chronic Disease Prevention and Health Promotion. Division of Nutrition and Physical Activity, 4770 Buford Highway, NE, Atlanta, GA 30341-3724. (888) CDC-4NRG ((888) 232-4674). <http://www.cdc.gov>.

The President's Council on Physical Fitness and Sports. Department W, 200 Independence Ave., SW, Room 738-H, Washington, DC 20004. (202) 690-9000; Fax: (202) 690-5211. <http://fitness.gov/index.html>.

Juli M. Berwald

F

Fabry disease

Definition

Fabry disease is a genetic condition that typically affects males. It is caused by deficiency of an enzyme, a chemical that speeds up another chemical reaction. Fabry disease can affect many parts of the body including the kidneys, eyes, brain, and heart. **Pain** in the hands and feet and a characteristic rash are classic features of this disease.

Description

The symptoms of Fabry disease were first described by Dr. Johann Fabry and Dr. William Anderson in 1898. The enzyme deficiency that leads to the disease was identified in the 1960s.

The symptoms of Fabry disease are variable. Some individuals with Fabry disease have severe complications, while others have very mild symptoms. The first sign of the disease may be a painful burning sensation in the hands and feet (acroparesthesias). A red rash, most commonly between the belly button and the knees (angiokeratoma) is also common. The outer portion of the eye (cornea) may also become clouded in individuals with Fabry disease. The progressive buildup of globotriaosylceramide can also lead to kidney problems and heart disease in adulthood.

Demographics

Fabry disease affects approximately one in 40,000 live births. It occurs evenly among all ethnic groups. Almost always, only male children are affected. Although female carriers of the disease occasionally develop symptoms of the disease, it is rare for a female carrier to be severely affected.

Causes and symptoms

Fabry disease is caused by a change (mutation) in the GLA gene. This gene is responsible for the production of the enzyme alpha-galactosidase A. Alpha-galactosidase A

normally breaks down globotriaosylceramide. Globotriaosylceramide is a natural substance in the body, made of sugar and fat. A mutation in the GLA gene leads to a decrease in alpha-galactosidase A activity which, in turn, leads to an excess of globotriaosylceramide. The excess globotriaosylceramide builds up in blood vessels (veins, arteries, and capillaries) and obstructs normal blood flow. It also builds up in parts of the skin, kidneys, heart, and brain. It is this buildup that inhibits normal function and leads to the symptoms associated with the disease.

The gene that produces alpha-galactosidase A is located on the X chromosome. It is called the GLA gene. Since the GLA gene is located on the X chromosome, Fabry disease is considered to be X-linked. This means that it generally affects males.

The signs and symptoms of Fabry disease vary. Some individuals with Fabry disease have many severe symptoms, while other individuals' symptoms may be few and mild. The symptoms typically increase or intensify over time. This progression is caused by the slow buildup of globotriaosylceramide as the person ages.

A painful burning sensation in the hands and feet (acroparesthesias) is one of the first symptoms of Fabry disease. This pain can be severe and may grow worse with **exercise**, stress, illness, extreme heat, or extreme cold. Another symptom of Fabry disease typically present during childhood is a red rash (angiokeratoma). This rash typically develops between the navel and the knees. Children with Fabry disease may also have a clouding of the outer most portion of the eye (cornea). This symptom is usually diagnosed by an eye doctor (ophthalmologist). The cloudiness may increase with time. A decreased ability to sweat is another common symptom of Fabry disease.

Due to the progressive nature of Fabry disease, most affected individuals develop additional symptoms by age 40. The buildup of globotriaosylceramide in the heart can lead to heart problems. These heart problems can include changes in the size of the heart (left ventricular enlargement), differences in the heart beat, and leaky heart valves.

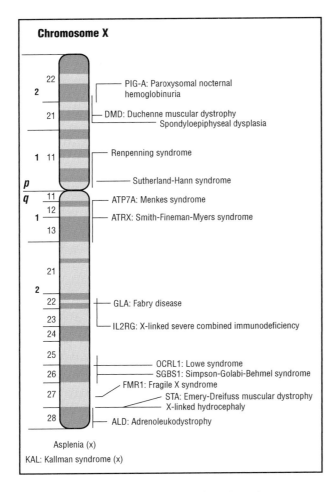

Fabry disease, on chromosome X. *(Gale Group.)*

Mitral valve prolapse is a particular type of leaky heart valve that is common in Fabry disease, even in childhood. The excess globotriaosylceramide can also disrupt normal blood flow in the brain. In some cases this can cause **dizziness**, **seizures**, and **stroke**. The kidneys are other organs affected by Fabry disease. Kidney problems can lead to an abnormal amount of protein in the urine (proteinuria). Severe kidney problems can lead to kidney failure.

Although the symptoms of Fabry disease usually occur in males, female carriers may occasionally exhibit symptoms of the disease. Some carriers experience pain in their hands and feet. Carrier females may also have proteinuria and clouding of their cornea. It is rare for a female to experience all of the symptoms associated with Fabry disease.

Diagnosis

Initially, the diagnosis of Fabry disease is based on the presence of the symptoms. It should also be suspected if there is a family history of the disorder. The diagnosis of Fabry disease is definitively made by measuring the activity of the alpha-galactosidase A enzyme. When the activity is very low, it is diagnostic of Fabry disease. This enzyme analysis can be performed through a blood test. Measuring the activity of the enzyme can also detect female carriers. Women who are carriers of Fabry disease have enzyme activity that is lower than normal.

Prenatal diagnosis is possible by measuring the alpha-galactosidase A activity in fetal tissue drawn by amniocentesis or chorionic villus sampling (CVS). Fetuses should be tested if the mother is a carrier. A woman is at risk of being a carrier if she has a son with Fabry disease or someone in her family has Fabry disease.

Treatment team

A number of specialized practitioners are necessary to care for patients with Fabry disease. Depending on the specific manifestations, these specialists may include a dermatologist to treat skin problems; a **neurologist** to treat such complications as dizziness, seizure, stroke; an ophthalmologist to treat eye problems; a nephrologist to treat kidney problems; a cardiologist to treat heart problems. A pain specialist may be helpful, as well.

Treatment

There is currently no cure for Fabry disease. Until such time as enzyme replacement therapy is proven to be safe and effective, individuals with Fabry disease must rely on traditional treatments. Pain can be treated with medications such as **carbamazepine** and dilantin. Individuals with Fabry disease are recommended to have routine evaluations of their heart and kidneys. Some individuals with kidney disease require a special diet that is low in sodium and protein. Dialysis and kidney transplantation may be necessary for patients with severe kidney disease. Certain medications may reduce the risk of stroke. Finally, individuals with Fabry disease are recommended to avoid the situations that cause the pain in their hands and feet to grow worse. In some situations medication may be required to reduce the pain.

Clinical trials

A number of **clinical trials** are underway. Some are studying the specific nervous system effects of the disase. Others are giving individuals with Fabry disease the alpha-galactosidase A enzyme (Replagal) as a form of enzyme replacement therapy. If successful, this enzyme replacement therapy may reduce or eliminate the symptoms associated with Fabry disease. Clopidogrel, a blood thinner, is also being studied to see if its administration may decrease the rate/severity of such complications as stroke and heart attack.

Key Terms

Acroparesthesias Painful burning sensation in hands and feet.

Amniocentesis A procedure performed at 16–18 weeks of pregnancy in which a needle is inserted through a woman's abdomen into her uterus to draw out a small sample of the amniotic fluid from around the baby. Either the fluid itself or cells from the fluid can be used for a variety of tests to obtain information about genetic disorders and other medical conditions in the fetus.

Angiokeratoma Skin rash comprised of red bumps. Rash most commonly occurs between the navel and the knees.

Blood vessels General term for arteries, veins, and capillaries that transport blood throughout the body.

Chorionic villus sampling (CVS) A procedure used for prenatal diagnosis at 10-12 weeks gestation. Under ultrasound guidance a needle is inserted either through the mother's vagina or abdominal wall and a sample of cells is collected from around the fetus. These cells are then tested for chromosome abnormalities or other genetic diseases.

Cornea The transparent structure of the eye over the lens that is continuous with the sclera in forming the outermost protective layer of the eye.

Dialysis Process by which special equipment purifies the blood of a patient whose kidneys have failed.

Enzyme replacement therapy Giving an enzyme to a person who needs it for normal body function. It is given through a needle that is inserted into the body.

Left ventricular enlargement Abnormal enlargement of the left lower chamber of the heart.

Mitral valve prolapse A heart defect in which one of the valves of the heart (which normally controls blood flow) becomes floppy. Mitral valve prolapse may be detected as a heart murmur, but there are usually no symptoms.

Mutation A permanent change in the genetic material that may alter a trait or characteristic of an individual, or manifest as disease, and can be transmitted to offspring.

Proteinuria Excess protein in the urine.

Prognosis

The prognosis for individuals with Fabry disease is good, especially with the arrival of enzyme replacement therapy. Currently, affected individuals survive into adulthood with the symptoms increasing over time.

Resources

BOOKS

Desnick, Robert J., Yiannis Ioannou, and Christine Eng. "Galactosidase A Deficiency: Fabry Disease." In *The Molecular Bases of Inherited Disease*. 8th ed. New York: McGraw Hill, 2001.

ORGANIZATIONS

Alliance of Genetic Support Groups. 4301 Connecticut Ave. NW, Suite 404, Washington, DC 20008. (202) 966-5557. Fax: (202) 966-8553. <http://www.geneticalliance.org>.

Deptartment of Human Genetics, International Center for Fabry Disease. Box 1497, Fifth Ave. at 100th St., New York, NY 10029. (866) 322-7963. <http://www.mssm.edu/genetics/fabry>.

Fabry Support and Information Group. PO Box 510, 108 NE 2nd St., Suite C, Concordia, MO 64020. (660) 463-1355. <http://www.cpgnet.com/fsig.nsf>.

National Institute of Neurological Disorders and Stroke. 31 Center Drive, MSC 2540, Bldg. 31, Room 8806, Bethesda, MD 20814. (301) 496-5751 or (800) 352-9424. <http://www.ninds.nih.gov>.

National Organization for Rare Disorders (NORD). PO Box 8923, New Fairfield, CT 06812-8923. (203) 746-6518 or (800) 999-6673. Fax: (203) 746-6481. <http://www.rarediseases.org>.

WEBSITES

Fabry Disease Home Page. <http://www.sci.ccny.cuny.edu/~fabry/>.

Online Mendelian Inheritance in Man (OMIM). <http://www.ncbi.nlm.nih.gov/htbin-post/Omim/dispmim?301500>.

Holly Ann Ishmael, MS, CGC
Rosalyn Carson-DeWitt, MD

Facial synkinesis

Definition

Facial synkinesis is the involuntary movement of facial muscles that accompanies purposeful movement of some other set of muscles; for example, facial synkinesis may result in the mouth involuntarily closing or grimacing when the eyes are purposefully closed.

Description

Facial synkinesis occurs during recuperation from conditions or injuries that affect the facial nerve, for example during recovery from **Bell's palsy**. During recovery, as the facial nerve tries to regenerate, some new nerve twigs may accidentally regrow in close proximity to muscles that they wouldn't normally innervate (stimulate). Facial synkinesis may occur transiently, during recovery, or may become a permanent disability.

As with all facial injuries or palsies, facial synkinesis can cause considerable emotional distress. Lack of control over one's facial expressions is known to be a serious psychological stressor.

Causes and symptoms

Facial synkinesis can follow any injury or condition causing palsy or paralysis of the facial nerve. The most common associated disorder is Bell's palsy; about 40% of all individuals who are recovering from Bell's palsy will experience facial synkinesis during recovery. Other conditions that may prompt the development of facial synkinesis include **stroke**, head injury, birth trauma, head injury, trauma following tumor removal (such as acoustic neuroma), infection, **Lyme disease**, diabetes, and **multiple sclerosis**.

Facial synkinesis can cause a number of abnormalities in the facial muscles. For example, when a patient with facial synkinesis tries to close his or her eyes, the muscles around the mouth may twitch or grimace. Conversely, when the patient tries to smile, the eyes may involuntarily close. The phenomenon of purposeful mouth movements resulting in involuntary eye closing is often referred to as "jaw winking." Unfortunately, as with any facial deformity or disability, facial synkinesis carries with it a high risk of concomitant **depression**, anxiety, and disruption of interpersonal relationships and employment.

Diagnosis

Diagnosis is usually apparent on physical examination. When the patient is asked to move certain facial muscles (i.e., smile), other facial muscles will be activated (e.g., the eyes may close involuntarily). When the underlying condition is unclear, a variety of tests may be required, such as **CT** or **MRI** scanning or EMG (electromyographic) testing to evaluate the functioning of the facial nerves and muscles.

Treatment team

Facial synkinesis may be treated by neurologists or otorhinolaryngologists.

Treatment

Treatment may include:

- surgery, to remove causative tumors or other sources of pressure on and damage to the facial nerve
- steroid medications, to decrease inflammation of the facial nerve
- facial exercises
- electrical stimulation (this remains controversial, and may, in fact, worsen facial synkinesis in some patients)
- intensive video-assisted, electromyographic feedback facial muscle retraining
- injections of the paralytic agent botox into the muscle groups that are contracting involuntarily

Prognosis

The prognosis of facial synkinesis is quite variable, depending largely on the prognosis of the underlying condition that caused its development.

Resources

BOOKS

Goetz, Christopher G., ed. *Textbook of Clinical Neurology.* Philadelphia: W. B. Saunders Company, 2003.

PERIODICALS

Armstrong, M. W., R. E. Mountain, and J. A. Murray. "Treatment of facial synkinesis and facial asymmetry with botulinum toxin type A following facial nerve palsy." *Clin Otolaryngol* 21, no. 1 (February 1996): 15–20.

Messé, S. R. "Oculomotor synkinesis following a midbrain stroke." *Neurology* 57, no. 6 (September 2001): 1106–1107.

Münevver, Çelik, Hulki Forta, and Çetin Vural. "The Development of Synkinesis after Facial Nerve Paralysis." *European Neurology* 43 (2000): 147–151.

Zalvan, C., B. Bentsianov, O. Gonzalez-Yanes, and A. Blitzer. "Noncosmetic uses of botulinum toxin." *Dermatol Clin* 22, no. 2 (April 2004): 187–195.

WEBSITES

Diels, H. Jacqueline. *New concepts in Non-Surgical Facial Nerve Rehabilitation.* Bell's Palsy Infosite. (June 2, 2004). <http://www.bellspalsy.ws/printretrain.htm>.

Rosalyn Carson-DeWitt, MD

Fainting

Definition

Fainting is a temporary loss of consciousness, weakness of muscles, and inability to stand up, all caused by sudden loss of blood flow to the brain. Fainting is a relatively common symptom caused by a variety of problems relating to changes in blood pressure. The American Heart Association reports that fainting is responsible for 3% of all visits to emergency rooms and 6% of all admissions to hospitals.

Description

Fainting is a common symptom, also called syncope, vasovagal attack, neurally mediated syncope (NMS), neurocardiogenic syncope, and vasodepressor or reflex mediated syncope. Most simple faints result from an over-stimulation of the autonomic nervous system that results in a drop in blood pressure and a slowed heart rate. Both of these conditions decrease blood flow to the brain, which causes a feeling of lightheadedness (presyncope) or a complete loss of consciousness (syncope). Fainting usually occurs in people who are standing or sitting upright. A person about to faint may also feel nauseated, weak, and warm. The person may experience temporary visual impairment, **headache**, ringing in the ears, shortness of breath, sensation of spinning, tingling in the extremities, and incontinence. A person experiencing presyncope may also appear pale or bluish. When consciousness is lost, a person usually falls down. This allows for more blood flow to the brain, resulting in a return to consciousness, usually within a few minutes.

Causes

Fainting is caused by a variety of factors, including stress, **pain**, overheating, dehydration, excessive sweating, exhaustion, hunger, alcohol, and drugs. Fainting may also be a side effect of some medications. A simple faint resulting from any of these factors is usually not a symptom of a neurological disorder.

Some people faint when changing positions, a condition known as postural hypotension. When people with this condition move from a lying position to a standing or sitting position, the sudden pooling of blood in the legs may cause a temporary decrease in blood circulation to the brain, causing a faint. This condition is common in elderly people who have been bedridden for some time and in people with poor muscle tone.

Some faints indicate serious disorders of the nervous or circulatory systems. Nervous system disorders that cause faints include acute or subacute dysautonomia, post-ganglionic autonomic insufficiency, and chronic preganglionic autonomic insufficiency. Fainting may also signal an irregular pattern of nervous stimulation such as micturition syncope (fainting while urinating), **glossopharyngeal neuralgia** (irritation of the ninth cranial nerve, causing pain in the tongue, throat, ear, and tonsils), cough syncope (fainting while coughing violently), and stretch syncope (fainting when stretching arms and neck). Faints

can also indicate problems with the regulation of blood pressure and heart rate, and with disorders such as diabetes, alcoholism, malnutrition, and amyloidosis. Fainting can signal circulatory problems, particularly those that disrupt blood flow to the brain, as well as problems with the electrical impulses that control the heart, problems with the sinus node of the heart, heart arrhythmia, blood clots in the lung, a narrowing of the aorta, or other anatomical irregularities in the heart. Additionally, hyperventilation, usually associated with anxiety or panic, can result in a faint.

Diagnosis

Patients visiting a doctor because of fainting will usually have their blood pressure checked when they are lying down and then again after they stand up. If there is a significant decrease in blood pressure, it may indicate postural hypotension. A more sophisticated form of this blood pressure test is a tilt test, during which a person is strapped to a board that is rotated from the horizontal to the vertical position. Blood pressure is measured in both positions; an extreme drop indicates postural hypotension.

To test for circulatory problems, a physician may also use an electrocardiogram (EKG) to test for abnormalities of the heart beat. **Exercise** stress tests or wearing a Holter monitor for a day may also be performed to check for disorders of the heart. Fainting suspected to be caused by neurological disorders requires additional tests and evaluation by a **neurologist**.

Treatment

If a person faints while sitting, the body weight should be supported and the head positioned between the knees. If a person faints while standing, the individual should be carefully lowered to the ground and the legs elevated. Any tight clothes, including belts and collars, should be loosened. The head should be turned to the side so that the tongue does not obstruct the trachea and any vomit can be cleared from the airway. If the person stops breathing, cardiopulmonary resuscitation (CPR) should be started and a call should be placed to emergency medical services. A person who has fainted may benefit from cold compresses to the head and neck. After the person regains consciousness, he or she should remain lying or sitting for some time and should stand up only if no feeling of lightheadedness persists.

A person who faints often will be treated for the underlying condition. Often, medications are used to control fainting; however, other methods may be helpful as well. In some people, changing to a high-salt diet or wearing support hose to keep blood from pooling in the legs prevents fainting. Some people may be able to prevent fainting by keeping glucose levels at a more constant level or

Key Terms

Autonomic nervous system   The part of the nervous system that controls so-called involuntary functions, such as heart rate, salivary gland secretion, respiratory function, and pupil dilation.

Postural hypotension   A drop in blood pressure that causes faintness or dizziness and occurs when an individual rises to a standing position. Also known as orthostatic hypotension.

Syncope   A loss of consciousness over a short period of time, caused by a temporary lack of oxygen in the brain.

by learning breathing techniques to prevent hyperventilation. Another technique for preventing faints is drinking enough fluid to keep blood volume high.

Resources

BOOKS

Icon Health Publications. *The Official Patient's Sourcebook on Syncope: A Revised and Updated Directory for the Internet Age.* San Diego, CA: ICON Group International, 2003.

OTHER

DeNoon, Daniel. *Fainting Is a Serious Symptom.* WebMD. January 14, 2002 (March 18, 2004). <http://my.webmd.com/content/Article/35/1728_96070.htm>.

Fainting. FamilyDoctor. March, 2002 (March 18, 2004). <http://familydoctor.org/x1682.xml?printxml>.

Grayson, Charlotte. *Understanding Fainting—The Basics.* WebMD. January 1, 2002 (March 18, 2004). <http://mywebmd.com/content/article/7/2951_478>.

The Mayo Clinic Staff. *Simple Faint (Vasovagal Syncope).* The Mayo Clinic. June 26, 2003 (March 18, 2004). <http://www.mayoclinic.com/invoke.cfm?id=AN00103>.

Syncope. American Heart Association. December 22, 2003 (March 18, 2004). <http://www.americanheart.org/presenter.jhtml?identifier=4749>.

ORGANIZATIONS

American Heart Association National Center. 7272 Greenville Avenue, Dallas, TX 75231. (800) AHA-USA1. <http://www.americanheart.org/presenter.jhtml?identifier=1200000>.

National Heart, Blood and Lung Institute. P.O. Box 30105, Bethesda, MD 20824-0105. (301) 592-8573; Fax: (301) 592-8563. <http://www.nhlbi.nih.gov/index.htm>.

National Institute of Neurological Disorders and Stroke. P.O. Box 5801, Bethesda, MD 20824. (301) 496-5751 or (800) 352-9424. <http://www.ninds.nih.gov/>.

Juli M. Berwald

Familial hemangioma *see* **Cerebral cavernous malformation**

Familial spastic paralysis *see* **Hereditary spastic paraplegia**

Fatigue

Definition

Fatigue may be defined as a subjective state in which one feels tired or exhausted, and in which the capacity for normal work or activity is reduced. There is, however, no commonly accepted definition of fatigue when it is considered in the context of health and illness. This lack of definition results from the fact that a person's experience of fatigue depends on a variety of factors. These factors include culture, personality, the physical environment (light, noise, vibration), availability of social support through networks of family members and friends, the nature of a particular fatiguing disease or disorder, and the type and duration of work or **exercise**. The experience of fatigue associated with disease will be different for someone who is clinically depressed, is socially isolated, and is out of shape, as compared to another person who is not depressed, has many friends, and is aerobically fit.

Description

Fatigue is sometimes characterized as normal or abnormal. For example, the feeling of tiredness or even exhaustion after exercising is a normal response and is relieved by resting; many people report that the experience of ordinary tiredness after exercise is pleasant. Moreover, this type of fatigue is called "acute" since the onset is sudden and the desired activity level returns after resting. On the other hand, there is fatigue that is not perceived as ordinary, that may develop insidiously over time, is unpleasant or seriously distressing, and is not resolved by rest. This kind of fatigue is abnormal and is called "chronic."

Some researchers regard fatigue as a defense mechanism that promotes the effective regulation of energy expenditures. According to this theory, when people feel tired they take steps to avoid further stress (physical or emotional) by resting or by avoiding the stressor. They are then conserving energy. Since chronic fatigue is not normal, however, it is a common symptom of some mental disorders, a variety of physical diseases with known etiologies (causes), and medical conditions that have no biological markers although they have recognizable syndromes (patterns of symptoms and signs).

Fatigue is sometimes described as being primary or secondary. Primary fatigue is a symptom of a disease or mental disorder, and may be part of a cluster of such symptoms as **pain**, fever, or nausea. As the disease or disorder progresses, however, the fatigue may be intensified by the patient's worsening condition, by the other disease symptoms, or by the surgical or medical treatment given to the patient. This subsequent fatigue is called secondary.

Risk factors

Fatigue is a common experience. It is one of the top ten symptoms that people mention when they visit the doctor. Some people, however, are at higher risk for developing fatigue. The risk for women is about 1.5 times the risk for men, and the risk for people who do not exercise is twice that of active people. Some researchers question whether women really are at higher risk, since women are more likely than men to go to the doctor with health problems; also, men are less likely to admit they feel fatigued. Other risk factors include obesity, smoking, use of alcohol, high stress levels, **depression**, anxiety, and low blood pressure. Having low blood pressure is usually considered desirable in the United States, but is regarded as a treatable condition in other countries. Low blood pressure or postural hypotension (sudden lowering of blood pressure caused by standing up) may cause fatigue, **dizziness**, or **fainting**.

Major sources of chronic fatigue
Disease

There are many diseases and disorders in which fatigue is a major symptom—for example, cancer, cardiovascular disease, emphysema, **multiple sclerosis**, rheumatic arthritis, systemic **lupus** erythematosus, HIV/AIDS, infectious mononucleosis, chronic fatigue syndrome, and fibromyalgia. The reasons for the fatigue, however, vary according to the organ system or body function affected by the disease.

Physical reasons for fatigue include:

- Circulatory and respiratory impairment. When the patient's breathing and blood circulation are impaired, or when the patient has anemia (low levels of red blood cells), body tissues do not receive as much oxygen and energy. Consequently, the patient experiences a general sense of fatigue. Fatigue is also an important warning sign of heart trouble; it precedes 30–55% of myocardial infarctions (heart attacks) and sudden cardiac deaths.

- Infection. Microorganisms that disturb body metabolism and produce toxic wastes cause disease and lead to fatigue. Fatigue is an early primary symptom of chronic, nonlocalized infections found in such diseases as acquired immune deficiency syndrome (**AIDS**), **Lyme disease**, and tuberculosis.

KEY TERMS

Biological marker An indicator or characteristic trait of a disease that facilitates differential diagnosis (the process of distinguishing one disorder from other, similar disorders).

Deconditioning Loss of physical strength or stamina resulting from bed rest or lack of exercise.

Electrolytes Substances or elements that dissociate into electrically charged particles (ions) when dissolved in the blood. The electrolytes in human blood include potassium, magnesium, and chloride.

Metabolism The group of biochemical processes within the body that release energy in support of life.

Stress A physical and psychological response that results from being exposed to a demand or pressure.

Syndrome A group of symptoms that together characterize a disease or disorder.

- Nutritional disorders or imbalances. Malnutrition is a disorder that promotes disease. It is caused by insufficient intake of important nutrients, vitamins, and minerals; by problems with absorption of food through the digestive system; or by inadequate calorie consumption. Protein-energy malnutrition (PEM) occurs when people do not consume enough protein or calories; this condition leads to wasting of muscles and commonly occurs in developing countries. In particular, young children who are starving are at risk of PEM, as are people recovering from major illness. In general, malnutrition damages the body's immune function and thereby encourages disease and fatigue. Taking in too many calories for the body's needs, on the other hand, results in obesity, which is a predictor of many diseases related to fatigue.

- Dehydration. Dehydration results from water and sodium imbalances in body tissues. The loss of total body water and sodium may be caused by diarrhea, vomiting, bed rest, overexposure to heat, or exercise. Dehydration contributes to muscle weakness and mental confusion; it is a common and overlooked source of fatigue. Once fatigued, people are less likely to consume enough fluids and nutrients, which makes the fatigue and confusion worse.

- Deconditioning. This term refers to generalized organ system deterioration resulting from bed rest and lack of exercise. In the 1950s and 1970s, the National Aeronautics and Space Administration (NASA) studied the effects

GALE ENCYCLOPEDIA OF NEUROLOGICAL DISORDERS

363

of bed rest on healthy athletes. The researchers found that deconditioning occurred rapidly (within 24 hours) and led to depression and weakness. Even mild exercise can counteract deconditioning, however, and it has become an important means of minimizing depression and fatigue resulting from disease and hospitalization.

- Pain. When pain is severe enough, it may disrupt sleep and lead to the development of such sleep disorders as insomnia or **hypersomnia**. (Insomnia is the term for having difficulty falling and/or staying asleep. Hypersomnia refers to excessive sleeping.) In general, disrupted sleep is not restorative; people wake up feeling tired, and as a result their pain is worsened and they may become depressed. Furthermore, pain may interfere with movement or lead to too much bed rest, which results in deconditioning. Sometimes pain leads to social isolation because the person cannot cope with the physical effort involved in maintaining social relationships, or because family members are unsympathetic or resentful of the ill or injured person's reduced capacity for work or participation in family life. All of these factors worsen pain, contributing to further sleep disruption, fatigue, and depression.

- Stress. When someone experiences ongoing pain and stress, organ systems and functional processes eventually break down. These include cardiovascular, digestive, and respiratory systems, as well as the efficient elimination of body wastes. According to the American Psychiatric Association, various chronic diseases are related to stress, including regional enteritis (intestinal inflammation), ulcerative colitis (a disease of the colon), gastric ulcers, rheumatoid arthritis, cardiac angina, and dysmenorrhea (painful menstruation). These diseases deplete the body's levels of serotonin (a neurotransmitter important in the regulation of sleep and wakefulness, as well as depression), and endorphins (opiate-like substances that moderate pain). Depletion of these body chemicals leads to insomnia and chronic fatigue.

- Sleep disorders. There are a variety of sleep disorders that cause fatigue, including insomnia, hypersomnia, **sleep apnea**, and **restless legs syndrome**. For example, hypersomnia may be the result of brain abnormalities caused by viral infections. Researchers studying the aftermath of infectious mononucleosis proposed that exposure to viral infections might change brain function with the effect of minimizing restorative sleep. Another common disorder is sleep apnea, in which the patient's breathing stops for at least 10 seconds, usually more than 20 times per hour. Snoring is common. People may experience choking and then wake up gasping for air; they may develop daytime hypersomnia (daytime sleepiness) to compensate. Sleep apnea is associated with aging, weight gain, and depression. It is also a risk factor for

stroke and myocardial infarctions. Restless legs syndrome is a condition in which very uncomfortable sensations in the patient's legs cause them to move and wake up from sleep, or keep them from falling asleep. All of these disorders reduce the quality of a person's sleep and are associated with fatigue.

Fibromyalgia and chronic fatigue syndrome

Fibromyalgia (also known as myofascial syndrome or fibrositis) is characterized by painful and achy muscles, tendons, and ligaments. There are 18 locations on the body where patients typically feel sore. These locations include areas on the lower back and along the spine, neck, and thighs. A diagnostic criterion for fibromyalgia (FM) is that at least 11 of the 18 sites are painful. In addition to pain, people with FM may experience sleep disorders, fatigue, anxiety, and irritable bowel syndrome. Some researchers maintain, however, that when fatigue is severe, chronic, and persistent, FM is indistinguishable from chronic fatigue syndrome (CFS). The care that patients receive for FM or CFS depends in large measure on whether they were referred to a rheumatologist (a doctor who specializes in treating diseases of the joints and muscles), **neurologist**, or psychiatrist.

Some doctors do not accept CFS (also known as myalgic encephalomyelitis) as a legitimate medical problem. This refusal is stigmatizing and distressing to the person who must cope with disabling pain and fatigue. Many people with CFS may see a number of different physicians before finding one who is willing to diagnose CFS. Nevertheless, major health agencies such as the Centers for Disease Control (CDC) in the United States have studied the syndrome. As a result, a revised CDC case definition for CFS was published in 1994 that lists major and minor criteria for diagnosis. The major criteria of CFS include the presence of chronic and persistent fatigue for at least six months; fatigue that does not improve with rest; and fatigue that causes significant interference with the patient's daily activities. Minor criteria include such flu-like symptoms as fever, sore throat, swollen lymph nodes, myalgia (muscle pain), difficulty with a level of physical exercise that the patient had performed easily before the illness, sleep disturbances, and headaches. Additionally, people often have difficulty concentrating and remembering information and they experience extreme frustration and depression as a result of the limitations imposed by CFS. The prognosis for recovery from CFS is poor, although the symptoms are manageable.

Psychological disorders

While fatigue may be caused by many organic diseases and medical conditions, it is a chief complaint for several mental disorders, including generalized anxiety disorder and clinical depression. Moreover, mental disorders may coexist with physical disease. When there is considerable symptom overlap, the differential diagnosis of fatigue is especially difficult.

GENERALIZED ANXIETY DISORDER

People are diagnosed as having generalized anxiety disorder (GAD) if they suffer from overwhelming worry or apprehension that persists, usually daily, for at least six months, and if they also experience some of the following symptoms: unusual tiredness, restlessness and irritability, problems with concentration, muscle tension, and disrupted sleep. Such stressful life events as divorce, unemployment, illness, or being the victim of a violent crime are associated with GAD, as is a history of psychiatric problems. Some evidence suggests that women who have been exposed to danger are at risk of developing GAD; women who suffer loss are at risk of developing depression, and women who experience danger and loss are at risk of developing a mix of both GAD and depression.

While the symptoms of CFS and GAD overlap, the disorders have different primary complaints. Patients with CFS complain primarily of tiredness, whereas people with GAD describe being excessively worried. In general, some researchers believe that anxiety contributes to fatigue by disrupting rest and restorative sleep.

DEPRESSION

In the fourth edition of the *Diagnostic and Statistical Manual of Mental Disorders* (DSM-IV), the presence of depressed mood or sadness, or loss of pleasure in life, is an important diagnostic criterion for depression. Daily fatigue, lack of energy, insomnia, and hypersomnia are indicators of a depressed mood. The symptoms of depression overlap with those of CFS; for example, some researchers report that 89% of people with depression are fatigued, as compared to 86–100% of people with CFS. The experience of fatigue, however, seems to be more disabling with CFS than with depression. Another difference between CFS and depression concerns the onset of the disorder. Most patients with CFS experience a sudden or acute onset, whereas depression may develop over a period of weeks or months. Also, while both types of patients experience sleep disorders, CFS patients tend to have difficulty falling asleep, whereas depressed patients tend to wake early in the morning.

Some researchers believe that there is a link between depression, fatigue, and exposure to too much REM sleep. There are five distinct phases in human sleep. The first two are characterized by light sleep; the second two by a deep restorative sleep called slow-wave sleep; and the last by rapid eye movement, or REM, sleep. Most dreams occur during REM sleep. Throughout the night, the intervals of REM sleep increase and usually peak around 8:30 A.M. A

sleep deprivation treatment for depression involves reducing patients' amount of REM sleep by waking them around 6:00 A.M. Researchers think that some fatigue associated with disease may be a form of mild depression and that reducing the amount of REM sleep will reduce fatigue by moderating depression.

Managing fatigue

The management of fatigue depends in large measure on its causes and the person's experience of it. For example, if fatigue is acute and normal, the person will recover from feeling tired after exertion by resting. In cases of fatigue associated with influenza or other infectious illnesses, the person will feel energy return as they recover from the illness. When fatigue is chronic and abnormal, however, the doctor will tailor a treatment program to the patient's needs. There are a variety of approaches that include:

• Aerobic exercise. Physical activity increases fitness and counteracts depression.

• Hydration (adding water). Water improves muscle turgor, or tension, and helps to carry electrolytes.

• Improving sleep patterns. The patient's sleep may be more restful when its timing and duration are controlled.

• Pharmacotherapy (treatment with medications). The patient may be given various medications to treat physical diseases or mental disorders, to control pain, or to manage sleeping patterns.

• Psychotherapy. There are several different treatment approaches that help patients manage stress, understand the motives that govern their behavior, or change maladaptive ideas and negative thinking patterns.

• Physical therapy. This form of treatment helps patients improve or manage functional impairments or disabilities.

In addition to seeking professional help, people can understand and manage fatigue by joining appropriate self-help groups, reading informative books, seeking information from clearinghouses on the Internet, and visiting websites maintained by national organizations for various diseases.

Resources
BOOKS

Beers, Mark H., and Robert Berkow, eds. *The Merck Manual of Diagnosis and Therapy*, 17th ed. Whitehouse Station, NJ: Merck Research Laboratories, 1999.

Glaus, A. *Fatigue in Patients with Cancer: Analysis and Assessment.* Recent Results in Cancer Research, no. 145. Berlin, Germany: Springer-Verlag, 1998.

Hubbard, John R., and Edward A. Workman, eds. *Handbook of Stress Medicine: An Organ System Approach.* Boca Raton, FL: CRC Press, 1998.

Natelson, Benjamin H. *Facing and Fighting Fatigue: A Practical Approach.* New Haven, CT: Yale University Press, 1998.

Winningham, Maryl L., and Margaret Barton-Burke, eds. *Fatigue in Cancer: A Multidimensional Approach.* Sudbury, MA: Jones and Bartlett Publishers, 2000.

PERIODICALS

Natelson, Benjamin H. "Chronic Fatigue Syndrome." *JAMA: Journal of the American Medical Association* 285, no. 20 (May 23–30 2001): 2557–59.

ORGANIZATIONS

MEDLINEplus Health Information. U.S. National Library of Medicine, 8600 Rockville Pike, Bethesda, MD 20894. (888) 346-3656. <http://www.medlineplus.gov>.

National Chronic Fatigue Syndrome and Fibromyalgia Association. P.O. Box 18426, Kansas City, MO 64133. (816) 313-2000.

Tanja Bekhuis, PhD
Rosalyn Carson-DeWitt, MD

Febrile seizures

Definition

Febrile **seizures** are the most common type of convulsions in infants or small children and are triggered by fever. It is not in the strict sense an **epilepsy** syndrome but rather a symptom of a febrile illness, and it normally affects children between three months and five years of age, mainly toddlers. During a febrile seizure, a child may lose consciousness and move or shake the limbs. The seizure itself is normally harmless and does not cause brain damage. A child who experiences a seizure in the setting of a fever should be taken to the hospital so that any serious causes of the fever can be evaluated.

Description

Febrile seizures (or convulsions) occur mainly in children between three months and five years of age and are associated with a fever of any cause. Toddlers are most commonly affected and there is a tendency for febrile seizures to run in families. These seizures are associated with fevers that rapidly rise to temperature up to or above 102°F, but they can also occur with lower temperatures.

There are two types of febrile seizures: simple (or benign) and complex. Benign febrile seizures account for 80–85% of all febrile seizures, and last less than 15 minutes. They usually do not recur within 24 hours. Complex febrile seizures, which suggest a more serious illness, account for 15–20% of all cases, last more than 15 minutes, and can recur within 24 hours.

Children with febrile seizures often lose consciousness and shake, moving limbs on both sides of the body. Less commonly, children become rigid or have twitches on only one side of the body.

Demographics

About 2–5% of all children experience a febrile seizure and about 25% of these children have a first-degree relative with history of febrile seizures. There is a slightly higher prevalence among boys, and no ethnic differences have been reported. Less than 5% of children with febrile seizures will eventually develop epilepsy.

Causes and symptoms

The exact role of the fever in the development of seizures is not clear. However, it is known that viral infections are the most common cause of fever in children with a first febrile seizure who are admitted to hospitals, mainly caused by viruses like herpes and influenza. Meningitis causes less than 1% of febrile seizures, but should be investigated to rule out this serious infection, especially in children less than one year old or those who continue to appear ill after the fever subsides. Seizures that occur after immunizations are likely to be the febrile type due to temperature elevation, particularly those after the DTP (diphtheria, pertussis, tetanus) and measles immunizations. Upper respiratory tract infections accompanied by high fever, in combination with a low seizure threshold, can often affect infants and young children and, thus, account for the most common cause of these convulsions.

In a few studies, children with febrile seizures have been found to have decreased zinc levels in both the serum and the cerebrospinal fluid, which is the fluid that bathes the brain and the spinal cord. Deprivation of zinc may play a role in the seizures. Children with iron-deficiency anemia have been shown to have febrile seizures at a higher rate than nonanemic children.

There is a positive family history in up to 31% of all cases of febrile seizures, although the exact mode of inheritance is not known and varies among families. It has long been recognized that there is a genetic component for the susceptibility to this type of seizure; this may be caused by mutations in several genes, especially the FB4 gene.

Febrile seizures typically begin with a sudden contraction of muscles on both sides of the body, usually facial muscles, trunk, arms, and legs. The force of the

Key Terms

Epilepsy A disorder of the central nervous system characterized by seizures.

Meningitis Inflammation of the meninges, the membranes that surround the brain and spinal cord.

Seizure Abnormal electrical discharge of neurons in the brain, often resulting in abnormal body movements or behaviors.

muscle contraction may cause the child to emit an involuntary cry or moan. The child falls, if standing, and may bite the tongue. Urinary incontinence and vomiting can occur. The child will not breathe, and may turn blue. Children cannot respond to any stimuli, and loss of consciousness, hallucinations, confusion, and feelings of fear or other emotions may occur. Focal seizures (those without loss of consciousness) involving only a part of the body are less common, and might become generalized, affecting the whole body.

Diagnosis

The first action of the physician is to stop the fever and find its cause(s). Physicians may ask about previous seizures without a fever, which can indicate that the child is more likely to have an underlying seizure disorder such as epilepsy rather than a febrile seizure. Physicians also consider the family history of seizures, febrile or otherwise, and must investigate any known nervous disorder in the child, such as developmental delay or severe head injury. Any medication the child has taken is suspicious, and the possibility of drug reaction or poisoning may also be considered.

It is important to rule out any infectious disease as the first cause of a seizure, especially meningitis. In the case of meningitis, the child appears particularly ill, shows neck rigidity, has an unusually long period of drowsiness after the seizure, and experiences a complex febrile seizure (often prolonged and repeated). Lumbar puncture (commonly known as a spinal tap) can be performed in this case to examine the cerebrospinal fluid for indications of meningitis. Other tests such as blood tests, urine tests, and x rays may be used in diagnosing the cause of fever.

Treatment team

A pediatrician is normally the first physician to be seen, and a **neurologist** should be considered for those cases in which a neurological disorder is thought to be the cause of the seizure rather than the fever.

Treatment

During the acute phase of the seizure, the main objective is to keep the child in a position on his or her side or stomach to avoid aspiration of saliva or vomit and avoid injuries. The child should be placed on the floor or in a safe area, and all dangerous objects must be removed. A child having a seizure should not be restrained. If the child vomits, or if saliva and mucus build up in the mouth, a side posture should be used. It is also important that parents do not force anything into the child's mouth, as this could result in breaking teeth. Also, tongue swallowing will not occur. If the child inadvertently bites the tongue, it will heal. Any tight clothing should be removed, especially around the neck. Because the seizure occurs in the setting of a fever, the main target of therapy is to bring the fever down. Removing the clothes and applying cool washcloths to the child's neck and face may help, and acetaminophen or ibuprofen suppositories, if available, may control the elevated temperature.

Rarely, a child may experience a persistent seizure, which could evolve into what is called **status epilepticus**. Airway management and anticonvulsivants are the first line of treatment during this medical emergency.

The most commonly used medication includes **benzodiazepines** such as lorazepan (Ativan) and **diazepam** (Valium). An intravenous line is usually placed in the vein because it is the fastest and most reliable means of drug administration.

Recovery and rehabilitation

Children are normally drowsy or in a state of confusion after a seizure, but become responsive within 15–30 minutes. A simple febrile seizure stops by itself within a few seconds to 10 minutes, usually followed by a brief period of drowsiness or confusion. In this case, an antiseizure medication may not be required. After a seizure, the child is twitchy, with jerks of the arms and legs.

Clinical trials

As of early 2004, there are no open **clinical trials** for febrile seizures at the National Institutes of Health (NIH). However, the National Institute of Neurological Disorders and Stroke (NINDS), a part of the NIH, often sponsors research on febrile seizures in medical centers throughout the United States.

Prognosis

About 35% of children who have had a febrile seizure will have another one with a subsequent fever. Of those who do, about 50% will have a third seizure. Few children have more than three seizure episodes. A child is more likely to fall in the group that has more than one febrile seizure if there is a family history, if the first seizure happened before 12 months of age, or if the seizure happened with a fever below 102°F.

Seizures occur at the time the brain is sensitive to the effects of temperature and often cause parents great anxiety. As the onset is dramatic, parents are afraid their children will die or undergo brain damage. However, simple febrile seizures are harmless and they do not cause death, brain damage, epilepsy, **mental retardation**, or learning difficulties.

Special concerns

Parental anxiety or other factors may cause a child to be placed on long-term anticonvulsant medicine. This will not benefit the patient. Children with the possibility of having a second seizure should not engage in activities that are potentially harmful, such as taking unsupervised baths or climbing higher than 5 ft (1.5 m) off the ground.

Resources

BOOKS

Baram, Tallie Z., and Shlomo Shinnar. *Febrile Seizures.* New York: Academic Press, 2001.

Icon Health Publications Staff. *The Official Parent's Sourcebook on Febrile Seizures: A Revised and Updated Directory for the Internet Age.* San Diego: Icon Group International, 2002.

PERIODICALS

Baumann, R. J., and P. K. Duffner. "Treatment of Children with Simple Febrile Seizures: The AAP Practice Parameter." *Pediatr Neurol 23* (2000): 11–17.

OTHER

"NINDS Febrile Seizures Information Page." *National Institute of Neurological Disorders and Stroke.* March 4, 2004 (April 27, 2004). <http://www.ninds.nih.gov/health_and_medical/disorders/febrile_seizures.htm>.

ORGANIZATIONS

Epilepsy Foundation. 4351 Garden City Drive, Landover, MD 20785-7223. (301) 459-3700 or (800) 332-1000; Fax: (301) 577-2684. postmaster@efa.org. <http://www.epilepsyfoundation.org>.

Marcos do Carmo Oyama
Iuri Drumond Louro, MD, PhD

Felbamate

Definition

Felbamate is an anticonvulsant indicated for the control of **seizures** in the treatment of **epilepsy**, a neurological dysfunction in which excessive surges of electrical energy are emitted in the brain.

Purpose

Felbamate is thought to decrease abnormal activity and excitement within the **central nervous system** (CNS) that may trigger seizures. While felbamate controls some types of seizures associated with epilepsy, there is no known cure for the disorder. Felbamate has shown effectiveness in controlling partial seizures in adults when prescribed alone. When prescribed with other antiepileptic medicines, felbamate has shown effectiveness in managing the intractable (difficult to control) seizures of **Lennox-Gastaut syndrome** in children.

Description

In the United States, felbamate is sold under the brand name Felbatol and FBM. Felbamate acts to depress CNS function; however the precise mechanisms by which it exerts its therapeutic effects in the prevention of seizures is unknown.

Recommended dosage

Felbamate is taken by mouth and is available in tablet or oral suspension form. Adult patients usually take felbamate three to four times daily. The typical total daily dose for an adult or teenager over 14-years-old ranges from 1200 mg to 3600 mg. Treatment including felbamate is appropriate for some children with intractable seizures. The typical total daily dosage formula for a child is between 15 mg and 45 mg per kilogram of body weight.

Beginning a course of treatment which includes felbamate requires a gradual dose-increasing regimen. Patients typically take a reduced dose at the beginning of treatment. The prescribing physician will determine the proper beginning dosage and may raise a patient's daily dosage gradually over the course of several weeks. It may take several weeks to realize the full benefits of felbamate.

It is important to not take a double dose of felbamate. If a daily dose is missed, take it as soon as possible. However, if it is almost time for the next dose, then skip the missed dose. When ending treatment for epilepsy that includes felbamate, physicians typically direct patients to gradually taper their daily dosages. Stopping the medicine suddenly may cause seizures to return or occur more frequently.

Precautions

Prior to initiating therapy with felbamate, blood tests to check for anemia, infection, and liver function will likely be performed. Periodic blood tests are necessary to monitor liver and bone marrow function while receiving felbamate therapy, and for a period after the drug is discontinued.

Key Terms

Epilepsy A disorder associated with disturbed electrical discharges in the central nervous system that cause seizures.

Seizure A convulsion, or uncontrolled discharge of nerve cells that may spread to other cells throughout the brain, resulting in abnormal body movements or behaviors.

Felbamate may not be suitable for persons with a history of **stroke**, anemia, liver or kidney disease, mental illness, diabetes, high blood presure, angina (chest **pain**), irregular heartbeats, or other heart problems.

Before beginning treatment with felbamate, patients should notify their physician if they consume a large amount of alcohol, have a history of drug use, are pregnant, nursing, or plan on becoming pregnant. Research in animals indicates that felbamate may inhibit fetal growth and development. Patients who become pregnant while taking felbamate should contact their physician.

Consult a physician before taking felbamate with certain non-perscription medications. Patients should avoid alcohol and CNS depressants (medicines that can make one drowsy or less alert, such as antihistimines, sleep medications, and some pain medications) while taking felbamate.

Side effects

Patients should discuss with their physicians the risks and benefits of treatment including felbamate before taking the medication. Dizziness and nausea are the most frequently reported side effects. Most mild side effects do not require medical treatment, and may diminish with continued use of the medication. Additional possible mild side effects include anorexia (loss of appetite), vomiting, insomnia, **headache**, and sleepiness. If any symptoms persist or become too uncomfortable, the prescribing physician should be consulted.

Felbamate has been implicated as the cause of serious side effects, including plastic anemia (bone marrow failure) and liver failure. It is estimated that one in every 3,600 to 5,000 patients taking felbamate will eventually develop aplastic anemia, and the fatality rate of complicating aplastic anemia is nearly 30%. For this reason, felbamate is prescribed seldomly, and only after other medications have failed to control seizures. Persons taking felbamate who experience any of the following symptoms should immediately contact a physician:

- rash or purple spots on skin
- nosebleed
- yellow tint to eyes or skin
- bruising easily
- signs of infection
- weakness and fatigue

Interactions

Felbamate should be used with other other seizure prevention medications (**anticonvulsants** or anti-epileptic drugs [AEDs]), only if prescribed by a physician. Felbamate increases blood levels of phenytoin (Dilantin) and valproic acid (Depekene), while reducing blood levels of **carbamazepine** (Tegretol).

Felbamate, like many other anticonvulsants, may decrease the effectiveness of oral contraceptives (birth control pills) or contraceptives containing estrogen.

Resources

BOOKS

Devinsky, Orrin, M.D. *Epilepsy: Patient and Family Guide,* 2nd. ed. Philadelphia: F. A. Davis Co., 2001.

Weaver, Donald F. *Epilepsy and Seizures: Everything You Need to Know.* Toronto: Firefly Books, 2001.

OTHER

Dodson, W. Edwin. M.D. *Hard Choices with Felbamate.* Washington University School of Medicine. (April 23, 2004). <http://www.neuro.wustl.edu/epilepsy/pediatric/articleFelbamate.html>

"Felbamate (Systemic)." *Medline Plus.* National Library of Medicine. (April 23, 2004). <http://www.nlm.nih.gov/medlineplus/druginfo/uspdi/202711.html>

ORGANIZATIONS

American Epilepsy Society. 342 North Main Street, West Hartford, CT 06117-2507, USA. <http://www.aesnet.org>.

Epilepsy Foundation. 4351 Garden City Drive, Landover, MD 20785-7223. (800) 332-1000. <http://www.epilepsyfoundation.org>.

Adrienne Wilmoth Lerner

Fisher syndrome

Definition

Fisher syndrome is a rare, acute neurological disorder characterized by a triad of clinical manifestations that includes brain-damage associated abnormal coordination (**ataxia**), a condition that involves the paralysis of the eyes called ophthalmoplegia, and a generalized absence of reflexes (areflexia).

Description

Fisher syndrome is also known as Miller Fisher syndrome, as was described in 1956 by Canadian physician Charles Miller Fisher. It is an acute, rare nerve disease that is considered to be a variant of **Guillain-Barré syndrome**. In both syndromes, the associated nerve disease can be acquired after viral illness. Once the disorder is diagnosed and treated, the physical and mental effects can be minimal or absent, thus emphasizing the importance of medically identifying affected individuals and treating them accordingly.

Fisher syndrome is also known as acute idiopathic ophthalmologic neuropathy syndrome of ophthalmoplegia, ataxia, and areflexia. Related conditions include disorders called Bickerstaff's brainstem **encephalopathy** and acute ophthalmoparesis.

Demographics

Fisher syndrome is an extremely rare disorder. It is reported to affect persons between the ages of 38 and 65 years old. The related Guillain-Barré syndrome is more common than Fisher syndrome. Age is not a factor, and anyone who produces specific antibodies can acquire it.

Causes and symptoms

The majority of affected individuals with Fisher syndrome produce an antibody by their immune system that is related to the susceptibility to develop the disease following a viral illness; it is unclear how. It is thought that the antibody anti-GQ1b IgG is associated with paralysis of the eye, or ophthalmoplegia. The cause of Fisher syndrome and Guillain-Barré syndrome in both cases is due to an autoimmune disease whereby antibodies produced by the body's immune system mistakenly attack a nerve insulator and impulse carrier called the myelin sheath. This causes inflammation and damage to the nervous system. Guillain-Barré syndrome differs from Fisher syndrome in that different nerve groups are targeted and paralysis in the former begins with the legs and moves upward. Fisher syndrome, on the other hand, begins in the head (paralysis of the eyes) and moves in the direction toward the neck and arms. Although the direct cause is unknown, 65% of cases are thought to be linked to herpes-related viral illness (although viruses other than herpes can also be involved).

The first symptoms appear to be related to a virus and include a **headache**, fever, and pneumonia. The characteristic triad of symptoms that result in individuals who acquire Fisher syndrome is in addition to generalized muscle atrophy (weakness) and respiratory complications that can involve respiratory failure if untreated. It is uncommon to observe a patient with Fisher syndrome that does not have some degree of generalized weakness. Damage to motor function is believed to be associated with damage sustained by the cranial nerves of the brain, with sensory nerve damage extending to the patient's arms and legs. In cases that also include abnormalities in the brainstem, it is more likely to be due to a related disorder called Bickerstaff's syndrome.

Diagnosis

Diagnosis is made clinically by detecting manifestations involving the characteristic trio of symptoms usually following a viral infection: paralysis of the eyes (ophthalmoplegia), abnormal coordination (ataxia), and absence of reflexes (areflexia).

Treatment team

Patients are usually treated by a physician that specializes in infectious diseases, and a **neurologist**. Diagnosis and treatment are usually made by these professionals.

Treatment

Treatment for Fisher syndrome involves removing the plasma from affected individuals, a procedure called plasmapheresis. In doing so, antibodies that cause the disease are also removed. In the alternative, patients can be treated with an intravenous injection of immunoglobulin (IVIg) to boost the immune system. Untreated patients can experience double vision, nausea, difficulty walking, and sensitivity to light that can continue for several months.

Recovery and rehabilitation

Once Fisher syndrome is identified, treatment can lead to recovery in as soon as two to four weeks after the symptoms are initially acquired. After six months, the symptoms are usually almost completely resolved. Although some individuals have secondary complications and relapses occur in 3% of cases, most individuals have a nearly complete recovery.

Clinical trials

As most affected individuals who are treated have a good prognosis, **clinical trials** to treat the disorder are not currently being investigated. There is research being conducted to find better ways to diagnose and ultimately cure the neurological damage that sometimes occurs in Fisher syndrome.

Prognosis

The prognosis is good for individuals who are detected and treated soon after the onset of symptoms. In these cases, affected individuals have a favorable prognosis and (on average) should expect to have a normal lifespan. This disorder is seldom life-threatening.

Key Terms

Areflexia   Absence of a reflex; a sign of possible nerve damage.

Ataxia   Loss of coordinated movement caused by disease of nervous system.

Ophthalmoplegia   Paralysis of the motor nerves of the eye.

Resources

BOOKS

Staff. *The Official Patient's Sourcebook on Miller Fisher Syndrome: A Revised and Updated Directory for the Internet Age.* San Diego: Icon Group International, 2002.

PERIODICALS

Derakhshan, I. "Recurrent Miller Fisher Syndrome." *Neurol India.* (June 2003): 283.

OTHER

NINDS Miller Fisher Syndrome Information Page. National Institute of Neurological Disorders and Stroke. March 4, 2004 (May 22, 2004). <http://www.ninds.nih.gov/health_and_medical/disorders/miller_fisher.htm>.

ORGANIZATIONS

Guillain-Barré Syndrome Foundation International. P.O. Box 262, Wynnewood, PA 19096. (610) 667-0131; Fax: (610) 667-7036. info@gbsfi.com. <http://www.gbsfi.com>.

Bryan Richard Cobb, PhD

Floppy infant syndrome *see* **Hypotonia**

Foot drop

Definition

Foot drop is a weakness of muscles that are involved in flexing the ankle and toes. As a result, the toes droop downward and impede the normal walking motion.

Description

The use of the term foot drop can make it seem as if the condition is rather simple and inconsequential. This is not the case. Foot drop can be a consequence of injury to muscles that are known as dorsiflexor muscles, injury to certain nerves, a **stroke**, brain injury, toxic effect of drugs, and even diabetes. Foot drop is likely not a new malady. Historical descriptions that match foot drop date back over 2000 years.

Foot drop can also be described as drop foot, steppage gait, and as equinovarus deformity.

Demographics

Foot drop affects both males and females. However, it is more common in males (the male to female ratio is approximately 2.8:1). Both feet are equally as prone to develop the problem. Some forms of foot drop occur in mid-aged people who put stress on that area of the body during athletics. Surgery to the knee or leg can lead to nerve damage that then leads to the development of foot drop. For example, approximately 0.3–4% of people who have a surgical procedure called a total knee arthroplasty develop foot drop. People who undergo surgery to the tibia (a leg bone) subsequently experience foot drop at a rate of 3–13%.

Causes and symptoms

Foot drop is caused by weakness that occurs in specific muscles of the ankle and the foot. The affected muscles participate in the downward and upward movement of the ankle and the foot. The specific muscles include the anterior tibialis, extensor hallucis longus, and the extensor digitorum longus. The normal function of these muscles is to allow the toes to swing up from the ground during the beginning of a stride and to control the movement of the foot following the planting of the heel towards the end of the stride. Abnormal muscle function makes it difficult to prevent the toes from clearing the ground during the stride. Some people with foot drop walk with a very exaggerated swinging hip motion to help prevent the toes from catching on the ground. Another symptom of foot drop, which occurs as the foot is planted, is an uncontrolled slapping of the foot on the ground.

There are three general causes of the muscle weakness. Damage to nerves can affect the transmission of impulses that help control muscle movement and function. **Motor neuron diseases** such as **amyotrophic lateral sclerosis** (ALS) or **post-polio syndrome**, tumors in the brain or spinal cord, or diseases of the nerve roots of the lumbar spine are all neurological conditions that may produce foot drop. Second, the muscles themselves may be damaged. Third, there can be some skeletal or other anatomical abnormality that affects the movement of the ankle or foot. A combination of these factors can also be involved, as is the case with the drop foot malady known as Charcot foot.

Diagnosis

Diagnosis of foot drop is based on the visual appearance of the altered behavior of the foot. Analysis of blood can be done to look for a metabolic cause, such as diabetes, alcoholism, or presence of a toxin. Among the tests

Key Terms

Gait Body position during and manner of walking.

Orthotic A device applied to or around the body to aid in positioning or mobility, commonly used to control foot mechanics.

commonly performed are fasting blood sugar, hemoglobin determination, and determination of the levels of nitrogen and creatinine.

Visual examination of the foot can include routine photographs, **magnetic resonance imaging** or magnetic resonance neurography (both of which are useful in visualizing areas surrounding damaged nerves). An electromyelogram can be useful in distinguishing between the different types of nerve damage that can be responsible for foot drop.

Treatment team

Treatment can involve the family physician, family members, and physical therapists. Physical therapists guide exercises that assist in maximizing muscular strength.

Treatment

Foot drop that cannot be treated by surgery is often treated using a special orthotic device that provides normal range of motion to the foot and ankle during walking. Other people with foot drop can benefit from the stimulation of the affected nerves. The stimulation is applied as the foot is raised during a stride and is stopped when the foot touches down on the ground.

When the cause of foot drop is a muscular or nerve difficulty, surgery can be beneficial. Surgery can relieve the pressure on a compacted nerve, repair a muscle, and even restore a normal gait by lengthening the Achilles tendon or replacing a defective tendon.

Recovery and rehabilitation

Depending on the nature of the cause of foot drop, recovery can be partial or complete. Physical therapy and an ankle foot orthotic device worn in the shoe are important aspects of rehabilitation.

Clinical trials

As of mid-2004, there were no **clinical trials** recruiting participants for the study or treatment of foot drop, although the National Institute of Neurological Disorders

and Stroke supports research into many of the neurological conditions that may result in foot drop.

Prognosis

When foot drop is due to a compressed nerve, corrective surgery can produce a complete recovery within several months. If the cause is a skeletal problem or other neurological problem, the prognosis for complete recovery is not as certain.

Resources

BOOKS

Ronthal, Michael. *Gait Disorders.* Boston: Butterworth-Heinemann, 2002.

OTHER

"Foot Drop." *eMedicine.com.* (May 5, 2004). <http://www.emedicine.com/orthoped/topic389.htm>
"Peroneal Neuropathy" *drkoop.com.* (May 1, 2004). <http://www.drkoop.com/template.asp?ap=93&page=ency&encyid=212>

ORGANIZATIONS

National Institute of Arthritis and Musculoskeletal and Skin Diseases (NIAMS)
National Institutes of Health. Bldg. 31, Rm. 4C05, Bethesda, MD 20892. (301) 496–8188; Fax: (540) 862–9485. ncpoa@cfw.com. <http://www.niams.nih.gov/index.htm>.

Brian Douglas Hoyle, PhD

Fourth nerve palsy

Definition

The sole function of the fourth nerve is innervation of the superior oblique muscle, which is one of the six muscles of eye movement. Fourth nerve palsy or trochlear nerve palsy is a neurological defect resulting from dysfunction of the fourth cranial nerve. Double vision, also known as diplopia, may occur because of the inability of the eyes to maintain proper alignment.

Description

Trochlear nerve palsy has been described since the mid-1800s. Bielchowsky was first to describe it as the leading cause of vertical (two images appearing one on top of the other or at angles) double vision.

Injury to the fourth cranial nerve can stem from congenital or acquired causes with one or both nerves being affected. It is unclear whether the congenital variant of this disorder is due to developmental abnormalities of the nerve itself or nucleus, which is an area of the brain where the nerve begins and receives signals for proper functioning. In addition the muscle and its tendon may also display abnormal laxity and muscle fiber weakness. Most cases of acquired fourth nerve palsy results from dysfunction of the nerve itself, although cerebrovascular accidents (**stroke**) may directly injure the nucleus.

Demographics

Fourth nerve palsies have no predilection for males or females. It is difficult to accurately predict the occurrence of congenital palsies since some go unnoticed throughout a person's life. Acquired nerve palsies are more likely to occur in older patients with diabetes or vascular disease versus the general population.

Causes and symptoms

Causes of fourth nerve palsy can be broadly classified as congenital or acquired. Isolated congenital palsies may be heralded by head-tilting to the opposite side of the affected nerve in early childhood. In others a congenital palsy may go unnoticed because of a compensatory mechanism allowing for alignment of the eyes when focusing on an image.

Isolated acquired trochlear nerve palsies can be the result of numerous disorders. Most commonly an underlying cause cannot be found and this is known as an idiopathic palsy. Due to its long course within the brain, the fourth nerve is susceptible to injury following severe head trauma. Depending on the site of **nerve compression** during trauma one or both nerves may be affected. **Aneurysms** or brain tumors may directly compress or result in an increase of intracranial pressure (the pressure within the skull) resulting in nerve palsies.

Disorders such as **myasthenia gravis**, diabetes, meningitis, microvascular disease (atherosclerotic vascular disease) or any cause of increased intracranial pressure may result in trochlear nerve palsy. A congenital palsy that has gone undetected may manifest itself in adulthood when the compensatory mechanism for ocular alignment is lost. Additionally the removal of a cataract may restore clear vision to both eyes allowing the patient to become aware of their double vision.

A child with a congenital palsy may be found doing a head tilt by his or her parents or relatives. Children will very rarely complain of double vision.

Adults with a new onset fourth nerve palsy will note two images, one on top of the other or angled in position when both eyes are open. Covering of one eye, no matter which one is covered, will resolve their diplopia. Their double vision will worsen when looking down or away from the affected side. If both nerves are affected he or she may experience a horizontal diplopia (two images side by

side) when looking downward. If a decompensated palsy is suspected, one should review old photographs to document a pre-existing head tilt to support the diagnosis.

Diagnosis

Diagnosing a fourth nerve palsy is for the most part a clinical diagnosis. Careful history taking and examination is the key to diagnosis. The Bielchowsky head-tilt test is one commonly used and reliable technique to diagnose isolated trochlear nerve palsies. Review of patient's old photographs can prove indispensable in diagnosing a decompensated palsy, obviating the need for additional testing.

Computed tomography or **magnetic resonance imaging** may be needed if the palsy is thought to be due to a structural brain lesion. Blood work or a lumbar puncture may be ordered if myasthenia gravis, meningitis or other systemic disorders are considered as potential causes.

Treatment team

Ophthalmologists, neuro-ophthalmologists, optometrists and neurologists are medical specialists who can evaluate and diagnose a patient with a fourth nerve palsy. Usually an optometrist or ophthalmologist will initially see a patient complaining of diplopia or displaying stigmata of trochlear nerve palsy. A referral will then likely be made to a **neurologist** or neuro-ophthalmologist for evaluation and workup.

Treatment

Since most fourth nerve palsies are idiopathic, treatment is conservative given the high rate of spontaneous resolution. Monitoring a patient for six months to one year for improvement can prove to be frustrating and disabling for the patient. A prism may resolve or greatly reduce a patient's diplopia during this period, allowing for return to normal daily activities, such as driving, shopping or reading.

Botulinum toxin used to weaken muscles that overact, causing ocular misalignment, in the presence of a trochlear nerve palsy has been disappointing thus far. Surgery aimed at weakening or strengthening one or more of the extraocular muscles has proven useful in many cases of persistent palsies. Indications for surgery include worsening diplopia, head-tilt resulting in neck **pain** and poor cosmetic appearance. Procedures performed include the Knapp, Plager or Harada-Ito techniques and are chosen based on the amount and type of ocular misalignment found on examination. These procedures weaken or strengthen extraocular muscles by relocating their attachments to the eye. Muscles may also be weakened by cutting across or removing a portion of the muscle.

Recovery and rehabilitation

A six-month to one-year waiting period is warranted to observe for spontaneous improvement. During this period the patient may benefit from prismatic lenses to eliminate or reduce their diplopia. Eye movement exercises have not proved useful for improving or expediting recovery.

Clinical trials

As of November, 2003 no **clinical trials** regarding trochlear nerve palsies were underway.

Prognosis

The prognosis for trochlear nerve palsies is dependent upon the underlying cause. Most cases of idiopathic or microvascular nerve palsies resolve within a several weeks to six-month time period without treatment. Traumatic nerve palsies may take up to one year to resolve, with less than half regaining any improvement. Palsies secondary to brain masses or aneurysms have the least likelihood of any recovery and may take up to one year to improve. If present, proper treatment of myasthenia gravis or other underlying systemic disease, excluding a cerebrovascular accident usually results in complete recovery in the vast majority of cases.

Special concerns

Patients afflicted with a fourth nerve palsy should refrain from driving unless an eye patch is used. In addition certain types of employment may warrant a medical leave or temporary change of duties.

Resources

BOOKS

Burde, Ronald M., Peter J. Savino, and Jonathan D. Trobe. *Clinical Decisions in Neuro-Ophthalmology,* 3rd ed. St. Louis: Mosby, 2002.

Liu, Grant T., Nicholas J. Volpe, and Steven L. Galetta. *Neuro-Ophthalmology Diagnosis and Management,* 1st ed. Philadelphia: W. B. Saunders Company, 2001.

Neuro-Ophthalmologic and Cranial Nerve Disorders; Section 14, Chapter 178. *The Merck Manual of Diagnosis and Therapy,* edited by Mark H. Beers and Robert Berkow. Whitehouse Station, NJ: Merck Research Laboratories, 1999.

Newman, Nancy J., ed. *Ophthamology Clinics of North America,* pp. 176-179. Philadelphia: W. B. Saunders Company, 2001.

PERIODICALS

Brazis, Paul W. "Palsies of the trochlear nerve: diagnosis and localization-recent concepts." *Mayo Clinic Proceedings* 68, no. 5 (May 1993): 501.

WEBSITES

Sheik, Zafar A., and Kelly A. Hutcheson. "Trochlear Nerve Palsy." *eMedicine.com.* <www.eMedicine.com>.

Adam J. Cohen, MD

Friedreich ataxia

Definition

Friedreich **ataxia** (FRDA or FA) is an inherited, degenerative nervous system disorder that results in muscle weakness and inability to coordinate voluntary muscle movements.

Description

Onset of FDRA is usually in childhood or early adolescence. The disorder is characterized by unsteady gait, slurred speech, absent knee and ankle jerks, Babinski responses, loss of position and vibrations senses, leg muscle weakness, loss of leg muscle mass, scoliosis, foot deformities, and heart disease. FRDA is a slowly progressive condition associated with a shortened life span, most often due to complications of heart disease.

FRDA is named for Nikolaus Friedreich, the German doctor who first described the condition in 1863. The most common form of the disorder, found in about three–quarters of patients, is referred to as "classic" or "typical" FDRA. Atypical forms of FDRA include: late onset Friedreich ataxia (LOFA), very late onset Friedreich ataxia (VLOFA), Friedreich ataxia with retained reflexes (FARR), Acadian type (Louisiana form), and spastic paraparesis without ataxia.

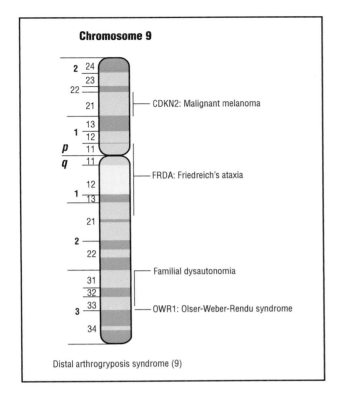

Chromosome 9

2 — 24
   — 23
22 —
   — 21 — CDKN2: Malignant melanoma
1 — 13
   — 12
p — 11
q — 11
1 — 12 — FRDA: Friedreich's ataxia
   — 13
   — 21
2 —
   — 22
   — 31 — Familial dysautonomia
   — 32
3 — 33 — OWR1: Olser-Weber-Rendu syndrome
   — 34

Distal arthrogryposis syndrome (9)

Friedreich ataxia, on chromosome 9. *(Gale Group.)*

Demographics

FRDA is the most common inherited ataxia and affects between 3,000–5,000 people in the United States. The prevalence of FDRA in the Caucasian population is approximately one in 50,000 to one in 25,000. Prevalence appears to be highest in French Canadians from Quebec, Acadians from Louisiana, and among certain populations in southern Italy and Cyprus. Approximately 1% of Caucasian individuals carry one defective copy of the gene responsible for FRDA, known as FRDA1. FRDA is rare in people of Asian or African descent.

Causes and symptoms

FRDA is an autosomal recessive condition, which means that an affected individual has two altered or non-functioning FRDA1 genes, one from each parent. The FRDA1 gene is located on chromosome 9 and codes for a protein called frataxin. The most common gene alteration (or mutation), which is found in greater than 95% of affected individuals, is a triplet repeat expansion. The triplet repeat is a sequence of DNA bases called GAA. Normally the GAA sequence is repeated five to 33 times but in people with FRDA, it is repeated between 66 to 1700 times. Longer GAA triplet repeats are associated with more severe disease, but the severity of disease in a given individual cannot be predicted from the repeat length. About

4% of patients have the triplet repeat expansion in one copy of the FDRA1 gene and a different type of mutation, a point mutation, in the other FRDA1 gene. There have been a few patients with classic FDRA in which the FRDA1 gene on chromosome 9 has been shown not to be the cause.

FRDA1 gene mutations lead to loss of function of the gene and subsequently to decreased production of frataxin. Frataxin plays a role in the balance of iron in the mitochondria, the cellular energy structures. Frataxin insufficiency leads to a number of effects including excessive iron accumulation in the mitochondria and, eventually, the production of chemicals called free radicals that can damage and kill the cell. The cells most affected in FRDA are those in the brain, spinal cord, nerves, heart, and pancreas.

FRDA is a slowly progressive, unremitting, ataxia. There is variability in age of onset, presence of symptoms, rate of progression, and severity. Although onset of FRDA usually occurs before age 25, symptoms may appear as early as age two or as late as 30 to 40 years. Gait ataxia, or difficulty walking, is often the first sign of the disease. For example, an affected child might trip frequently over low obstacles. The ataxia eventually spreads to the arms within several years, resulting in decreased hand-eye coordination. Unsteadiness when standing still and deterioration of position sense is common. Other symptoms that appear early in the course of the disease are loss of knee and ankle tendon reflexes and **dysarthria** (slowness and slurring of speech). Over time, individuals with FRDA experience loss of sensation that begins in their hands and feet and may spread to other parts of the body. Abnormal muscle control and tone leads to problems such as scoliosis (curvature of the spine) and foot deformities such as *pes cavus* (high-arched feet) with extensor plantar response. Arm weakness, if it occurs, develops later in the course of the disorder. Loss of muscle control eventually necessitates use a wheelchair.

Heart disease represents a potentially significant complication of FRDA. Heart muscle enlargement with or without an abnormal heartbeat is present in about two–thirds of cases and represents a major cause of death. About one–third of patients develop diabetes, most of whom will require insulin. Other medical findings in FRDA include optic nerve atrophy, nystagmus (eye tremor), tremor, amyotrophy (loss of muscle mass), hearing loss, difficulty swallowing, and incontinence.

Diagnosis

A diagnosis of FDRA is based on clinical findings and results of genetic testing. The clinical diagnosis of Friedreich ataxia is made through physical exam and medical history. The presence of progressive ataxia, loss of position and/or vibration sense, and loss of lower limb

Key Terms

Amniocentesis A procedure performed at 16-18 weeks of pregnancy in which a needle is inserted through a woman's abdomen into her uterus to draw out a small sample of the amniotic fluid from around the baby for analysis. Either the fluid itself or cells from the fluid can be used for a variety of tests to obtain information about genetic disorders and other medical conditions in the fetus.

Chorionic villus sampling (CVS) A procedure used for prenatal diagnosis at 10–12 weeks gestation. Under ultrasound guidance a needle is inserted either through the mother's vagina or abdominal wall to draw out a sample of the chorionic membrane. These cells are then tested for chromosome abnormalities or other genetic diseases.

Chromosome A microscopic thread-like structure found within each cell of the human body and consisting of a complex of proteins and DNA. Humans have 46 chromosomes arranged into 23 pairs. Chromosomes contain the genetic information necessary to direct the development and functioning of all cells and systems in the body. They pass on hereditary traits from parents to child (like eye color) and determine whether the child will be male or female.

DNA Deoxyribonucleic acid; the genetic material in cells that holds the inherited instructions for growth, development, and cellular functioning.

Gene A building block of inheritance, which contains the instructions for the production of a particular protein, and is made up of a molecular sequence found on a section of DNA. Each gene is found on a precise location on a chromosome.

---

tendon reflexes in a child or adolescent is suspicious of the diagnosis. Tests that may aid in diagnosis include **electromyography**, nerve conduction studies, an electrocardiogram, an echocardiogram, **magnetic resonance imaging (MRI)**, computed tomography (CT) scan, a spinal tap, and glucose analysis of blood and urine. Genetic testing is recommended for all individuals in whom the diagnosis of FRDA is suspected.

Genetic testing is accomplished by counting the number of GAA repeats in the FRDA gene to see if there is an expansion (66 or more repeats). For those cases in which only one FRDA gene has a triplet repeat expansion, the same genetic test may be used to determine the presence of the genetic defect in the carrier state (i.e., one normal copy and one defective copy of the frataxin gene) in unaffected individuals, such as adult siblings, who would like to learn their chances of producing an affected child. During pregnancy, the DNA of a fetus can be tested using cells obtained from chorionic villus sampling (CVS) or amniocentesis.

Treatment team

Management of FRDA requires a multidisciplinary approach. In addition to the patient's primary health care professionals, medical professionals involved in the care of patients with FRDA generally include a **neurologist**, a cardiologist, an orthopedic surgeon, an ophthalmologist, a speech therapist, a physical therapist, an occupational therapist, and a physiatrist. Additional specialists in endocrinology and urology may be needed. Some patients with FRDA may receive comprehensive services through a **muscular dystrophy** association (MDA) clinic and/or a Shriner's Hospital for Children. A genetic specialist, such as a clinical geneticist or a genetic counselor, may be helpful to the patient and family, especially at the time of diagnosis or prior to genetic testing. Psychological counseling and support groups may also assist families in coping with this condition.

Treatment

As of 2003, there is no cure for FRDA. The purpose of treatment, which is largely supportive, is to help patients optimize function and to manage any associated medical complications of the disorder. Treatment includes most if not all of the following options:

• Orthopedic intervention. Braces or surgery may be necessary to treat scoliosis and foot deformities. For example, a surgical procedure known as spinal fusion may be considered in patients with significant curvature.

• Medications. Some antioxidants (chemicals that capture free radicals) have shown benefits in patients with FRDA. Vitamin E and coenzyme Q10, which are naturally occurring substances, may be prescribed. Patients should discuss the current recommendations with their physician.

• Cardiac and diabetes care. Since cardiac disease is the most common cause of death, proper cardiac care is essential. For those cases in which there is heart disease, medications can be effective for many years. Of those individuals with diabetes mellitus, most will require insulin therapy.

Recovery and rehabilitation

Rehabilitation for Friedreich ataxia consists of speech, physical, and occupational therapy. The goal of these therapies is to make full use of the patient's existing muscular functions. For example, physical therapy can help stretch muscles to improve or maintain flexibility. Speech therapy can help to retrain certain muscles in order to improve speech and swallowing. Occupational therapy can teach patients to use adaptive techniques and devices that may help compensate for loss of coordination and strength. For example, prostheses, walking aids, and wheelchairs may be recommended to help the individual with FRDA to remain ambulatory or mobile.

Clinical trials

Research studies of idebenone, a synthetic antioxidant, have shown it to reduce hypertrophy (overgrowth) of the left ventricle of the heart in patients with FRDA. A phase I clinical trial will be conducted in the United States to establish the maximum tolerated dose of idebenone in children, adolescents, and adults with Friedreich's ataxia; as of November 2003, active patient recruitment was underway. Information on this trial can be found at <http://www.clinicaltrials.gov> or by contacting the National Institute of Neurological Disorders and Stroke patient recruitment and public liason office at 1-800-411-1222. Another substance that is being researched is an antioxidant known as mitoquinone or "MitoQ" which is a synthetic form of coenzyme Q10 that has the potential to protect the mitochondria from free radical damage. As of 2003, mitoquinone was in the developmental phase of study and not yet available to patients.

Prognosis

The rate of progression of FRDA varies. Most patients lose the ability to walk within 15 years of symptom onset, and 95% require a wheelchair for mobility by age 45. Shortened life span from FRDA complications, usually cardiac, is also quite variable. Average age at death, usually from heart problems, is in the mid-30s, but may be as late as the mid-60s.

Special concerns

A child with a diagnosis of Friedreich ataxia is eligible to have an Individual Education Plan (IEP). An IEP provides a framework from which administrators, teachers, and parents can meet the educational needs of a child with FRDA.

Resources

BOOKS

Nance, Martha A. *Living with Ataxia,* 2nd ed. Minneapolis: National Ataxia Foundation, 1997.

Parker, James N., and Philip M. Parker, eds. *The Official Parent's Sourcebook on Friedreich's Ataxia: A Revised and Updated Directory for the Internet Age.* San Diego, CA: ICON Health Publications, 2002.

Ruzicka, Evzen, Mark Hallett, and Joseph Jankovic, eds. *Gait Disorders.* Philadelphia, PA: Lippincott Williams and Wilkins, 2001.

PERIODICALS

Alper, G., and V. Narayanan. "Friedreich's Ataxia." *Pediatric Neurology* 28 (May 2003): 335–341.

Pilch, J., E. Jamroz, and E. Marza. "Friedreich's Ataxia." *Journal of Child Neurology* 17 (May 2002): 315–319.

WEBSITES

Friedreich's Ataxia Parents Group (FAPG). <http://www.fortnet.org/fapg/>.

The Muscular Dystrophy Association (MDA). *Facts about Friedreich's Ataxia (FA).* <http://www.mdausa.org/publications/fa-fried-qa.html>.

The National Institute of Neurological Disorders and Stroke (NINDS). *Friedreich's Ataxia Fact Sheet.* <http://www.ninds.nih.gov/health_and_medical/pubs/friedreich_ataxia.htm>.

ORGANIZATIONS

Friedreich's Ataxia Research Alliance (FARA). 2001 Jefferson Davis Highway, Suite 209, Arlington, VA 22202. (703) 413-4468; Fax: (703) 413-4467. fara@frda.org. <http://www.frda.org>.

Muscular Dystrophy Association. 3300 East Sunrise Drive, Tucson, AZ 85718. (520) 529-2000 or (800) 572-1717; Fax: (520) 529-5300. mda@mdausa.org. <http://www.mdausa.org>.

National Ataxia Foundation (NAF). 2600 Fernbrook Lane, Suite 119, Minneapolis, MN 55447. (763) 553-0020; Fax: (763) 553-0167. naf@ataxia.org. <http://www.ataxia.org>.

Dawn J. Cardeiro, MS, CGC

G

Gabapentin

Definition

Gabapentin is a prescription drug that was initially approved to help manage **epilepsy**. The Food and Drug Administration (FDA) has also approved gabapentin for treatment of the nerve **pain** that sometimes accompanies herpes infections. Gabapentin is available in the United States under the trade name Neurontin.

Purpose

Although the FDA has only approved gabapentin for managing epilepsy and treating nerve pain associated with herpes infections, doctors often prescribe the medication for managing other conditions, including **tremors** associated with **multiple sclerosis**, nerve pain, bipolar disorder, and migraine prevention.

Description

As an antiepileptic drug, gabapentin may be used in conjunction with other drugs to prevent partial **seizures**. Partial seizures are caused by brief abnormal electrical activity in localized areas of the brain. Partial seizures usually do not cause unconsciousness, but may cause rhythmic contractions in one area of the body or abnormal numbness or tingling sensations.

Although gabapentin was originally approved by the FDA in 1993, it is still not understood how gabapentin prevents seizures. However, the drug is related to gamma-aminobutyric acid (GABA), a neurochemical that possesses inhibitory properties. In brain cells, these inhibitory actions prevent excitatory electrical impulses from spreading to neighboring cells. As a result, gabapentin probably prevents the spread of abnormal excitatory activity in the brain at least in part, by mimicking the actions of GABA.

By preventing excitatory communication between cells, gabapentin may also inhibit the electrical impulses involved in pain conduction. This may account for the drug's ability to alleviate pain, especially nerve pain.

When gabapentin is used along with other therapies for managing epileptic partial seizures, improvements should be observed within 12 weeks. On the other hand, pain relief may be evident within one week when the drug is used for pain associated with herpes infections.

Recommended dosage

For adults, the initial dose of gabapentin is 300 mg taken by mouth three times each day. The dosage may be increased if necessary. Dosages as high as 800–1,200 mg three times daily have been well tolerated.

In children three to 12 years of age, the starting dose should be 10–15 mg/2.2 lb (1 kg)/day given in three equal doses. This dose can be increased until an effective dosage is reached, typically 25–40 mg/2.2 lb (1 kg)/day. Lower dosages are required for patients that have kidney disease.

Precautions

In children, gabapentin may cause behavioral and emotional disorders. The drug should be used cautiously and the dosage should be reduced in those with severe kidney disease. In experimental animals, gabapentin caused tumors to develop; however, it is not known if this occurs in humans.

Patients should take gabapentin only as prescribed. The drug should never be stopped abruptly because doing so increases the likelihood of having a seizure. Since gabapentin can cause **dizziness** and **fatigue**, patients should avoid driving or operating complex machinery until they know whether the drug adversely affects their reaction time or impairs their judgment.

Side effects

The most common side effects that cause adults to stop taking gabapentin are dizziness, sleepiness, fatigue, shaky movements, difficulty walking, or swelling in the ankles.

Key Terms

Antiepileptic   A drug that prevents or limits the spread of epileptic seizures.

Bipolar disorder   A mental illness that causes episodes of depression and mania; also known as manic-depressive illness.

Epilepsy   A chronic nervous system disorder that typically causes temporary behavior changes, uncontrolled shaking, loss of attention, or unconsciousness.

Gamma-aminobutyric acid (GABA)   The major inhibitory neurotransmitter in the brain.

Herpes   A virus that causes cold sores, sexually transmitted diseases, shingles, or chicken pox.

Kilogram (kg)   One thousand grams, or about the equivalent of 2.2 pounds (lb).

Migraine   A recurrent headache, often accompanied by vomiting, that typically affects just one side of the head.

Milligram (mg)   One-thousandth of a gram, or about the equivalent of 0.035 ounces (oz).

Multiple sclerosis   A chronic disease of the central nervous system in which the tissues surrounding the brain and spinal cord are damaged.

Neurotransmitter   A chemical in the brain that transmits messages between neurons or nerve cells.

Partial seizures   Brief, temporary alterations in movement or sensory nerve function cause by abnormal electrical activities in localized regions of the brain.

In children, the side effects the drug may cause include emotional problems, hostility, and hyperactivity.

Interactions

Unlike many other drugs that are used to treat epilepsy, there are few drug interactions associated with gabapentin. It is recommended, however, that antacids not be used sooner than two hours after gabapentin to avoid compromising gabapentin's effectiveness.

Resources

BOOKS

Drug Facts and Comparisons, 6th edition. St. Louis, MO: A Wolter Kluwer Company, 2002.

Mosby's Medical Drug Reference. St. Louis, MO: Mosby, Inc, 1999.

Neurontin Package Insert. Vega Baja, PR: Parke-Davis Pharmaceuticals, Ltd., 2002.

Kelly Karpa, PhD, RPh

Galantamine *see* **Cholinesterase inhibitors**

Gaucher disease

Definition

Gaucher disease is a rare, inherited disorder in which a deficient or missing enzyme causes an abnormal buildup of a fatty substance called glucosylceramide throughout the body. Abnormal accumulations of this substance are toxic to organs and tissues, resulting in progressive, permanent damage.

Description

Gaucher disease belongs to a group of conditions called lipid storage diseases. Lipids are fatty substances used throughout the body. In lipid storage diseases, enzymes that would ordinarily break down lipids so that they can be appropriately used are absent. This results in the progressive accumulation of large quantities of these lipids.

In Gaucher disease, the specific type of lipid that accumulates is called a glucosylceramide. Deficient activity of an enzyme called beta-glucosidase results in glucosylceramide accumulation throughout the body and damage to normal tissues and organs.

There are three types of Gaucher disease. Type 1 is the most common. Each type has a characteristic age of onset and constellation of symptoms.

Demographics

In the general population, one in 50,000–100,000 develop Gaucher disease. However, Gaucher type 1 disease is considerably more common among Jewish people from eastern and central Europe (Ashkenazi Jews), affecting one in 500–1,000 individuals.

Causes and symptoms

Gaucher disease is an inherited disease, caused by a defective GBA gene. The disease is recessive, meaning that a child has to inherit a defective gene from both the mother and the father in order to have the actual condition.

Type 1 affects both children and adults. Its major manifestations include easy bruising, anemia, **fatigue,**

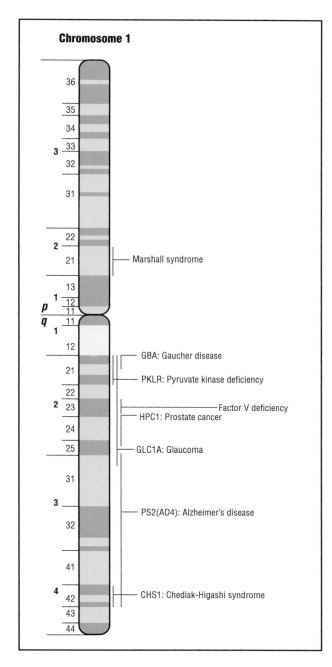

Chromosome 1

36
35
34
3   33
32

31

2   22
21   — Marshall syndrome

13
1   12
p   11
q   11
1

12
                      — GBA: Gaucher disease
21
                      — PKLR: Pyruvate kinase deficiency
22
2   23   — Factor V deficiency
                      — HPC1: Prostate cancer
24

25   — GLC1A: Glaucoma

31

3
                      — PS2(AD4): Alzheimer's disease
32

41

4   — CHS1: Chediak-Higashi syndrome
42
43
44

Gaucher disease, on chromosome 1. *(Gale Group.)*

liver and/or spleen enlargement, bone and joint **pain**, joint problems, and increased risk of bone fractures.

Type 2 usually begins to show symptoms during infancy. This type causes many of the same symptoms seen in type 1 (easy bruising, anemia, liver and/or spleen enlargement), but it also results in severe and progressive neurological problems. Damage to the **central nervous system** results in **seizures**, difficulty walking, paralyzed eye muscles, and progressive **dementia**. Most patients with type 2 disease die by about age two.

Type 3 causes the same kinds of symptoms seen in type 2, but the neurological involvement is more mild and the progression is more gradual.

Diagnosis

Diagnosis of Gaucher disease can be made by performing a bone marrow examination, and identifying specific "Gaucher cells" within the specimen. Other cells can be examined to demonstrate decreased activity of the enzyme beta-glucosidase. DNA testing can also reveal the specific mutation responsible for the disease, particularly within Ashkenazi Jewish populations.

Treatment team

The treatment team may vary, depending on the patient's specific symptoms. Early in the diagnostic phase, a geneticist may be helpful. If neurological problems predominate, a **neurologist** will be necessary. A hematologist may be consulted to handle the blood-related complications such as anemia. Other specialists may include an ophthalmologist, orthopedic surgeon, physical and occupational therapists, and speech and language therapist.

Treatment

Symptomatic treatment may include blood transfusions to treat anemia, removal of the enlarged spleen, and joint replacement. Some patients have been cured via bone marrow transplant, but this procedure carries a very high risk of complications and death, and requires a carefully matched donor, which can be difficult to find.

Newer treatments include enzyme replacement therapy. While not curative, intravenous enzyme replacement can decrease the severity of, or reverse, many of the complications of type 1 disease, including liver/spleen enlargement, anemia, neurologic problems, and bone abnormalities. Severe brain damage cannot be reversed, however.

Clinical trials

A variety of **clinical trials** on Gaucher disease are being conducted, including testing of a medicine called OGT918 that may slow or decrease the accumulation of lipids, hopefully with improved neurological outcomes. Other clinical trials are evaluating the outcome of treatment with enzyme replacement therapy in Gaucher disease types 2 and 3, the effect of alendronate sodium on bone disease in Gaucher disease, and the short- and longer-term outcome of bone marrow or umbilical cord blood transplantation in children with Gaucher disease.

Key Terms

Beta-glucosidase An enzyme responsible for breaking down glucosylceramide.

Glucosylceramide A chemical substance composed of glucose (sugar) and lipid (fat).

Lipid A fatty substance in use throughout the body.

Prognosis

The prognosis of Gaucher disease depends on the specific type. Because type 1 has no neurologic manifestations, it has the best prognosis. Lifespan depends on the severity of the complications, but some patients live into the 70s or 80s. Type 2 is universally fatal, generally by about age two. Patients with type 3 generally survive until about age 20 or 30.

Special concerns

Carriers of the defective gene may be identified during genetic counseling, and prenatal diagnosis is also possible.

Resources

BOOKS

"Nutritional Disorders of the Neuromuscular Transmission and of Motor Neurons." In *Nelson Textbook of Pediatrics*, edited by Richard E. Behrman, et al. Philadelphia: W. B. Saunders Company, 2004.

Maertens, Paul, and Paul Richard Dyken. "Storage Diseases: Neuronal Ceroid-Lipofuscinoses, Lipidoses, Glycogenoses, and Leukodystrophies." In *Textbook of Clinical Neurology*, edited by Christopher G. Goetz. Philadelphia: W. B. Saunders Company, 2003.

McGovern, Margaret M., and Robert J. Desnick. "Lysosomal Storage Diseases." In *Textbook of Clinical Neurology*, edited by Christopher G. Goetz. Philadelphia: W. B. Saunders Company, 2003.

WEBSITES

Genetics Home Reference. National Library of Medicine, National Institutes of Health. (April 27, 2004). <http://ghr.nlm.nih.gov/ghr/page/Home;jsessionid=52A6DA98F1237CEFE8E49B215F316502>.

National Institute of Neurological Disorders and Stroke (NINDS). (April 27, 2004). *Gaucher Disease Fact Sheet.* <http://www.ninds.nih.gov>.

ORGANIZATIONS

Center for Jewish Diseases, Department of Human Genetics, Mount Sinai Medical Center. Fifth Avenue at 100th Street, New York, NY 10029. (212) 659-6774 or (212) 241-6947. <http://www.mssm.edu/jewish_genetics/overview.shtml>.

Children's Gaucher Research Fund. PO Box 2123, Granite Bay, CA 95746. (916) 797-3700; Fax: (916) 797-3707. research@childrensgaucher.org. <http://www.childrensgaucher.org>.

National Gaucher Foundation. 5410 Edson Lane, Suite 260, Rockville, MD 20852-3130. (301) 816-1515 or 800-GAUCHER (428-2437); Fax: (301) 816-1516. ngf@gaucherdisease.org. <http://www.gaucherdisease.org>.

Rosalyn Carson-DeWitt, MD

Gene therapy

Definition

Classic gene therapy is the direct use of genetic material in the treatment of disease. This usually involves inserting a functional gene or DNA fragment into key cells to mitigate, or cure, a disease. A broader definition of gene therapy includes all applications of DNA technology to treat disease. For people with certain neurological conditions such as **Parkinson's disease** and **Canavan disease**, initial gene therapy trials have shown promise. Developing gene therapies for treating disorders of the nervous system poses unique challenges, such as how to introduce the therapeutic gene across the blood-brain barrier or how to target the therapeutic gene to one specific area of the brain.

Purpose

Genes play a role in every function of the human body. Defects or mutations within a gene can lead to malfunction or disease of cells, tissues, and/or organs. Although standard drug therapy is usually effective in treating the symptoms of a disorder, a patient may be required to take the drugs for an extended time and there may be serious or unpleasant side effects. However, a patient may be cured with few negative consequences if treatment can be targeted directly at the specific cause of the disease (the gene defect), or if that cause can be neutralized or reversed. Therefore, gene therapy provides an attractive alternative to drug therapy as it seeks to provide treatment strategies that will be more complete and less toxic to the patient. Furthermore, gene therapy may provide a way of treating diseases that cannot be managed by standard therapies.

Description

There are many diverse approaches to gene therapy since the biological basis of each disease is unique, presenting a different set of parameters and challenges. However, in each case, a basic set of criteria must be met. First, it is essential to fully understand the disease to be treated. The cells or tissues associated with the disease must be well defined and accessible. The gene and the specific mutation or mutations causing the disease must be known, and it must be possible to isolate or synthesize a normal, functional copy of that gene and to incorporate it into a vector. The vector then transfers the new gene to the target cells where, hopefully, the gene will become fully active. The most common roles for the expressed gene include replacing a defective gene, inhibiting or degrading a deleterious DNA, RNA, or protein, or directly or indirectly killing the cell.

Single gene disorders resulting in a loss of gene function in one specific target tissue provide the easiest options for gene therapy, though strategies for many types of mutations have been investigated. A broad spectrum of diseases has been considered for gene therapy, including:

• neurological disorders, e.g., Parkinson disease, Huntington disease

• muscular dystrophies

• immunological disorders, e.g., severe combined immunodeficiency syndrome (SCIDS)

• blood abnormalities, e.g., thalassemias, hemophilia

• cancer

Unfortunately, many of the more commonly occurring disorders, including heart disease, diabetes, and high blood pressure, result from defects in multiple genes making them unlikely candidates for gene therapy using existing technologies.

For each disease, it must be determined if *ex vivo* or *in vitro* technology is the best approach. In *ex vivo* technology, patient cell samples are collected and cultured in the laboratory. The new gene is incorporated into the growing cells, and these are subsequently transferred back into the patient. Not all of the cultured cells will include the new gene, and not all will survive the transfer. The hope is that a sufficient number of the modified cells will be functional in the patient such that the therapy will reverse the disease. *In vitro* therapy involves injecting the new gene directly into the target tissue where the individual cells must pick it up. Of the two, this method is technically easier and cheaper, but it is harder to determine how many of the target cells actually acquire the new gene. *Ex vivo* therapy is more expensive and time consuming, but allows greater control of the conditions.

Both processes require the use of a vector to get the new gene across the cell membrane and into a cell. Viruses have proven to be highly effective as vectors since these are biological entities with a natural function of infecting host cells. DNA technology allows viruses to be manipulated to replace the normal payload of disease-causing genetic material with therapeutic genes. The virus will retain its ability to infect a host cell but, instead of causing a disease, it will deposit the new gene into the cell.

Other mechanisms of gene transfer have also been investigated. Artificial chromosomes have been developed, but these are often too large to move across cell membranes. Liposomes, structures with lipid membranes, that encompass genetic material can be successfully used as vectors if the liposome is absorbed by the cell or if its membrane fuses with the cell membrane releasing the new gene inside the cell.

Once the gene enters the cell, one of two things occurs. It may be degraded and lost, which is an unfavorable outcome. Preferably, the gene will stably incorporate into the DNA of the target cell so that it can be processed as a normal part of that genome. If the gene therapy is designed to replace a defective gene, the best-case scenario is for the new gene to integrate into a completely renewable cell such as a stem cell. Theoretically, in this situation, the gene will be permanently incorporated into the patient's body and no further therapy will be required. Alternatively, if the gene integrates into a genome of a cell with a finite lifespan, the beneficial effects of the gene will only exist while that cell lives, requiring the gene therapy to be repeated at a later time.

One of the early successes of gene therapy was for a four-year-old girl with adenine deaminase (ADA) deficiency. This is a form of SCIDS that results in malfunction of the immune system and can lead to death as a result of severe infection. Conventional treatment had failed for this patient, making her a candidate for gene therapy. A normal ADA gene was incorporated into a retroviral vector that transferred the gene into the patient's lymphocytes *in vitro*. The modified cells were returned to her circulation by transfusion. After five months, her levels of ADA activity had risen from less than 1% to 50%. With additional therapies over the next two years, her health improved as the enzyme activity stabilized, and she was able to begin a normal life. Twelve years later, she still demonstrates reasonable levels of ADA activity, but the gene therapy was not a cure as she must continue to receive the standard enzyme replacement therapy to maintain her health.

Acquired diseases can also be treated with gene therapy as demonstrated by a novel strategy for treating brain cancer. The thymidine kinase (TK) gene from the herpes simplex virus (HSV) has an enzymatic property that converts the drug ganciclovir into a toxic substance that can kill human cells. It was postulated that this could be used as a targeted killing tool. To investigate, cloned HSV TK

Key Terms

DNA Deoxyribonucleic acid; the genetic material in cells that holds the inherited instructions for growth, development, and cellular functioning.

Gene A building block of inheritance, which contains the instructions for the production of a particular protein, and is made up of a molecular sequence found on a section of DNA. Each gene is found on a precise location on a chromosome.

Mutation A permanent change in the genetic material that may alter a trait or characteristic of an individual, or manifest as disease. This change can be transmitted to offspring.

Recombinant DNA DNA that has been altered by joining genetic material from two different sources. It usually involves putting a gene from one organism into the genome of a different organism.

RNA Ribonucleic acid, a nucleic acid that transmits messages in the DNA to other elements in the cell.

Severe combined immunodeficiency syndrome (SCIDS) A group of rare, life-threatening diseases present at birth, that cause a child to have little or no immune system. As a result, the child's body is unable to fight infections.

Vector A carrier organism (such as a fly or mosquito) that serves to deliver a virus (or other agent of infection) to a host. Also refers to a retrovirus that had been modified and is used to introduce specific genes into the genome of an organism.

Virus A small infectious agent consisting of a core of genetic material (DNA or RNA) surrounded by a shell of protein. A virus needs a living cell to reproduce.

genes were injected into brain tumors. In the brain, only the tumor cells are dividing, so these are the only cells that will be infected by the viral vector, and are thus the only cells that will receive the HSV TK gene. When the patient is subsequently treated with ganciclovir, the tumor cells that have incorporated the HSV TK gene will be selectively killed. **Clinical trials** proved that tumor cells could be selectively eliminated by demonstrating a reduction in the size of the brain tumors in seven of nine patients.

A completely different set of therapies is possible if the idea of gene therapy includes the use of DNA for patient treatment in ways other than inserting new genes into cells. One example is the drug Gleevec that was approved in 2001 for use in patients with chronic myelogenous leukemia (CML). Gleevec is a substance that binds to the defective protein produced in CML, blocking that protein's activity and alleviating the symptoms of the disease. This is a targeted therapy that affects only the cells with the CML mutation, so there are very few side effects. Recombinant DNA technology has also been utilized to generate genetically engineered copies of vaccines (Recombivax HB), antibodies, and normal gene products (insulin).

Aftercare

If the new DNA can be stably incorporated into the proper regenerative target cells, the patient may be cured of disease. No additional care should be required, although periodic monitoring of the patient is appropriate.

For gene therapies in which the new DNA is inserted into cells with a finite lifespan, the therapeutic effect will be lost when those cells die. In these situations, the patient will require continuing treatments. Monitoring of patients who receive drugs and substances arising from recombinant DNA technology is the same as standard drug therapy.

Precautions

Currently classic gene therapy is still experimental. Although many patients have shown significant improvement following their treatment, at least two individuals have died as a result of this type of therapy. Therefore, experts carefully review all protocols before any studies are undertaken. Initial research is done in an animal model system, and any problems detected are carefully evaluated before the same treatments are attempted in humans.

Risks

A patient who is receiving gene therapy may face a number of potential problems. The viral vectors used may cause infection and/or inflammation of tissues, and artificial introduction of viruses into the body may initiate other disease processes. Functional gene therapy relies on stable incorporation of a new gene into an individual's own DNA. As the integration is random, occasionally the new gene may insert within another normally functioning gene, causing its damage or inactivation. This, in turn, could lead to cancer or other disease. It is also critical that the new gene have the proper regulatory controls so that the gene product is produced in the proper amount. Over-expression of certain genes can have deleterious results. Any of these problems could render the gene therapy ineffective, or, at worst, cause the death of the subject.

Normal results

Classic gene therapy seeks to treat or cure a defined disease by incorporating a functional gene or gene product into target cells of an affected individual.

Resources
BOOKS

George, Linda. *Gene Therapy.* Woodbridge, CT: Blackbirch Marketing, 2003.

Nussbaum, Robert L., Roderick R. McInnes, and Huntington F. Willard. *Thompson and Thompson Genetics in Medicine*, 6th edition. Philadelphia, PA: W. B. Saunders Company, 2001.

Strachan, T., and Andrew P. Read. *Human Molecular Genetics*, 2nd edition. New York, NY: John Wiley and Sons, 1999.

OTHER

National Cancer Institute. *Questions and Answers about Gene Therapy.* Cited January 4, 2004 (March 23, 2004). <http://cis.nci.nih.gov/fact/7_18.htm>.

Constance K. Stein

Gerstmann-Straussler-Scheinker disease

Definition

Gerstmann-Straussler-Scheinker disease is a progressively disabling and ultimately fatal brain infection caused by a unique protein particle called a prion. Gerstmann-Straussler-Scheinker disease is an inherited disorder, and occurs in familial clusters.

Description

Gerstmann-Straussler-Scheinker disease belongs to a group of diseases originally known as slow virus infections. Currently, slow virus infections are classed together as transmissible spongiform encephalopathies (TSE), or **prion diseases**. Other TSEs include **kuru**, **Creutzfeldt-Jakob disease**, and fatal familial insomnia. The TSE called new variant Creutzfeldt-Jakob disease (also known colloquially as "Mad Cow Disease") has received a great

deal of public attention. The TSEs, including Gerstmann-Straussler-Scheinker disease, involve abnormal clumps of protein that accumulate throughout the brain, destroying brain tissue and leaving spongy holes.

Demographics

About 10% of all transmissible spongiform encephalopathies are inherited. Gerstmann-Straussler-Scheinker disease occurs worldwide, but because of its pattern of familial transmission, cases tend to occur in specific geographic clusters. Only a few families have been identified as carrying the mutation that causes Gerstmann-Straussler-Scheinker disease.

Gerstmann-Straussler-Scheinker disease is caused by a genetic mutation caused by an infectious protein particle called a prion, which stands for proteinaceous infectious particle. A prion is similar to a virus, except that it lacks any nucleic acid, which prevents it from reproducing. Prions are abnormal versions of proteins that are found in the membranes of normal cells. These abnormal proteins can be passed directly to individuals through the ingestion of prion-infected tissue or when open sores on the recipient's skin are exposed to prion-infected tissue. In addition to being transmissible (as are other infectious agents like viruses or bacteria), prions are unique because they can also be acquired through genetic inheritance. This is the case with Gerstmann-Straussler-Scheinker disease.

In Gerstmann-Straussler-Scheinker disease, one of several possible specific gene mutations is present, leading to the abnormal deposition of tangled masses of a protein called amyloid throughout the brain. The spinocerebellar tracts (nerves that run from the brain's **cerebellum** throughout the spinal cord) become increasingly atrophied (shrunken) and dysfunctional over time.

Symptoms of Gerstmann-Straussler-Scheinker disease tend to begin in later middle age, usually between the ages of 40 and 55. Early symptoms include unsteady gait and difficulty walking, discoordination, clumsiness. As the disease progresses, the individual experiences difficulty speaking; abnormal, involuntary, rapid darting eye movements; paralyzed eye movement; deafness; blindness; and **dementia**. Death often occurs within five to 10 years of the initial symptoms.

Diagnosis

Diagnosis of Gerstmann-Straussler-Scheinker disease is arrived at through characteristic abnormalities found on the electroencephalogram (EEG), a test of brain waves and electricity. **MRI** studies and biopsies (tissue samples) from the brain may also show changes that are characteristic of

Key Terms

Classic Creutzfeldt-Jakob disease A rare, progressive neurological disease that is believed to be transmitted via an abnormal protein called a prion.

Fatal familial insomnia A rare, progressive neurological disease that is believed to be transmitted via an abnormal protein called a prion.

Gerstmann-Sträussler-Scheinker syndrome A rare, progressive neurological disease that is believed to be transmitted via an abnormal protein called a prion.

New variant Creutzfeldt-Jakob disease A more newly identified type of Creutzfeldt-Jakob disease that has been traced to the ingestion of beef from cows infected with bovine spongiform encephalopathy. Known in the popular press as Mad Cow Disease.

Transmissible spongiform encephalopathy A term that refers to a group of diseases, including kuru, Creutzfeldt-Jakob disease, Gerstmann-Sträussler-Scheinker syndrome, fatal familial insomnia, and new variant Creutzfeldt-Jakob disease. These diseases share a common origin as prion diseases, caused by abnormal proteins that accumulate within the brain and destroy brain tissue, leaving spongy holes.

prion disease. Like certain forms of CJD, Gerstmann-Straussler-Scheinker disease can be analyzed with DNA testing; specifically, the white blood cells are examined in order to identify one of the mutations associated with the disease.

Treatment team

Diagnosis of slow virus infection is usually made by a **neurologist**.

Treatment

There are no available treatments for Gerstmann-Straussler-Scheinker disease. It is relentlessly progressive, incurable, and fatal. Supportive care for the patient and his or her family is the only treatment.

Prognosis

Gerstmann-Straussler-Scheinker disease is always fatal.

Special Concrns

Gerstmann-Straussler-Scheinker disease is unique among transmissible spongiform encephalopathies, because mutations can be identified through DNA analysis of a sufferer's white blood cells. This allows other family members to be counseled regarding their personal risk of disease inheritance, projected age of disease onset, and potential illness duration. While some mutations sentence an individual to certain disease, other locations of mutations have only a 50% chance of leading to actual disease. Additionally, in families known to carry a mutation of Gerstmann-Straussler-Scheinker disease, amniocentesis can identify fetuses affected by the mutation, allowing families to make decisions about whether or not to continue a pregnancy.

Resources

BOOKS

Berger, Joseph R., and Avindra Nath. "Slow virus infections." In *Cecil Textbook of Medicine*, edited by Thomas E. Andreoli, et al. Philadelphia: W. B. Saunders Company, 2000.

Brown, Paul. "Transmissible Spongiform Encephalopathy." In *Textbook of Clinical Neurology*, edited by Christopher G. Goetz. Philadelphia: W. B. Saunders Company, 2003.

Murray, T. Jock, and William Pryse-Phillips. "Infectious diseases of the nervous system." In *Noble: Textbook of Primary Care Medicine*, edited by John Noble, et al. St. Louis: W. B. Saunders Company, 2001.

PERIODICALS

Sy, Man-Sun, Pierluigi Gambetti, and Wong Boon-Seng. "Human Prion Diseases." *Medical Clinics of North America* 86 (May 2002): 551–571.

WEBSITES

National Institute of Neurological Disorders and Stroke (NINDS). *NINDS Gerstmann-Straussler-Scheinker Disease Information Page.* March 26, 2003 (June 4, 2004). <http://www.ninds.nih.gov/health_and_medical/disorders/gss.htm>.

Rosalyn Carson-DeWitt, MD

Gerstmann syndrome

Definition

Gerstmann syndrome is a cluster of neurological symptoms that includes difficulty writing (dysgraphia or agraphia), difficulty with arithmetic (dyscalculia or acalculia), an inability to distinguish left from right, and difficulty identifying fingers (finger **agnosia**).

Description

Two types of Gerstmann syndrome have been identified: an acquired form that occurs in adults who have suffered brain injury through **stroke** or trauma, and a developmental form that has been noted in children.

The brain area that seems to be primarily responsible for the deficits seen in Gerstmann syndrome appears to be the parietal lobe, which is located behind the frontal lobe. Current research has not identified a tendency for the developmental form of Gerstmann syndrome to be inherited.

Although both adults and children with Gerstmann syndrome may have considerable impairment, they do not necessarily have abnormal intelligence.

Demographics

Gerstmann syndrome is usually identified in adult patients who have a history of brain injury or stroke. A very small group of children have also been identified as having the developmental form of the condition. Although the diagnosis tends to be made in school-aged children (usually at the point when writing and calculating become central classroom tasks), the condition may well be congenital. There are no reports clarifying the frequency or incidence of either the acquired or the developmental forms of Gerstmann syndrome.

Causes and symptoms

In adults, Gerstmann syndrome may be acquired when bleeding into the brain during a stroke or after a traumatic head injury occurs in an area of the left parietal lobe called the angular gyrus. A few adult cases of Gerstmann syndrome have also been described after viral encephalitis, tumor, or toxic exposure has caused injury to this same area of the brain. A specific cause for developmental Gerstmann syndrome has not been identified, although the fact that both parietal lobes are affected suggests that the problem occurs some time during early brain development.

The core symptoms in Gerstmann syndrome include:

• dysgraphia or agraphia: an inability or impairment in the ability to express oneself through the written word.

• dyscalculia or acalculia: an inability to perform basic calculations.

• left-right confusion: difficulty identifying the left or right of one's body or of other objects.

• finger agnosia: an inability to identify one's own or someone else's finger on the basis of a verbal command to hold up a particular finger.

Adults with Gerstmann syndrome may also display some degree of **aphasia**, which is an impaired ability to

---

Key Terms

Acalculia The inability to perform basic calculation (addition, subtraction, multiplication, division).

Agraphia The inability to write.

Angular gyrus A particular ridge (outfolding) in the parietal lobe of the brain.

Aphasia Difficulty using or understanding language.

Apraxia Difficulty performing a voluntary movement, although the muscles necessary are all functional.

Constructional apraxia Difficulty or inability to copy a drawing.

Dyscalculia Difficulty with basic arithmetic and calculations.

Dysgraphis Difficulty writing.

Finger agnosia Inability to identify a particular finger.

Parietal lobes The brain lobes on top of the brain, behind the frontal lobes.

---

communicate verbally, to understand verbal communication, and to understand written language. Children with developmental Gerstmann syndrome may also exhibit poor handwriting, difficulty spelling, reading problems, and difficulty copying simple drawings (called constructional **apraxia**).

Diagnosis

Diagnosis is through a comprehensive neurological exam and through psychoeducational testing.

Treatment team

The treatment team may include a **neurologist**, behavioral pediatrician, psychologist, psychiatrist, occupational therapist, physical therapist, and educational specialist.

Treatment

There is no cure for Gerstmann syndrome. Neither children nor adults with this disorder will recover completely from its effects. Instead, supportive therapy may teach some skills, but will also help identify bypass strategies that can be used. For example, if the arithmetic facts cannot be learned, then the use of calculators and other resources should be encouraged. Word processing programs on computers, including those that have voice-recognition capability, can greatly assist someone with Gerstmann syndrome with the tasks of writing. Classroom accommodations for children with Gerstmann syndrome can help assure success.

Prognosis

Gerstmann syndrome is a permanent disorder. It will last an individual's lifetime. However, the prognosis can be very good if the patient is helped to understand his or her deficits, supported in using effective bypass strategies, and encouraged to continue developing his or her areas of strength.

Special concerns

Good diagnosis and support is necessary so that individuals with Gerstmann syndrome can maintain the strongest possible self-esteem. Care must be taken not to suggest that the individual's failed efforts are due to laziness or lack of caring. Instead, the neurological basis of the disorder should be clearly explained, and reasonable bypass strategies should be immediately identified and implemented.

Resources

BOOKS

Cummings, Jeffrey L. "Disorders of Cognition." In *Cecil Textbook of Internal Medicine*, edited by Lee Goldman, et al. Philadelphia: W. B. Saunders Company, 2000.

Mesulam, M. Marsel. "Aphasias and Other Focal Cerebral Disorders." In *Harrison's Principles of Internal Medicine*, edited by Eugene Braunwald, et al. New York: McGraw-Hill Professional, 2001.

Swanberg, Margaret M., et al. "Speech and Language." In *Textbook of Clinical Neurology*, edited by Christopher G. Goetz. Philadelphia: W. B. Saunders Company, 2003.

PERIODICALS

Roux, F. E. "Writing, Calculating, and Finger Recognition in the Region of the Angular Gyrus: A Cortical Stimulation Study of Gerstmann Syndrome." *Journal of Neurosurgery* 99 (November 2003): 716–727.

Kronenberger, William G., and David W. Dunn. "Learning Disorders." *Neurologic Clinics* 21 (November 2003): 941–952.

OTHER

National Institute of Neurological Disorders and Stroke (NINDS). *NINDS Gerstmann's Syndrome Information Page.* March 21, 2003 (June 9, 2004). <http://www.ninds.nih.gov/health_and_medical/disorders/gerstmanns.htm>.

Rosalyn Carson-DeWitt, MD

Giant cell arteritis *see* **Temporal arteritis**

Giant cell inclusion disease *see* **Cytomegalic inclusion body disease**

Gilles de la Tourette syndrome *see* **Tourette syndrome**

Globoid cell leukodystrophy *see* **Krabbe disease**

▌Glossopharyngeal neuralgia

Definition

Glossopharyngeal neuralgia is a chronic **pain** syndrome that causes intense, shooting pains in the back of the tongue and throat, tonsillar areas, and middle ear.

Description

Glossopharyngeal neuralgia may be due to inflammation or compression of either the glossopharyngeal nerve or the vagus nerve, another nerve that innervates (stimulates) the same basic areas. The condition usually comes on quite suddenly, and may wax and wane in severity over time. This condition may occur in conjunction with **trigeminal neuralgia** (a pain syndrome affecting the face).

Demographics

Glossopharyngeal neuralgia usually strikes people over the age of 40. It is a relatively rare condition, affecting about 0.7/100,000 individuals per year.

Causes and symptoms

The cause of glossopharyngeal neuralgia is not completely understood, although it seems that conditions (tumors, infections, injuries, or blood vessels located close to the glossopharyngeal nerve) that put pressure on the glossopharyngeal nerve may sometimes be responsible for its development. Individuals with diabetes or **multiple sclerosis** may also develop glossopharyngeal neuralgia. Episodes of pain may be brought on by swallowing, sneezing, chewing, clearing the throat, eating spicy foods, drinking cold liquids, speaking, laughing, or coughing.

Glossopharyngeal neuralgia causes sudden, intense pains in the throat, mouth, tongue, jaw, ear, and neck. The pains have been described as excruciating and electric shock-like, and usually last from seconds to several minutes. Because the glossopharyngeal nerve also affects heart rate and blood pressure, some patients experience abnormal heart rhythms during episodes of pain. The heart rate may become so slow, in fact, that the patient faints.

Diagnosis

The diagnosis is usually strongly suspected from the patient's characteristic description of the pain episodes. Often, the doctor can trigger an episode by gently touching the back of the throat with a cotton swab. The test is then repeated after application of a topical anesthetic has been used to numb the throat. If the pain episodes are caused by glossopharyngeal neuralgia, touching the back of the anesthetized throat with a cotton swab will not trigger an episode of pain.

CT or **MRI** may reveal inflammation of the glossopharyngeal nerve or the presence of an abnormality (such as a tumor) that is exerting pressure on the nerve. **Angiography** involves introducing dye into the vascular system, in order to take x-ray, CT, or MRI images that may reveal the location of a blood vessel that is exerting pressure on the glossopharyngeal nerve.

Treatment team

Neurologists and otorhinolaryngologists treat glossopharyngeal neuralgia.

Treatment

Carbamazepine, phenytoin, **gabapentin**, baclofen, and tricyclic antidepressants may be used to ameliorate the pain of glossopharyngeal neuralgia. When a blood vessel is identified as compressing the glossopharyngeal nerve, surgery may be performed to move the vessel or to position a Teflon felt pad between the blood vessel and the nerve, in order to attempt to mitigate any pressure that is exerted on the nerve. In severe cases of glossopharyngeal neuralgia that don't respond to other treatments, surgery that severs the glossopharyngeal nerve may be the only treatment that relieves the sufferer's pain.

Prognosis

The prognosis of glossopharyngeal neuralgia varies, depending on the underlying cause of the disorder. Some individuals are completely relieved of the pain episodes after surgery; others continue to have periodic exacerbations throughout their lives.

Resources

BOOKS

Cutrer, F. Michael, and Michael A. Moskowitz. "Headaches and Other Head Pain." In *Cecil Textbook of Internal Medicine*, edited by Lee Goldman, et al. Philadelphia: W. B. Saunders Company, 2000.

Hermanowicz, Neal. "Cranial Nerves IX (Glossopharyngeal) and X (Vagus)." In *Textbook of Clinical Neurology*, edited by Christopher G. Goetz. Philadelphia: W. B. Saunders Company, 2003.

PERIODICALS

Rozen, Todd D. "Trigeminal neuralgia and glossopharyngeal neuralgia." *Neurologic Clinics* 22, no. 1 (February 2004).

WEBSITES

NINDS Glossopharyngeal Neuralgia Information Page. National Institute of Neurological Disorders and Stroke (NINDS). November 6, 2002 (June 2, 2004). <http://www.ninds.nih.gov/health_and_medical/disorders/glossopharyngeal_neuralgia.htm>

Rosalyn Carson-DeWitt, MD

Glucocorticoids

Definition

Glucocorticoids are naturally-produced steroid hormones, or synthetic compounds, that inhibit the process of inflammation.

Purpose

The target of glucocorticoids: inflammation

Glucocorticoids are used to stop the inflammation process. The inflammatory process has evolved in the body for a useful purpose; namely as a defensive reaction to the damage or injury to tissue. By a series of reactions, inflammation is designed to isolate whatever is causing the irritation, help eradicate the presumed invader, and help repair the surrounding damaged tissue.

The hallmarks of inflammation are redness, heat, swelling, and **pain**. These reactions arise from the various steps in the inflammation pathway. The inflammatory response begins with the expansion of the capillaries, which allows more blood to flow to the target site. Various proteins from the blood then exit the blood and gather at the target site. Ultimately, white blood cells called leukocytes also accumulate at the site of injury. When these processes occur in response to an invader such as a microorganism, this is beneficial for the body, as it can rid the body of a potential problem. However, sometimes the inflammatory response can persist long after the actual problem is gone, or can be maintained if an infection itself becomes chronic, or can be activated by some malfunction in the body's defense mechanisms. Chronic inflammation of this type can cause damage to host tissue. Examples of processes that can produce chronic inflammation are tuberculosis, inflammatory bowel diseases such as ulcerative

Key Terms

Osteoporosis A disorder involving loss of calcium and density in the bones, resulting in brittle bones and changes in posture.

Steroid A naturally-occurring hormone, and a large class of drugs that chemically resemble cholesterol. Among the more common types of steroids, anabolic steroids are sometimes used illegally in athletics, and glucocorticoid steroids are used to reduce inflammation.

colitis and Crohn's disease, silicosis, and the continued presence of a foreign body in a wound.

Glucocorticoids can be prescribed to dampen or stop entirely this chronic inflammatory chain of events. Depending on the particular glucocorticoid that is used, inflammation can be affected at different points in the inflammatory pathway.

Description

Some of the various glucocorticoids can be naturally produced in the body. Chemically, these are steroid hormones. They are different from the infamous anabolic steroids that some athletes use to increase muscle mass and strength. Rather, glucocorticoids are catabolic steroids, meaning they are designed to break down compounds. Natural glucocorticoids are produced in the adrenal glands located immediately above the kidneys (the word adrenal derives from "ad," meaning top of, and "renal," meaning kidney). The region of the adrenal glands called the cortex is the site of glucocorticoid manufacture.

Glucocorticoids can also be artificially made, and are usually referred to as glucocorticoid drugs. Examples of glucocorticoids are prednisone, prednisilone, methylprednisilone, dexamethasone, and hydrocortisone. Glucocorticoids are usually taken orally as tablets, capsules, syrup, and liquid, with the exception of hydrocortisone (which is applied as a cream). Most can also be used in cream form, and some can be applied as drops to relieve eye irritations.

Prednisone is the commonly prescribed glucocorticoid because of its high activity. In the body prednisone is transformed by the liver into prednisolone. Prednisolone is equally as effective and is often prescribed by physicians instead of prednisone. Dexamethasone can be prescribed in higher doses than the other glucocorticoids. A common use for this compound is the reduction of nerve swelling following nerve damage or neurosurgery. Depending on

the manufacturer, dexamethasone is marketed as Decadron, Dexameth, Dexone, and Hexadrol.

Glucocorticoids and metabolism

As well as affecting the inflammatory process, glucocorticoids have an effect on the utilization of compounds in the body (metabolism). Indeed, the designation glucocorticoid arose from observations that the hormones played a role in the utilization of glucose. In an absence of food, which can be broken down to supply glucose, glucocorticoids act to increase and maintain the normal levels of glucose in the blood. They accomplish this by stimulating glucose production by cells, particularly in the liver, and by enhancing the breakdown of fat in fat tissue. As well, glucocorticoids curb the storage of glucose in cells of the body, which leaves the sugar ready for use.

Glucocorticoids and inflammation

Glucocorticoids are global in their inhibition of the inflammatory response. That is, they act at different stages in the process, and affect all types of inflammatory responses no matter what stimulated the response. The action of glucocorticoids has to do with their structure. Their shape permits them to move across the membrane that surrounds cells in the body, and to be recognized by molecules inside the cell called glucocorticoid receptors. Binding of the particular glucocorticoid to a receptor forms a complex between the two molecules. This complex can enter the nucleus of the cell (the zone where the genetic material is located, and where the two-step process whereby nucleic acid forms the blueprint for the manufacture of the protein building blocks of the cell takes place). Within the nucleus, the complex affects the manufacture of the proteins. The production of some proteins is enhanced while the manufacture of other protein species is diminished. The latter are proteins involved in inflammation and in the release of a normally membrane-bound molecule that acts as a signal for inflammation to begin. The end result is the suppression of inflammation.

Recommended dosage

The prescribed dosages of glucocorticoids vary depending on the compound used and the nature of the patient's condition. Depending on the glucocorticoid, the dose may be taken once a day, over the course of several doses spaced evenly throughout the day, or even every other day.

Precautions

As with any prescription drug, the recommended daily dosage and schedule for the drugs should not be changed independent of a physician's notification. As well, side effects associated with the long-term use of glucocorticoids can occur.

Side effects

Prolonged use of glucocorticoids may cause a number of adverse effects. These include the suppression of the immune system (which makes the person more susceptible to infections), osteoporosis, shifts in the body's fluid balance, skin changes, changes in brain chemistry, and altered behavior.

Dexamethasone can cause loss of appetite, weight loss, stomach upset, vomiting, drowsiness, **headache**, confusion, fever, joint pain, and peeling skin. Not all side effects will be present in everyone taking dexamethasone.

More severe side effects of glucocorticoid use include development of diabetes (which can occur transiently even with short-term use of the drugs), glaucoma, cataract formation, peptic ulcer, convulsions, and inhibited growth of children. A physician determines whether the potential risks of the particular glucocorticoid outweigh the advantages of its use, and prescribes the minimum dose necessary to achieve the desired effect.

Interactions

Interactions between glucocorticoids and other medications can occur. These include anticoagulants (such as aspirin), digoxin, estrogen, oral contraceptives, **phenobarbital**, some antibiotics, and even some vitamins.

Resources

BOOKS

Goulding, N. J. *Glucocorticoids (Milestones in Drug Therapy).* Birkhauser, 2001.

Zuckerman, Eugenia, and Julie R. Inglefinger. *Coping with Prednisone and Other Cortisone-Related Medicines: It May Work Miracles, but How Do You Handle the Side Effects?* St. Martin's Press, 1998.

OTHER

"Dexamethasone oral." *Medline Plus.* National Library of Medicine. (May 6, 2004). <http://www.nlm.nih.gov/medlineplus/druginfo/medmaster/a682792.html>.

"Glucocorticoids Disease Mechanism II: Inflammation." Stanford University. (May 6, 2004). <http://www.stanford.edu/group/hopes/treatmts/antiinflam/I_glucocorticoids.html>

Brian Douglas Hoyle, PhD

Guillain-Barré syndrome

Definition

Guillain-Barré syndrome (GBS) is an inflammation of the covering that surrounds nerve cells of the brain and spinal cord. The basis of the inflammation is not conclusively known, but is generally considered to arise from a malfunctioning immune system that recognizes host tissues as being foreign. The inflammation reaction damages the nerves of the brain and spinal cord, producing weakness in the muscles, loss of sensation (such as the sense of touch in the fingers), or outright paralysis.

GBS is termed a syndrome rather than a disease because there is no conclusive evidence to support the possibility that a specific disease-causing agent such as a bacteria or a virus is the direct cause of the malady. Infections may be a trigger to the development of GBS, however.

Description

The syndrome is named after George Charles Guillen and Jean-Alexandre Barré, French co-authors of a classic paper on the syndrome that was published in 1916. A third author, André Strohl, was not subsequently associated with the syndrome that was the subject of the paper.

GBS is a rare and acute disorder. An acute disorder displays a rapid appearance of symptoms, and a rapid worsening of the symptoms. In the case of GBS, symptoms typically appear over just a single day. Most often, symptoms are first noticed in the feet and legs. The symptoms often progress to involve different parts of the body over the next several days to several weeks. In addition, during that time other more severe symptoms can appear. In more than 90% of cases, the symptoms reach their peak by four weeks.

The syndrome is an inflammatory disorder, in which a person's own immune system attacks the nerves outside the brain and the spinal cord. These nerves are known as peripheral nerves. The nerve inflammation that occurs can damage the nerve cells. The covering (sheath) of a fatty material called myelin that surrounds the cells can be lost. This loss is called demyelination.

Additionally, the elongated portion of the nerve cell called the axon can be killed. This phenomenon is called denervation. The axon conveys electrical impulses to more distant areas of muscles, and from one nerve cell to another. Demyelination and denervation bring about muscle weakness, loss of sensation, or paralysis because the affected nerves cannot transmit signals to muscles. This loss of signal transmission inhibits the muscles from being able to respond to nerve signals. As well, the brain receives fewer signals and the person can become unable to feel heat, cold, or **pain**.

GBS is also known as Landry-Guillain-Barré syndrome, acute idiopathic polyneuritis, infectious polyneuritis, and acute inflammatory demyelinating polyneuropathy (AIDP). Another malady called chronic inflammatory demyelinating polyradicalneuropathy is possibly related to GBS. It is far less common than GBS (which itself is rare) and persists longer.

Demographics

GBS can occur at any age. However, the syndrome tends to be more prevalent in men and women aged 15–35 years and 50–75 years (a bimodal pattern of age distribution), respectively. Males are slightly more susceptible than females (the ratio of those affected is approximately 1.5 male per female). There is no known racial group that is any more susceptible to GBS, nor any known geographical localization of the syndrome.

In the United States, the syndrome is rare. For example, the annual incidence of GBS in the United States ranges from 0.6 to 2.4 cases per 100,000 people. Nonetheless, GBS is the most common cause of neuromuscular paralysis among Americans.

Causes and symptoms

Causes

The exact cause of GBS is not known. However, bacterial or viral infections may be a trigger for its development. Almost 70% of those who develop GBS have had an infectious illness in the preceding two to four weeks. Examples of infections include sore throat, cold, flu, and diarrhea. Bacteria that have been associated with the subsequent development of GBS include chlamydia, *Mycoplasma pneumoniae*, and *Campylobacter jejuni.*

The suspected involvement of Campylobacter is noteworthy, as this bacterium is a common contaminant of poultry. Inadequate cooking can allow the microbe to survive and cause an infection in those who consume the food. Thus, there may be a connection between GBS and food quality. The form of GBS that may be associated with the presence of Campylobacter may be particularly severe. For reasons that are unclear, the peripheral nerves can themselves be directly attacked, rather than just the myelin sheath around the nerves.

Usually, infections such as those caused by Campylobacter have abated before the onset of GBS. As well, chronic infection with the viruses responsible for mononucleosis, herpes, and acquired immunodeficiency syndrome can prelude the appearance of GBS. The latter is also known as HIV-1 associated acute inflammatory demyelinating polyneuropathy.

Other possible associated factors include vaccination (rabies, swine flu, influenza, Group A streptococci), surgery, pregnancy, and maladies such as Hodgkin's disease and systematic **lupus** erythematosus.

Whether there is direct (causal) connection between infections and maladies and the subsequent development of GBS, or whether the events are only coincidental, is not known. For example, vaccination of Americans against the swine flu in 1976 increased the rate of GBS by less than one case per 100,000 people. Whether this increase was directly due to the vaccine is impossible to determine. Furthermore, more than 99% of people suffering from GBS who have been surveyed by the United States Centers for Disease Control and Prevention (CDC) have not recently been vaccinated. According to the CDC, the chance of developing GBS as a result of vaccination is remote.

It is conceivable that the infections or illnesses disrupt the body's immune system such that autoimmune destruction of nerve cell components occurs. Although this intriguing possibility is favored among many scientists, it remains unsubstantiated.

There is no evidence to indicate that GBS is an infection or that it is a genetically linked (heritable) disorder.

Symptoms

The initial sensation of weakness or paralysis in the toes spreads upward within days to a few weeks to the arms and the central part of the body. In medical terminology, this represents an ascending pattern of spread. The weakness and paralysis can also be accompanied by a tingling sensation, and a cramping or more constant pain in the feet, hands, thighs, shoulders, lower back, and buttocks. Use of the hands and feet can become impaired. More serious development of paralysis can make breathing difficult, even to the point that mechanical ventilation becomes necessary.

Other, less typical symptoms include blurred vision, clumsiness, difficulty in moving facial muscles, involuntary muscle contractions, and a pronounced heartbeat. Symptoms that are indicative of an emergency include difficulty in swallowing, drooling, breathing difficulty, and **fainting**.

Progression from the early symptoms to the more severe symptoms can occur very quickly (i.e., 24–72 hours). Typically, the exacerbated condition persists for several weeks. Recovery then typically occurs gradually, and can take anywhere from days to six months or more.

In very mild cases, an individual may just have a general feeling of weakness. As the symptoms abate after a few weeks, the person may dismiss the incident as a viral infection, without ever knowing the true nature of the illness.

Diagnosis

GBS is suspected if a patient displays muscle weakness or paralysis that has been increasing in severity, especially if an illness has occurred recently. Loss of reflexes such as the knee jerk reaction can be an early clue to a clinician.

Clinical data can be useful in diagnosis. For example, a hormone that is involved in maintaining the proper chemical balance of urine can be affected in GBS. The result is

Key Terms

Autonomic nervous system The part of the nervous system that is concerned with the control of involuntary bodily functions such as breathing, sweating, blinking, and the heartbeat.

Axon The long, hairlike extension of a nerve cell that carries a message to a nearby nerve cell.

Demyelination Loss of the myelin (a fatty substance) sheath that surrounds and insulates the axons of nerve cells and is necessary for the proper conduction of neural impulses.

Neuropathy A disorder of the nervous system or a nerve.

called the syndrome of inappropriate antidiuretic hormone. Antibodies to nerve cells may be present as a result of the body's immune reaction against its own constituents.

Another clue to the diagnosis of GBS can be the finding of muscle weakness by neurological examination. One such test is known as nerve conduction velocity. In this test, the selected nerve is stimulated, usually with surface electrodes contained in a patch that is applied to the surface of the skin. The nerve can be stimulated using a very mild electrical current put out from one electrode, and the resulting electrical activity is recorded by the other electrodes in the patch. The nerve conduction velocity is calculated knowing the distance between electrodes and measuring the time it takes for the impulses to travel from the generating to the measuring electrodes. A person with GBS whose nerves have usually lost some or most of the myelin sheath will display a slower conduction velocity than that displayed by an unaffected person. Electrical impulses travel along the damaged nerve slower than along an undamaged nerve.

Muscle response to electrical stimulation can also be measured by **electromyography** (EMG). In this test, a needle electrode is inserted through the skin into the muscle. When the muscle is stimulated, for example, by contracting it, the resulting visual or audio pattern carries the information about the muscle's response. The characteristic pattern of wavelengths produced by a healthy muscle (the action potential) can be compared to a muscle in someone suspected of having GBS.

When paralysis of the heart muscle is suspected, an electrocardiogram can be used to record the electrical activity of the heart. GBS muscle paralysis can alter the normal pattern of the heartbeat.

Finally, an examination of the cerebrospinal fluid by means of a spinal tap (also known as a lumbar puncture)

may detect a higher-than-normal level of protein in the absence of an increase in the number of white blood cells (WBCs). An increase in WBCs is a hallmark of an infection.

Treatment team

Neurologists, immunologists, physical therapists, occupational therapists, and nurses figure prominently in GBS treatment. The assistance of support groups such as the Guillen-Barré Syndrome Foundation International can also be a useful adjunct to treatment.

Treatment

As recently as the 1980s, treatment for GBS consisted of letting the syndrome run its course. While most people recovered completely with time, some people were not as lucky. Those who develop severe symptoms such as breathing difficulty are routinely hospitalized.

One medical procedure that can be useful in the treatment of GBS is called plasmaphoresis. It is also known as plasma exchange. In plasmapheresis, antibody-laden blood plasma (the liquid portion of the blood) is removed from the body. Red blood cells are separated and put back into the body with antibody-free plasma or intravenous fluid. The treatment can lessen the symptoms of GBS and hasten recovery time. As of December 2003, it is not known why plasmapheresis works. It is suspected that the removal of antibodies may lessen the effects of the body's immune attack on the nerve cells.

Another procedure that produces similar results involves the administration of intravenous immune globulin (IVIG). Both treatments have been shown to speed up recovery time by up to 50%. IVIG has been shown to be an effective treatment for immune-system-related neuropathies in general. IVIG may act by reducing the amount of anti-myelin antibodies through the binding of the defective antibodies by healthy antibodies contained in the IVIG solution, and in suppressing the immune response.

Other treatments are designed to prevent or lessen complications of GBS. For example, choking during eating, because of throat muscle weakness or paralysis, can be prevented using a feeding tube, and formation of blood clots can be lessened by the use of chemicals that thin the blood. The pain associated with GBS can be treated with anti-inflammatory drugs or, if necessary, stronger-acting narcotic medication. For patients who have breathing difficulties, clinicians may first need to supply oxygen, install a breathing tube (intubation), and/or use a mechanical device that helps in breathing.

Physical therapy is helpful. Caregivers can move a patient's arms and legs to help maintain the flexibility and strength of the muscles. Later in recovery, sessions in a whirlpool (hydrotherapy) can help restore function to arms and legs. Often, therapists will design a series of exercises to be performed when the patient returns home.

Recovery and rehabilitation

More than 95% of people afflicted with GBS survive. In about 20% of people, however, muscle weakness and **fatigue** may remain. Some people find that wearing highly elastic gradient compression stockings beneficial. The stockings produce the greatest compression at the toes, with a tapering-off upwards to the thigh. The effect is to reduce the volume of veins, which increases the rate of blood flow through the veins. The increased blood flow can reduce the feeling of numbness in the toes.

Clinical trials

As of early 2004, three **clinical trials** were recruiting patients, including:

• Assessment of chronic Guillain-Barré syndrome improvement with use of 4-aminopyridine. The study, funded by the United States Food and Drug Administration Office of Orphan Products Development, seeks to assess the potential of 4-aminopyridine in increasing the transmission of impulses in damaged nerves. It is hoped that increased nerve activity could restore some lost muscle activity, as has occurred using the drug with those afflicted with **multiple sclerosis**. The contact is the Spain Rehabilitation Center, University of Alabama at Birmingham, 35249-7330; Jay Meythaler, M.D. (205) 934-2088, (email: Jmeythal@uab.edu).

• Safety, tolerability, and efficacy of rituximab in patients with anti-glycoconjugate antibody-mediated demyelinating neuropathy: a double-blind placebo-controlled randomized trial. While not directly related to GBS, the study concerns the loss of the myelin sheath of nerves and so is relevant. The study, sponsored by the National Institute of Neurological Disorders and Stroke (NINDS), is designed to evaluate the usefulness of rituximab in preventing the antibody damage to nerves. The contact is the National Institutes of Health Patient Recruitment and Public Liaison Office, Building 61, 10 Cloister Court, Bethesda, MD, 20892-4754; (800) 411-1222; prpl@mail.cc.nih.gov.

• Diagnostic evaluation of patients with neuromuscular diseases. This NINDS-sponsored study is designed to screen patients for other studies and to help train clinicians in the diagnosis of maladies including GBS. The contact information is the same as the above item.

Prognosis

Most of those afflicted with GBS recover completely, although the recovery can in some cases be slow (months to years). Complete recovery usually occurs when the symptoms fade within three weeks of appearing. The typical scenario is for a patient to experience the most weakness from 10–14 days after the appearance of symptoms, with complete recovery occurring within weeks or a few months. In contrast, a poor prognosis can be associated with a rapid appearance of symptoms, use of assisted ventilation for a month or more, severe nerve damage, and with advancing age.

While recovery is complete for most of those afflicted with GBS, in 10–20% of cases the symptoms reappear, in 15–20% the neurologic complications can persist and can cause a long-term disability, and 5–10% of those who are afflicted die. The main cause of death historically was from respiratory failure due to muscle paralysis. With mechanical ventilation, respiratory failure in GBS is less often fatal. Currently the main cause of death is malfunctioning of the autonomic nervous system, which controls involuntary processes such as heart rate, blood pressure, and body temperature.

Resources

PERIODICALS

Quarles, R. H., and M. D. Weiss. "Autoantibodies Associated with Peripheral Neuropathy." *Muscle Nerve* (July 1999): 800–822.

OTHER

Guillain-Barré Syndrome (GBS) and Influenzae Vaccine. Centers for Disease Control and Prevention. CDC. December 15, 2003 (April 4, 2004). <http://www.cdc.gov/nip/vacsafe/concerns/GBS/default.htm>.

Fanion, David, and Daniel M. Joyce. "Guillain-Barré Syndrome." *eMedicine.* December 12, 2003 (April 4, 2004). <http://www.emedicine.com/EMERG/topic222.htm>.

Mayo Foundation for Medical Education and Research. "Guillain-Barré Syndrome." *MayoClinic.com.* December 13, 2003 (April 4, 2004). <http://www.mayoclinic.com/invoke.cfm?id=DS00413>.

National Institutes of Health. "Guillain-Barré Syndrome." *MEDLINEplus Medical Encyclopedia.* December 13, 2003 (April 4, 2004). <http://www.nlm.nih.gov/medlineplus/ency/article/000684.htm>.

NINDS Guillain-Barré Syndrome Information Page. National Institute of Neurological Disorders and Stroke. December 10, 2003 (April 4, 2004). <http://www.ninds.nih.gov/health_and_medical/disorders/gbs.htm>.

ORGANIZATIONS

Centers for Disease Control and Prevention. 1600 Clifton Road, Atlanta, GA 30333. (404) 639-3311 or (800) 311-3435. <http://www.cdc.gov/>.

Guillain-Barré Syndrome Foundation International. P.O. Box 262, Wynnewood, PA 19096. (610) 667-0131; Fax: (610) 667-7036. info@gbsfi.com. <http://www.gbsfi.com>.

National Institutes of Health. 9000 Rockville Pike, Bethesda, MD 20892. (301) 496-4000. NIHInfo@od.nih.gov. <http://www.nih.gov>.

National Institute for Neurological Disorders and Stroke. P.O. Box 5801, Bethesda, MD 20824. (301) 496-5761 or (800) 352-9424. <http://www.ninds.nih. gov>.

Brian Douglas Hoyle, PhD

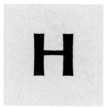

H

Hallervorden-Spatz disease *see*
Pantothenate kinase-associated neurodegeneration (PKAN)

Hallucination

Definitions

A hallucination is a sensory perception without a source in the external world. The English word "hallucination" comes from the Latin verb *hallucinari*, which means "to wander in the mind." Hallucinations can affect any of the senses, although certain diseases or disorders are associated with specific types of hallucinations.

It is important to distinguish between hallucinations and illusions or delusions, as the terms are often confused in conversation and popular journalism. A hallucination is a distorted sensory experience that appears to be a perception of something real even though it is *not* caused by an external stimulus. For example, some elderly people who have been recently bereaved may have hallucinations in which they "see" the dead loved one. An illusion, by contrast, is a mistaken or false interpretation of a real sensory experience, as when a traveler in the desert sees what looks like a pool of water, but in fact is a mirage caused by the refraction of light as it passes through layers of air of different densities. The bluish-colored light is a real sensory stimulus, but mistaking it for water is an illusion. A delusion is a false belief that a person maintains in spite of evidence to the contrary and in spite of proof that other members of their culture do not share the belief. For example, some people insist that they have seen flying saucers or unidentified flying objects (UFOs) even though the objects they have filmed or photographed can be shown to be ordinary aircraft, weather balloons, satellites, etc.

Description

It would be difficult to describe a "typical" hallucination, as these experiences vary considerably in length of time, quality, and sense or senses affected. Some hallucinations last only a few seconds; however, some people diagnosed with Charles Bonnet syndrome (CBS) have reported visual hallucinations lasting over several days, while people who have taken certain drugs have experienced hallucinations involving colors, sounds, and smells lasting for hours. Albert Hoffman, the Swiss chemist who first synthesized lysergic acid diethylamide (LSD), experienced nine hours of hallucinations after taking a small amount of the drug in 1943. In 1896, the American **neurologist** S. Weir Mitchell published an account of the six hours of hallucinations that followed his experimental swallowing of peyote buttons.

There is not always a close connection between the cause of a person's hallucinations and the emotional response to them. One study of patients diagnosed with CBS found that 30% of the patients were upset by their hallucinations, while 13% found them amusing or pleasant. The environment in which LSD and other hallucinogens are taken may affect an individual's psychological constitution and personal reactions. The writer Peter Matthiessen, for example, noted that his 1960s experiences with LSD "were magic shows, mysterious, enthralling," while his wife "... freaked out; that is the drug term, and there is no better.... her armor had cracked, and all the night winds of the world went howling through." In contrast to those who take hallucinogens, however, a majority of patients with **narcolepsy**, alcoholic hallucinosis, or post-traumatic disorders finds their hallucinations frightening.

Demographics

The demographics of hallucinations vary depending on their cause; however, many researchers think that they are underreported for several reasons:

• Fear of being thought "crazy" or mentally ill

- Gaps in research. For example, some types of hallucinations are associated with disorders that primarily affect the elderly, who are often underrepresented in health surveys

- Fear of being reported to law enforcement for illegal drug use

In 2000, one of the few studies of hallucinations in a general Western population reported the following statistics:

- Of a total sample of 13,000 adults, 38.7% reported hallucinations: 6.4% had hallucinations once a month, 2.7% once a week, and 2.4% more than once a week.

- Of the subjects, 27% reported having hallucinations in the daytime. In this group, visual (3.2%) and auditory (0.6%) hallucinations were closely associated with diagnoses of psychotic or anxiety disorders.

- Of the subjects, 3.1% reported haptic (tactile) hallucinations; most of these subjects were current drug users.

There is currently no evidence that hallucinations occur more frequently in some racial or ethnic groups than in others. In addition, gender does not appear to make a difference. The demographics of hallucinations associated with some specific age groups, conditions, or disorders are as follows:

- Children. Hallucinations are rare in children below the age of eight. About 40% of children diagnosed with **schizophrenia**, however, have visual or auditory hallucinations.

- Eye disorders. About 14% of patients treated in eye clinics for glaucoma or age-related macular degeneration report visual hallucinations.

- Alzheimer's disease (AD). About 40–50% of patients diagnosed with AD develop hallucinations in the later stages of the disease.

- Drug use. Hallucinogens are the third most frequently abused class of drugs (after alcohol and marijuana) among high school and college students. Various surveys report that about 7% of people in the United States over the age of 12 have taken LSD at least once; that 5% of high school seniors admit to using MDMA (Ecstasy); and that 20–24% of college students use MDMA. The highest rate of hallucinogen abuse is found in Caucasian males between the ages of 18 and 25.

- Normal sleep/wake cycles. Sleep researchers in Great Britain and the United States have reported that 30–37% of adults experience hypnagogic hallucinations, which occur during the passage from wakefulness into sleep, while about 10–12% report hypnopompic hallucinations, which occur as a person awakens. Hallucinations related to ordinary sleeping and waking are not considered an indication of a mental or physical disorder.

- Migraine headaches. About 10% of patients diagnosed with migraine headaches experience visual hallucinations prior to the onset of an acute attack.

- Adult-onset schizophrenia. According to the National Institute of Mental Health (NIMH), about 75% of adults diagnosed with schizophrenia experience hallucinations, most commonly auditory or visual. The auditory hallucinations may be command hallucinations, in which the person hears voices ordering him or her to do something. For example, the man who killed a Swedish politician in September 2003 told the police that voices in his head told him "to attack."

- Temporal lobe **epilepsy** (TLE). About 80% of patients diagnosed with TLE report gustatory and olfactory hallucinations as well as auditory and visual hallucinations.

- Narcolepsy. Frequent hypnagogic hallucinations are considered one of four classic symptoms of narcolepsy, and are experienced by 60% of patients diagnosed with the disorder.

- Post-traumatic stress disorder (PTSD). Studies of combat veterans diagnosed with PTSD have found that 50–65% have experienced auditory hallucinations. Visual, olfactory, and haptic hallucinations have been reported by survivors of rape and childhood sexual abuse.

Causes

The neurologic causes of hallucinations are not currently completely understood, although researchers have identified some factors in the context of specific disorders, and have proposed various hypotheses to explain hallucinations in others. There does not appear to be a single causal factor that accounts for hallucinations in all people who experience them.

Sleep deprivation

Research subjects who have undergone sleep deprivation experiments typically begin to hallucinate after 72–96 hours without sleep. It is thought that these hallucinations result from the malfunctioning of nerve cells within the prefrontal cortex of the brain. This area of the brain is associated with judgment, impulse control, attention, and visual association, and is refreshed during the early stages of sleep. When a person is sleep-deprived, the nerve cells in the prefrontal cortex must work harder than usual without an opportunity to recover. The hallucinations that develop on the third day of wakefulness are thought to be hypnagogic hallucinations that occur during "microsleeps," or short periods of light sleep lasting about one to ten seconds.

Amygdala   An almond-shaped brain structure in the limbic system that is activated in stressful situations to trigger the emotion of fear. Hallucinations related to post-traumatic stress are thought to be caused by the activation of memory traces in the amygdala that have not been integrated and modified by other parts of the brain.

Auditory   Pertaining to the sense of hearing.

Charles Bonnet syndrome (CBS)   A disorder characterized by visual hallucinations following a sudden age-related deterioration in a person's vision, most commonly glaucoma or macular degeneration. CBS is named for a Swiss doctor who first described it in his visually impaired grandfather in 1780.

Command hallucination   A type of auditory hallucination in which the person hears voices ordering him or her to perform a specific act.

Corollary discharge   A mechanism in the brain that allows one to distinguish between self-generated and external stimuli or perceptions.

Delusion   A false belief that a person maintains in spite of obvious proof or evidence to the contrary.

Flashback   A vivid sensory or emotional experience that happens independently of the initial event or experience. Flashbacks resulting from the use of LSD are sometimes referred to as hallucinogen persisting perception disorder, or HPPD.

Gustatory   Pertaining to the sense of taste.

Hallucinogen   A drug or other substance that induces hallucinations.

Haptic   Pertaining to the sense of touch; sometimes called tactile hallucinations.

Hippocampus   A part of the brain that is involved in memory formation and learning. The hippocampus is shaped like a curved ridge and belongs to an organ system called the limbic system.

Hypnagogic   Pertaining to drowsiness; refers to hallucinations that occur as a person falls asleep.

Hypnopompic   Persisting after sleep; refers to hallucinations that occur as a person awakens.

Illusion   A false interpretation of a real sensory image or impression.

Irritative hallucinations   Hallucinations caused by abnormal electrical activity in the brain.

Lysergic acid diethylamide (LSD)   The first synthetic hallucinogen, discovered in 1938.

Neuroleptic   Another name for an antipsychotic medication.

Neurotransmitters   Chemicals that carry nerve impulses from one nerve cell to another.

Olfactory   Pertaining to the sense of smell.

Psychosis   A severe mental disorder characterized by loss of contact with reality. Hallucinations are associated with such psychotic disorders as schizophrenia and brief psychotic disorder.

Release hallucinations   Hallucinations that develop after partial loss of sight or hearing, and represent images or sounds formed from memory traces rather than present sensory input. They are called "release" hallucinations because they would ordinarily be blocked by incoming sensory data.

Post-traumatic memory formation

Hallucinations in trauma survivors are caused by abnormal patterns of memory formation during the traumatic experience. In normal situations, memories are formed from sensory data, organized in a part of the brain known as the hippocampus, and integrated with previous memories in the frontal cortex. People then "make sense" of their memories through the use of language, which helps them to describe their experiences to others and to themselves. In traumatic situations, however, bits and pieces of memory are stored in the amygdala, an almond-shaped structure in the brain that ordinarily attaches emotional significance to memories, without being integrated by the

hippocampus and interpreted in the frontal cortex. In addition, the region of the brain that governs speech (Broca's area) often shuts down under extreme stress. The result is that memories of the traumatic event remain in the amygdala as a chaotic wordless jumble of physical sensations or sensory images that can re-emerge as hallucinations during stressful situations at later points in the patient's life.

Irritative hallucinations

In 1973, a British researcher named Cogan categorized hallucinations into two major groups that he called "irritative" and "release" hallucinations. Irritative hallucinations result from abnormal electrical discharges in the brain, and are associated with such disorders as migraine **headaches** and epilepsy. Brain tumors and traumatic damage to the brain are other possible causes of abnormal electrical activity manifesting as visual hallucinations.

Hallucinations have also been reported with a number of infectious diseases that affect the brain, including bacterial meningitis, rabies, herpes virus infections, **Lyme disease**, HIV infection, toxoplasmosis, Jakob-Creuzfeldt disease, and late-stage syphilis.

Release hallucinations

Release hallucinations are most common in people with impaired eyesight or hearing. They are produced by the spontaneous activity of nerve cells in the visual or auditory cortex of the brain in the absence of actual sensory data from the eyes or ears. These experiences differ from the hallucinations of schizophrenia in that those patients experiencing release hallucinations are often able to recognize them as unreal. Release hallucinations are also more elaborate and usually longer in duration than irritative hallucinations. The visual hallucinations of patients with CBS are an example of release hallucinations.

Neurotransmitter imbalances

Neurotransmitters are chemicals produced by the body that carry electrical impulses across the gaps (synapses) between adjoining nerve cells. Some neurotransmitters inhibit the transmission of nerve impulses, while others excite or intensify them. Hallucinations in some conditions or disorders result from imbalances among these various chemicals.

NARCOLEPSY Narcolepsy is a disorder characterized by uncontrollable brief episodes of sleep, frequent hypnagogic or hypnopompic hallucinations, and sleep paralysis. Between 1999 and 2000, researchers discovered that people with narcolepsy have a much lower than normal number of hypocretin neurons, which are nerve cells in the hypothalamus that secrete a neurotransmitter known as hypocretin. Low levels of this chemical are thought to be responsible for the daytime sleepiness and hallucinations of narcolepsy.

PRESCRIPTION MEDICATIONS Hallucinations have been reported as side effects of such drugs as ketamine (Ketalar), which is sometimes used as an anesthetic but has also been used illegally to commit date rape; paroxetine (Paxil), an SSRI antidepressant; mirtazapine (Remeron), a serotonin-specific antidepressant; and zolpidem (Ambien), a sleep medication. Ketamine prevents brain cells from taking up glutamate, a neurotransmitter that governs perception of **pain** and of one's relationship to the environment. Paroxetine alters the balance between the neurotransmitters serotonin and acetylcholine.

Hallucinations in patients with Alzheimer's disease are thought to be a side effect of treatment with neuroleptics (antipsychotic medications), although they may also result from inadequate blood flow in certain regions of the brain. The antiretroviral drugs used to treat HIV infection may also produce hallucinations in some patients.

HALLUCINOGENS AND DRUGS OF ABUSE Like the hallucinations caused by prescription drugs, hallucinations caused by drugs of abuse result from disruption of the normal balance of neurotransmitters in the brain. Hallucinations in cocaine and amphetamine users, for example, are associated with the overproduction of dopamine, a neurotransmitter associated with arousal and motor excitability. LSD appears to produce hallucinations by blocking the action of the neurotransmitters serotonin (particularly serotonin-2) and norepinephrine. Phencyclidine (PCP) acts like ketamine in producing hallucinations by blocking the reception of glutamate.

People who have used LSD sometimes experience flashbacks, which are spontaneous recurrences of the hallucinations and other distorted perceptions caused by the drug. Some doctors refer to this condition as hallucinogen persisting perception disorder, or HPPD.

There are two types of alcohol withdrawal syndromes characterized by hallucinations. Alcoholic hallucinosis typically occurs after abrupt withdrawal from alcohol after a long period of excessive drinking. The patient hears threatening or accusing voices rather than "seeing things," and his or her consciousness is otherwise normal. **Delirium** tremens (DTs), on the other hand, is a withdrawal syndrome that begins several days after drinking stops. A patient with the DTs is disoriented, confused, depressed, feverish, and sweating heavily as well as hallucinating, and the hallucinations are usually visual.

MOOD DISORDERS Visual hallucinations occasionally occur in patients diagnosed with **depression**, particularly the elderly. These hallucinations are thought to result from low levels of the neurotransmitter serotonin. The hallucinations that occur in patients with **Parkinson's disease** appear to result from a combination of medication side effects, depressed mood, and impaired eyesight.

Schizophrenia

The auditory hallucinations associated with schizophrenia may be the end result of a combination of factors. These hallucinations have sometimes been attributed to unusually high levels of the neurotransmitter dopamine in the patient's brain. Other researchers have noted abnormal patterns of brain activity in patients with schizophrenia. In particular, these patients suffer from dysfunction of a mechanism known as corollary discharge, which allows people to distinguish between stimuli outside the self and internal intentions and thoughts. Electroencephalograms (EEGs) of patients with schizophrenia that were taken while the patients were talking showed that corollary discharges from the frontal cortex of the brain (where thoughts are produced) failed to inform the auditory cortex (where sounds are interpreted) that the talking was self-generated. This failure would lead the patients to interpret internal speech as coming from external sources, thus producing auditory hallucinations. In addition, the brains of patients with schizophrenia appear to suffer tissue loss in certain regions. In early 2004, some German researchers reported a direct correlation between the severity of auditory hallucinations in patients with schizophrenia and the amount of brain tissue that had been lost from the primary auditory cortex.

Diagnosis

The differential diagnosis of hallucinations can be complicated, but in most cases taking the patient's medical history will help the doctor narrow the list of possible diagnoses. If the patient has been taken to a hospital emergency room, the doctor may ask those who accompanied the patient for information. The doctor may also need to perform a medical evaluation before a psychiatric assessment of the hallucinations can be made. The medical evaluation may include laboratory tests and imaging studies as well as a physical examination, depending on the patient's other symptoms. If it is suspected that the patient is suffering from delirium, **dementia**, or a psychotic disorder, the doctor may assess the patient's mental status by using a standard instrument known as the mini-mental status examination (MMSE) or the Folstein (after the clinician who devised it). The MMSE yields a total score based on the patient's appearance, mood, cognitive skills, thought content, judgment, and speech patterns. A score of 20 or lower usually indicates delirium, dementia, schizophrenia, or severe depression.

Hallucinations in elderly patients may require specialized evaluation because of the possibility of overlapping causes. The American Association for Geriatric Psychiatry lists hallucinations as an indication for consulting a geriatric psychiatrist. In addition, elderly patients should be routinely screened for visual or hearing impairments.

Treatment

Hallucinations are treated with regard to the underlying disorder. Depending on the disorder, treatment may involve antipsychotic, anticonvulsant, or antidepressant medications; psychotherapy; brain or ear surgery; or therapy for drug dependence. Hallucinations related to normal sleeping and waking are not a cause for concern.

Prognosis

The prognosis of hallucinations depends on the underlying cause or disorder.

Resources

BOOKS

Altman, Lawrence K., MD. *Who Goes First? The Story of Self-Experimentation in Medicine.* Berkeley, CA: University of California Press, 1998.

American Psychiatric Association. *Diagnostic and Statistical Manual of Mental Disorders,* 4th edition, text revision. Washington, DC: American Psychiatric Association, 2000.

Beers, Mark H., MD. "Behavior Disorders in Dementia." *The Merck Manual of Geriatrics*, edited by Mark H. Beers, MD, and Robert Berkow, MD. Whitehouse Station, NJ: Merck Research Laboratories, 2002.

"Drug Use and Dependence." *The Merck Manual of Diagnosis and Therapy*, edited by Mark H. Beers, MD, and Robert Berkow, MD. Whitehouse Station, NJ: Merck Research Laboratories, 2002.

Matthiessen, Peter. *The Snow Leopard.* New York: Penguin Books USA, 1987.

"Psychiatric Emergencies." *The Merck Manual of Diagnosis and Therapy*, edited by Mark H. Beers, MD, and Robert Berkow, MD. Whitehouse Station, NJ: Merck Research Laboratories, 2002.

"Schizophrenia and Related Disorders." Section 15, Chapter 193 in *The Merck Manual of Diagnosis and Therapy*, edited by Mark H. Beers, MD, and Robert Berkow, MD. Whitehouse Station, NJ: Merck Research Laboratories, 2002.

PERIODICALS

Braun, Claude M. J., Mathieu Dumont, Julie Duval, et al. "Brain Modules of Hallucination: An Analysis of Multiple Patients with Brain Lesions." *Journal of Psychiatry and Neuroscience* 28 (November 2003): 432–439.

Cameron, Scott, MD, and Michael Richards, MD. "Hallucinogens." *eMedicine.* Cited January 9, 2004 (March 23, 2004). <http://www.emedicine.com/med/topic3407.htm>.

Chuang, Linda, MD, and Nancy Forman, MD. "Mental Disorders Secondary to General Medical Conditions." *eMedicine.* Cited January 30, 2003 (March 23, 2004). <http://www.emedicine.com/med/topic3447.htm>.

Cowell, Alan. "Swedish Foreign Minister's Killer Blames 'Voices' in His Head." *New York Times.* Cited January 15, 2004.

Ford, J. M., and D. H. Mathalon. "Electrophysiological Evidence of Corollary Discharge Dysfunction in Schizophrenia During Talking and Thinking." *Journal of Psychiatric Research* 38 (January-February 2004): 37–46.

Gaser, C., I. Nenadic, H. P. Volz, et al. "Neuroanatomy of 'Hearing Voices': A Frontotemporal Brain Structural Abnormality Associated with Auditory Hallucinations in Schizophrenia." *Cerebral Cortex* 14 (January 2004): 91–96.

Gleason, Ondria C., MD. "Delirium." *American Family Physician* 67 (March 1, 2003): 1027–1034.

Ohayon, M. M. "Prevalence of Hallucinations and Their Pathological Associations in the General Population." *Psychiatry Research* 97 (December 27, 2000): 153–164.

Pelak, V. S., and G. T. Liu. "Visual Hallucinations." *Current Treatment Options in Neurology* 6 (January 2004): 75–83.

Rovner, Barry R., MD. "The Charles Bonnet Syndrome: Visual Hallucinations Caused by Vision Impairment." *Geriatrics* 57 (June 2002): 45–46.

Schneider, L. S., and K. S. Dagerman. "Psychosis of Alzheimer's Disease: Clinical Characteristics and History." *Journal of Psychiatric Research* 38 (January-February 2004): 105–111.

Tsai, M. J., Y. B. Huang, and P. C. Wu. "A Novel Clinical Pattern of Visual Hallucination After Zolpidem Use." *Journal of Toxicology: Clinical Toxicology* 41 (June 2003): 869–872.

OTHER

National Institute of Mental Health (NIMH). *Schizophrenia.* NIH Publication No. 02-3517. Bethesda, MD: NIMH, 2002. (March 23, 2004). <http://www.nimh.nih.gov/publicat/schizoph.cfm>.

National Institute on Drug Abuse (NIDA). *Research Report: Hallucinogens and Dissociative Drugs.* NIH Publication No. 01-4209. Bethesda, MD: NIDA, 2001.

ORGANIZATIONS

American Academy of Neurology (AAN). 1080 Montreal Avenue, Saint Paul, MN 55116. (651) 695-2717 or (800) 879-1960; Fax: (651) 695-2791. memberservices@aan.com. <http://www.aan.com>.

American Association for Geriatric Psychiatry. 7910 Woodmont Avenue, Suite 1050, Bethesda, MD 20814-3004. (301) 654-7850; Fax: (301) 654-4137. main@aagponline.org. <http://www.aagponline.org>.

American Psychiatric Association (APA). 1000 Wilson Boulevard, Suite 1825, Arlington, VA 22209-3901. (703) 907-7300. apa@psych.org. <http://www.psych.org>.

National Institute of Mental Health (NIMH) Office of Communications. 6001 Executive Boulevard, Room 8184, MSC 9663, Bethesda, MD 20892-9663. (301) 443-4513 or (866) 615-NIMH; Fax: (301) 443-5158. nimhinfo@nih.gov. <http://www.nimh.nih.gov>.

National Schizophrenia Foundation. 403 Seymour Avenue, Suite 202, Lansing, MI 48933. (517) 485-7168 or (800) 482-9534; Fax: (517) 485-7180. inquiries@nsfoundation.org. <http://www.nsfoundation.org>.

National Sleep Foundation (NSF). 1522 K Street NW, Suite 500, Washington, DC 20005. (202) 347-3471; Fax: (202) 347-3472. nsf@sleepfoundation.org. <http://www.sleepfoundation.org>.

Rebecca Frey, PhD

Head injury *see* **Traumatic brain injury**

Headache

Definition

Headache is a **pain** in the head and neck region that may be either a disorder in its own right or a symptom of an underlying medical condition or disease. The medical term for headache is cephalalgia. Headaches are one of the most common and universal human ailments, described in the Bible as well as in medical writings from ancient Egypt, Babylonia, Greece, Rome, India, and China. Severe chronic headaches were once treated by the oldest known surgical procedure, known as trepanning or trephining, in which the surgeon drilled a hole as large as 1–2 in diameter in the patient's skull without benefit of anesthesia. Evidence of trepanning has been found in skulls from Cro-Magnon people that are about 40,000 years old.

Description

Contemporary doctors divide headaches into two large categories, primary and secondary, according to guidelines established by the International Headache Society (IHS) in 1988 and revised for republication in 2004. Primary headaches are those that are not caused by an underlying medical condition. There are three types of primary headaches: migraine, cluster, and tension headaches. More than 90% of all headaches are primary headaches. Secondary headaches are caused by disease or medical condition; they account for fewer than 10% of all headaches.

Primary headaches

MIGRAINE HEADACHES Migraine headaches are characterized by throbbing or pulsating pain of moderate or severe intensity lasting from four hours to as long as three days. The pain is typically felt on one side of the head; in fact, the English word "migraine" is a combination of two Greek words that mean "half" and "head." Migraine headaches become worse with physical activity and are often accompanied by nausea and vomiting. In addition, patients with migraine headaches are hypersensitive to lights, sounds, and odors.

The two most common types of migraines are known as classic and common migraine, respectively. Classic migraine, which accounts for 10–20% of the cases of migraine, is distinguished by a brief period of warning symptoms 10–60 minutes before an acute attack. This prodrome, which is known as an aura, may include such symptoms as seeing flashing lights or zigzag patterns, temporary loss of vision, difficulty speaking, weakness in an arm or leg, and tingling sensations in the face or hands. Common migraine is not preceded by an aura, although some patients experience mood changes, unusual tiredness, or fluid retention shortly before an attack. An attack of common migraine may include diarrhea and frequent urination, as well as nausea and vomiting.

Less common types of migraines include hemiplegic migraine, characterized by temporary paralysis on one side of the body; ophthalmoplegic migraine, in which the pain is felt in the area around the eye; basilar artery migraine, which involves a major artery at the base of the brain and primarily affects young women; and headache-free migraine, which is characterized by the gastrointestinal and visual symptoms of classic migraine, but does not involve head pain.

CLUSTER HEADACHES Cluster headaches are recurrent brief attacks of sudden and severe pain on one side of the head, usually most intense in the area around the eye. Other names for these headaches include histamine cephalalgia, Horton neuralgia, or erythromelalgia. Cluster headaches may last between five minutes and three hours; they may occur once every other day or as often as eight times per day. The IHS classifies cluster headaches as either episodic or chronic. Episodic cluster headaches occur over periods lasting from seven days to one year, with the clusters separated by headache-free intervals of at least two weeks. The average length of a cluster ranges between two weeks and three months. Chronic cluster headaches occur over a period longer than a year without a headache-free interval, or with pain-free intervals that are shorter than two weeks.

The pain of a cluster headache is excruciating; some patients describe it as severe enough to make them consider suicide. Patients with cluster headaches are restless; they may pace the floor, weep, rock back and forth, or bang their heads against a wall in desperation to stop the pain. In addition to severe pain, patients with cluster headaches often have a runny or congested nose, watery or inflamed eyes, drooping eyelids, swelling in the area of the eyebrows, and heavy facial perspiration. Because of the nasal symptoms and the relative rarity of cluster headaches, these episodes have sometimes been misdiagnosed as sinusitis.

TENSION HEADACHES Tension headaches are the most common headaches in the general population; other names for them include muscle contraction headache, ordinary headache, psychomyogenic headache, and stress headache. The IHS classifies tension headaches as either episodic or chronic; episodic tension headaches occur 15 or fewer times per month, whereas chronic tension headaches occur on 15 or more days per month over a period of six months or longer.

Tension headaches rarely last more than a few hours; 82% resolve in less than a day. The patient will usually describe the pain of a tension headache as mild to moderate in severity. The doctor will not find anything abnormal in the course of a general physical or neurological examination, although sore or tense areas (trigger points) in the

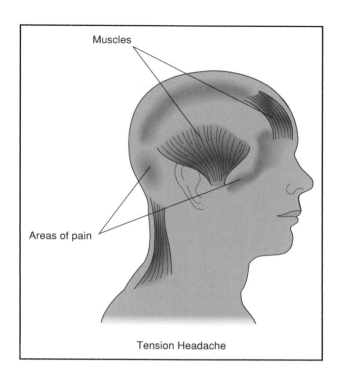

Muscles

Areas of pain

Tension Headache

Tension headaches are caused by severe muscle contractions triggered by stress or exertion. Tension headaches usually occur in the front of the head, although they may also appear at the top or the back of the skull. *(Illustration by Electronic Illustrators Group.)*

muscles of the patient's forehead, neck, or upper shoulder area may be detected.

REBOUND HEADACHES Rebound headaches, which are also known as analgesic-abuse headaches, are a subtype of primary headache caused by overuse of headache drugs. They may be associated with medications taken for tension and migraine headaches.

Secondary headaches

Secondary headaches, which are caused by diseases or disorders, are categorized as either traction or inflammatory headaches. Traction headaches result from the pulling, stretching, or displacing of structures that are sensitive to pain, as when a brain tumor presses on the outer layer of nerve tissue that covers the brain. Inflammatory headaches are caused by infectious diseases of the ears, teeth, sinuses, or other parts of the head.

Major causes of secondary headaches include the following:

- Brain tumors. Headaches associated with brain tumors usually begin as episodic nighttime headaches that are accompanied by projectile vomiting. The headaches may become continuous over time, and usually get worse if the patient coughs, sneezes, bears down while using the toilet, or does something else that increases the pressure inside the head.

- Meningitis. Meningitis is an inflammation of the **meninges**, the three layers of membranes that cover the brain and spinal cord. Meningitis is usually caused by bacteria or viruses, and may produce chronic headaches.

- Head trauma. Patients may complain of headaches as well as memory problems, general irritability, and **fatigue** for months or even years after a head injury. These symptoms are sometimes grouped together as post-concussion syndrome. In some cases, a blow on the head may cause some blood vessels to rupture and produce a hematoma, or mass of blood that displaces brain tissue, and can cause **seizures** or weakness as well as headaches.

- **Temporal arteritis**. First described in 1890, temporal arteritis is an inflammation of the temporal artery that most commonly affects people over 50. In addition to headache, patients with temporal arteritis may have fever, loss of appetite, and blurring or loss of vision. Temporal arteritis is treated with steroid medications.

- **Stroke**. Headaches may be associated with several conditions that may lead to stroke, including high blood pressure and heart disease. Headaches may also result from completed stroke or from the mini-strokes known as transient ischemic attacks, or TIAs.

- Lumbar puncture. About 25% of patients who undergo a lumbar puncture (spinal tap) develop a headache from the lowered cerebrospinal fluid pressure around the brain and spinal cord. Lumbar puncture headaches usually go away on their own after a few hours.

- Sinus infections. Acute sinusitis is characterized by fluid buildup inside sinus cavities inflamed by a bacterial or viral infection. Chronic sinusitis usually results from an allergic reaction to smoke, dust, animal fur, or similar irritants.

- Referred pain. This type of pain is felt in a part of the body at a distance from the injured or diseased area. Headache pain may be referred from diseased teeth; disks in the cervical spine that have been damaged by spondylosis (degeneration of the spinal vertebrae caused by osteoarthritis); or the temporomandibular joint, the small joint in front of the ear where the lower jaw is attached to the skull.

- Idiopathic intracranial hypertension. Also known as **pseudotumor cerebri**, this disorder is caused by increased pressure inside the skull in the absence of any abnormality of the **central nervous system** or blockage in the flow of the cerebrospinal fluid. In addition to headache, patients with this disorder experience diplopia (seeing double) and other visual symptoms.

Demographics

Headaches in general are very common in the adult population in North America. The American Council for Headache Education (ACHE) estimates that 95% of women and 90% of men in the United States and Canada have had at least one headache in the past 12 months. Most of these are tension headaches. Tension headaches may begin in childhood in some patients, but most commonly start in adolescence or the early 20s. The gender ratio for episodic tension headaches is about 1.4 F:1 M; for chronic tension headaches, 1.9 F:1 M.

Migraine and cluster headaches have distinctive demographic patterns. Migraine headaches are less common than tension headaches, affecting about 11% of the population in the United States and 15% in Canada. Several studies done in the United Kingdom and the United States, however, indicate that doctors tend to underdiagnose migraine headache; thus the true number of patients with migraine may be considerably higher than the usual statistics indicate. Migraines are a major economic burden; it is estimated that the annual cost of time lost from work due to migraines in the United States alone is $17.2 billion. Most people who experience migraines have their first episode in childhood or adolescence, although some experience their first migraine after age 20. Migraines occur most frequently in adults between the ages of 25 and 55; the gender ratio is about 3 F:1 M. Although migraine headaches occur in people of all races and ethnic groups, they are thought to affect Caucasians more often than African or Asian Americans.

Currently, migraine is the only type of primary headache known to run in families. A child with one parent affected by migraines has a 50% chance of developing migraines as an adult; if both parents are affected, the risk rises to 70%. Although geneticists think that a number of different genes are involved in transmitting a susceptibility to migraine, they have recently identified two specific loci on human chromosomes 1 and 14, respectively, that are linked to migraine headaches. The locus on chromosome 1q23 has been linked to familial hemiplegic migraine type 2, while the locus on chromosome 14q21 is associated with common migraine.

Cluster headaches are the least common type of primary headaches, affecting about 0.4% of adult males in the United States and 0.08% of adult females. The gender ratio is 5–7.5 M:1 F. Cluster headaches occur most commonly in adults between the ages of 20 and 40. It is not currently known whether cluster headaches are more common in some racial or ethnic groups than in others; however, many patients with cluster headaches have a history of face or head trauma.

The demographics of secondary headaches vary depending on the disease or disorder that causes the headache.

Key Terms

Analgesic A medication that relieves pain without causing loss of consciousness; over-the-counter analgesics include aspirin and NSAIDs.

Aura A group of visual or other sensations that precedes the onset of a migraine attack.

Cephalalgia The medical term for headache.

Dura mater The outermost and toughest of the three membranes or meninges that cover the brain and spinal cord. The arteries that supply the dura mater and the portion of the dura mater at the base of the skull are sensitive to pain.

Endodontist A dentist who specializes in the treatment of diseases and injuries that affect the tooth root, dental pulp, and the tissues surrounding the tooth root.

Idiopathic Of unknown cause or spontaneous origin. Some headaches are considered idiopathic.

Neurotransmitter Any of a group of chemicals that transmit nerve impulses across the gap (synapse) between two nerve cells.

Nociceptor A specialized type of nerve cell that senses pain.

Open-label study A type of study in which both the researchers and the subjects are aware of the drug or therapy that is being tested.

Pathophysiology The changes in body functions associated with a disorder or disease.

Primary headache A headache that is not caused by another disease or medical condition.

Prodrome A symptom or group of symptoms that appears shortly before an acute attack of illness. The term comes from a Greek word that means "running ahead of."

Projectile vomiting Forceful vomiting that is not preceded by nausea. It is usually associated with increased pressure inside the head.

Prophylaxis A measure taken to prevent disease or an acute attack of a chronic disorder. Migraine prophylaxis refers to medications taken to reduce the frequency of migraine attacks.

Rebound headache A type of primary headache caused by overuse of migraine medications or pain relievers. It is also known as analgesic abuse headache.

Secondary headache A headache that is caused by another disease or disorder.

Somatoform disorders A group of psychiatric disorders in the DSM-IV classification that are characterized by external physical symptoms or complaints related to psychological problems rather than organic illness.

Spondylosis A general medical term for degenerative changes in the spinal vertebrae caused by osteoarthritis.

Status migrainosus The medical term for an acute migraine headache that lasts 72 hours or longer.

Temporomandibular joint (TMJ) The small joint in front of the ear in humans where the mandible (lower jaw) is attached to the skull.

Causes and symptoms

Causes

PHYSICAL A person feels headache pain when specialized nerve endings known as nociceptors are stimulated by pressure on or injury to any of the pain-sensitive structures of the head. Most nociceptors in humans are located in the skin or in the walls of blood vessels and internal organs; the bones of the skull and the brain itself do not contain nociceptors.

The specific parts of the head that are sensitive to pain include:

• the skin that covers the skull and cervical spine

• the 5th, 9th, and 10th cranial nerves and the nerves that supply the upper part of the neck

• the venous sinuses inside the head

• the large arteries at the base of the brain

• the large arteries that supply the dura mater, which is the outermost of the three meninges (membranes) that cover the brain and spinal cord

• the portion of the dura mater at the base of the skull

Tension headaches typically result from tightening of the muscles of the face, neck, and scalp as a result of emotional stress; physical postures that cause the head and neck muscles to tense (e.g., holding a phone against the ear with one's shoulder); **depression** or anxiety; temporomandibular joint dysfunction (TMJ); or degenerative arthritis of the neck. The tense muscles put pressure on the walls of the blood vessels that supply the neck and head, which stimulates the nociceptors in the tissues that line the blood vessels. In addition, the nociceptors in patients with chronic tension headaches appear to be abnormally sensitive to stimulation.

The pathophysiology of migraine headaches has been debated among doctors since the 1940s. Some researchers think that migraines are the end result of a magnesium deficiency in the brain or of hypersensitivity to a neurotransmitter known as dopamine. Another theory holds that certain nerve cells in the brain cortex become unusually excitable and depolarize (lose their electrical potential) spontaneously, releasing potassium and glutamate, an amino acid. These substances then depolarize nearby nerve cells, resulting in a chain reaction known as cortical-spreading depression (CSD). CSD then leads to changes in the amount of blood flowing through the blood vessels and stimulation of their nociceptors, resulting in severe headache. More recently, the discovery of specific genes associated with migraine indicates that genetic mutations are responsible for the abnormal excitability of the nerve cells in the brains of patients with migraine.

Little is known about the causes of cluster headaches or changes in the central nervous system that produce them.

PSYCHOLOGICAL Chronic headaches are often associated with anxiety, depression, or a specific group of mental disorders known as somatoform disorders. These disorders include hypochondriasis and pain disorder; they are characterized by physical symptoms (frequently headache) that suggest that the patient has a general medical condition, but there is no diagnosable disease or disorder that fully accounts for the patient's symptoms. The relationship between psychological and physical factors in headaches is complex in that headaches may be either the cause or result of emotional disturbances, or both. Some patients find that chronic headaches disappear completely after a stressful family- or job-related situation has been resolved.

Warning symptoms

Most headaches are not associated with serious or life-threatening illnesses. Patients should, however, immediately call their primary physician if they have any of the following symptoms:

- three or more headaches per week
- need for a pain reliever every day or almost every day
- need for greater than recommended doses of over-the-counter medications (OTCs)
- stiff neck or fever accompanying the headache
- shortness of breath, hearing problems, blurry vision, or severe sore throat
- dizziness, weakness, slurred speech, mental confusion, or drowsiness

- headache following a head injury that is not relieved by OTCs
- headache triggered by **exercise**, coughing, sexual activity, or bending over
- persistent or violent vomiting
- change in the character of the headaches—for example, persistent severe headaches in a person who has previously had only mild headaches of brief duration
- recurrent headaches in a child
- recurrent severe headaches, beginning after age 50

Diagnosis
Patient history

The differential diagnosis of headaches begins with a complete patient history, including a family history. In many cases, a primary care physician can make the diagnosis on the basis of the history. The doctor will ask the patient about head injuries or surgery on the head; eye problems or disorders; sinus infections; dental problems or extensive oral surgery; and medications that the patient is taking regularly.

After taking the history, the doctor will ask the patient to describe the location and type of pain that he or she experiences during the headache. People who have tension headaches will typically describe the pain as "viselike," "tightening," "pressing," or as a steady or constant ache. Patients with migraine headaches, on the other hand, will usually say that the pain has a "throbbing" or "pulsating" character, while patients with cluster headaches describe the pain as "penetrating" or "piercing." About 85% of patients with tension headaches experience pain on both sides of the head, most commonly in the area around the forehead and temples. Patients with migraine or cluster headaches, however, are more likely to feel pain on only one side of the head.

Some primary care physicians give the patient a printed questionnaire that consists of 50–55 brief yes/no questions that cover such matters as the timing and frequency of the headaches; whether other family members have the same type of headache; whether the patient feels depressed; whether the headaches are related to changes in the weather; and so on. The answers to the questions will usually fall into a pattern that tells the doctor whether the patient has migraines, tension headaches, cluster headaches, or headaches with other causes. The doctor may also ask the patient to keep a headache diary to help identify foods, stress, lack of sleep, weather, and other factors that may trigger headaches.

It is possible for patients to have more than one type of headache. For example, patients with chronic tension headaches often have migraine headaches as well.

Physical examination

The physical examination helps the doctor identify other symptoms and signs that may be relevant to the diagnosis, such as fever; difficulty breathing; nausea or vomiting; stiff neck; changes in vision or hearing; watering or inflammation of the nose and eyes; evidence of head trauma; skin rashes or other indications of an infectious disease; and abnormalities in the structure or alignment of the patient's spinal column, teeth or jaw. In some cases, the doctor may refer the patient to a dentist, oral surgeon, or endodontist for a more detailed evaluation of the patient's mouth and jaw.

Special studies

Some laboratory tests are useful in identifying headaches caused by infections or by such disorders as anemia or thyroid disease. These tests include a complete blood count (CBC); erythrocyte sedimentation rate (ESR); and blood serum chemistry profile.

Patients who report **visual disturbances** and other neurologic symptoms may be given visual field tests and have the pressure of the fluid inside their eyes (intraocular pressure) tested to check for glaucoma. A lumbar puncture (spinal tap) may be done to confirm a diagnosis of idiopathic intracranial hypertension.

Imaging studies may include x rays of the sinuses to check for sinus infections; and CT or **MRI** scans, which are done to rule out brain tumors and cerebral **aneurysms**.

Patients whose symptoms cannot be fully explained by the results of physical examinations and tests may be referred to a psychiatrist for evaluation of psychological factors related to their headaches.

Treatment

Medical

TENSION HEADACHES Episodic tension headaches are usually relieved fairly rapidly by such over-the-counter analgesics as aspirin (300–600 mg every four hours), acetaminophen (650 mg every four hours), or another non-steroidal anti-inflammatory drug (NSAID), usually ibuprofen (Advil) or naproxen (Naprosyn, Aleve). The doctor may prescribe a tricyclic antidepressant or benzodiazepine tranquilizer in addition to a pain reliever for patients with chronic tension headaches. A newer treatment for chronic tension headaches is **botulinum toxin** (Botox type A), which appears to work very well for some patients. As of 2003, however, Botox has not yet been evaluated in controlled multicenter studies as a treatment for chronic headaches; the data obtained so far are derived from case reports and open-label studies.

MIGRAINE HEADACHES Medications can be prescribed to prevent migraines as well as to treat the symptoms of an acute attack. Drugs that are given for migraine prophylaxis (to prevent or lower the frequency of migraine attacks) include tricyclic antidepressants, beta-blockers, and anti-epileptic drugs, which are also known as **anticonvulsants**. As of 2003, sodium valproate (Epilim) is the only anticonvulsant approved by the Food and Drug Administration (FDA) for prevention of migraine. Such newer anticonvulsants as **gabapentin** (Neurontin) and **topiramate** (Topamax) are presently being evaluated as migraine preventives. Moreover, a new study reported that three drugs currently used to treat disorders of muscle tone are being explored as possible preventives for migraine— Botox, baclofen (Lioresal), and tizanidine (Zanaflex). Early results of open trials of these medications are positive.

Nonsteroidal anti-inflammatory drugs acetaminophen (Tylenol), ibuprofen (Motrin), and naproxen (Aleve) are helpful for early or mild migraines. More severe or unresponsive attacks may be treated with dihydroergotamine; a group of drugs known as triptans; beta-blockers and calcium channel-blockers; antiseizure drugs; antidepressants (SSRIs); meperidine (Demerol); or metoclopramide (Reglan). Some of these are also available as nasal sprays, intramuscular injections, or rectal suppositories for patients with severe vomiting. Sumatriptan and the other triptan drugs (zolmitriptan, rizatriptan, naratriptan, almotriptan, and frovatriptan) should not be taken by patients with vascular disease, however, because they cause narrowing of the coronary arteries.

About 40% of all migraine attacks do not respond to treatment with triptans or any other medication. If the headache lasts longer than 72 hours—a condition known as status migrainosus—the patient may be given narcotic medications to bring on sleep and stop the attack. Patients with status migrainosus are often hospitalized because they are likely to be dehydrated from severe nausea and vomiting.

CLUSTER HEADACHES Medications that are given as prophylaxis for cluster headaches include verapamil (Calan, Isoptin, Verelan), which is a calcium channel blocker, and methysergide (Sansert), which is a derivative of ergot. A new study indicates that topiramate (Topamax), an anticonvulsant, is also effective in preventing cluster headaches. Sumatriptan (Imitrex) or indomethacin (Indameth, Indocin) may be prescribed to suppress an attack.

REBOUND HEADACHES Continued use of some pain relievers or **antimigraine** drugs can lead to rebound headaches, which may be frequent or chronic and often occur in the early morning hours. Rebound headache can be avoided by using antimigraine drugs or analgesics under a doctor's supervision, using only the minimum dose necessary to treat symptoms. Tizanidine (Zanaflex) has been reported to be effective in treating rebound headaches when taken together with an NSAID; Botox has also been used successfully in some patients.

Diet and lifestyle modifications

One measure that people can take to lower the risk of episodic tension headaches is to get enough sleep and eat nutritious meals at regular times. Skipping meals, using unbalanced fad diets to lose weight, and having insufficient or poor-quality sleep can bring on tension headaches. In fact, the common association of tension headaches with hunger, lack of sleep, heat, and sudden temperature extremes has led some researchers to suggest that headaches developed over the course of human evolution as an internal protective response to stress from the environment.

Changes in diet may be helpful to some patients with migraine, although some experts think that the role of foods in triggering migraines has been exaggerated. Women with migraines, however, often benefit by switching from oral contraceptives to another method of birth control or by discontinuing estrogen replacement therapy.

Patients with cluster headaches are advised to quit smoking and minimize their use of alcohol, because nicotine and alcohol appear to trigger cluster headaches. Currently, the precise connection between these chemicals and cluster attacks, however, is not completely understood.

Surgical

Headaches that are caused by brain tumors, post-injury hematomas, dental problems, or disorders affecting the spinal disks usually require surgical treatment. Surgery may also be used to treat cases of idiopathic intracranial hypertension that do not respond to treatment with steroids, repeated lumbar punctures, or weight reduction.

Some plastic surgeons have reported success in treating patients with chronic migraines by removing some muscle tissue near the eyebrows, cutting a branch of the trigeminal nerve, and repositioning the soft tissue around the temples.

Psychotherapy

Psychotherapy may be helpful to patients with chronic headaches by interrupting the "feedback loop" between emotional upset and the physical symptoms of headaches. One type of psychotherapy that has been shown to be effective is cognitive restructuring, an approach that teaches people to reframe the problems in their lives—that is, to change their conscious attitudes and responses to these stressors. Some psychotherapists teach relaxation techniques, biofeedback, or other approaches to stress management as well as cognitive restructuring.

Complementary and alternative (CAM) treatments

There are a number of different CAM treatments for headache, but most fall into two major groups: those intended as prophylaxis or pain relief, and those that reduce the patient's stress level.

CAM therapies intended to prevent headaches or relieve discomfort include:

- Feverfew (*Tanacetum parthenium*). Feverfew is an herb related to the daisy that is traditionally used in England to prevent migraines. Published studies indicate that feverfew can reduce the frequency and intensity of migraines. It does not, however, relieve pain once the headache has begun.

- Butterbur root (*Petasites hybridus*). Petadolex is a natural preparation made from butterbur root that has been sold in Germany since the 1970s as a migraine preventive. Petadolex has been available in the United States since December 1998.

- Brahmi (*Bacopa monnieri*). Brahmi is a herb used in Ayurvedic medicine to treat headaches related to anxiety.

- **Acupuncture**. Studies funded by the National Center for Complementary and Alternative Medicine (NCCAM) have found that acupuncture is an effective treatment for headache pain in many patients.

- Naturopathy. Naturopaths include dietary advice and nutritional therapy in their approach to treatment, which is often effective for patients with episodic or chronic tension headaches.

- Chiropractic. Some patients with tension or migraine headaches find spinal manipulation effective in relieving their pain; however, no controlled studies of the long-term effectiveness of chiropractic in treating headaches have been done as of 2003.

CAM therapies that are reported to be effective in reducing emotional stress related to headaches include:

- yoga and t'ai chi
- prayer and meditation
- aromatherapy
- hydrotherapy, particularly whirlpool baths
- Swedish massage and shiatsu
- pet therapy
- humor therapy
- music therapy

Clinical trials

As of late 2003, there were three National Institutes of Health (NIH) trials recruiting patients with headaches: a study evaluating a new intranasal drug (civamide) for cluster headaches; a study of the effectiveness of biofeedback and relaxation training in patients with chronic migraine or tension headaches; and a study of migraine headaches in children.

Prognosis

The prognosis of primary headaches varies. Episodic tension headaches usually resolve completely in less than a day without affecting the patient's overall health. According to NIH statistics, 90% of patients with chronic tension or cluster headaches can be helped. The prognosis for patients with migraines, however, depends on whether the patient has one or more of the other disorders that are associated with migraine. These disorders include Tourette's syndrome, **epilepsy**, ischemic stroke, hereditary essential tremor, depression, anxiety, and others. For example, migraine with aura increases a person's risk of ischemic stroke by a factor of six.

The prognosis of secondary headaches depends on the seriousness and severity of their cause.

Resources

BOOKS

American Psychiatric Association. *Diagnostic and Statistical Manual of Mental Disorders*, 4th edition, text revision. Washington, DC: American Psychiatric Association, 2000.

"Headache." *The Merck Manual of Diagnosis and Therapy.* Edited by Mark H. Beers and Robert Berkow. Whitehouse Station, NJ: Merck Research Laboratories, 2002.

Pelletier, Kenneth R. *The Best Alternative Medicine*, Part II, "CAM Therapies for Specific Conditions: Headache." New York: Simon & Schuster, 2002.

"Psychogenic Pain Syndromes." *The Merck Manual of Diagnosis and Therapy.* Edited by Mark H. Beers and Robert Berkow. Whitehouse Station, NJ: Merck Research Laboratories, 2002.

PERIODICALS

Argoff, C. E. "The Use of Botulinum Toxins for Chronic Pain and Headaches." *Current Treatment Options in Neurology* 5 (November 2003): 483–492.

Astin, J. A., and E. Ernst. "The Effectiveness of Spinal Manipulation for the Treatment of Headache Disorders: A Systematic Review of Randomized Clinical Trials." *Cephalalgia* 22 (October 2002): 617–623.

Corbo, J. "The Role of Anticonvulsants in Preventive Migraine Therapy." *Current Pain and Headache Reports* 7 (February 2003): 63–66.

Freitag, F. G. "Preventative Treatment for Migraine and Tension-Type Headaches: Do Drugs Having Effects on Muscle Spasm and Tone Have a Role?" *CNS Drugs* 17 (2003): 373–381.

Guyuron, B., T. Tucker, and J. Davis. "Surgical Treatment of Migraine Headaches." *Plastic and Reconstructive Surgery* 109 (June 2002): 2183–2189.

Headache Classification Subcommittee of the International Headache Society. "The International Classification of Headache Disorders," 2nd ed. *Cephalalgia* 24 (2004) (Supplement 1): 1–150.

Lainez, M. J., J. Pascual, A. M. Pascual, et al. "Topiramate in the Prophylactic Treatment of Cluster Headache." *Headache* 43 (July-August 2003): 784–789.

Lenaerts, M. E. "Cluster Headaches and Cluster Variants." *Current Treatment Options in Neurology* 5 (November 2003): 455–466.

Lipton, R. B., A. I. Scher, T. J. Steiner, et al. "Patterns of Health Care Utilization for Migraine in England and in the United States." *Neurology* 60 (February 11, 2003): 441–448.

Marconi, R., M. De Fusco, P. Aridon, et al. "Familial Hemiplegic Migraine Type 2 is Linked to 0.9Mb Region on Chromosome 1q23." *Annals of Neurology* 53 (March 2003): 376–381.

Mendizabai, Jorge, MD. "Cluster Headache." *eMedicine*, 26 September 2003. <http://www.emedicine.com/neuro/topic70.htm>.

Sahai, Soma, MD, Robert Cowan, MD, and David Y. Ko, MD. "Pathophysiology and Treatment of Migraine and Related Headache." *eMedicine*, April 30, 2002 (February 16, 2004). <http://www.emedicine.com/neuro/topic517.htm>.

Singh, Manish K., MD. "Muscle Contraction Tension Headache." *eMedicine*, October 5, 2001 (February 16, 2004). <http://www.emedicine.com/neuro/topic231.htm>.

Soragna, D., A. Vettori, G. Carraro, et al. "A Locus for Migraine Without Aura Maps on Chromosome 14q21.2–q22.3." *American Journal of Human Genetics* 72 (January 2003): 161–167.

Tepper, S. J., and D. Millson. "Safety Profile of the Triptans." *Expert Opinion on Drug Safety* 2 (March 2003): 123–132.

OTHER

Migraine Information Page. NINDS. 2003 (February 16, 2004). <http://www.ninds.nih.gov/health_and_medical/pubs/migraineupdate.htm>.

National Institute of Neurological Disorders and Stroke (NINDS). "Headache—Hope Through Research." Bethesda, MD: NINDS, 2001. (February 16, 2004.) <http://www.ninds.nih.gov/health_and_medical/pubs/headache_htr>.

ORGANIZATIONS

American Academy of Neurology (AAN). 1080 Montreal Avenue, Saint Paul, MN 55116. (651) 695-2717 or (800) 879-1960; Fax: (651) 695-2791. memberservices@aan.com. <http://www.aan.com>.

American Council for Headache Education (ACHE). 19 Mantua Road, Mt. Royal, NJ 08061. (856) 423-0258; Fax: (856) 423-0082. achehq@talley.com. <http://www.achenet.org>.

International Headache Society (IHS). Oakwood, 9 Willowmead Drive, Prestbury, Cheshire SK10 4BU, United Kingdom. +44 (0) 1625 828663; Fax: +44 (0) 1625 828494. rosemary@ihs.u-net.com. <http://216.25.100.131>.

National Headache Foundation. 820 North Orleans, Suite 217, Chicago, IL 60610. (773) 525-7357 or (888) NHF-5552. <http://www.headaches.org>.

NIH Neurological Institute. P. O. Box 5801, Bethesda, MD 20824. (301) 496-5751 or (800) 352-9424. <http://www.ninds.nih.gov>.

Rebecca J. Frey, PhD

Hearing disorders

Definition

Hearing disorders range from a temporary, partial loss of hearing to the permanent loss of hearing known as deafness.

Description

The variety of hearing disorders includes a loss or decrease in the ability to discern certain frequencies of sound, a ringing or other noise that is unrelated to any actual external sound, damage due to physical trauma or infection, and genetically determined structural malformation.

Demographics

Hearing disorders occur worldwide in all races. The hearing loss that occurs with age is very common, affecting an estimated 30% of Americans over 60 years of age and 50% of those older than 75.

Tinnitus, a ringing or noisy sensation in the ears, is quite common with an estimated 20% of people affected worldwide. In the United States alone, some 36 million people experience tinnitus.

For hearing loss caused by otosclerosis, middle-aged Caucasian women are more prone than others, perhaps as a consequence of hormonal changes. In otosclerosis, abnormal bone development occurs in the middle ear, resulting in progressive hearing loss. Sudden hearing loss happens more often to people ages 30–60 for unknown reasons.

Causes and symptoms

Presbycusis

Presbycusis (or sensorineural hearing loss) is the loss of hearing that occurs with age. The condition results from the long-term assault on the ear structures, particularly on the inner ear, from a lifetime of noise, ear infections, or growths on bones of the outer or middle ear. The inner ear is where the vibrational sound waves are converted to electrical signals, courtesy of thousands of tiny hairs that are in a fluid-enclosed space called the cochlea. The hairs are connected to nerve cells, which send the electrical signals to the brain.

Most age-related hearing loss is due to damage to the cochlea. The tiny hairs can bend or even break, and the attached nerve cells can degenerate. The resulting less-efficient transmission of the electrical signal, particularly of higher-pitched tones, causes hearing loss.

Symptoms of presbycusis typically include increased difficulty in making out sounds of a certain volume or tone, especially when background sounds are present.

Conductive hearing loss

In conductive hearing loss, sound is not transmitted efficiently through the outer and middle ears. These regions house the eardrum, ear canal, and the trio of tiny bones (ossicles) in the middle ear that transmits sound energy to the inner ear. The hearing loss can be due to malformation of structures like the canal or the ossicles, dense buildup of ear wax, or fluid in the ear due to colds, allergies, or infections like otitis media. Symptoms include a decreased ability to detect fainter sounds and a general lowering of the sound level that can be detected.

Otitis media

Otitis media is an inflammation in the middle ear that is usually accompanied by fluid buildup. The condition may be transient in some children, but persistent in others to the point of requiring surgical correction. In developed countries, otitis media is second to the common cold as the most common health problem in preschool-aged children. Hearing loss occurs because of the fluid accumulation and the resulting suppression of sound waves moving to the inner ear.

Central auditory processing disorders

Central auditory processing disorders result in hearing loss when the areas of the brain involved in hearing are damaged. Sources of damage include disease, injury, and tumor growth. Consistent with the variety of causes, the symptoms of the disorders include the inability to hear certain sounds, inability to tell one sound from another, and the inability to recognize a pattern such as speech in sounds.

Congenital hearing loss

Congenital hearing loss is present from birth and is caused by a genetic defect or disturbance during fetal development. Genetic factors cause more than half of all such disorders. Depending on the nature of the genetic defect, the occurrence of the hearing loss may be common or rare. For example, if both parents have a genetically determined hearing deficiency, the chance of passing the trait to their children is high. In other cases, people who have normal hearing carry a second, defective copy of a crucial gene. The chance of passing on the hearing loss is 25%.

Hearing loss at birth can also be caused by pre-birth infections such as measles, cytomegalovirus, or herpes simplex virus.

Otosclerosis

The abnormal growth of the bone of the middle ear prevents the ossicles, particularly the last of the trio of bones (the stapes), from properly transmitting sound

Key Terms

Cochlear implant A device used for treating deafness that consists of one or more electrodes surgically implanted inside or outside the cochlea, an organ in the inner ear that transforms sound vibrations in the inner ear into nerve impulses for transmission to the brain.

Ossicles Tiny bones in the middle ear, the incus, malleus, and stapes, that convey sound impulses from the eardrum to the inner ear.

Otitis media Inflammation, usually with infection, of the middle ear.

Otosclerosis Abnormal bone development in the middle ear, resulting in progressive hearing loss.

Presbycusis Loss of hearing that gradually occurs because of age-related changes in the inner or middle ear.

Tinnitus Ringing or noisy sensations in the ears when no external sound is present, often associated with hearing impairment and excess noise exposure.

waves to the inner ear in otosclerosis. The cause(s) of otosclerosis are not clear, although observations that the disorder spans family generations make a genetic source likely.

The diminished hearing that occurs is not sudden. Rather, the change is gradual and is usually recognized when the person becomes aware that she or he can no longer hear a low-pitched sound such as a whisper.

Other genetically based hearing losses

Usher syndrome affects both the ears and eyes. The defective genes that are at the heart of the malady are passed from parents to children. Depending on the nature of the syndrome, children can be born with moderate to severe hearing loss, or can be totally deaf. Others begin life essentially normal, with hearing loss progressively worsening to deafness by the teenage years.

Waardenburg syndrome affects both the ears and the color of the skin, eyes, or hair. Eyes can be different colors and hair can have a patch of white or become prematurely gray. Hearing can range from normal to severely impaired. At least four genes can produce the syndrome when they undergo mutation.

Ménière's disease

Ménière's disease is a change in the volume of the inner ear that produces swelling, pressure, **pain**, intermittent hearing loss, **dizziness**, and tinnitus. Swelling may be so pronounced that membranes like the eardrum can rupture. As well, some people report that their voice sounds louder than normal. The disease may be caused by a viral or bacterial infection.

Tinnitus

Tinnitus is a ringing noise or other sound that occurs in the absence of an external source of sound. For some, tinnitus is an infrequent occurrence. Others are very inconvenienced by near-constant tinnitus. The noises experienced in tinnitus range in description and include electronic noise, hissing steam, chirping crickets, bells, breaking glass, buzzing, and even the noise of a chainsaw. The noises can be constant or may rise and fall in volume with head motion or with the planting of feet during running.

Tinnitus has various known triggers. Foods such as red wine, cheese, and chocolate have been implicated. Over-the-counter drugs such as ibuprofen and extra-strength aspirin, and prescribed drugs, including oral contraceptives and aminoglycoside antibiotics, can cause tinnitus. Drug-related tinnitus disappears when the dosage is reduced or the drug stopped. The growth of certain tumors can cause tinnitus.

The aging of the inner ear is also a factor in tinnitus. As nerve cells deteriorate and the many hairs in the cochlea that transmit sound waves to the nerves become damaged and broken with time, the signaling of sound impulses to the brain becomes faulty. Nerves may fire when there has been no stimulus. The brain interprets the signal as actual noise.

Sudden deafness or sudden sensorineural hearing loss

This rapid decrease or complete loss of hearing can occur within minutes or over the course of several days. The hearing loss typically affects one ear and often resolves with time. Sudden deafness is much more serious and should be treated as a medical emergency requiring immediate medical attention. Causes are unclear and may involve an infection, head injury, reaction to a drug, problems with circulation, and other disorders such as **multiple sclerosis**.

Deafness

The complete loss of hearing can be due to genetically determined developmental difficulties, a trauma such as a loud noise, physical damage to structures in the ear, nerves, or relevant areas of the brain, and infection during pregnancy (such as rubella). In a great many cases, deafness is permanent. Childhood deafness typically becomes apparent when a child appears inattentive and fails to meet language milestones.

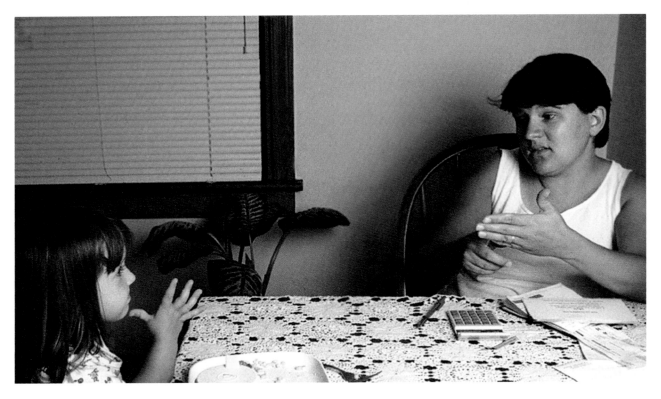

A mother and young daughter communicate with sign language. *(© Custom Medical Stock Photo. Reproduced by permission.)*

Diagnosis

Presbycusis is usually first detected by a family physician. Diagnosis is subsequently made by a hearing specialist or an audiologist, and involves a hearing test in which sounds of differing frequencies and gradually decreasing volume are sent to one ear at a time.

Tinnitus is self-evident, as the ringing or other sensation is impossible to ignore. In contrast, otitis media can be difficult to diagnose, as it is often not accompanied by pain or a fever. Fluid in the ear can be a sign of otitis media. Also, changes in children's behavior such as playing the television louder, misunderstanding directions, and pulling at the ears can all be indicators of otitis media.

Imaging of the inside of the ear using the technique of **magnetic resonance imaging (MRI)** can be useful in diagnosing Ménière's disease. Usher syndrome is diagnosed by the simultaneous appearance of ear and eye problems.

Treatment team

The varied treatment can involve the family physician and more specialized doctors, including audiologists and otolaryngologists (specialists in ear, nose, and throat disorders). As well, speech-language pathologists can be involved in the treatment of hearing loss-related speech disorders in children.

Treatment

Treatment for presbycusis can be as simple as keeping the ear canals free from sound-muffling wax buildup. Another fairly common treatment for older people is the use of a hearing aid, which amplifies sound and directs the sound into the ear canal. About 20% of those with age-related hearing loss can benefit from an aid. More severe presbycusis can be treated using a cochlear implant. The device actually compensates for the nonworking parts of the inner ear. Conductive hearing loss can usually be fully corrected by medication or surgery. Similarly, when tinnitus is caused by overmedication, the condition is alleviated by modifying or eliminating the dosage of the drug.

Ménière's disease and Usher syndrome cannot be cured, however, the symptoms can be greatly relieved by release of the buildup of pressure in the inner ear and the use of hearing aids or implants, respectively. Coping strategies and increased knowledge of the conditions can then help a person lead an essentially normal life.

Otosclerosis that is more pronounced can be treated by a surgical procedure called a stapedectomy, in which the damaged portion of the middle ear, the stapes, one of the three bones of the middle ear, is bypassed by an implanted device that routes sound to the inner ear. Milder otosclerosis may be lessened by the use of a hearing aid.

Recovery and rehabilitation

Some conditions that can be addressed by surgery or the use of a hearing aid or an implant have varying levels of recovery. Other conditions involving permanent deafness cannot be cured.

Clinical trials

As of April 2004, at least eight **clinical trials** were active in the United States. Most focus on deafness, in particular the determination of the genetic factors that contribute to or cause deafness. Updated information on these studies can be found at the National Institutes of Health Web site for clinical trials at <http://www.clinicaltrials.gov>.

Prognosis

Age-related hearing loss can be partially or almost completely compensated for by a change in lifestyle and the development of coping skills (listening to the radio at higher volume, different conversational behavior in crowds, use of hearing aids or implants). Otitis media can cause delayed speech development, if undiagnosed, because of the child's impaired ability to hear. Sudden hearing loss usually resolves on its own within a few days to several weeks. However, in about 15% of cases, the condition worsens with time.

Special concerns

The various surgeries that can be performed all carry some risk, and the quality of sound that is provided by cochlear implants varies greatly among recipients.

Additionally, tinnitus can be caused by the buildup of cholesterol in arteries around the ear, high blood pressure, and by malformed arteries or veins. Tinnitus, therefore, may be an indication of a more serious health problem.

Resources

BOOKS

Dugan, Marcia B. *Living with Hearing Loss.* Baltimore: Gallaudet Press, 2003.

Schwartz, Sue. *Choices in Deafness: A Parents' Guide to Communication Options.* Bethesda, MD: Woodbine House, 2003.

PERIODICALS

DeJonckere, P. H., and G. G. de Surgeres. "Acute Tinnitus and Permanent Audiovestibular Damage after Hepatitis B Vaccination." *International Tinnitus Journal* (July 2001): 59–61.

Waddell, A., and R. Canter. "Tinnitus." *American Family Physician* (February 2004): 591–592.

OTHER

"Hearing Loss." *MayoClinic.com.* April 8, 2004 (May 30, 2004). <http://www.mayoclinic.com/invoke.cfm?id=DS00172>.

"Tinnitus." *MayoClinic.com.* April 8, 2004 (May 30, 2004). <http://www.mayoclinic.com/invoke.cfm?id=DS00365>.

ORGANIZATIONS

American Academy of Audiology. 8300 Greensboro Drive, Suite 750, McLean, VA 22102. (703) 790-8466 or (800) 222-2336; Fax: (703) 790-8631. info@audiology.org. <http://www.audiology.org>.

American Speech-Language-Hearing Association. 10801 Rockville Pike, Rockville, MD 20852. (301) 638-8255 or (800) 638-8255; Fax: (301) 571-0457. actioncenter@asha.org. <http://www.asha.org>.

American Tinnitus Association. PO Box 5, Portland, OR 97207-0005. (503) 248-9985 or (800) 634-8978; Fax: (503) 248-0024. tinnitus@ata.org. <http://www.ata.org>.

Deafness Research Foundation. 1050 17th Street NW, Suite 701, Washington, DC 20036. (202) 289-5850. <http://www.drf.org>.

National Center on Deafness. 18111 Nordhoff Street, Northridge, CA 91330-8267. (818) 677-2145; Fax: (818) 677-7693. ncod@csun.edu. <http://ncod.csun.edu>.

National Institute on Deafness and Other Communication Disorders, National Institutes of Health. 31 Center Drive, MSC 2320, Bethesda, MD 20892-2320. (301) 496-7243 or (800) 241-1044; Fax: (301) 402-0018. nidcdinfo@nidcd.nih.gov. <http://www.nidcd.nih.gov>.

Brian Douglas Hoyle, PhD

Hemianopsia

Definition

Hemianopsia is a term that describes a loss of vision that affects half of the visual field of one eye or both eyes.

Description

Hemianopsia prevents an individual from seeing objects in half of the visual field of a particular eye. As a result, an individual suffering from hemianopsia will not see objects that are in the affected visual field.

Causes and symptoms

Conditions or injuries that affect the optic nerve can cause hemianopsia. The sequelae (aftereffects) of **stroke**, brain aneurysm, occlusion of the optic artery, brain tumors, or traumatic head injuries can all result in hemianopsia. Occasionally, individuals who suffer from migraine headaches may experience hemianopsia during a migrainous episode or as part of the prodromal aura that precedes the actual **headache**; this type of hemianopsia resolves completely upon resolution of the headache. Transient hemianopsia can result from bouts of extremely high blood pressure (as occurs in eclampsia) or during or after a seizure. Other rare causes of hemianopsia include infections, such as encephalitis, brain abscess, **progressive multifocal leukoencephalopathy**, and **Creutzfeldt-Jakob disease**.

Symptoms of hemianopsia involve the inability to see objects in half of the visual field of one or both eyes, which may be manifested by reading difficulties, problems walking through crowded areas, frequent accidents (bumping into objects that are located in the lost visual field), or being startled at what seems to be the sudden emergence of people or objects in the visual field.

Diagnosis

Diagnosis is usually evident when basic testing reveals a blind area in half of the visual field of one or both eyes. Further testing will be necessary to uncover the underlying causative condition: CT or **MRI** scanning may reveal the presence of a stroke, aneurysm, or brain tumor.

Treatment team

Neurologists, ophthalmologists, and neuroophthalmologists all work with patients with hemianopsia. Occupational therapists and vision rehabilitation specialists can be integral in teaching the individual how to compensate for their vision loss.

Treatment

Treatment includes therapy to practice techniques that may help an individual overcome the obstacles of hemianopsia. For example, changing reading techniques (looking at the last part of the word, rather than the first) may improve an individual's ability to read and enjoy reading. Special scanning techniques may be taught, using a machine called a Dynavision, which will help an individual learn how to turn the head in certain ways to scan the environment and compensate for the lost visual field.

Special glasses lenses, some with mirrors or prisms incorporated, may allow an individual with hemianopsia to view a greater visual field.

Prognosis

Recovery of vision after stroke or head injury is usually maximal within the first three to six months; hemianopsia persisting after that point is usually permanent.

Special concerns

Driving can be a particular concern for people with hemianopsia. By learning new techniques for scanning the environment, some individuals can safely return to driving; others will not be able to drive safely, and will no longer be able to obtain a driver's license. This can result in significant changes in an individual's lifestyle, independence, and employability.

Resources
BOOKS

Liu, Grant T., and Nancy J. Newman. "Cranial Nerve II and Afferent Visual Pathways." In *Textbook of Clinical Neurology*, edited by Christopher G. Goetz. Philadelphia: W. B. Saunders Company, 2003.

Pulsinelli, William A. "Ischemic Cerebrovascular Disease." In *Cecil Textbook of Internal Medicine*, edited by Lee Goldman, et al. Philadelphia: W. B. Saunders Company, 2000.

ORGANIZATIONS

Lighthouse International. 111 East 59th Street, New York, NY 10022. 212-821-9200 or 800-829-0500. info@lighthouse.org. <http://www.lighthouse.org/Default.htm>.

Rosalyn Carson-DeWitt, MD

Hemifacial spasm

Definition

A hemifacial spasm is an involuntary contraction of the muscles of facial expression, resulting in eyelid closure and upturning of the corner of the mouth and accompanied by facial weakness.

Description

Hemifacial spasm results in involuntary contraction of the facial muscles limited to one side of the face. The eyelids are involved, and upturning of the corner of the mouth is observed. The patient may have facial twitching during periods of sleep. If left untreated, the twitching may worsen and extend to other facial muscles.

Demographics

Females are affected more than males, regardless of race. Typically, patients afflicted with hemifacial spasm are in their 40s or 50s.

Causes and symptoms

The cause of hemifacial spasm has been linked to overactivity of the seventh cranial nerve nucleus that signals facial muscle movement. In other instances, hemifacial spasm may be caused by compression by a mass or abnormal blood vessel or by a lack of blood supply (ischemia) of the seventh cranial nerve at its origin or by the nucleus itself. It is thought that compression by a convoluted cerebral artery is the most common cause. In some patients, no underlying cause can be detected, which is termed an idiopathic hemifacial spasm. In younger patients, **multiple sclerosis** may be the cause.

Patients will usually report involuntary twitching of one side of the face (hemifacial), lasting seconds to minutes. Family members may observe facial twitching while the patient sleeps. **Pain** or numbness is usually not reported.

Diagnosis

When a clinical diagnosis has been established, imaging of the brain is required to rule out ischemia, mass lesions, or abnormal vasculature. **Magnetic resonance imaging (MRI)** of the brain, with and without contrast, as well as MRI-angiography, are advised. Blood tests are not required for patients believed to have hemifacial spasm.

Treatment team

Ophthalmologists, neuro-ophthalmologists, and neurologists are physicians who can diagnose and treat hemifacial spasm. If surgery is indicated as a form of treatment, it is usually performed by a neurological surgeon.

Treatment

The mainstay of treatment is injection of **botulinum toxin** to the face, which results in temporary paralysis of selected muscles of facial expression. Botulinum toxin, commonly known as Botox (Allergen Inc.), is a neurotoxin produced by the bacterium, *Clostridium botulinum*. This toxin weakens facial muscles by inhibiting the release of a neurotransmitter, acetylcholine, which results in temporary and partial muscle paralysis. Botulinum toxin has become an accepted and widely used treatment for hemifacial spasm. Although its use is relatively safe and easily injected, the effect of botulinum toxin is temporary, lasting approximately six months. This necessitates the need for re-injection or increased doses of the toxin, depending on the patient's response.

If botulinum toxin fails to be effective or the patient does not tolerate it well, decompression of the seventh cranial nerve can be attempted. This procedure, performed by a neurosurgeon, entails placing a sponge between the seventh nerve and the vessel compressing the nerve.

Other treatment options include severing branches of the seventh nerve, destruction of eyelid and facial musculature, and oral anti-seizure medications. However, oral medications have proven to be limited in their efficacy and have significant side effects.

Recovery and rehabilitation

There is usually no recovery period following the injection of botulinum toxin. The maximal effects are usually seen four to seven days following injection.

Clinical trials

Currently there are no clinical trials scheduled to study this disorder.

Prognosis

The vast majority of patients responds favorably to injections with a low rate of complications. A small percentage of patients improves spontaneously, and benefits from psychotherapy, surgery, or oral medications.

Special concerns

Support groups and information for patients and families are excellent resources that may improve treatment outcomes and psychosocial ramifications.

Resources
BOOKS
Beers, Mark H., and Robert Berkow, editors. "Cranial Nerve Disorders." *The Merck Manual of Diagnosis and Therapy.* Whitehouse Station, NJ: Merck Research Laboratories, 1999.
Burde, Ronald M., Peter J. Savino, and Jonathan D. Trobe. *Clinical Decisions in Neuro-Ophthalmology*, 3rd ed. St. Louis, MO: Mosby, 2002.
Liu, Grant T., Nicholas J. Volpe, and Steven L. Galetta. *Neuro-Ophthalmology Diagnosis and Management*, 1st ed. Philadelphia: W.B. Saunders Company, 2001.

OTHER
Gulevich, Steven. *Hemifacial Spasm.* <http://www.eMedicine.com>.
Cohen, Adam J., and M. Mercandetti. *Oculopfacial Applications of Botulinum Toxin.* <http://www.Ophthamichyperguides.com>.

ORGANIZATIONS
Hemifacial Spasm Association. <http://www.hfs-assn.org>.

Adam J. Cohen, MD

Hemiplegia alterans *see* **Alternating hemiplegia**

Hereditary spastic paraplegia
Definition

Hereditary spastic paraplegia (HSP) is a hereditary degenerative disorder affecting the corticospinal tracts (long never fibers that supply the upper and lower limbs) within the spinal cord. The disease frequently results in progressive **spasticity** (involuntary movement) of leg muscles with varying degrees of stiffness and weakness of other muscle groups in the thighs, lumbar spinal area, and muscles responsible for up and down feet movements. The extent of degeneration and severity of symptoms varies among the affected people, even those among the same family group. The age of onset for the disease also varies. Some families show a pattern of disease, with symptoms developing earlier in each new generation. In most individuals, however, the disease onset occurs between the second and the fourth decades of life, with a few cases beginning later, or as early as infancy and early childhood.

Description

Other names of this disorder are hereditary spastic paraparesis, Strumpell-Lorrain syndrome, Strumpell disease, familial spastic paraparesis, spastic spinal familial paralysis, and Troyer syndrome. When the only manifested symptom is progressive spasticity, HSP is also known as Pure Hereditary Spastic Paraplegia.

HSP presents three forms of inheritance: autosomal dominant HSP, autosomal recessive HSP, and X-linked HSP. Autosomal dominant HSP requires the presence of an inherited mutation in only one copy of the gene responsible for the disease, whereas autosomal recessive HSP requires mutation in the two copies (maternal and paternal) to manifest the disease. X-linked HSP is rare and the mutated gene is located in the X chromosome, which is transmitted by the mother. HSP is also divided into two categories, uncomplicated HSP and complicated HSP.

Demographics

As usually happens with other rare neurological diseases, the HSP symptoms may overlap or be mistaken with other neurodegenerative disorders. Consequently, HSP incidence is only estimated, with approximately three cases out of 100,000 individuals as an average estimate for the United States and Europe. Ninety percent of HSP cases are uncomplicated and do not affect life expectancy.

Causes and symptoms

Hereditary spastic paraplegia (HSP) belongs to a group of neurodegenerative (progressive nervous system dysfunction) disorders with common symptoms of progressive and usually severe weakness and spasticity of the lower limbs. However, mutations in different genes may result in HSP, a phenomenon known as genetic heterogeneity. For instance, uncomplicated HSP may be inherited as an autosomal dominant mutation in about 70% of cases; but the involved mutated gene may be a different one, located in a different chromosome, from one family

Key Terms

Ataxia A condition marked by impaired muscular coordination, most frequently resulting from disorders in the brain or spinal cord.

Autosomal Relating to any chromosome besides the X and Y sex chromosomes. Human cells contain 22 pairs of autosomes and one pair of sex chromosomes.

Corticospinal tract A tract of nerve cells that carries motor commands from the brain to the spinal cord.

Neurodegenerative disease A disease in which the nervous system progressively and irreversibly deteriorates.

Neuropathy A disease or abnormality of the peripheral nerves (the nerves outside the brain and spinal cord). Major symptoms include weakness, numbness, paralysis, or pain in the affected area.

Spinal cord The elongated nerve bundles that lie in the spinal canal and from which the spinal nerves emerge.

to another. Any of these genes is generically known as spastic paraplegia gene or SPG.

SPGs responsible for the uncomplicated form of the disease have been identified in chromosomes 2, 8, 12, 14, 15, 19, and 20; and an autosomal dominant complicated HSP gene has been found in chromosome 10. Autosomal recessive HSP may be caused by other than the above-mentioned SPGs, also located either in chromosome 8 or 15, or yet in chromosome 16. One form of autosomal recessive HSP, the Troyer syndrome, is associated with a SPG located in chromosome 13. Two different genes associated with autosomal recessive HSP have also been identified on the X chromosome. Approximately 40–50% of all cases of autosomal dominant HSP are caused by SPG located on chromosome 2.

Uncomplicated autosomal dominant HSP may start at any phase of life, from infancy or early childhood to adulthood or old age. In children, uncomplicated HSP progresses until adolescence and then stabilizes, resulting in partial walking disability. However, complete paralysis of the legs is rare in uncomplicated HSP, whatever the age of onset.

Autosomal recessive HSP is the complicated form of the disease with onset between two and 16 years of age. Complicated HSP symptoms continually progress and may be associated with other neurological conditions, such as **epilepsy**, **mental retardation**, **peripheral neuropathy** (numbness, **pain**, and sensory changes in nerves of limb extremities), ocular (eye) degenerations, such as retinopathy and/or the destruction of optic nerve tissues (ocular neuropathy). Other clinical complications are **ataxia** (motor coordination disorders), **dysarthria** (speech disorders), nystagmus (repetitive and involuntary eye movements), and ichthyosis (abnormal dryness, scaling, and thickening of the skin). However, these neurological symptoms may be caused by other disorders present at the same time. For instance, a person with uncomplicated HSP may have peripheral neuropathy due to diabetes.

Diagnosis

Family clinical history and physical and neurological examinations are the first tools in HSP diagnosis. The physician will conduct comparative examination of muscle tone and strength between arms and legs and look for signs of weakness in specific muscle groups of the thigh, presence of abnormal increase of deep tendon brisk reflexes in the lower extremities, loss of ankle flexibility, and decrease of sensation in the lower extremities. Genetic screening for SPG is the definitive test to avoid misdiagnosis.

Treatment

There is no curable or preventive treatment for HSP, except for antispasmodic drugs to reduce muscle spasms. However, symptomatic treatment for sensitive neuropathy may also be necessary in recessive HSP. Supportive care includes physical therapy and devices to assist with walking.

Resources

BOOKS

Fenichel, Gerald M. *Clinical Pediatric Neurology: A Signs and Symptoms Approach,* 4th ed. Philadelphia: W. B. Saunders Company, 2001.

ORGANIZATIONS

Genetic Alliance. 4301 Connecticut Avenue, N.W., Suite 404, Washington, DC 20008-2369. (202) 966-5557 or (800) 336-GENE (4363); Fax: (202) 966-8553. info@geneticalliance.org. <http://www.geneticalliance.org>.

National Ataxia Foundation (NAF). 2600 Fernbrook Lane, Suite 119, Minneapolis, MN 55447-4752. (763) 553-0020; Fax: (763) 553-0167. naf@ataxia.org. <http://www.ataxia.org>.

Spastic Paraplegia Foundation. P.O. Box 1208, Forston, GA 31808. (978) 256-2673. info@sp-foundation.org. <http://www.sp-foundation.org>.

Worldwide Education & Awareness for Movement Disorders (WE MOVE). 204 West 84th Street, New York, NY 10024. (212) 875-8312 or (800) 437-MOV2

(6682); Fax: (212) 875-8389. wemove@wemove.org. <http://www.wemove.org>.

Sandra Galeotti

Heredopathia atactica polyneuritiform *see* **Refsum disease**

Herpes zoster *see* **Shingles**

Hirayama syndrome *see* **Monomelic amyotrophy**

Holoprosencephaly

Definition

Holoprosencephaly is a birth defect caused by failure of the forebrain (prosencephalon) to grow as two separate hemispheres in the first few weeks of fetal life. The more complete the failure to divide, the worse the resulting abnormalities of brain, skull, and face. In its most severe form, holoprosencephaly entails the development of a tiny, undivided forebrain and is fatal before birth. Equivalent terms are arhinencephaly, holotelencephaly, and telencephalosynapsis. The prefix *holo* means undivided.

Description

There are three degrees of severity of holoprosencephaly: (1) *alobar* holoprosencephaly, in which a tiny, single-lobed, nonfunctional forebrain brain develops, along with other severe cerebral abnormalities and severe facial deformities including cyclopism, or formation of a single, nonfunctional eye where the bridge of the nose should be; (2) *semilobar* holoprosencephaly, in which the brain is partly divided and there may be significant facial deformities such as cleft palate; and (3) *lobar* holoprosencephaly, in which the brain is partly divided, but there is some fusion of structures along the midline. Some authorities distinguish a fourth category to include various mild abnormalities of prosencephalic division, namely olfactory aplasia (absence of olfactory bulbs and tracts) and middle interhemispheric variant, in which the posterior frontal and parietal lobes of the brain are not well-separated.

Demographics

Holoprosencephaly occurs in a small number of live births, with estimates varying from one in 5,000 to one in 31,000. However, its actual incidence is much higher, since many fetuses with holoprosencephaly, approximately 97%, are either stillborn or spontaneously aborted (miscarried). The rate of holoprosencephaly among all

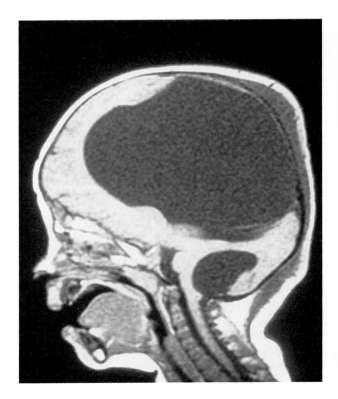

MRI of a 20-month-old girl with holoprosencephaly. The dark area represents the abnormally large fluid-filled ventrical typical of this disease. *(Simon Fraser / Neuroradiology Dept. / Newcastle General Hospital / Science Photo Library.)*

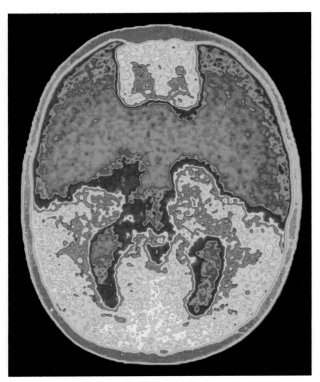

MRI of a brain with holoprosencephaly. The red area represents the large, fluid-filled cavity that develops where the forebrain would normally be. *(Mehau Kulyk / Photo Researchers, Inc.)*

pregnancies may therefore be as high as 1:200 or 1:250. As of 2004, the medical literature did not note a higher prevalence of holoprosencephaly in any particular racial group or geographic area.

Causes and symptoms

Holoprosencephaly has no single cause, but about half of all cases are associated with abnormal karyotype (abnormal numbers of chromosomes), especially trisomy 13 (extra copy of chromosome 13) and trisomy 15 (extra copy of chromosome 15). It can also run in families as an autosomal dominant, autosomal recessive, or X-linked recessive trait. Currently, researchers believe that holoprosencephaly might be linked to as many as 12 chromosomal regions on 11 chromosomes.

Risk is increased if the mother has diabetes or has an infection during pregnancy such as syphilis, herpes, cytomegalovirus, rubella, or toxoplasmosis. Use of certain drugs or other substances during pregnancy (e.g., alcohol, aspirin, lithium, thorazine, **anticonvulsants**, hormones, retinoic acid) has also been suggested as a risk factor. Women who have had previous miscarriages and bleeding in the first trimester are also more likely to have fetuses with holoprosencephaly.

Alobar holoprosencephaly causes death, either before or soon after birth. Cyclopia or formation of a single eye often occurs, with the nose being absent, having only a single nostril, or being replaced by a proboscis (small, tubular nose) either above or below the eye. Less severe degrees of holoprosencephaly cause **mental retardation** ranging from profound to mild. The eyes may be closely set together, the nose may be malformed, and there may be cleft lip (premaxillary agenesis). Children who survive birth generally have facial deformities, **spasticity**, **seizures**, problems with regulating body temperature, apneic attacks (spells of stopped breathing), psychomotor retardation, sleep disorders, gastroesophageal reflux, and other problems. However, holoprosencephaly occurs along a continuum, and at the mild end of the spectrum development may be essentially normal.

Diagnosis

Ultrasonic examination of the fetal brain has made early detection of holoprosencephaly common. In infants born live, a preliminary diagnosis may be based on extremely small head size (**microcephaly**) and on examination of the face, which is often deformed by the

Key Terms

Autosomal dominant disorder   A genetic disorder caused by a dominant mutant gene that can be inherited by either parent.

Autosomal recessive disorder   A genetic disorder that is inherited from parents that are both carriers, but do not have the disorder. Parents with an affected recessive gene have a 25% chance of passing on the disorder to their offspring with each pregnancy.

Microcephaly   An abnormally small head and underdeveloped brain.

Prosencephalon   The part of the brain that develops from the front portion of the neural tube.

X-linked disorder   Disorders caused by genes located on the X chromosome.

underlying developmental defects of the brain and skull. In particular, midfacial hypoplasia (subnormal growth of the features along the midline of the face) is strongly correlated with holoprosencephaly. Half of all cases of agnathia (total or virtual absence of a lower jaw) are also associated with holoprosencephaly. However, about 30% of cases of severe holoprosencephaly occur with normal development of the face. Ultrasound may give early warning of holoprosencephaly during fetal development; **magnetic resonance imaging** is the definitive method for diagnosing holoprosencephaly in non-severe cases.

Treatment team

If holoprosencephaly is known to have occurred in the family, consultation with a geneticist before or during pregnancy may help a woman determine if she is at higher risk for conceiving infants with holoprosencephaly. If a woman has diabetes, she should see a doctor with expertise in diabetes care to obtain the best possible care before and during pregnancy, including help in achieving tight blood-glucose control, as this can reduce a diabetic woman's risk of having a child with birth defects to near normal.

Treatment

There is no cure for holoprosencephaly. Severe forms are fatal. For children with milder forms, treatment is directed at the symptoms rather than the disease. For example, drugs such as **diazepam** (Valium) and baclofen can be used to moderate spasticity (involuntary muscle tightening). Dorsal rhizotomy (cutting of the sensory spinal

nerve roots), often done for the relief of intractable **pain**, can also be used to treat spasticity. Difficulty sleeping, common in children with holoprosencephaly, may be helped by such medications as Valium, chloral hydrate, or Melatonin. Low muscle tone in the esophageal sphincter, leading to gastroesophageal reflux ("spitting up" of the stomach contents into the esophagus and possibly out of the mouth, as occurs normally in small infants), can be treated with drugs that increase the speed with which the stomach and intestines pass material along and with antacids, which decrease the acidity of stomach contents and make gastroesophageal reflux less harmful. Emotional and intellectual care must be adjusted to the degree of retardation in each case.

Prognosis

The prognosis for an infant born with holoprosencephaly depends on the severity of the cerebral and other defects. The prognosis for an infant with severe holoprosencephaly is poor; most do not survive past six months, and those that do are likely to suffer profound mental retardation. At the mild end of the spectrum, where brain development may be nearly normal, a normal lifespan is likely.

Resources

BOOKS

Graham, David I., and Peter L. Lantos. *Greenfield's Neuropathology,* 6th edition. Bath, UK: Arnold, 1997.

OTHER

"Information about Holoprosencephaly." *Carter Centers for Brain Research in Holoprosencephaly and Related Malformations.* (March 6, 2004). <http://www.stanford.edu/group/hpe/about/>.

"NINDS Holoprosencephaly Information Page." *National Institute of Neurological Disorders and Stroke.* (March 6, 2004). <http://www.ninds.nih.gov/health_and_medical/disorders/holoprosencephaly.htm>.

ORGANIZATIONS

Carter Centers for Research in Holoprosencephaly. c/o Texas Scottish Rite Hospital, P.O. Box 190567, 2222 Welborn Street, Dallas, TX 75219-9982. (214) 559-8411; Fax: (214) 559-7835. hpe@tsrh.org. <http://www.stanford.edu/group/hpe>.

Larry Gilman, Ph.D.

▌ HTLV-1 associated myelopathy

Definition

Damage to the nerves (myelopathy) of the spinal cord caused by infection with the human T lymphotrophic virus type-1 is termed HTLV-1 associated myelopathy.

Description

HTLV-1 associated myelopathy is evident mainly as a chronic weakening of muscles, especially those in the legs. Weakening can be so severe as to produce partial paralysis. The myelin covering of spinal cord nerve cells can become damaged, as can the elongated part of the cell termed the axon.

HTLV-1 associated myelopathy is also known as **tropical spastic paraparesis** and additionally as HTLV-1 associated myelopathy/tropical spastic paraparesis.

Demographics

Myelopathy occurs in approximately 0.25 % of those infected with HTLV-1, typically in adults aged 40–60. The viral infection is associated with diseases including adult T-cell leukaemia, Acquired Immunodeficiency Syndrome (**AIDS**), various neurological disorders, inflammation of the uveal tract of the eye, and degenerative or arthritic **pain**.

HTLV-1 is common in Japan, the Caribbean, and some areas of Africa. Correspondingly, the associated myelopathy is more prominent in these regions, compared to other areas of the globe.

Causes and symptoms

HTLV-1 associated myelopathy is the result of infection with the HTLV-1 virus. The common routes of transmission are through breast milk, transfused blood (especially prior to 1989 when donated blood was not tested for HTLV-1), sexual intercourse, and drug injection.

Until the viral link was established in the mid-1980s, HTLV-1 associated myelopathy was thought to result in the inflammation of the **central nervous system** caused by infection by the bacteria *Treponema pallidum* (the cause of syphilis) or *Treponema pertenue* (the cause of yaws), or by a nutritional deficiency.

In addition to the damage to nerve myelin and axon, the white and grey matter of the spinal cord sometimes becomes infiltrated with certain white blood cells, along with nerve cell astrocytes. White lesions can develop along the length of the spinal cord. Occasionally, the entire cord can become swollen.

Along with the progressively increasing muscle weakness, patients also can display impaired sense of touch and pain receptivity, and malfunction of muscles called sphincters, which can contract to restrict the flow of some body fluids and relax to resume flow. Leakage of urine is a problem in over 90% of those with this form of myelopathy. Patients can also develop eye inflammation, arthritis, dryness of the cornea and conjunctiva, and skin inflammation.

Key Terms

Myelopathy   A disorder in which the tissue of the spinal cord is diseased or damaged.

Diagnosis

Diagnosis can be made using several clinical observations. A medical history will show that the current symptoms were not present during childhood. Within two years of the first appearance of symptoms, a person will likely have experienced an increase in the frequency of urination, and weakness, numbness, pains, or cramps in both legs. In a physical examination, an increased knee-jerk reaction is seen. Difficulty using both legs is evident. Finally, eye abnormalities such as changes in the appearance of the pupil are present.

The visualization of spinal cord nerve damage can also aid in diagnosis. Lesions and swelling associated with the spinal cord can be visualized by **magnetic resonance imaging (MRI)**.

Demonstration of the presence of HTLV-1 is an important part of the diagnosis. Antibodies to several viral proteins can be detected shortly after an infection begins. But, within a few months, an infection can become undetectable using antibody detection techniques. Thus, the absence of HTLV-1 antibodies does not necessarily rule out an infection. HTLV-1 genetic material can be detected from lymphocyte cells using a sensitive technique called polymerase chain reaction.

A more reliable diagnostic finding can be an increased level of a compound called neopterin in the cerebrospinal fluid (CSF) that is obtained by a lumbar puncture. Neopterin is released by immune cells called macrophages when they are stimulated as part of an immune response to the infecting virus. As well, lymphocyte cells in the CSF can adopt a characteristic flower-like appearance.

Treatment team

Family physicians, neurologists and other specialized clinicians, physical therapists, and caregivers are all part of the treatment team.

Treatment

Currently, there is no specific treatment regimen for HTLV-1 associated myelopathy. Steroid medications help lessen symptoms and discomfort in many people. Drug therapy with lioresal or tizanidine can help relieve muscle spasms. The leakage of urine due to malfunction of the urinary sphincter muscle can be treated using oxybutynin, or managed by use of a catheter.

The use of plasmapheresis, in which plasma is withdrawn, antibodies removed, and the antibody-free liquid put back into the person, has not shown promise for HTLV-1 myelopathy. Interestingly, this technique is useful in treating myelin damage caused in other disorders such as **Guillain-Barré syndrome**.

Recovery and rehabilitation

Physical and occupational therapy is useful in maintaining muscle function.

Clinical trials

A clinical trial sponsored by the National Institute of Neurological Disorders and Stroke has been underway since 1997 in which blood samples are collected from patients in order to evaluate the functioning of the immune system and the levels of the virus during the course of the disease.

Prognosis

While the disorder may become progressively worse, HTLV-1 associated myelopathy is seldom fatal. People with the disorder normally live for several more decades after being diagnosed. A better outcome typically results when steps are taken to lessen the chance of urinary tract infection (which can commonly occur when a catheter is used), and skin inflammation.

Resources
PERIODICALS

Zaninovic, V. "On the etiology of tropical spastic paraparesis and human T-cell lymphotropic virus-I-associated myelopathy." *Int J Infect Dis.* 3, no. 3 (Spring 1999): 168–76.

OTHER

National Institute of Neurological Disorders and Stroke. *NINDS Tropical Spastic Paraparesis Information Page.* (December 24, 2003). http://www.ninds.nih.gov/health_and_medical/disorders/tropical_spastic_paraparesis.htm>.

ORGANIZATIONS

National Institute for Allergy and Infectious Diseases. National Institutes of Health, 31 Center Drive, Room 7A50, MSC 2520, Bethesda, MD 20892-2520. (301) 435-3848. <http://www.niaid.nih.gov>.

National Institute for Neurological Disorders and Stroke. P.O. Box 5801, Bethesda, MD 20824. (301) 496-5761 or (800) 352-9424. <http://www.ninds.nih.gov>.

National Organization for Rare Disorders. P.O. Box 1968, Danbury, CT 06813-1968. (203) 744-0100 or (800) 999-6673; Fax: (203) 798-2291. orphan@rarediseases.org. <http://www.rarediseases.org>.

Brian Douglas Hoyle, PhD

Huntington chorea *see* **Huntington disease**

Huntington disease
Definition

First described by Dr. George Huntington in 1872, Huntington disease (HD) is a relatively common hereditary neurological condition that most commonly affects people in their adult years. HD is a progressive disorder that often involves thinking and learning problems, psychological disturbances, and abnormal movements. HD has been well studied and documented in family histories across the world. This ultimately led to the discovery of the HD gene, now known to be responsible for the disorder.

Description

Huntington disease is also known by the name Huntington (or Huntington's) **chorea**; "chorea" refers to neurological diseases that are characterized by spasmodic movements of the limbs and facial muscles. This is because about 90% of people with HD have chorea. These movements may be mild at first, but can worsen and become more involuntary with time.

About two-thirds of people with HD first present with neurological signs, while others first have psychiatric changes. Other neurological signs include various abnormal movements, changes in eye movements, difficulty speaking, difficulty swallowing, and increased reflexes.

A general decline in thinking skills occurs in essentially everyone with HD. This may begin as general forgetfulness and progress to difficulty gathering thoughts or keeping and using new knowledge. People with HD often also have psychiatric changes, including significant personality and behavior changes.

The majority of those with HD first develops symptoms between the ages of 35 and 50 years. Symptoms vary considerably between people and sometimes within families, so it is difficult to predict an individual's exact experience with HD if he or she is diagnosed with the condition. Disease progression occurs in everyone, with death usually seen 10–30 years after its onset.

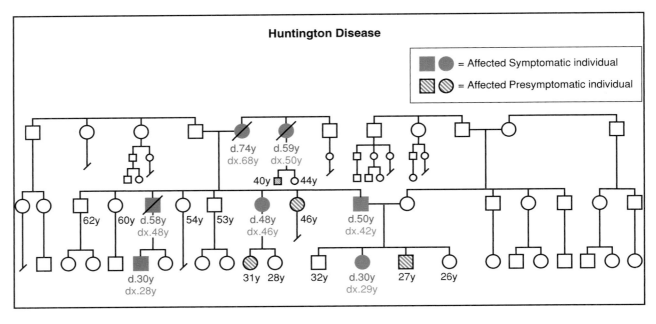

Huntington Disease

☐ ● = Affected Symptomatic individual

▨ ◨ = Affected Presymptomatic individual

See Symbol Guide for Pedigree Charts. *(Gale Group.)*

Demographics

HD is estimated to occur in the United States and most of Europe at a rate of about five cases per 100,000 people. Pockets of populations exist where the prevalence may be a bit higher, such as those with western European ancestors. Conversely, HD is estimated to have a much lower prevalence in Japan, China, Finland, and Africa. For example, the frequency of HD in Japan has been estimated at between 0.1 and 0.38 per 100,000 people.

Symptoms of HD typically begin after about age 35 years. However, in some families a juvenile form of HD has been seen with an onset of symptoms in the first or second decades of life. About a quarter of people with the condition are diagnosed past the age of 50 years. HD is a disease that affects males and females equally.

Currently, genetic testing is widely available to identify a well-documented mutation in the HD gene. Testing is available for confirmation of a clinical diagnosis, or for those at risk but who, as yet, have no symptoms. Predictive genetic testing (for those who are asymptomatic) typically involves a specialized protocol with pretest and post-test counseling, requiring coordinated care with various medical professionals.

Causes and symptoms

Some neurological changes have been seen in HD. However, the connection of many of these changes to the disease's symptoms is still not understood. Atrophy of the

basal ganglia and corpus striatum are common neurological findings in HD, which may worsen over time. Cortical atrophy is often present, and this may be seen with **magnetic resonance imaging (MRI)** or computed tomography (**CT**) scans. From pathology studies after death, brain atrophy is most prominent in the caudate, putamen, and cerebral cortex in people with HD. Total brain weight may be reduced by as much as 25–30% in people who have advanced cases of HD.

A specific mutation in the HD gene called a triplet expansion causes symptoms of the condition to occur. The four different deoxyribonucleic acid (DNA) bases that make up genes are abbreviated as A, C, T, and G. Three DNA bases, CAG, are naturally repeated in the HD gene; a certain number of repeats is considered normal. People with symptoms of HD have a higher number of repeats than the usual range. Unfortunately, the number of CAG repeats can increase (or expand) from generation to generation, and this usually occurs in men. This genetic process is called anticipation; it cannot be predicted when and how the CAG repeats will expand in someone when they have children. A larger CAG repeat size is generally associated with developing symptoms at a younger age.

HD is inherited in an autosomal dominant manner, which means that an affected individual has a one in two chance to pass the disease-causing mutation to his or her children, regardless of the gender. Children who inherit a disease-causing mutation will develop signs of HD at some point in their lives. On the other side of that, children who do not inherit the mutation should not develop the disease. Strong family histories of HD have been well documented and studied across the globe.

HD is usually first suspected with the observation or progression of abnormal movements. The initial reasons for seeking medical attention are often clumsiness, tremor, balance trouble, or jerkiness. Chorea is a frequent symptom.

The areas of the body most commonly affected by chorea are the face, limbs, and trunk. As the chorea progresses, breathing, swallowing, and the mouth and nasal muscles may become involved. Muscles may become extremely rigid and gait may show signs of **ataxia**. Chorea may also be mixed with other **movement disorders** such as **dystonia**. Visual muscles may also be affected, and this can eventually lead to difficulties with vision, speech, swallowing, and breathing.

Weight loss is a common symptom in HD, which may occur despite a proper intake of calories and nutrients. Because people with HD are frequently moving, it is thought this continual activity increases metabolic rates and may explain the weight loss. However, the exact cause for weight loss in HD is still not well understood.

Mental impairment is an eventual sign of HD. This may begin at about the same time as movement abnormalities. If a diagnosis of HD is made, cognitive decline may have actually begun earlier, but might have gone unnoticed until other symptoms of the condition began to develop.

General forgetfulness, loss of mental flexibility, difficulty with mental planning, and organization of sequential activities may be early signs of HD. Reduced attention and concentration spans are common, and this may lead to one being quite distractible. **Aphasia** and **agnosia** are less evident than in Alzheimer's disease, but overall cognitive speed and efficiency are usually affected. The ability to speak is usually maintained, but people with HD may eventually have difficulty with complex words or finding the correct words to express their thoughts. Late-stage symptoms may include difficulty with visual and spatial relations.

The last category of symptoms in HD is that involving psychological disturbances. Irritability and **depression** are common early signs of HD. People may initially be incorrectly diagnosed with psychiatric diseases like **schizophrenia** and delusional disorder, particularly if they have no other symptoms of HD. This is probably because a large percentage of people with HD have significant personality changes or affective psychosis. Behavioral issues can include intermittent explosiveness, apathy, aggression, alcohol abuse, sexual problems and deviations, paranoid delusions, and an increased appetite.

Suicide occurs in 5–12% of people with HD. Late-stage disease is often quite significant and can be disabling. Weight loss, sleep problems, and incontinence are common signs of advanced HD.

Juvenile HD occurs when someone develops symptoms in the first two decades of life; this occurs in about 5–10% of all HD cases. Symptoms are distinct from those associated with adult-onset forms of HD. For example, chorea rarely occurs in people who develop HD in their first decade of life. However, dystonia and rigidity can be very significant for those individuals. Common characteristics of people with juvenile HD diagnosed before age 10 include declining performance in school, mouth muscle abnormalities, rigidity, and problems with their gait. **Seizures** are also a somewhat unique characteristic of juvenile HD.

Complications related to immobility are often the cause of death in people with HD. Abnormal muscular movements, particularly those related to swallowing and breathing, may cause someone to die from aspiration pneumonia and other infections; such a cause of death occurs years after the onset of the disease.

People with juvenile HD diagnosed between the age of 10 and 20 may have symptoms similar to adult-onset HD. Others may have more severe behavioral and psychiatric problems noticed before anything else. Common among people with juvenile HD is a father with adult-onset HD.

Diagnosis

Until the discovery of the HD gene on chromosome 4 in 1993, the diagnosis of the condition was made purely on a clinical basis. This can be somewhat challenging because of similarities with other hereditary and non-hereditary conditions involving chorea.

A careful neurological examination and documentation of abnormal movements are important to diagnose HD. **Sydenham's chorea** is a nonhereditary, infectious cause of chorea. It most often occurs in children and adolescents following a streptococcal infection, and the chorea associated is slightly different than that with HD. About 30% of people with rheumatic fever or polyarthritis develop Sydenham's chorea two to three months later. Symptoms may even come back in pregnancy, or in people taking oral contraceptives. The chorea in Sydenham's chorea is brisk and abrupt, but it is more flowing and somewhat slower in HD. Treatment for Sydenham's chorea usually involves bed rest, sedation, and antibiotic therapy with medications like penicillin.

Movements with characteristics of dystonia and athetosis, called choreoathetosis, are also common in HD.

Key Terms

Affective psychosis Abnormalities in mood, emotions, feelings, sensibility, or mental state.

Agnosia Inability to notice or process sensory stimuli.

Anticipation Genetic phenomenon in which a triple repeat DNA mutation expands in a future generation, causing symptoms to develop earlier.

Aphasia Inability to communicate by speaking, writing, or signing.

Aspiration pneumonia Infection of the lungs, caused by the presence of foreign material like food.

Ataxia Uncoordinated muscular movement; often causes difficulty with walking and other voluntary movements.

Athetosis Slow, writhing involuntary movements that involve muscle flexing and extension.

Atrophy Wasting or loss of tissue.

Basal ganglia Large masses of gray matter at the base of the brain; typically describes the corpus striatum and cell groups around it.

Bradykinesia Slowness in movement.

Caudate A region of gray matter near the lateral ventricle of the brain; also called caudate nucleus.

Cerebral cortex Grey material covering the entire surface of the brain.

Chorea Irregular, unpredictable, brief, jerky movements that randomly affect the body.

Corpus striatum Region of the brain that contains the caudate nucleus and putamen.

Cortical Related to a cortex, such as the cerebral cortex.

Dementia General decline in cognitive function.

Deoxyribonucleic acid (DNA) The chemical bases that make up genes.

Dopamine Neurotransmitter chemical, typically found in the basal ganglia of the brain.

Dystonia State of abnormal muscle tone, with either too much or too little.

Gait The way in which one walks.

Mutation A change in the order of DNA bases that make up genes, akin to a misspelling.

Neuropathy Term for any disorder affecting the nervous system or cranial nerves.

Polyarthritis Inflammation of several joints at the same time.

Putamen Structure in the brain that is connected to the caudate nucleus and a component of the corpus striatum.

Rheumatic fever Fever following a throat infection with group A Streptococcus, typically affecting children and young adults.

Tremor An involuntary trembling movement.

People with HD may be able to more easily mask their movements at first, because they are not that intrusive in the early stages. Tardive **dyskinesia** is a nonhereditary cause of chorea that may be mistaken for HD in an individual on antipsychotic medications.

Chorea occurs in 1–7% of people with **lupus**, and in a proportion of people with drug-related problems. It is important to rule out nonhereditary causes of chorea because treatments may exist for them, which may increase quality of life for the affected person.

Although very useful for many other neurological conditions, looking at the brain with techniques like **magnetic resonance imaging (MRI)** or computed tomography (CT) scans currently are not as helpful in diagnosing HD. These techniques may help find some typical brain changes in HD. For example, caudate atrophy is typically associated with advanced HD. Studies have shown that serial CT scans of the basal ganglia in at-risk individuals without symptoms may show signs of caudate atrophy before the disease even shows symptoms. These types of imaging studies can be useful to rule out other diagnoses that may mimic HD, because those may involve other specific brain changes.

An important step in diagnosing HD is to take a careful family history. Strong family histories with multiple generations affected, with roughly equal males and females affected, are common in HD.

Many hereditary conditions mimic HD. People who are diagnosed with HD much later in life may seem similar to people with **Parkinson's disease**, because abnormal movements may be the primary symptom. Neuroacanthocytosis is a hereditary condition with chorea, but it should be considered if muscle loss, absent lower limb tendon reflexes, neuropathy, and specific results on a blood test are present. Benign hereditary chorea is an autosomal dominant condition in which the chorea is not progressive, and does not involve any cognitive decline. Dentatorubropallidoluysian atrophy (DRPLA) is another hereditary condition that mimics HD; it typically affects adults and involves **dementia**, ataxia, and seizures, along with chorea. As a group, the hereditary spinocerebellar ataxias (SCAs) may mimic some of the movement abnormalities seen in HD. However, the psychological and cognitive components may not be present in the SCAs.

Often, diagnosis is most clearly made with genetic testing, which is done to confirm a suspected clinical diagnosis. Genetic testing identifies the exact number of CAG repeats in each copy of a person's HD gene.

There are several CAG repeat ranges that may be found through testing. Each genetic laboratory may use slightly different ranges, so test results should be interpreted carefully. Generally, a range of 10–27 CAG repeats is considered to be normal. If someone has results in these ranges, this person does not have HD, and will not develop signs of it.

A range of 27–35 CAG repeats will not cause symptoms of HD in the person. In this range, the repeat size may rarely increase when passed on to children. In other words, the person with this test result will not develop symptoms of HD, but he or she may have a child who develops symptoms. This would particularly be the case if the person were a man, because of the anticipation phenomenon.

A range of 36–39 CAG repeats is considered a range where the person may or may not develop HD symptoms at some point in his or her life. Additionally, the repeat may or may not expand to his or her children.

People with an HD gene that has greater than 39 CAG repeats will develop symptoms of HD at some point in their lives. They would have a 50% chance of passing this gene on to future children.

People with juvenile HD usually have much larger CAG repeat sizes than those who have the typical form of HD. Despite this, it is still impossible to predict exactly when someone may develop symptoms, or to predict the exact symptoms they will experience.

Genetic testing for those who have symptoms is fairly straightforward, and often ordered with the aid of a **neurologist**. Predictive testing for HD, as it is called when the person does not have symptoms, is a bit more complicated. This is because there are many complex factors in the testing process.

Ideally, at-risk asymptomatic individuals have several appointments before genetic testing is performed. They should see a neurologist for a thorough examination to identify any subtle signs of HD. They should also see a **neuropsychologist** for an evaluation. The neuropsychologist can help assess whether a person is a good candidate for genetic testing, potentially reducing the risk for poor

outcomes, like suicide, following positive results. Individuals should also see a medical geneticist and genetic counselor to receive thorough information about the risks, benefits, and limitations of genetic testing.

Much has been studied about the myriad of issues with genetic testing in HD. Risks from any outcome can be considerable, and these may include a sudden change in family dynamics, self-image, or serious emotional and psychological harms.

Health, life, or disability insurance discrimination from HD testing may be a possibility, especially related to positive results. Employment may also be an issue. In October 2003, a young teacher in Germany was refused a permanent job because members of her family have HD; she was found to be at risk for the condition during a required governmental medical examination. Currently, there is not enough documentation in the medical literature to know what the actual risks are related to these issues. Awareness and discussion of these issues are important in pretest counseling.

Limitations and benefits from genetic testing should be given equal weight as well. Results may not be easily understood, simply identifying one and one's children to be potentially at risk. These types of vague results can cause great angst to an at-risk individual. However, benefits from testing may include relief from years of worry, empowerment from medical knowledge, and the ability to make life plans or tailor medical care based upon more accurate information.

Generally, at-risk asymptomatic children under age 18 are not tested for HD. The decision to learn their genetic status should be theirs, and at a time they feel is appropriate. Along the same lines, prenatal genetic testing for HD is not done, except in cases involving special circumstances or assistive reproductive techniques.

Treatment team

Treatment for people with HD is highly dependent on their symptoms. A multidisciplinary team and approach can be very helpful. A treatment team may include a neurologist, neuropsychologist, medical geneticist, genetic counselor, physical therapist, occupational therapist, speech therapist, registered dietitian, social worker, psychotherapist, psychiatrist, ophthalmologist, and a primary care provider. Some hospitals offer day clinics devoted to people with HD, which makes things much easier in terms of coordinating appointments. Pediatric specialists in these fields may help in the care for children.

Treatment

Currently, there is no known cure for Huntington disease. No specific treatment is known to slow, stop, or reverse the progressive nature of the disease. Current treatment for HD is mainly focused on relieving symptoms and reducing the impact of physical and mental complications related to the disease.

Medications are available to help treat chorea in HD, including therapies for blocking dopamine receptors, or those that deplete dopamine from its natural storage sites in the brain. Medications like these are tetrabenazine, pimozide, and haloperidol. They can have side effects, like drowsiness and a lessened ability to make voluntary movements. Some find the side effects to be more troublesome than the chorea, so medications should be prescribed under careful supervision.

Psychiatric problems in HD are often treated with medications as well. Some selective serotonin reuptake inhibitors (SSRIs) with trade names like Celexa, Paxil, Prozac, and others have been effective. Some tricyclic antidepressants like Nordil, Marplan, and Eldepryl have been effective. Lastly, some monoamine oxidase inhibitors (MAOIs) like Elavil, Tofranil, and Anafranil have been useful in treating depression.

Benzodiazepine and antipsychotic drugs can be used to treat anxiety, irritability, and agitation in HD. It is rare to find a medication without side effects, and drug interactions are also important to consider. As yet, no medications have been found helpful to treat the cognitive problems in HD.

Other therapies have been tested through **clinical trials** to see whether the disease progression may be slowed in any way. A combination of coenzyme Q10 and remacemide has been tested in mice, showing it to be helpful in reducing weight loss and brain loss. In a study by The Huntington Study Group in 2001, people with early-stage HD were given coenzyme Q10 or remacemide, but neither had significant effects. A 2000 study found that minocycline, an antibiotic, delayed motor decline in mice by 14%.

Riluzole is a drug currently used to treat people with **amyotrophic lateral sclerosis** (ALS, or Lou Gehrig's disease). In clinical trials with HD patients in 1999, the drug reduced chorea in about a third of people over six weeks. Behavior was improved by about 61% after 12 months.

Studies are under way to see whether transplanting fetal cells from the corpus striatum will be helpful to treat people with HD. This follows closely on the heels of similar trials with people who have Parkinson's disease. As of early 2004, preliminary results seem promising but much more time is needed to fully study and interpret them.

Recovery and rehabilitation

Supportive therapy for people with HD is very helpful, and often greatly needed as time goes on. It may begin shortly after diagnosis and continue for years, until the disease becomes advanced and supportive care is needed.

Physical therapy, speech therapy, and dietary advice can be extremely important and most effective when in tandem. Special consideration should be given to nursing and supportive care, home health care options, diet, special adaptive equipment, and eligibility for governmental benefits. A practical approach with common sense, emotional support, and careful attention to a family's needs is effective for many people with HD.

Clinical trials

As of early 2004, many clinical trials were under way to study Huntington disease:

- Family Health after Predictive Huntington Disease (HD) Testing, sponsored by National Institute of Nursing Research (NINR).

- Minocycline in Patients with Huntington's Disease, sponsored by FDA Office of Orphan Products Development.

- Prospective Huntington At-Risk Observational Study (PHAROS), sponsored by National Institute of Neurological Disorders and Stroke (NINDS) and National Human Genome Research Institute (NHGRI).

- Neurobiological Predictors of Huntington's Disease (PREDICT-HD), sponsored by NINDS.

- Brain Tissue Collection for Neuropathological Studies, sponsored by National Institute of Mental Health (NIMH).

Prognosis

Prognosis has historically been somewhat bleak for people with HD. Complications related to movement abnormalities and immobility, such as pneumonia and respiratory complications, are a common cause of death in HD. Though no cure is currently available, treatments or therapies may be available in the future to maintain a better quality of life, and these continue to offer hope.

Resources
BOOKS
Parker, James N., and Philip M. Parker. *The Official Patient's Sourcebook on Huntington's Disease: A Revised and Updated Directory for the Internet Age.* San Diego: Icon Health Publishers, 2002.

Quarrell, Oliver. *Huntington's Disease: The Facts.* Oxford: Oxford University Press, 1999.

PERIODICALS
Burgermeister, Jane. "Teacher Was Refused Job because Relatives Have Huntington's Disease." *British Medical Journal* (October 11, 2003) 327 (7419): 827.

Grimbergen, Yvette A. M., and Raymond A. C. Roos. "Therapeutic Options for Huntington's Disease." *Current Opinion in Investigational Drugs* (2003) 4(1): 51–54.

Margolis, Russell L., and Christopher A. Ross. "Diagnosis of Huntington Disease." *Clinical Chemistry* (2003) 49(10): 1726–1732.

Sutton Brown, M., and O. Suchowersky. "Clinical and Research Advances in Huntington's Disease." *The Canadian Journal of Neurological Sciences* (2003) 30 (Suppl. 1): S45–S52.

WEBSITES

Caring for People with Huntington's Disease. (June 2, 2004). <http://www.kumc.edu/hospital/huntingtons/index.html>.

GeneTests/GeneReviews. (June 2, 2004). <http://www.genetests.org>.

National Institute of Neurological Disorders and Stroke. (June 2, 2004). <http://www.ninds.nih.gov/index.htm>.

Testing for Huntington Disease: Making an Informed Choice. (June 2, 2004). <http://depts.washington.edu/neurogen/HuntingtonDis.pdf>.

Testing Guidelines in Huntington's Disease. (June 2, 2004). <http://www.hdfoundation.org/testread/hdsatest.htm>.

ORGANIZATIONS

Huntington's Disease Society of America. 158 West 29th Street, 7th Floor, New York, NY 10001-5300. (212) 242-1968 or (800) 345-HDSA (4372); Fax: (212) 239-3430. hdsainfo@hdsa.org. <http://www.hdsa.org>.

Huntington Society of Canada. 151 Frederick Street, Suite 400, Kitchener, Ontario N2H 2M2, Canada. (519) 749-7063 or (800) 998-7398; Fax: (519) 749-8965. info@hsc-ca.org. <http://www.hsc-ca.org>.

International Huntington Association. Callunahof 8, 7217 St Harfsen, The Netherlands. + 31-573-431595. iha@huntington-assoc.com. <http://www.huntington-assoc.com>.

Deepti Babu, MS, CGC

Hydantoins

Definition

Hydantoin **anticonvulsants** are most commonly used in the treatment of **seizures** associated with **epilepsy**, a neurological dysfunction in which excessive surges of electrical energy are emitted in the brain. Some hydantoins, such as phenytoin, are also indicated for use as skeletal muscle relaxants and in the treatment of severe nerve **pain**, as in **trigeminal neuralgia**.

Purpose

While hydantoins control the seizures associated with epilepsy, there is no known cure for the disorder. The precise mechanisms by which hydantoins work are unknown, but they are thought to exert their therapeutic effect by depressing abnormal neuronal discharges in the **central nervous system** (CNS).

Description

For the treatment of seizures, hydantoins may be used alone or in combination with other anti-epileptic drugs (AEDs) or anticonvulsants. However, the use of multiple anticonvulsants and AEDs should be carefully monitored by the prescribing physician. Phenytoin, mephenytoin, ethotoin, and fosphenytoin are the individual hydantoin anticonvulsants. They are marketed under several brand names, including Cerebyx, Dilantin, Mesantoin, Peganone, and Phentek.

Recommended dosage

Hydantoins anticonvulsants are available in oral and injectable (phenytoin and fosphenytoin only) forms. Orally-administered hydantoins are available in the form of tablets, capsules, or oral suspension. Hydantoins are prescribed by physicians in varying daily dosages.

Some hydantoin anticonvulsants are taken in divided daily doses, twice daily. Others are administered in a single daily dose. A double dose of any hydantoin should not be taken. If a dose is missed, it should be taken as soon as possible. However, if it is almost time for the next dose, the missed dose should be skipped.

It may take several weeks to realize the full benefits of hydantoins. Beginning any course of treatment including hydantoins requires a gradual dose-increasing regimen. Children and adults typically take a smaller daily dose for the first two weeks. Daily dosages of hydantoins may then be slowly increased over time. When ending a course of treatment that includes hydantoin anticonvulsants, physicians typically taper the patient's daily dose over a period of several weeks. Suddenly stopping treatment with hydantoins may cause seizures or pain to occur or return with greater frequency.

Precautions

Persons taking hydantoins should consult the prescribing physician before taking non-perscription medications. Patients should avoid alcohol and CNS depressants (medications that make one drowsy such as antihistimines, sleep medications, and some pain medications) while taking hydantoins. These medications may increase the frequency and severity of the side effects of hydantoins. Hydantoins may also potentiate the action of alcohol, and alcohol can increase the risk or frequency of seizures.

Hydantoins may not be suitable for persons with a history of thyroid, liver, or kidney disease, depressed renal function, diabetes mellitus, porphyria, **lupus**, mental illness, high blood presure, angina (chest pain), or irregular heartbeats and other heart problems. Before beginning treatment with hydantoins, patients should notify their

Key Terms

Epilepsy A disorder associated with disturbed electrical discharges in the central nervous system that cause seizures.

Neurogenic pain Pain originating in the nerves or nervous tissue.

Trigeminal neuralgia A disorder affecting the trigeminal nerve (the 5th cranial nerve), causing episodes of sudden, severe pain on one side of the face.

physician if they consume a large amount of alcohol, have a history of drug use, are nursing, pregnant, or plan to become pregnant.

Physicians usually advise women of child-bearing age to use effective birth control while taking hydantoin anticonvulsants. Many anticonvulsant medications, including hydantoins, have been shown to increase the risk of birth defects. Patients who become pregnant while taking hydantoins should contact their physician.

Some hydantoin anticonvulsant medications may be prescribed for children; however, children sometimes experience increased side effects. Research indicates that some children who take high doses of hydantoins for an extended period of time may experience mild learning difficulties or not perform as well in school.

Side effects

In some patients, hydantoins may produce some mild side effects. Drowsiness and **dizziness** are the most frequently reported side effects of anticonvulsants. Other general side effects of hydantoins that usually resolve without medical attention include:

- mild coordination problems
- constipation
- muscle twitching
- unpleasant taste in mouth or dry mouth
- unusual or excessive hair growth on face or body.

Many of these side effects disappear or occur less frequently during treatment as the body adjusts to the medication. However, if any symptoms persist or become too uncomfortable, the perscribing physician should be consulted.

Other, uncommon side effects of hydantoins may indicate an allergic reaction or other potentially serious condition. A patient taking hydantoin who experiencs any of the following symptoms should contact their physician immediately:

- rash, excessive bruising, or bluish patches on the skin
- bleeding in the gums or mouth
- ringing or vibrations in the ears
- general loss of motor skills
- severe lack of appetite
- altered vision
- difficulty breathing
- chest pain or irregular heartbeat
- faintness or loss of consciousness
- persistent fever or pain

Interactions

Hydantoins may have negative interactions with some antacids, anticoagulants, antihistimines, antidepressants, antibiotics, pain killers and monoamine oxidase inhibitors (MAOIs). Other medications such as amiodarone, diazoxide, **felbamate**, phenybutazone, sulfonamides (sulfa drugs), corticosteroids, sucralfate, rifampin, and warfarin may also adversely react with hydantoins.

Some hydantoins should not be used with other anticonvulsants. For example, phenytoin (a hydantoin) when used with valproic acid (a non-hydantoin anticonvulsant) may increase the seizure frequency. However, some patients may use hydantoins with other seizure prevention medications if carefully monitored by a physician.

Hydantoins may decrease the effectiveness of contraceptives, including oral contraceptives (birth control pills), progesterone implants (Norplant), and progesterone injections (Depo-Provera).

Resources

BOOKS

Weaver, Donald F. *Epilepsy and Seizures: Everything You Need to Know.* Firefly Books, 2001.

PERIODICALS

"Risk of birth defects with anticonvulsants evaluated." *Psychopharmacology Update* 12, no. 5 (May 2001): 3.

OTHER

"Anticonvulsants, Hydantoin (Systemic)." *Medline Plus.* National Library of Medicine. (April 20, 2004). <http://www.nlm.nih.gov/medlineplus/druginfo/uspdi/202052.html>.

ORGANIZATIONS

Epilepsy Foundation. 4351 Garden City Drive, Landover, MD 20785-7223. (800) 332-1000. <http://www.epilepsy foundation.org>.

American Epilepsy Society. 342 North Main Street, West Hartford, CT 06117-2507. <http://www.aesnet.org>.

Adrienne Wilmoth Lerner

Hydranencephaly

Definition

Hydranencephaly is a rare congenital deformity (a deformity that occurs during fetal development) that is characterized by the absence of the cerebral hemispheres of the brain. Instead, the regions of the brain known as the left and right cerebral hemispheres are replaced by sacs that are filled with cerebrospinal fluid.

Description

The absence of the cerebral hemispheres may not be apparent in the first days following birth. The normal and involuntary actions of a newborn such as sucking, swallowing, and crying all occur, as the brainstem controls these actions, and it is usually normal. Moreover, the baby with hydranencephaly appears physically normal, including the size of the head.

The normal behaviors of a growing infant reflect the functions of the left and right cerebral hemispheres. The left hemisphere is normally associated with the acquisition of language. The right hemisphere participates in the perception of space and distance. These sorts of skills are not yet developed in a newborn. Within several weeks to months of birth, the symptoms of hydranencephaly can become apparent.

Demographics

Hydranencephaly is a rare occurrence. It is estimated that one or two babies are born with hydranencephaly worldwide for every 10,000 births. There is no indication that any gender or race is any more susceptible to the disorder.

Causes and symptoms

Within a few weeks of birth, the infant typically becomes irritable and the contraction of the muscles (muscle tone) becomes more pronounced. Muscles may spasm. **Seizures** can occur. Other symptoms that can develop with time include poor vision or the total loss of vision, poor or no growth, deafness, paralysis, and impaired intellectual development (such as language difficulty).

Hydranencephaly may be caused by a genetic defect, infection associated with vessels, or a trauma that occurs after the twelfth week of pregnancy. Maternal exposure to carbon monoxide early in pregnancy has also been implicated as a possible cause, along with the possibility of early **stroke** in the developing fetus, or as a result of infection with some viruses.

Diagnosis

Diagnosis is based on the appearance of symptoms noted above. Diagnosis may not be made for weeks or months following birth, because of the initial normal appearance and behavior of the newborn. Prior to birth, ultrasound can reveal hydranencephaly, although techniques for surgical correction in the fetus have not been developed.

Treatment team

A range of medical help, from a family practitioner to pediatric surgeon, can be involved. As well, nurses and family members are part of the care-giving team. Social service workers can refer parents of children with hydranencephaly to community support organizations.

Treatment

There is no definitive treatment for hydranencephaly. Usually, symptoms are treated as they occur and support is provided to make the child as comfortable and happy as possible. Medications are given to control seizures and if excess cerebrospinal fluid collects near the brainstem, a shunt is usually surgically inserted to facilitate redirection of the excess fluid.

Recovery and rehabilitation

Rehabilitation is not stressed for the infant with hydranencephaly, as the long-term prognosis is poor. Physical and occupational therapists may assist in providing treatment to maintain muscle tone for as long as possible, and positioning aids when necessary. Medications are given to control seizures and for comfort.

Clinical trials

As of January, 2004, there were no **clinical trials** underway or planned in the United States for the study of hydranencephaly. Organizations such as the National Institute for Neurological Disorders and Stroke undertake and fund studies designed to reveal more about the normal development patterns of the brain. By understanding how development can be disrupted, scientists attempt to learn strategies for detecting defects and methods to correct them.

Prognosis

The long-term outlook for children with hydranencephaly is poor. Most children die in their first year of life, although survival past the age of 10 can rarely occur.

Key Terms

Brainstem The stalk of the brain that connects the two cerebral hemispheres with the spinal cord. It is involved in controlling vital functions, movement, sensation, and nerves supplying the head and neck.

Seizure A sudden attack, spasm, or convulsion.

Currently, the oldest known survivor was 20 years, 6 months old.

Special concerns

Providing support for parents of babies born with hydranencephaly includes genetic counseling and referrals to support groups, where parents can learn practical advice and share information with other parents of children similarly affected. Additionally, mothers who have given birth to a baby with hydranencephaly may be tested for some of the viruses suspected in playing a part in the fetal development of hydranencephaly, including toxoplasmosis, cytomegalovirus, and Herpes simplex virus.

Resources

PERIODICALS

Covington, C., H. Taylor, C. Gill, B. Padaliya, W. Newman, J. R. Smart III, and P. D. Charles. "Prolonged survival in hydranencephaly: a case report." *Tennessee Medicine* (September 2003): 423–424.

Lam, Y. H., and M. H. Tang. "Serial sonographic features of a fetus with hydranencephaly from 11 weeks to term." *Ultrasound Obstetrics and Gynecology* (July 2000): 77–79.

OTHER

"NINDS Hydranencephaly Information Page." *National Institute for Neurological Diseases and Stroke.* (January 20, 2004). <www.ninds.nih.gov/health_and_medical/disorders/hydranen_doc.htm>.

ORGANIZATIONS

March of Dimes Birth Defects Foundation. 1275 Mamaroneck Avenue, White Plains, NY 10605. (914) 428-7100 or (888) 663-4637; Fax: (914) 428-8203. askus@marchofdimes.com. <http://www.marchofdimes.com>.

National Information Center for Children and Youth with Disabilities. P.O. Box 1492, Washington, DC 20013-1492. (202) 884-8200 or (800) 695-0285; Fax: (202) 884-8441. nichcy@ead.org. <http://www.nichcy.org>.

National Institute for Neurological Diseases and Stroke (NINDS). 6001 Executive Boulevard, Bethesda, MD 20892. (301) 496-5751 or (800) 352-9424. <http://www.ninds.nih.gov>.

National Organization for Rare Disorders. 55 Kenosia Avenue, Danbury, CT 06813-1968. (203) 744-0100 or (800) 999-6673; Fax: (203) 798-2291. orphan@rarediseases.org. <http://www.rarediseases.org>.

Brian Douglas Hoyle, PhD

Hydrocephalus

Definition

The word hydrocephalus derives from the Greek words *hydro*, meaning water, and *cephalus*, meaning head. Hydrocephalus is the result of the excessive accumulation of fluid in the brain. Traditionally, hydrocephalus has been described as a disease characterized by increased intracranial pressure (ICP), increased cerebrospinal fluid (CSF) volume, and dilatation of the CSF spaces known as cerebral ventricles.

Description

Hydrocephalus is the result of an imbalance between the formation and drainage of cerebrospinal fluid. This imbalance appears when an injury or illness alters the circulation of CSF; one or more of the ventricles of the brain become enlarged as CSF accumulates. However, hydrocephalus is not a single disease entity, as a wide number of underlying diseases are responsible for causing retention of CSF, resulting in ventricular dilatation and increased intracranial pressure (ICP). In infants and children, for example, hydrocephalus usually results from a birth defect, viral infection, head injury, hemorrhage, meningitis, or tumor.

In adults, the causes of hydrocephalus include brain damage due to **stroke** or injury, Alzheimer's disease, or obstruction of the ventricles. Often, the cause is unknown. Conditions responsible for hydrocephalus in a fetus include infantile congenital (present at birth) hydrocephalus, hydrocephalus associated with encephalocele or myelomeningocele, posthemorrhagic hydrocephalus in newborns, and postmeningitic hydrocephalus. Conditions responsible for hydrocephalus in adults include hydrocephalus following subarachnoid hemorrhage, idiopathic adult hydrocephalus, and posttraumatic hydrocephalus. Tumors can also result in hydrocephalus in both children and adults. Based on the different kind of CSF circulation in the brain, hydrocephalus can be divided into two types: communicating and non-communicating. In communicating hydrocephalus, the CSF circulation pathways are competent from the ventricles inside of the brain to the fluid spaces just below the third ventricle. Non-communicating (obstructive) hydrocephalus refers to hydrocephalus that

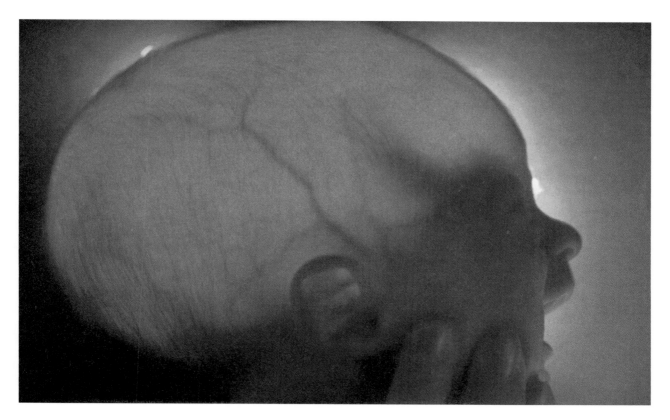

Sideview of the skull of infant suffering from hydrocephalus. *(© Lester V. Bergman/Corbis. Reproduced by permission.)*

develops from a blockage of the normal circulation of CSF within the brain. In most cases, it refers to a blockage between the third and fourth ventricles.

Demographics

Overall incidence of infantile hydrocephalus is approximately one to two per 1,000 live births. The overall prevalence of hydrocephalus in the United States is about 0.5%. When cases of **spina bifida** are included, congenital hydrocephalus occurs in two to five births per 1,000 births. The incidence of acquired hydrocephalus in adults is not known because it occurs as a result of injury, illness, or environmental factors. Normal pressure hydrocephalus was found to be significantly more prevalent in males, and can occur in adults of any age group. The age distribution in children and teenagers is disputed.

Causes and symptoms

Approximately 16 oz (500 ml) of CSF are formed within the brain each day, by cells located on the wall of the four ventricles in the brain. Once formed, CSF circulates among all the ventricles before it is absorbed. The normal adult volume of circulating CSF is about 2 oz (150 ml). The CSF turnover rate is more than three times per day. Because production is independent of absorption, reduced absorption causes CSF to accumulate within the ventricles.

Hydrocephalus can be subdivided into three forms, involving the following:

• Disorders of cerebrospinal fluid circulation. Tumors, hemorrhages, congenital malformations, and infections can cause such obstructions in the circulation of cerebrospinal fluid.

• Disorders of cerebrospinal fluid absorption, resulting from diseases such as the superior vena cava syndrome and sinus thrombosis.

• Disorders of cerebrospinal fluid production: This is the less common form of hydrocephalus resulting from tumors that secrete cerebrospinal fluid in excess of its absorption.

Congenital hydrocephalus is thought to be caused by a complex interaction of genetic and environmental factors. The origin of hydrocephalus in congenital cases is unknown. Very few cases (less than 2%) are inherited (X-linked hydrocephalus). The most common causes of hydrocephalus in acquired cases are tumor obstruction, trauma, intracranial hemorrhage, and infection.

The two most common adult forms of hydrocephalus are hydrocephalus ex-vacuo and normal pressure hydrocephalus. Hydrocephalus ex-vacuo occurs when a stroke or injury damages the brain, yielding a brain substance. Although there is more CSF than usual, the CSF pressure may or may not be elevated. Normal pressure hydrocephalus is an abnormal increase of CSF in the brain's ventricles due to the gradual blockage of the CSF-draining pathways. This may result from a subarachnoid hemorrhage, head trauma, infection, tumor, or complications of surgery. The ventricles enlarge to handle the increased volume of the CSF, and the compression of the brain from within by the fluid-filled ventricles destroys or damages brain tissue. Fluctuation of CSF pressure from high to normal to low can also be present.

For congenital-onset hydrocephalus, early symptoms include enlargement of the head (increased head circumference), bulging fontanelles (soft spots) with or without enlargement of the head size, separation of sutures (the flexible and fibrous joints between the skull bones of an infant), and vomiting. Symptoms of continued hydrocephalus include irritability and muscle **spasticity**. Late symptoms of congenital-onset hydrocephalus seen in children up to five years of age include decreased mental function, delayed development, slow or restricted movement, difficulty feeding, lethargy, and delayed growth.

In children, symptoms depend on the amount of damage caused by ICP. Symptoms may be similar to many of those in infants or may include **headache**, vomiting, vision changes such as crossed eyes, uncontrolled eye movements, loss of coordination, poor gait (walking pattern), mental confusion, or psychosis. For adult-onset hydrocephalus, headaches and nausea are the most common symptoms. Other signs of the condition include difficulty focusing the eyes, unsteady gait, weakness of the legs, sudden falls, and a distinctive inability to walk forward. As hydrocephalus progresses, decreased mental activity appears, including lethargy, apathy, impaired memory, and speech problems. Urinary and bowel incontinence can also occur. During the final stage, **dementia** involving loss of movement, sensory functions, and cognitive abilities may result.

Diagnosis

Ultrasound can be used to diagnose prenatal hydrocephalus. Although fetal hydrocephalus may be an isolated finding, it is more frequently found along with other cerebral anomalies, including neural tube defects. Diagnosis after birth may be suggested by symptoms; however, imaging studies of the brain are the mainstay of diagnosis. Computed tomography (**CT**) and **magnetic resonance**

imaging (**MRI**) reveal enlarged ventricles and may indicate a specific cause of hydrocephalus, such as a tumor or hemorrhage. The presence of papilledema (elevation or swelling of the optic disc) also indicates that hydrocephalus that is well developed. In rare cases, long-standing hydrocephalus causes blindness.

Small abnormalities that may not be seen with CT scanning, such as cysts and abscesses, are often seen with **MRI**. These studies can also help the neurosurgeon differentiate between communicating and non-communicating hydrocephalus. In cases of suspected normal pressure hydrocephalus, a lumbar puncture (spinal tap) may help determine CSF pressure. Also, a cisternagram can be useful to evaluate the dynamics of CSF flow in the brain and spinal chord. Cisternography can reveal CSF concentration, obstruction, leakage, and pressure. Also, certain biochemical markers in the blood have been described in the disease. They include increased neurofilament light protein (NFL) and tau protein, both markers of neuronal degeneration; increased myeline basic protein (a marker of demyelination; and albumin); and a marker of the blood-brain barrier function.

Treatment team

Treatment of hydrocephalus for children or adults will likely involve a **neurologist**, neurosurgeon, obstetrician, pediatrician, and specialty nurses and physical therapists.

Treatment

Medical treatment is first aimed at reducing intracranial pressure, while the need for a more permanent solution is determined. Reduction of fluid intake and administration of drugs such as mannitol, glycerol, urea (drugs with an osmotic effect), or furosemide (a diuretic) are able to reduce ICP and CSF production.

External drainage of the CSF is useful for urgent reduction of intracranial pressure, as well as of ventricular or subarachnoid hemorrhage. Complications include overdrainage, blocked tube, or bacterial contamination. The placement of a permanent **ventricular shunt** (internal shunting) is a common procedure. Around 33,000 shunts are placed in the United States each year; almost half of them to replace previous shunt devices. CSF from the ventricles in the brain is usually shunted to the peritoneum, pleura, ureter, bladder, or vascular spaces such as the jugular or subclavian veins. Most shunts are connected to the peritoneum. Some shunts operate according to intracranial pressure by using a valve system able to regulate the flow at a pressure close to the normal values of ICP. Others are programmable and can be adjusted to open at a given ICP. Complications include overdrainage that may cause intracranial hypotension, **subdural hematoma**,

Key Terms

Cerebrospinal fluid (CSF)   The clear fluid made in the ventricular cavities of the brain that bathes the brain and spinal cord.

Gait   Posture and manner of walking.

Hydrocephalus   A condition characterized by the abnormal accumulation of cerebrospinal fluid within the ventricles of the brain.

Increased intracranial pressure (ICP)   Increased pressure within the skull caused by extra tissue or fluid in the brain.

Papilledema   Swelling of the optic disc, where the optic nerve enters the eyeball, or elevation of the optic nerve, and indication of increased intracranial pressure.

Ventricle   The cavities or chambers within the brain that contain the cerebrospinal fluid.

shunt occlusion, and infection. The risk of shunt failure is greater within the first year (between 25–40% of shunts must be replaced). The subsequent failure rate is around 5% for each year.

Other surgical procedures include, in some cases, choroid plexectomy, third ventriculostomy, and ventricular reservoir. Ventricular reservoir is basically a catheter inserted into a ventricle of the brain to draw CSF. This procedure is much simpler than placing a full shunt system and is used to provide temporary control of ICP until a full shunt can be placed.

Recovery and rehabilitation

Hydrocephalus is a chronic condition, and clinical symptoms are based on the time of insurgence of the disease. With appropriate, early treatment, a normal lifespan with few limitations can be reached. After surgery, specially trained medical professionals carefully monitor the patient. Some symptoms such as headaches may disappear immediately due to the release of excess pressure. The symptoms associated with normal pressure hydrocephalus (walking difficulties, mild dementia, poor bladder control) may improve quickly, or may take weeks to months to improve. In some patients, little or no improvement is also possible.

The length of the patient's hospital stay will be determined by the rate of recovery. If neurological problems persist, rehabilitation may be required to further the patient's improvement. However, recovery may be limited by

the extent of the damage already caused by the hydrocephalus. Because hydrocephalus is an ongoing condition, patients do require long-term follow up. Follow-up diagnostic tests, including CT scans, MRI, and x rays, may be performed to determine if the shunt is working correctly.

Clinical trials

Ventricular shunts are the most common surgical treatment for hydrocephalus and appear to be the safest. It is possible that choroid plexectomy and third ventriculostomy may become more feasible in the future if better procedures and equipment are developed.

As of mid-2004, several **clinical trials** to study hydrocephalus were underway, including a trial to evaluate the efficacy and safety of endoscopic choroid plexus coagulation with third ventriculostomy in the treatment of idiopathic normal pressure hydrocephalus, sponsored by the Frenchay Hydrocephalus Research Fund. The National Institute of Neurological Disorders and Stroke is sponsoring a study to establish the physiology of **syringomyelia**. Updated information on these and other ongoing clinical trials may be found at the National Institutes of Health website for clinical trials at <http://www.clinicaltrials.gov>.

Prognosis

Untreated hydrocephalus has a survival rate of 40–50%, with the survivors having varying degrees of intellectual, physical, and neurological disabilities. Prognosis for treated hydrocephalus varies, depending on the cause. If the child survives for one year, more than 80% will have a fairly normal lifespan. Approximately one-third will have normal intellectual function, but neurological difficulties may persist. Hydrocephalus not associated with infection has the best prognosis, and hydrocephalus caused by tumors has a very poor prognosis. About 50% of all children who receive appropriate treatment and follow up will develop IQs in the near-normal or normal range.

Resources
BOOKS

Matsumoto, Satoshi. *Hydrocephalus: Pathogenesis and Treatment.* New York: Springer-Verlag, 1991.

The Official Parent's Sourcebook on Hydrocephalus: A Revised and Updated Directory for the Internet Age. San Diego: Icon Group International, 2002.

Toporek, Chuck, and Kellie Robinson. *Hydrocephalus: A Guide for Patients, Families and Friends.* Sebastopol, CA: Patient-Centered Guides, 1999.

PERIODICALS

Arriada, N., and J. Sotelo. "Review: Treatment of Hydrocephalus in Adults." *Surg Neurol.* (2002) Dec 58 (6): 377–84.

Davis, G. H. "Fetal Hydrocephalus." *Clin Perinatol.* (2003) Sep 30 (3): 531–9.

Meier, U., and C. Miethke. "Predictors of Outcome in Patients with Normal-Pressure Hydrocephalus." *J Clin Neurosci.* (2003) Jul 10 (4): 453–9.

OTHER

"NINDS Hydrocephalus Information Page." *National Institute of Neurological Disorders and Stroke.* May 15, 2004 (May 22, 2004). <http://www.ninds.nih.gov/health_and_medical/disorders/hydrocephalus.htm>.

"What is Hydrocephalus?" *Hydrocephalus Foundation, Inc.* May 15, 2004 (May 22, 2004). <http://www.hydrocephalus.org/>.

ORGANIZATIONS

Hydrocephalus Association. 870 Market Street, Suite 705, San Francisco, CA 94102. (415) 732-7040 or (888) 598-3789; Fax: (415) 732-7044. info@hydroassoc.org. <http://www.hydroassoc.org>.

National Hydrocephalus Foundation. 12413 Centralia Road, Lakewood, CA 90715-1623. (562) 402-3523 or (888) 857-3434; Fax: (562) 924-6666. hydrobrat@earthlink.net. <http://nhfonline.org>.

Antonio Farina, MD, PhD

Hydromyelia

Definition

Hydromyelia (HM) is a condition characterized by widening of the central canal of the spinal cord. Fluid can accumulate in this space, creating increased pressure on the spinal cord. The term hydromyelia is sometimes used interchangeably with a closely related condition, **syringomyelia** (or syringohydromyelia). Syringomyelia (SM) is a condition in which fluid collects in the area of the spinal cord that is outside the central canal. The end result of hydromyelia and syringomyelia is essentially the same: an abnormal cyst (collection of fluid) in the spinal cord that is associated with a wide range of neurological complaints and signs. For simplicity, the term syringomyelia is used to refer to a fluid-filled cyst in the spinal cord that is inside or outside of the central canal.

Description

Syringomyelia is a variable condition in which the symptoms depend on the location and extent of the cavitation (hollowing out) of the cord. Over time, the expansion and elongation of the fluid-filled cavity (or cyst) can destroy the center of the spinal cord. This damage to the spinal cord results in **pain**, weakness, and loss of sensation for the affected individual. Syringomyelia may be an isolated finding or may be found in association with a syndrome that disrupts the flow of cerebral spinal fluid (CSF), such as the **Arnold-Chiari malformation** or the **Dandy-Walker** malformation.

The earliest known description of cystic dilatation (widening) of the spinal cord dates back to the sixteenth century. The terms syringomyelia and hydromyelia were first used in published reports in 1827 and 1859, respectively.

Demographics

Syringomyelia occurs across all races and ethnic groups and affects both children and adults. Although syringomyelia usually appears in midlife, it can occur at any age. Estimates of the incidence of syringomyelia vary and range from 1 in 18,000 to as high as 1 in 1,300 people in the United States.

Causes and symptoms

The causes of syringomyelia are not well understood. It is thought that syringomyelia occurs when one or more factors interfere with the normal development of the spinal canal during formation of the embryo or when factors such as trauma to the spinal cord, infection, or a mass (such as tumor) interfere with the fluid dynamics in the spinal cord. Arnold-Chiari malformation is the leading cause of syringomyelia. Syringomyelia occurs in as many as one-quarter of people who have a **spinal cord injury**. Various theories have been postulated to explain how movement of cerebrospinal fluid and pressure in the **central nervous system** (the brain and spinal cord) interact to produce this defect. In some cases, genetic factors may play a role in the development of this condition.

The symptoms of syringomyelia can be quite variable and depend upon the location and extent of the cyst. Common symptoms of syringomyelia in affected individuals include:

- extreme pain or "heavy" feeling in the neck; shoulders are usually numb
- headaches
- leg or hand weakness
- numbness or loss of sensation in the hands and feet
- problems with walking
- loss of bowel and bladder control
- spasticity and paralysis of the legs
- visual disturbances
- ataxia

- speech problems
- scoliosis (curvature of the spine)

Diagnosis

Diagnosis of syringomyelia is based on neurological exam and results of neuroradiological imaging studies. The neurological exam of an affected individual will show loss of sensation in the hands, balance problems, decreased strength, difficulty walking or an abnormal gait, and abnormal reflexes. Some people with no symptoms or mild symptoms are diagnosed with syringomyelia incidentally in the course of evaluation for another condition. Imaging studies used to diagnose syringomyelia include **magnetic resonance imaging (MRI)**, CINE **MRI** (a type of MRI that shows the flow of cerebrospinal fluid), and **electromyography** (EMG). In some cases it may be technically difficult to distinguish hydromyelia from syringomyelia.

Treatment

Currently, there is no cure for syringomyelia. Neurosurgery is the primary method of treatment for this condition. Surgery tends to be reserved for those individuals with moderate or severe neurological problems. The goal of the various neurosurgical techniques is to restore normal flow of cerebral spinal fluid. There are four main categories of procedures:

- decompression procedures
- laminectomy and syringostomy
- terminal ventriculostomy
- percutaneous aspiration

Surgical interventions for syringomyelia have limitations and carry risks for potentially severe complications. The decision to operate is generally based on the severity of symptoms and the findings on MRI or other imaging studies. Patients are followed closely after surgery for signs of further neurological impairment. Some patients will need to undergo more than one surgery.

Treatment team

Management of syringomyelia requires a multidisciplinary approach. In addition to the patient's primary health care professionals, medical professionals involved in the care of patients with syringomyelia generally include a **neurologist** and a neurosurgeon. Additional specialists in pain management and rehabilitation may also be needed.

Recovery and rehabilitation

Patients with syringomyelia may require a wide range of rehabilitation services including physical therapy, occupational therapy, and speech therapy to help them compensate for weakness and loss of function. Chronic pain can pose a significant problem for some patients. Management of chronic pain may include prescription and non-prescription medications, physical therapy, occupational therapy, medical procedures such as nerve blocks or trigger point injections, psychological therapy, and chiropractics.

Clinical trials

As of early 2004, there were three **clinical trials** for patients with syringomyelia, all of which are sponsored by the National Institute of Neurological Disorders and **Stroke** (NINDS). There is a study (Study and Surgical Treatment of Syringomyelia) to establish the mechanism(s) of progression of primarily spinal syringomyelia (PSS). More information on this study can be obtained at http://clinicalstudies.info.nih.gov/detail/A_2001-N-0085.html or by contacting the patient recruitment and public liaison office at (800) 411-1222 or prpl@mail.cc.nih.gov. In another study (Establishing the Physiology of Syringomyelia), researchers would like to learn more about how the CSF pressure and flow contribute to the progression of syringomyelia. More information can be obtained at http://clinicalstudies.info.nih.gov/detail/A_1992-N-0226.html or by contacting the patient recruitment and public liaison office. Finally, there is a study (Genetic Analysis of the Chiari I Malformation) whose purpose is to better understand the genetic factors related to the Chiari I malformation. More information can be found at http://clinicalstudies.info.nih.gov/detail/A_2000-N-0089.html or by contacting the patient recruitment and public liaison office. There is also an ongoing genetic research study for Chiari type I malformation and syringomyelia (CMI/S) to determine whether or not there is a genetic component to CMI/S. Interested patients and families may find more information at the Center for Human Genetics at Duke University at http://wwwchg.mc.duke.edu/patients/cms.html or by contacting the center at (800) 283-4316 or syringo@dnadoc.mc.duke.edu.

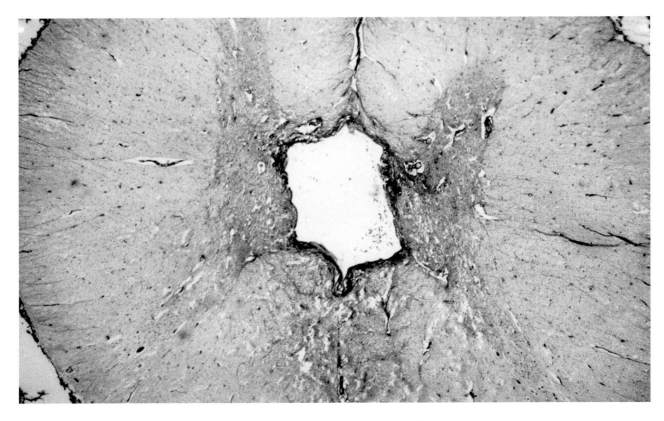

The widened spinal cord canal associated with hydromyelia. *(Custom Medical Stock Photo. All Rights Reserved.)*

Prognosis

The course of syringomyelia is not well defined. Some untreated patients will experience a spontaneous remission of symptoms. Among treated patients, some will have a permanent end to their neurological deficits whereas others will only experience temporary relief of symptoms. Long-term studies of affected patients are needed to better understand the natural history and prognosis of this condition.

Resources

BOOKS

Graham, D. I., and P. L. Lantos, eds. *Greenfield's Neuropathology*, volume I, 7th edition. London: Arnold, 2002.

Parker, James N., MD, and Philip M. Parker, PhD, eds. *The Official Parent's Sourcebook on Syringomyelia: A Revised and Updated Directory for the Internet Age.* San Diego, CA: ICON Health Publications, 2002.

Klekamp, Joerg, and Madjid Samii. *Syringomyelia: Diagnosis and Treatment*, 1st edition. New York: Springer Verlag, 2001.

PERIODICALS

Caldarelli, M., and C. Di Rocco. "Diagnosis of Chiari I Malformation and Related Syringomyelia: Radiological and Neurophysiological Studies." *Child's Nervous System* 53 (March 2004): epublication, ahead of print.

Kyoshima K., and E. I. Bogdanov. "Spontaneous Resolution of Syringomyelia: Report of Two Cases and Review of the Literature." *Neurosurgery* 53 (Sept 2003): 762–9.

Wisoff, J. H. "Hydromyelia: A Critical Review." *Child's Nervous System* 4 (1988): 1–8.

WEBSITES

American Syringomyelia Alliance Project, Inc. Home Page. (June 2, 2004). <http://www.asap.org.html>.

Chiari and Syringomyelia News Home Page. (June 2, 2004). <http://www.chiari-syringo-news.com/.html>.

The National Institute of Neurological Disorders and Stroke (NINDS). *Hydromyelia Information Page.* (June 2, 2004). <http://www.ninds.nih.gov/health_and_medical/disorders/hydromyelia.htm>.

The National Institute of Neurological Disorders and Stroke (NINDS). *Syringomyelia Information Page.* (June 2, 2004). <http://www.ninds.nih.gov/health_and_medical/disorders/syringomyelia_short.htm>.

ORGANIZATIONS

American Syringomyelia Alliance Project, Inc. P. O. Box 1586, Longview, TX 75606-1586. (903) 236-7079 or (800) ASAP-282; Fax: (903) 757-7456. info@ASAP.org. <http://www.asap.org>.

American Chronic Pain Association (ACPA). P.O. Box 850, Rocklin, CA 95677-0850. (916) 632-0922 or (800) 533-3231; Fax: (916) 632-3208. ACPA@pacbell.net. <http://www.theacpa.org>.

National Spinal Cord Injury Association. 6701 Democracy Blvd. #300-9, Bethesda, MD 20817. (301) 214-4006 or (800) 962-9629; Fax: (301) 881-9817. info@spinalcord.org. <http://www.spinalcord.org>.

Dawn J. Cardeiro, MS, CGC

Hypercortisolism *see* **Cushing syndrome**

Hypersomnia

Definition

Hypersomnia refers to a set of related disorders that involve excessive daytime sleepiness.

Description

There are two main categories of hypersomnia: primary hypersomnia (sometimes called idiopathic hypersomnia) and recurrent hypersomnia (sometimes called recurrent primary hypersomnia). Both are characterized by the same signs and symptoms and differ only in the frequency and regularity with which the symptoms occur.

Primary hypersomnia is characterized by excessive daytime sleepiness over a long period of time. The symptoms are present all, or nearly all, of the time. Recurring hypersomnia involves periods of excessive daytime sleepiness that can last from one to many days, and recur over the course of a year or more. The primary difference between this and primary hypersomnia is that persons experiencing recurring hypersomnia will have prolonged periods where they do not exhibit any signs of hypersomnia, whereas persons experiencing primary hypersomnia are affected by it nearly all the time. One of the best documented forms of recurrent hypersomnia is Kleine-Levin syndrome, although there are other forms as well.

There are many different causes for daytime sleepiness that are not considered hypersomnia, and there are many diseases and disorders in which excessive daytime sleepiness is a primary or secondary symptom. Feelings of daytime sleepiness are often associated with the use of common substances such as caffeine, alcohol, and many medications. Other common factors that can lead to excessive daytime sleepiness that is not considered hypersomnia include shift work and insomnia. Shift work can disrupt the body's natural sleep rhythms. Insomnia can

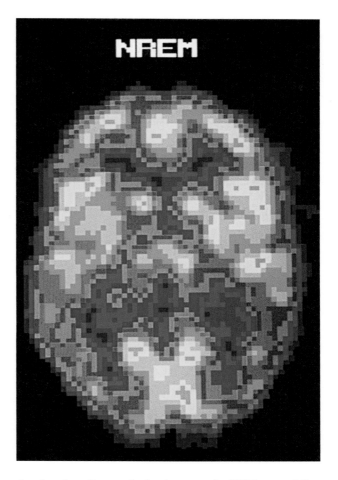

A colored positron emission tomography (PET) scan of the human brain during deep, non-REM sleep; the brain is active but not as active as during REM sleep. Active areas are red and yellow, inactive areas are blue. *(© Hank Morgan/ Science Source/Photo Researchers, Inc. Reproduced by permission.)*

cause excessive daytime sleepiness because of lack of nighttime sleep, and is a separate disorder.

Demographics

Hypersomnia is an uncommon disorder. In general, 5% or fewer of adults complain of excessive sleepiness during the daytime. That does not mean all those who complain of excessive sleepiness have hypersomnia. There are many other possible causes of daytime sleepiness. Of all the people who visit sleep clinics because they feel they are too sleepy during the day, only about 5–10% are diagnosed with primary hypersomnia. Kleine-Levin syndrome is present in about three times more males than females, but it is a very rare syndrome.

Hypersomnia generally appears when the patient is between 15 and 30 years old. It does not begin suddenly, but becomes apparent slowly, sometimes over years.

Causes and symptoms

People experiencing hypersomnia do not get abnormal amounts of nighttime sleep. However, they often have problems waking up in the morning and staying awake during the day. People with hypersomnia nap frequently, and upon waking from the nap, do not feel refreshed. Hypersomnia is sometimes misdiagnosed as **narcolepsy**. In many ways the two are similar. One significant difference is that people with narcolepsy experience a sudden onset of sleepiness, while people with hypersomnia experience increasing sleepiness over time. Also, people with narcolepsy find daytime sleep refreshing, while people with hypersomnia do not.

People with Kleine-Levin syndrome have symptoms that differ from the symptoms of other forms of hypersomnia. These people may sleep for 18 or more hours a day. In addition, they are often irritable, uninhibited, and make indiscriminate sexual advances. People with Kleine-Levin syndrome often eat uncontrollably and rapidly gain weight, unlike people with other forms of hypersomnia. This form of recurrent hypersomnia is very rare.

The causes of hypersomnia remain unclear. There is some speculation that in many cases it can be attributed to problems involving the hypothalamus, but there is little evidence to support that claim.

Diagnosis

Hypersomnia is characterized by excessive daytime sleepiness, and daytime naps that do not result in a more refreshed or alert feeling. Hypersomnia does not include lack of nighttime sleep. People experiencing problems with nighttime sleep may have insomnia, a separate sleep disorder. In people with insomnia, excessive daytime sleepiness may be a side effect.

The Diagnostic and Statistical Manual of Mental Disorders which presents the guidelines used by the American Psychiatric Association for diagnosis of disorders, states that symptoms must be present for at least a month, and must interfere with a person's normal activities. Also, the symptoms cannot be attributed to failure to get enough sleep at night or to another sleep disorder. The symptoms cannot be caused by another significant psychological disorder, nor can they be a side effect of a medicinal or illicit drug or a side effect of a general medical condition. For a diagnosis of recurrent hypersomnia, the symptoms must occur for at least three days at a time, and the symptoms have to be present for at least two years.

Treatment team

A number of specialists deal with sleep problems, including internal medicine physicians, psychiatrists, neurologists, and sleep disorder specialists.

Key Terms

Hypothalamus   A part of the forebrain that controls heartbeat, body temperature, thirst, hunger, blood pressure, blood sugar levels, and other functions.

Narcolepsy   A disorder characterized by frequent and uncontrollable attacks of deep sleep.

Treatments

There have been some attempts at using drugs to treat hypersomnia. No substantial body of evidence supports the effectiveness of these treatments. Stimulants are not generally recommended to treat hypersomnia as they treat the symptoms but not the base problem. Some researchers believe that treatment of the hypothalamus may be a possible treatment for hypersomnia.

Prognosis

Kleine-Levin syndrome has been reported to occasionally resolve by itself around middle age. Except for that syndrome, hypersomnia is considered both a lifelong disorder and one that can be significantly disabling. There is no body of evidence that concludes there is a way to treat the majority of hypersomnia cases successfully.

Resources

BOOKS

Aldrich, Michael S. *Sleep Medicines.* New York: Oxford University Press, 1999.

American Psychiatric Association *Diagnostic and Statistical Manual of Mental Disorders.* 4th edition, text revised. Washington DC: American Psychiatric Association, 2000.

Chokroverty, Susan, ed. *Sleep Disorders Medicine: Basic Science, Technical Considerations, and Clinical Aspects.* 2nd ed. Boston: Butterworth-Heinemann, 1999.

Sadock, Benjamin J. and Virginia A. Sadock, eds. *Comprehensive Textbook of Psychiatry.* 7th edition, vol. 2. Philadelphia: Lippincott Williams and Wilkins, 2000.

Thorpy, Michael J, ed. *Handbook of Sleep Disorders.* New York: Marcel Dekker Inc, 1990.

PERIODICALS

Boris, Neil W., Owen R. Hagina, Gregory P. Steiner. "Case Study: hypersomnolence and precocious puberty in a child with pica and chronic lead intoxication." *Journal of the American Academy of Child and Adolescent Psychiatry* 35, no. 8 (August 1996): 1050-1055.

National Center on Sleep Disorders Research Working Group, Bethesda, Maryland. "Recognizing Problem Sleepiness in Your People." *American Family Physician* (February 15, 1999): 937-38.

ORGANIZATIONS

American Academy of Sleep Medicine. 6301 Bandel Road NW, Suite 101, Rochester, MN 55901. (507) 287-6006. <www.asda.org>.

Tish Davidson, AM
Rosalyn Carson-DeWitt, MD

Hypertonia *see* **Spasticity**

Hypotonia

Definition

Hypotonia means "low tone," and refers to a physiological state in which a muscle has decreased tone, or tension. A muscle's tone is a measure of its ability to resist passive elongation or stretching.

Description

Hypotonia is more a description than a diagnosis. It is most often seen in newborns (congenital) and infants, but it may persist through adolescence into adulthood. Another name for infantile hypotonia is "floppy baby syndrome." This refers to the tendency of a hypotonic infant's arms, legs, and head to "flop," or dangle loosely, when they are picked up or moved. In the past, the term "benign congenital hypotonia" was used for many cases in which no obvious cause for the hypotonia could be detected. Better diagnostic techniques and increased knowledge of neuromuscular disorders, however, have resulted in much less frequent use of this term.

Demographics

Hypotonia is the most common muscular abnormality seen in neonatal (newborn) neurological disorders. It affects males and females equally, and shows no preponderance in any particular ethnic group or race. An increase in the occurrence of hypotonia in recent years is correlated with increased survival rates of infants born significantly premature, since these children are at increased risk for neurological problems.

Causes and symptoms

The causes of hypotonia are varied and numerous. Some involve trauma to, or diseases of, the brain or spinal cord (CNS), while others affect the peripheral nerves, neuromuscular junction, or the muscles themselves. A disorder of the nervous system is a neuropathy, while a muscle disease is a **myopathy**. A neuromuscular condition is one

---

Key Terms

Congenital   Present at birth.

Muscle tone   Also termed tonus; the normal state of balanced tension in the tissues of the body, especially the muscles.

Myopathy   Any abnormal condition or disease of muscle tissue, characterized by muscle weakness and wasting.

Neuromuscular   Involving both the muscles and the nerves that control them.

Neuropathy   A disease or abnormality of the peripheral nerves (the nerves outside the brain and spinal cord). Major symptoms include weakness, numbness, paralysis, or pain in the affected area.

---

in which a neurological disorder results in associated muscular symptoms.

CNS trauma and infection are perhaps the most common cause of hypotonia, both in infants and in children. Insult to the brain may occur prenatally (before birth), perinatally (around the time of birth), or postnatally (after birth).

Prenatal CNS damage may be caused by certain maternal/fetal infections, maternal diseases, problems with the placenta or umbilical cord, or maternal use of harmful substances such as alcohol or certain drugs. Most congenital brain malformations, however, have no discernible cause and are likely due to chance maldevelopment of a very complex organ. Perinatal asphyxia/hypoxia (lack of oxygen to the baby's brain) occurs less frequently than is commonly believed, but does present a risk for CNS damage that can result in hypotonia. The greatest risk for asphyxia/hypoxia is from complicated and/or premature deliveries. Infants who are born healthy may sustain postnatal brain injury if they suffer from breathing difficulties, develop an infection in the lining of the brain (see Meningitis), or suffer some other type of physical trauma or abuse.

While it is less common, hypotonia may develop in an adult. This is again most often the result of CNS trauma or disease, usually affecting the **cerebellum**. The primary function of the cerebellum is control of balance and coordination, including maintaining passive tension/tone of the muscles, such as muscular control required for standing.

A number of different genetic disorders are associated with hypotonia, and may affect the nerves (and by extension the muscles), or the muscles only. Most genetic conditions are generalized (affecting multiple muscle groups) and progressive. Some genetic conditions are hereditary

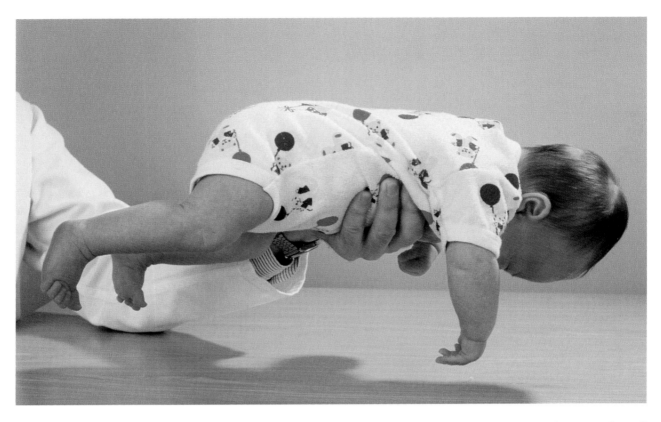

A six-week-old baby girl is held horizontally by the trunk in a test for hypotonia, sometimes called "floppy infant syndrome." *(Saturn Stills / Science Photo Library.)*

(autosomal recessive or X-linked recessive) and some are sporadic (chromosomal disorders). Hereditary conditions would typically imply a 25% recurrence risk for siblings on the affected child, while the chance for another child with the same chromosomal abnormality is usually about 2–3%.

In addition to low muscle tone, infants with hypotonia may also exhibit excessive flexibility of the joints (hypermobility), decreased deep tendon reflexes (e.g., tapping the knee joint produces little or no muscle jerk), and difficulties with sucking and swallowing. Children in whom hypotonia persists often show delays in gross motor skills such as sitting up, crawling, and walking. They may also have difficulties with coordination and exhibit speech delays. In some cases, symptoms may persist into adulthood. Hypotonia itself is not associated with decreased intellectual development, but the underlying cause may pose significant risks for developmental delay and **mental retardation**.

Diagnosis

Diagnosis of the cause of hypotonia may involve a number of different medical methods, procedures, and tests. These include:

- A complete prenatal (before birth) and perinatal (around the time of birth) history. Along with this a complete family medical history should be obtained.

- A physical examination to determine the degree of hypotonia and the muscles affected

- An electromyelograph (EMG), measures muscle response to electrical stimulation

- A nerve conduction velocity (NCV), measures a nerve's ability to transmit electrical impulses to and from the muscle

- Electroencephalogram (EEG), a test that measures the electrical activity in the brain

- A muscle **biopsy** to analyze the microscopic structure of affected muscle

- Biochemical tests on muscle tissue and blood

- Genetic tests to look for possible sporadic (chance occurrence) or hereditary genetic errors affecting the brain, nerves, and/or muscles

- Imaging studies (**CT scan** or **MRI**) of the brain and spinal cord

Determining which tests to use depends on the clinician's judgment of what is most likely to be the underlying cause of the hypotonia. This in turn is based upon the history and physical findings. In some cases, different doctors will order different tests based upon their area of expertise. There is always a possibility that a diagnosis will not be determined. The term for hypotonia without a diagnosis is "idiopathic," which literally means "unknown cause."

Treatment team

Along with normal pediatric care, specialists who may be involved in the care of a child with hypotonia include developmental pediatricians (specialize in child development), neurologists, neonatologists (specialize in the care of newborns), geneticists, occupational therapists, physical therapists, speech therapists, orthopedists, pathologists (conduct and interpret biochemical tests and tissue analysis), and specialized nursing care. Depending on the cause and progression of hypotonia, treatment and evaluation may be needed throughout life.

Treatment

Unlike the wide array of potential causes of hypotonia, treatment options for low muscle tone are somewhat limited. In very severe cases, treatment may be primarily supportive, such as mechanical assistance with basic life functions like breathing and feeding, physical therapy to prevent muscle atrophy and maintain joint mobility, and measures to try and prevent opportunistic infections such as pneumonia. Treatments to improve neurological status might involve such things as medication for a seizure disorder, medicines or supplements to stabilize a metabolic disorder, or surgery to help relieve the pressure from **hydrocephalus** (increased fluid in the brain). If the neurologic condition is untreatable, physical and occupational therapy may help to improve muscle tone, strength, and coordination.

Recovery and rehabilitation

In all cases, frequent or periodic monitoring of muscle tone and performance, along with neurological status, should be done to determine if the hypotonia is worsening, static, or improving. Effective recovery and rehabilitation can only be achieved if an accurate status of the condition is known. Since muscle weakness often accompanies hypotonia, efforts to improve muscle strength may also improve low muscle tone. Some individuals with persistent symptoms may need assistance with mobility, such as a walker or wheelchair. Occupational and physical therapy can assist individuals in developing alternative methods for accomplishing some everyday tasks they may find difficult. Speech therapy is primarily directed at young children to help them develop language skills early, but can be beneficial at any age if the muscles of the face and throat are hypotonic.

Clinical trials
Prognosis

Determining a prognosis depends on determining a diagnosis for hypotonia. Some genetic conditions are fatal in infancy, while others result in permanent disability and mental retardation. For those few genetic metabolic disorders that are treatable, improvement may be dramatic, or minimal. Outcomes for hypotonia caused by CNS trauma or infection depend on the severity of neurologic damage. Mild trauma obviously has the best chance for improvement and recovery, but even significant neurologic deficits may improve over time.

Most individuals with a nongenetic form of hypotonia will improve to some degree. From a broad perspective, some individuals with hypotonia will respond very little or not at all to any treatment method attempted, while in others the condition will resolve on its own; each case is unique.

Resources
BOOKS

Volpe, Joseph J. *Neurology of the Newborn,* 4th ed. Philadelphia: W. B. Saunders Company, 2001.

Weiner, William J. and Christopher G. Goetz, eds. *Neurology for the Non-Neurologist,* 4th ed. Philadelphia: Lippincott Williams & Wilkins, 1999.

OTHER

The National Institute of Neurological Disorders and Stroke. *NINDS Hypotonia Information Page.* (March 26, 2003). <http://www.ninds.nih.gov/health_and_medical/disorders/hypotonia.htm>.

Thompson, Charlotte E. "Hypotonia, Benign Congenital" *National Organization for Rare Disorders Report.* (2003). <http://www.rarediseases.org>.

ORGANIZATIONS

March of Dimes Birth Defects Foundation. 1275 Mamaroneck Avenue, White Plains, NY 10605. 888-663-4637; Fax: 914-428-8203. <http://www.marchofdimes.com>.

Muscular Dystrophy Association. 3300 East Sunrise Drive, Tucson, AZ 85718-3208. 800-572-1717; Fax: 520-529-5300. <http://www.mdausa.org/>.

National Institute of Child Health and Human Development Clearinghouse. PO Box 3006, Rockville, MD 20847. 800-370-2943. <http://www.nichd.nih.gov>.

National Organization for Rare Disorders (NORD) . P.O. Box 1968, 55 Kenosia Avenue, Danbury, CT 06813-1968. 203-744-0100; Fax: 203-798-2291. <http://www.rarediseases.org>.

Scott J. Polzin, MS, CGC

Hypoxia

Definition

Hypoxia generally refers to a lack of oxygen in any part of the body. In a neurological context, it refers to a reduction of oxygen to the brain despite adequate amounts of blood.

Description

A decrease in oxygen supply to the brain can occur due to choking, strangling, suffocation, head trauma, carbon monoxide poisoning, cardiac arrest, and as a complication of general anesthesia. A failure to deliver oxygen and glucose to the brain causes a cascade of abnormal events. The extent of damage is directly proportional to the severity of the injury. The severity of cerebral ischemia, a low-oxygen state caused by arterial obstruction or lack of blood supply, and the duration of blood-flow loss in the brain determine the extent of brain damage. The neurons can suffer temporary dysfunction, or there may be irreversible damage to nerve cells that are sensitive to minute changes in oxygen levels. Severe damage involving extensive areas can occur (cerebral infarction). Cerebral hypoxia/ischemia can be caused by a broad spectrum of diseases that affect the cardiovascular pumping system or the respiratory system. There are four types of disorders to consider: focal cerebral ischemia, global cerebral ischemia, diffuse cerebral hypoxia, and cerebral infarction.

Focal cerebral ischemia

Focal cerebral ischemia (FCI) is often results from a blood clot in the brain. The blood flow in the affected area is reduced. The reduction could be severe or mild but usually FCI causes irreversible injury to sensitive neurons. The clinical signs and symptoms last approximately 15–30 minutes.

Global cerebral ischemia

Global cerebral ischemia (GCI) is a serious condition caused by ventricular fibrillation or cardiac asystole, which stops all blood flow to the brain. If the GCI lasts more than five to ten minutes, then it is likely the person will have suffered a loss of consciousness that makes recovery doubtful.

Diffuse cerebral hypoxia

Diffuse cerebral hypoxia (DCH) is limited to conditions that cause mild to moderate hypoxemia, or low arterial-oxygen content due to deficient blood oxygenation. Pure cerebral hypoxia causes cerebral dysfunction but not irreversible brain damage. Pure cerebral hypoxia can

---

occur due to pulmonary disease, altitude sickness, or severe anemia.

Cerebral infarction

Cerebral infarction (CI) is a severe condition caused by a focal vascular occlusion in an area of the brain. This causes an area of destruction resulting from a lack of oxygen delivery.

Pathology of cerebral ischemia

Lack of oxygen causes neurons in the brain to die in several ways. Autolysis can occur, which results from the digestion of nerve tissues by enzymes. Cerebral infarction causes the death of neurons; transient cessation of the **cerebral circulation** for a few minutes causes selective areas of ischemic necrosis. This type of necrosis is especially evident in highly vulnerable neurons that are sensitive to abrupt oxygen deprivation. More prolonged periods of moderate-to-severe hypoxemia or carbon monoxide poisoning can cause a loss of the outer sheath of neurons.

Molecular mechanisms of cerebral hypoxia

In cases of severe ischemia to brain tissue, the tissue loses structural integrity within a few seconds or a few minutes. Soon after there is an abnormal exchange of ions in neurons through a process called depolarization; this is characterized by an influx of sodium and calcium ions inside the neuron, and a simultaneous efflux of potassium ions outside the neuron.

Cerebral edema

Cerebral edema refers to abnormal increases in water content in the brain and occurs with all types of cerebral ischemia and hemorrhagic **stroke**. Increased water retention in the brain causes an increase in intracranial pressure. This pressure causes the brain to be pushed against the skull, resulting in neurologic deterioration and death due to herniation. Cerebral edema and herniation of the brain is the cause of death for approximately 75% of all fatal stroke victims and 33% of fatalities for all ischemic events to the brain.

GALE ENCYCLOPEDIA OF NEUROLOGICAL DISORDERS

Symptoms

Symptoms vary depending on the severity of damage. Symptoms of mild cerebral hypoxia can include poor judgment, memory loss, inattentiveness, and a decrease in motor coordination. In more severe cases, there can be permanent neurologic deficits, coma, **seizures**, or death.

Treatment

Treatment depends on the cause and availability of equipment. Treatment is urgent and includes basic and advanced life-support measures. It is important to maintain breathing, dispense intravenous fluids and medications, and maintain stability with blood products and medications that control blood pressure and seizures. The outlook depends on the extent of cerebral ischemia.

Resources

BOOKS

Goldman, Lee, et al. *Cecil's Textbook of Medicine*, 21st ed. Philadelphia: W. B. Saunders Company, 2000.

ORGANIZATIONS

Brain Injury Association. 8201 Greensboro Drive, Suite 611, McLean, VA 22102. (703) 761-0750 or (800) 444-6443; Fax: (703) 761-0755. FamilyHelpline@biausa.org. <http://www.biausa.org>.

National Rehabilitation Information Center (NARIC). 4200 Forbes Boulevard, Suite 202, Lanham, MD 20706-4829. (301) 562-2400 or (800) 346-2742; Fax: (301) 562-2401. naricinfo@heitechservices.com. <http://www.naric.com>.

Laith Farid Gulli, MD
Robert Ramirez, DO

I

Idiopathic neuropathy

Definition

Idiopathic neuropathy is a disorder that affects the peripheral nerves and has no identifiable primary cause. According to this definition, a third of all neuropathies can be classified as idiopathic neuropathies.

Description

The nervous system is divided into two parts: the **central nervous system** (CNS) and the **peripheral nervous system** (PNS). The brain and spinal cord compose the CNS, and the nerves that lead to or branch off the CNS compose the PNS.

Peripheral neuropathies encompass a wide range of disorders in which peripheral nerves are damaged. It may also be referred to as peripheral neuritis (inflammation of peripheral nerves), or if many nerves are involved, the terms polyneuropathy or polyneuritis may be used.

Some of the causes of peripheral neuropathies are common, such as diabetes, and others are extremely rare, such as acrylamide poisoning and certain inherited disorders. Sometimes peripheral neuropathies seem to happen for no particular reason. In such cases, they are called idiopathic, meaning of unknown cause. Idiopathic neuropathies can be classified as idiopathic mononeuropathies and polyneuropathies. An idiopathic mononeuropathy, or **radiculopathy**, refers to the involvement of a single nerve or nerve root, respectively. A polyneuropathy usually refers to the diffuse involvement of peripheral nerves.

Clinical manifestations depend on the type and distribution of the affected nerve population, the degree to which they are damaged, and the course of the disease. For example, if a motor nerve is damaged, the neuropathy manifests as weakness and muscle atrophy, whereas if the damage involves sensory nerves, it may cause loss of sensation, **pain**, and sensory **ataxia**.

Demographics

Idiopathic peripheral neuropathies occur typically in middle-aged and elderly individuals and affect two million people in the United States. However, epidemiological studies are scarce. Available studies suggest that 2.4–8% of all adults may have some form of neuropathy. The most common cause is diabetes, which accounts for approximately one-third of all neuropathies; the remaining two-thirds are idiopathic and of all other known causes.

Causes and symptoms

There are no known causes for idiopathic neuropathies, and therefore they are considered primary diseases. If a cause is detected, then the neuropathy is secondary to that, and not idiopathic.

Nonetheless, there are many different peripheral neuropathies, among them the idiopathic type, which demonstrates the functional diversity of PNS activities. Symptoms may involve sensory, motor, or autonomic functions. Symptoms are classified based on the affected nerve type and the duration of disease development. Acute development refers to symptoms that have appeared within days, and subacute refers to those that have evolved over a number of weeks. Early chronic symptoms are those that take months to a few years to develop, and late chronic are the ones that have been present for several years.

Most times, the first symptoms include numbness, tingling and pain, unsteadiness when standing or walking, muscle weakness (including weak ankles), or cramps and faintness. Depending on the affected group of nerves, secondary symptoms may vary from loss of vibratory sensation at the toes to loss of temperature perception to muscle atrophy.

Diagnosis

Several tests are necessary in order to eliminate all the possible primary causes of the disease, after which idiopathic neuropathy may be defined as a diagnosis; hence it

Key Terms

Electromyography A test that detects electric activity in muscle that is used to determine nerve or muscle damage.

Idiopathic A disease or condition of unknown cause or origin.

Neuropathy A disease or condition of the nervous system or a nerve.

Paresthesia Abnormal numbness or tingling sensation, whether spontaneous or evoked.

is a diagnosis of exclusion. The patient's history plays a major role in the diagnosis and has to include all symptoms, date of onset, duration, extension of affected area, and amount of discomfort and pain. Specific details about tingling, numbness, weakness, or other symptoms are also very important.

During the neurological evaluation, a physical examination will test for loss of vibratory sensation, ankle jerks, and other reflexes. Sensations in the feet and hands will be evaluated. The purpose of these tests is to assess the neurological function, including muscle strength, autonomic nerve function, and the ability to feel different sensations.

An **electromyography** may be performed to measure the electrical activity of muscles and nerves. Through this measurement, the physician is able to detect the presence of nerve damage, the possible cause of the damage, and if damaged nerves are responding to treatment. If necessary, other tests can be used, such as a nerve **biopsy**, a lumbar puncture (spinal fluid analysis), and **magnetic resonance imaging (MRI)**, which creates images of the body and its organs that may be used in the confirmation or exclusion of disorders with similar symptoms.

Blood tests are commonly employed to check for vitamin deficiencies, toxic elements, and evidences of abnormal immune responses. The quantitative sensory test (QST) is a method used to assess damage to small nerve endings (temperature changes) and large nerve endings (vibration changes). Autonomic tests measure how autonomic nerves respond to stimulation. Data collected will indicate if the autonomic nervous system is functioning adequately, or if nerve damage is present. The quantitative sudomotor axon reflex test (QSART) is used to assess small nerve fibers linked to sweat glands. QSART is used to diagnose painful, small fiber neuropathies when nerve conduction test results are normal.

Treatment

Treatment for idiopathic neuropathies is mostly symptomatic, including pain therapy for paresthesias, physical and occupational therapy to help improve mobility and function, supportive measures to maintain blood pressure, and bowel and bladder function if the autonomic system is involved.

Treatment options for reducing pain include medication, injection therapy, and physical therapy. Surgery may be needed to treat some causes of neuropathy (e.g., **carpal tunnel syndrome**, radiculopathy).

Because analgesics (aspirin, ibuprofen) are usually ineffective against pain caused by neuropathy, treatment often involves medications that target nerve cells. Antidepressants such as **gabapentin** and amitriptyline are usually the first medications prescribed. Side effects of these drugs include drowsiness, **dizziness**, low blood pressure, and **fatigue**. Other medications include **anticonvulsants** (**carbamazepine** and **lamotrigine**), local anesthetics (lidocaine), and antiarrhythmics (mexiletine). Anticonvulsants may cause low white blood cell counts, nausea, vomiting, and dizziness. Side effects of lidocaine and mexiletine include nervousness, lightheadedness, drowsiness, and double vision.

Topical treatment with capsaicin cream may be prescribed for patients with focal neuropathy. Capsaicin causes stinging upon application and is often combined with a local anesthetic to reduce this side effect.

Injection therapy involves injecting a nerve block (lidocaine) into the area surrounding affected nerves, preventing the nerve from carrying impulses to the brain and temporarily reducing symptoms. Injection therapy is often used with other treatments such as medication and physical therapy.

Discontinuing medication or exposure to toxic substances may eliminate neuropathy caused by drugs or toxins. Vitamin supplements may be used to treat nutritional neuropathy. Physical therapy, including **exercise**, massage, and heat, and **acupuncture** (insertion of fine needles into specific points on the body) may be used to treat symptoms.

Treatment for the causes of neuropathy include antibiotics or antiviral agents for infectious neuropathies, immunomodulating agents for immune-mediated neuropathies, improved glycemic control for diabetic neuropathies, and surgery for compressive neuropathies.

Over-the-counter pain relievers can help treat mild-to-moderate pain associated with **peripheral neuropathy**. There are two main types of over-the-counter pain relievers: acetaminophen and nonsteroidal anti-inflammatory drugs (NSAIDs). Acetaminophen is used to treat mild-to-moderate pain and reduce fever, but it is not very effective at reducing inflammation. Acetaminophen provides relief from pain by increasing the pain threshold. Nonsteroidal anti-inflammatory drugs (NSAIDs) reduce pain, swelling, stiffness, and inflammation. Two drugs in this category, ibuprofen and naproxen, also reduce fever. When these drugs are taken regularly, they build up in the blood to levels that fight pain caused by inflammation and swelling, and also provide general pain relief.

Support groups often help patients cope with feelings of isolation and frustration and improve their quality of life.

Clinical trials

As of 2004, there were no **clinical trials** for idiopathic neuropathies; however, there are several that aim at other types of neuropathies, such as the diabetic neuropathy.

Prognosis

Prognosis and complications depend on the type and severity of the neuropathy. Idiopathic neuropathies range from a reversible problem to a potentially fatal complication. In the best-case scenario, a damaged nerve regenerates. Nerve cells cannot be replaced if they are killed, but they are capable of recovering from damage. The extent of recovery is tied to the extent of the damage, to the patient's age, and to the general health status. Recovery can take weeks to years due to the slow neuronal regrowth rate. Full recovery may not be achieved in some cases.

Special concerns

Complementary and alternative therapies can help manage pain caused by neuropathies. These are noninvasive, drug-free treatments that support natural body healing. They may be used alone or combined with other medications and treatments. Some alternative therapies are biofeedback, acupuncture, and relaxation techniques.

Resources
PERIODICALS
Donofrio, P. D. "Immunotherapy of Idiopathic Inflammatory Neuropathies." *Muscle Nerve* 28 (2003): 273–292.

Lacomis, D. "Small-Fiber Neuropathy." *Muscle Nerve* 26 (2002): 173–188.

Low, P. A., S. Vernino, and G. Suarez. "Autonomic Dysfunction in Peripheral Nerve Disease." *Muscle Nerve* 27 (2003): 646–661.

Kelkar, P., W. R. Mcdermott, and G. J. Parry. "Sensory-Predominant, Painful, Idiopathic Neuropathy: Inflammatory Changes in Sural Nerves." *Muscle Nerve* 26 (2002): 413–416.

OTHER
Neurology Channel. *Neuropathy.* January 4, 2004 (April 4, 2004). <http://www.neurologychannel.com/neuropathy>.

The Jack Miller Center for Peripheral Neuropathy, University of Chicago. *Idiopathic Neuropathy.* January 4, 2004 (April 4, 2004). <http://millercenter.uchicago.edu/learnaboutpn/typesofpn/idiopathic/index.shtml>.

ORGANIZATIONS
The Jack Miller Center for Peripheral Neuropathy, University of Chicago. 5841 South Maryland Avenue, MC2030, Chicago, IL 60637. (773) 702-5546. maa@myositis.org. <http://millercenter.uchicago.edu/index.shtml>.

The Neuropathy Association. 60 East 42nd Street, New York, NY 10165-0999. (212) 692-0662 or (800) 247-6968; Fax: (212) 696-0668. info@neuropathy.org. <http://www.neuropathy.org>.

Bruno Marcos Verbeno
Iuri Drumond Louro

Immune-mediated encephalomyelitis *see* **Acute disseminated encephalomyelitis**

Inclusion body myositis
Definition

Inclusion body myositis (IBM) is an inflammatory muscle disease characterized by progressive muscle weakness and wasting. The common feature of IBM is the abnormal finding of inclusion bodies, or granular material, in muscle fibers. The onset generally occurs gradually over months or years, and persons often experience falling and tripping as the first symptoms. Inclusion body myositis affects both proximal (closest to the center of the body) and distal (farthest from the center of the body) muscles.

Description

Sporadic inclusion body myositis is the most common muscle disease in people aged 50 years and older with an unknown cause. The disease was named in 1971, when scientists noted a case of myositis (muscle inflammation) that showed granular material in muscle fibers called inclusion bodies. The inclusion bodies are now recognized to contain abnormal deposits of amyloid proteins, similar to those found in the brain of patients with Alzheimer's disease. The deposits may represent a protein product left within the muscle fibers as they degenerate.

The onset of IBM is insidious, with symptoms often having been present for more than five years before diagnosis. The course of the disease is progressive over months or years, leading to severe disability. IBM may appear identical to another inflammatory myositis called **polymyositis**, although differences are clear in more than half of cases.

Weakness and impairment of muscle function are the hallmarks of IBM, and weakness distribution is variable, with both proximal (closest to the center of the body) and distal (farthest from the center of the body) muscles affected. Diminished deep-tendon reflexes and wasting (atrophy) of the involved musculature occur. Thus, loss of finger dexterity and grip strength may be present, while falling and tripping appear as the first signs. Patients often suffer from **fatigue** and reduced tolerance to exertion, and consequently become out of breath easily.

Demographics

There are no data currently available for the incidence of IBM internationally, although it has been reported in Europe and Asia. IBM is thought to account for approximately 15–20% of all cases of inflammatory myositis in the United States. Mortality rate (rate of deaths) is difficult to assess, as most people with IBM are older and may die of other coexisting medical problems. There is no race prevalence, but it is uncommon among African Americans. The male/female ratio is 3:1 and most affected individuals are 50 years or older. Nevertheless, IBM does not seem to affect life expectancy.

Causes and symptoms

The causes of IBM remain unknown and it is thought to be a multifactorial disease. Aging factors may play an important role as pathogenic (disease-causing) components. Research has been made to establish whether IBM might be influenced by environmental factors. Thus, inflammation may be a secondary component occurring in response to foreign proteins called antigens, such as viral proteins or altered muscle proteins, and perhaps induces an autoimmune response (a reaction of the organism against itself).

A possibility that excessive accumulation of certain proteins within muscle fibers can induce inflammation is supported by the findings in transgenic mice studies in which mice were modified to express these human proteins. The results have shown that when synthesizing large amounts of the protein in the muscles, mice developed an age-related motor deficit with muscle inflammation. Also, aging muscle fiber was shown to promote accumulation of abnormal proteins, suggesting an aging-based degenerative process. It has been shown that muscle can secrete this protein and thus, it might cause inflammation by stimulating the immune system to react against the affected muscle.

Key Terms

Autoimmune   An immune response by the body against its own tissues or cells.

Inclusion bodies   Small intracellular bodies found within another intracellular body, characteristic of certain diseases.

Myositis   Inflammation of a muscle.

The stimulus for excessive amyloid production is unknown, and whether this precedes inflammation, or vice-versa, remains to be determined.

Genetic causes of IBM have also been proposed, and studies focused on human leukocyte antigen genes that encode for proteins that influence immune response. They were found related to the development of IBM, but their role is not clear.

As an acquired process, weakness or impairment of muscle function in the area(s) affected is the primary symptom of IBM. The distribution of weakness is variable, but most muscles are affected, including those in the neck, hip, quadriceps, back, shoulder, wrist, and finger. Many people with IBM notice shrinking, or atrophy, in the arms and thighs as the muscles become weaker. As thighs are affected by atrophy, sudden falls may occur.

Lower leg weakness can cause difficulty lifting up the foot, which can lead to tripping. Difficult swallowing, or dysphagia, is a common problem in up to 40% of persons with IBM, and choking may become a problem when ingesting some types of food or liquids. Weakness of facial muscles is sometimes seen. Fatigue and reduced tolerance to exertion are common, and cardiac disease is also present in those with IBM, although its relation to IBM has not been demonstrated. The disease itself does not cause **pain**; however, weakened muscles can predispose to injuries affecting bones, joints and soft tissues. Elderly patients normally die of other clinical problems rather than of IBM, and most suffer some degree of disability as disease progresses.

Diagnosis

The IBM diagnosis is carried out according to clinical features and laboratory studies. The illness lasts longer than six months and the age of onset is greater than 30 years old. People with IBM have considerable quadriceps and wrist and finger flexor weakness. Blood tests show high levels of creatine kinase, a muscle enzyme released by damaged muscle. **Electromyography** (EMG) can be used to detect the electrical impulses of muscle contraction, which exhibit a different pattern in IBM patients. Although useful, EMG cannot be taken as a definite diagnosis.

As IBM muscles are damaged, muscle **biopsy** is the definitive test. In a muscle biopsy, a small sample of the muscle is taken under local anesthesia. Laboratory analysis can identify the inclusion bodies within muscle fibers and the invasion of the damaged tissue by immune cells featuring the inflammation with muscle destruction. This appearance will allow the pathologist and clinician to confirm the diagnosis of IBM. None of the other clinical or laboratory features are mandatory if muscle biopsy features are diagnostic. Muscle biopsy is also important for the exclusion of other neuromuscular diseases.

It has been suggested that **magnetic resonance imaging (MRI)** may be useful detecting active myositis and recognizing selective patterns of muscle involvement in IBM. **MRI** is also helpful in selecting an appropriate biopsy site. The results of such studies are also useful to guide therapeutic decisions when a biopsy is not possible or the biopsy findings are inconclusive.

Because of the imprecise nature of muscle weakness in IBM, a diagnosis is sometimes delayed for years after the onset of weakness. In some patients, the initial biopsy may not disclose the diagnosis, and a second biopsy may be necessary.

Treatment team

A **neurologist** or rheumatologist is the primary consultant for IBM treatment, along with allied health care areas including but not limited to physical therapists and otolaryngologists (ear, larynx, and upper respiratory tract specialists).

Treatment

Currently, no treatment has been shown to be effective against the different forms of IBM. Some moderate success has been obtained with the drug therapy combination of corticosteroids and methotrexate or human intravenous immunoglobulins. New therapeutic protocols are currently being tested. Physical therapy, occupational therapy, and ergotherapy (treatment of disease by muscular **exercise**) are commonly prescribed.

Recovery and rehabilitation

In most cases of IBM, there is continued deterioration in spite of the treatment reduction of muscle inflammation and immune cells invasion of muscle tissue. Because of the slow progression, any treatment trial should last for at least six months (possibly 12–18 months) to evaluate benefits. Physical therapy and occupational therapy may help patients as disability increases.

Clinical trials

No treatment has shown to be effective against IBM; however, new therapies are currently being tested. The National Institute of Neurological Disorders and Stroke (NINDS) is sponsoring a study entitled "Immune Abnormalities in Sporadic Inclusion Body Myositis." This is an investigative study intended to better define the pathogenesis of IBM. The National Institute of Arthritis and Musculoskeletal and Skin Diseases (NIAMS) is recruiting patients to a study, "Study and Treatment of Inflammatory Muscle Diseases," which intends to obtain useful material for immunological studies and to sponsor standard therapies for patients. It is likely that in the future more therapeutic trials of drugs in IBM will be organized.

Prognosis

IBM generally worsens progressively and slowly. Some observations of stabilizations and remissions, spontaneous or under treatment, have been reported but are usually only temporary.

Special concerns

Exercise is generally helpful by getting the most out of diseased muscles. Falls and injuries, however, can cause substantial disability. Patients, therefore, have the difficult task of undertaking regular exercise within their capability, but avoiding injury through accident. Because weakened muscles cannot carry an excessive load, keeping to an ideal weight is helpful. A well-balanced diet is also helpful. Patients with severe inflammation of the muscles may need extra protein to balance their loss.

Resources

BOOKS

Askanas, Valerie, Georges Serratrice, and W. Engel. *Inclusion Body Myositis and Myopathies.* New York: Cambridge University Press, 1998.

Parker, James N., and Philip M. Parker. *The Official Patient's Sourcebook on Inclusion Body Myositis.* San Diego: Icon Group International, 2002.

PERIODICALS

Mastaglia, F. L., M. J. Garllep, B. A. Phillips, and P. J. Zilko. "Inflammatory Myopathies: Clinical, Diagnostic and Therapeutic Aspects." *Muscle & Nerve* (April 2003): 407–425.

OTHER

"Inclusion Body Myositis." *The Myositis Association.* March 4, 2004 (April 27, 2004). <http://myositis.org>.

"NINDS Inclusion Body Myositis Information Page." *National Institute of Neurological Disorders and Stroke.* March 4, 2004 (April 27, 2004). <http://www.ninds.nih.gov/health_and_medical/disorders/inclusion_doc.htm>.

ORGANIZATIONS

Myositis Association of America. 755 Cantrell Ave., Suite C, Harrisonburg, VA 22801. (540) 433-7686; Fax: (540) 432-0206. maa@myositis.org. <http://www.myositis.org>.

Marcos do Carmo Oyama
Iuri Drumond Louro, MD, PhD

Incontinentia pigmenti

Definition

Incontinentia pigmenti is a rare genetic disease resulting in a neurocutaneous disorder. Neurocutaneous means that the disorder affects the nervous system and that clinical abnormalities can involve the skin, hair, and teeth of affected individuals.

Description

Incontinentia pigmenti patients develop discolored, abnormally pigmented skin that is distributed randomly and asymmetrically. Occasionally, persons with incontinentia pigmenti experience cognitive delays (including **mental retardation**), but most have normal intelligence. Muscle weakness in one or both sides of the body is also characteristic of the disorder. Incontinentia pigmenti is also known as Bloch-Sulzberger syndrome, as well as incontinentia pigmenti, type 2.

Demographics

Incontinentia pigmenti is considered rare, with only about 1,000 affected individuals reported in medical literature. The gene that is defective in this disease is located on the X chromosome and is inherited as a dominant disorder, meaning that each child of an affected mother has a 50% risk of inheriting the faulty gene and the disorder. Most male fetuses affected with incontinentia pigmenti die before birth; more females are affected with the disorder.

Causes and symptoms

Incontinentia pigmenti results in defects in the skin, nails, hair, and teeth. The disorder is caused by mutations in the IKBKG gene, located on the X chromosome. This gene encodes a protein that is important during human development. Approximately 80% of affected individuals have mutations in this gene. Cases can be caused by inherited mutations or spontaneous mutation that occur randomly in families; therefore, there is an absence of a family history.

Defects in the skin usually develop at birth in four distinct stages. The first stage usually occurs before four months old when the blisters appear in the skin. The second stage involves a wart-like rash that eventually turns into the third stage, in which regions of swirling, darkened pigmentation (skin color) appear after six month of age (and into adulthood). The last stage is characterized by linear hypopigmentation, or areas of the body that are less darkly pigmented.

Neurological problems associated with incontinentia pigmenti occur in about 25% of cases and include cerebral atrophy (deterioration and loss of brain cells), leading to poor muscle control and weakness. Mental retardation and **seizures** are also similarly present.

Other symptoms include defects in the teeth, with too few or too many present. The finger and toenails can often be brittle or pitted, often resembling fungal infections. Patients often have alopecia (hair loss) that occurs on the scalp or body trunk and extremities. Hair can appear patchy and hair loss can occur in areas that blistered during the first stage of the disease. Some patients have been reported to have defects in blood flow in the retina of the eye, predisposing them to retinal detachment during childhood.

Diagnosis

Diagnosis is achieved first by a clinical diagnosis from a clinical geneticist, followed by molecular genetic testing in a CLIA-approved diagnostic laboratory. This test usually supports DNA sequencing of the IKBKG gene. A mutation in this gene can confirm the clinical diagnosis. The clinical diagnosis requires the presence of involved skin that displays any or all the following symptoms, including blisters anywhere on the body except the face, usually before four months of age, hyperpigmentation (increased areas of pigment) occurring on the trunk of the body that fades during adolescence, and/or hairless streaks or patches that occur after adolescence.

Treatment team

The treatment team consists of a **neurologist**, clinical geneticist, genetic counselor, speech pathologist, ophthalmologist, and a dermatologist. A specialist that deals with **learning disorders** or developmentally delayed children may be necessary in certain cases.

Treatment

As there is no cure for incontinentia pigmenti, treatment is based on symptoms. The risk of infection from blisters is a consideration, and topical medications can often be used to lessen the associated **pain**. Corrective dentistry might be necessary to help with eating and talking.

Key Terms

Cognitive delay Impairment or slowing of the mental processes of thinking and acquiring knowledge.

Dominant disorder A disorder resulting from an inheritance pattern where one parent has a single, faulty dominant gene, and has a 50% chance of passing on that faulty gene to offspring with each pregnancy.

Hyperpigmentation An excess of melanin, leading to abnormal areas of increased dark skin color.

Hypopigmentation A deficiency of melanin, leading to abnormal areas of lighter skin color.

Neurocutaneous Conditions involving unique manifestations of the skin, hair, teeth, and nervous system, usually with familial tendencies.

Recovery and rehabilitation

There is no cure for incontinentia pigmenti. A speech pathologist and a nutritionist can often help with rehabilitation to address problems associated with speech difficulties and difficulties eating.

Clinical trials

As of mid-2004, there were no ongoing **clinical trials** specific for the study or treatment of incontinentia pigmenti.

Prognosis

The skin abnormalities can improve with age and in some instances disappear completely. The prognosis for neurological abnormalities depends on each case, but is often permanent and significant. Life expectancy, however, is considered normal.

Special concerns

Genetic counseling is important in cases in which there is a family history of incontinentia pigmenti, or in which there is a clinical diagnosis.

Resources

BOOKS

Staff. *The Official Parent's Sourcebook on Incontinentia Pigmenti: A Revised and Updated Directory for the Internet Age.* San Diego: Icon Group International, 2002.

OTHER

"Incontinentia Pigmenti." *Incontinentia Pigmenti International Foundation (IPIF).* April 23, 2004 (June 2, 2004). <http://imgen.bcm.tmc.edu/IPIF/nipfchar.htm#Top%20of%20page>.

"NINDS Incontinentia Pigmenti Information Page." *National Institute of Neurological Disorders and Stroke.* April 23, 2004 (June 2, 2004). <http://www.ninds.nih.gov/health_and_medical/disorders/inconpig_doc.htm>.

ORGANIZATIONS

Incontinentia Pigmenti International Foundation (IPIF). 30 East 72nd Street, 16th Floor, New York, NY 10021. (212) 452-1231; Fax: (212)452-1406. ipif@ipif.org. <http://www.imgen.bcm.tmc.edu/IPIF>.

Bryan Richard Cobb, PhD

Infantile hypotonia *see* **Hypotonia**

Infantile phytanic acid storage disease *see* **Refsum disease**

Infantile Refsum disease *see* **Refsum disease**

Infantile spasms

Definition

Infantile spasms (IS) are **seizures** seen in **epilepsy** of infancy and early childhood. The typical pattern of an infantile spasm occurs soon after arousal from sleep, and involves a sudden bending forward and stiffening of the body, arms, and legs. Additionally, arching of the torso can also be seen during an infantile spasm. Infantile spasms typically last for one to five seconds and occur in clusters, ranging from two to 100 spasms at a time.

Description

Infantile spasms were first described by the English physician W.J. West (1794–1848) in 1841. West's paper, published in the first volume of the medical journal *Lancet,* was a landmark in the development of pediatric neurology, and the seizure syndrome also became known as West syndrome. West observed the condition in his own infant son, giving a precise and complete description of the symptoms, along with the gradual mental deterioration, and intractability of the syndrome. Other neurological disorders, such as **cerebral palsy**, may be seen in almost half of infants with infantile spasms.

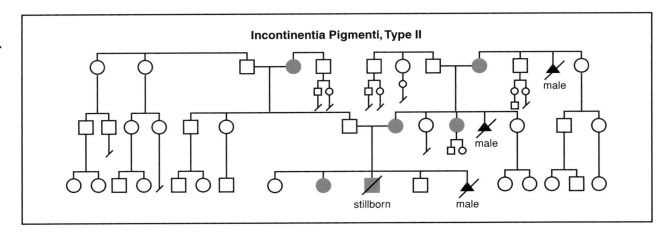

Incontinentia Pigmenti, Type II

male

male

stillborn   male

See Symbol Guide for Pedigree Charts. *(Gale Group.)*

Infantile spasms may have variable features, but have been categorized primarily into three subtypes based on manifestations of posture and patterns of muscle involvement during the seizure. Flexor spasms involve flexion of the neck, trunk, and extremities. Extensor spasms consist of extension of the neck, trunk, and extremities. Mixed flexor-extensor spasms involve combinations of the above.

In many patients, spasms exhibit characteristic patterns involving time. Fifty to eighty percent of the epileptic spasms occur in clusters of two to more than 100 seizures. Patients may have dozens of clusters and several hundred spasms per day, but individual variability in seizure frequency is often large. Although spasms rarely occur during sleep, clusters of spasms are frequently activated after awakening from sleep. Spasms are occasionally triggered by loud noises with associated arousal from drowsiness and sleep, but are generally not sensitive to stimulation by human voices.

Demographics

In the United States, infantile spasms constitute 2% of childhood epilepsies, and 25% of epilepsies with onset in the first year of life. The rate of IS is 1.6–5.0 cases per 10,000 live births. As many as 5% of infants with this condition eventually die from complications of the seizures. Although males are affected slightly more often than females, no significant gender difference is noted.

Causes and Symptoms

The number of neurological diseases that can result in infantile spasms is very large, but some of the major categories include intrauterine injury and infection, disorders caused by lack of blood flow to the fetal brain, developmental malformations of the cerebral cortex, metabolic

disorders, other genetic or chromosomal defects, meningitis, and tumors. These seizures are assumed to reflect abnormal interactions between the cortex and brainstem structures. The frequent onset of the spasms in infancy suggests that an immature **central nervous system** may be important in the formation of infantile spasm syndrome. One theory states that the effect of different stressors in the immature brain produces an abnormal excessive secretion of corticotropin-releasing hormone, which causes spasms.

In 90% of children with the condition, infantile spasms occur in the first year of life, typically between three to six months of age. Often, in the beginning, the attacks are brief, infrequent and not typical, so it is quite common for the diagnosis to be delayed. Frequently, because of the pattern of attacks and the cry that a child gives during or after an attack, they are initially thought to be due to colic, or gastric distress.

The typical pattern is of a sudden flexion (bending forward) in a tonic (stiffening) fashion of the body, arms, and legs. Sometimes, however, the episodes are of the extensor type (arching). Usually, they are symmetrical, but sometimes one side is affected more than the other.

Typically, each episode lasts a few seconds, followed by a pause of a few seconds, and a further spasm. While single spasms may occur, infantile spasms usually occur in sets of several spasms in a row. It is common for babies with infantile spasms to become irritable and for their development to slow down or even regress until the spasms are controlled.

Diagnosis

Information about the child's seizures and about the pregnancy, birth, and progress since birth, will help the physician in making the diagnosis. The diagnosis of infantile spasms is made by a combination of the typical features, along with a characteristic electroencephalogram (EEG), which shows a very disorganized pattern termed hypsarrhythmia.

Most children with infantile spasms will need a number of tests, such as blood, urine, and cerebrospinal fluid (fluid which circulates around the brain and spinal cord) sampling, in an attempt to screen for any infection or metabolic abnormality. X-ray studies such as CT scans, ultrasound, or **MRI** will be performed to evaluate the structure of the brain.

Treatment Team

The treatment team usually includes pediatric neurologists, neurosurgeons, nurses specializing in epilepsy care, and dietitians. In addition to conventional therapies, the team provides the latest in diagnostic and therapeutic approaches, including such innovations as the ketogenic diet, diagnostic video telemetry, and epilepsy surgery for intractable seizures. New epilepsy studies focus in investigating promising new drugs and other novel therapies.

Treatment

Due to the poor prognosis of infantile spasms, treatment is usually initiated quickly and aggressively after diagnosis, often at the risk of serious side effects, with the hope of changing the natural history of the disease. Antiepileptic medications are the mainstay of therapy for infants with infantile spasms. Unfortunately, no one medical treatment gives satisfactory relief for all patients. In most open-label or retrospective studies, adrenocorticotrophic hormone ACTH or prednisone induces a reduction or complete cessation of spasms, as well as an

improvement in the EEG, in approximately 50–75% of patients. This effect is usually achieved within a couple weeks. Patients unresponsive to ACTH may respond to prednisone and vice-versa. A large variety of ACTH doses have been used, but there is no evidence that larger doses (150 units/day) are more effective than lower doses (20–30 units/day). While relapses occur in about one-third to one-half of patients, a second course of ACTH is often effective.

Among conventional anti-seizure drugs, valproate and nitrazepam have been shown to be effective as first-line therapy. In addition to medication, there are some potential surgical options for infantile spasms, although they may only be applicable to a small percentage of patients. Although in most patients the precise source of the spasms in the brain cannot be localized, there is a small minority of patients who have secondarily generalized spasms from lesions in the brain that can be surgically removed.

Newer anti-seizure medicines such as Vigabatrin, although not yet approved in the United States, have shown promise in reducing the frequency of infantile spasms by increasing the brain's available amount of GABA, a neurotransmitter that helps transmit information as it bridges the gaps between nerve cells.

Recovery and rehabilitation

Infantile spasms usually cease spontaneously by age five, but are often replaced by seizures of other types. Therefore, emphasis is placed on lifelong seizure prevention rather than recovery. Maintaining control of seizures in infancy can sometimes reduce developmental delays and **mental retardation**, although most infants will already have significant neurological impairment before the onset of symptoms.

Clinical trials

Although as of early 2004, there were no ongoing **clinical trials** for infantile spasms, the National Institutes of Health (NIH) sponsors research related to many seizure disorders. Information on the numerous current clinical trials for the study and treatment of seizure disorders can be found at the NIH website: <http://clinicaltrials.gov/search/term=Seizure+Disorder>.

Prognosis

Infantile spasms usually resolve with or without treatment in the majority of patients, generally by mid-childhood. However, other seizure types arise in 50–70% of patients. Similarly, on long-term follow-up, chronic intractable (unable to respond to treatment) epilepsy is present in approximately 50% of patients with a history of infantile spasms.

Mental retardation occurs in 70–90% of persons with infantile spasms, usually involving severe to profound retardation. Other neurological deficits, such as cerebral palsy, may be seen in about 30–50% of patients. By far, the most important factor in predicting neurological prognosis, including developmental outcome and long-term epilepsy, is the underlying cause of the seizures.

Factors that have been associated with a good prognosis include normal neurological exam and development at onset, absence of other seizure types at onset, older age of onset, short duration of spasms, and early effective treatment of spasms (reported with ACTH).

Special concerns

Once infants begin to have infantile spasms, they often fail to meet new milestones and may even regress, losing mental or physical skills previously learned. When the seizures begin, parents may notice a loss of interest in people and objects in the child's environment. Social interaction may diminish, smiling may cease, sleep may become disrupted, and the child may seem irritable or indifferent to surroundings. A child who had learned to sit may stop sitting or even lose the ability to roll over; a child who had been babbling happily may become silent or fussy.

Resources

BOOKS

Frost, James D., Jr., and Richard A. Hrachovy. *Infantile Spasms: Diagnosis, Management and Prognosis.* New York: Kluwer Academic Publishers, 2003.

PERIODICALS

Shields, W. D. "West's syndrome." *J. Child Neurol* 17 (2002): S76–79.

West, W. J. "On a peculiar form of infantile convulsions." *Lancet* (1840–1841) I: 724–725.

OTHER

National Institute of Neurological Disorders and Stroke. *NINDS Infantile Spasms Information Page.* (April 5, 2004). <http://www.ninds.nih.gov/health_and_medical/disorders/infantilespasms.htm>.

ORGANIZATIONS

Epilepsy Foundation. 4351 Garden City Drive, Landover, MD 20785-7223. (301) 459-3700 or (800) 332-1000. (301) 577-2684. postmaster@efa.org. <http://www.epilepsyfoundation.org>.

National Organization for Rare Disorders (NORD). 55 Kenosia Avenue, Danbury, CT 06813-1968. (203) 744-0100; Fax: (203) 798-2291. orphan@rarediseases.org. <http://www.rarediseases.org>.

Francisco de Paula Careta
Iuri Drumond Louro

Inflammatory myopathy

Definition

Inflammatory **myopathy** is a term that defines a group of muscle diseases involving inflammation and degeneration of skeletal muscle tissues. They are thought to be autoimmune disorders. In inflammatory myopathies, inflammatory cells surround, invade, and destroy normal muscle fibers as though they were defective or foreign to the body. This eventually results in discernible muscle weakness. This muscle weakness is usually symmetrical and develops slowly over weeks to months or even years.

When using the term inflammatory myopathy, one is actually considering three separate disease entities, namely **dermatomyositis** (DM), **polymyositis** (PM), and **inclusion body myositis** (IBM). Although all of these diseases result in muscle weakness, each is unique in its development and treatment.

Description

Inflammatory myopathies include a diverse group of disorders ranging from localized varieties confined to a single muscle or group of muscles, to diffuse forms in which there is widespread involvement of the skeletal muscles.

Inclusion body myositis (IBM) mainly affects individuals over the age of 50. The onset is truly insidious with symptoms often having been present for more than five years before diagnosis. Clinically and histologically, IBM may appear identical to another inflammatory myositis called polymyositis, although differences are clear in more than half the patients.

Weakness in (IBM) may be localized in the extremities, or asymmetric, and it may be accompanied by diminished deep-tendon reflexes. Disease progression is usually slow and steady in some, while it seems to plateau in others, leaving them with fixed weakness and atrophy (muscle wasting) of the involved musculature. In the muscle tissue, a characteristic change in IBM is the presence of intracellular rimmed vacuoles (pockets). The muscle fibers with pockets are now recognized to contain abnormal deposits of amyloid proteins.

Polymyositis usually occurs after the second decade of life and is a subacute myopathy (one that occurs over time) that evolves over weeks or months, and presents with weakness of the arm and leg muscles. PM mimics many other myopathies. It should be viewed as a syndrome of diverse causes that occurs separately or in association with other autoimmune disorders. In PM, muscle fibers are found to be in varying stages of necrosis (tissue death) and regeneration.

Key Terms

Amyloid A waxy, translucent, starch-like protein that is deposited in tissues during the course of certain chronic diseases such as rheumatoid arthritis and Alzheimer's disease.

Autoimmune Pertaining to an immune response by the body against its own tissues or types of cells.

Dermatomyositis (DM) is identified by a characteristic skin rash accompanying or, more commonly, preceding muscle weakness. DM affects children and adults and presents a varying degree of muscle weakness that develops slowly, over weeks to months.

Demographics

In the United States and Canada, IBM accounts for approximately 15–28% of all cases of inflammatory myopathies. IBM most frequently affects men with a male to female ratio of 3:1. No race predilection for IBM is known, but it is uncommon among African-Americans and has been reported in Europe and Asia. Assessing demographic data is difficult due to the fact that IBM patients often exhibit other medical problems.

Polymyositis (PM) is most common among black people and is most prevalent in women, with a male to female ratio of 1:2. In the United States, its incidence is one per 100,000 persons per year. Dermatomyositis (DM) affects mainly white people and is more prevalent in women, with a male to female ratio of 1:2. In the United States, the estimated incidence is 5.5 cases of DM per one million people.

Causes and symptoms

Inclusion body myositis (IBM) is thought to be a sporadic disease, meaning one that is not hereditary. The cause of IBM remains unknown, but is thought to be a form of autoimmune disease, where the immune system responds in a harmful manner to the rest of the body. Very rarely, IBM can be present within families, and it is not known whether this form is inherited or if family members have another susceptibility to whatever causes the sporadic form of the disease.

The trigger mechanism for all inflammatory myopathies remains unknown. Some scientists maintain that a viral illness causes an injury that activates a flawed immune response. Other scientists, noting that cancer sometimes occurs along side some types of inflammatory myopathy, are investigating the relationship between the two diseases. A genetic predisposition may exist for DM, and abnormal activities of certain white blood cells may be involved in the cause of both the skin and the muscle disease.

Weakness of muscle function in the area affected is usually the first symptom of inflammatory myopathy. The distribution of weakness is variable, and involvement of the knee extensor muscle and the wrist and finger flexor muscles are common. **Fatigue** is common, along with reduced tolerance to exertion, difficulty swallowing (dysphagia), and some forms of heart disease.

In polymyositis (PM), weakness and muscle **pain** on both sides of the body at rest or with use are the first signs of the disease. The weakness becomes chronic, lasting for weeks or months. If swallowing muscles are involved, dysphagia may occur. Joint pain and difficulty kneeling, climbing, or descending stairs, raising arms, and arising from a sitting or lying position are also noticeable.

People often present with skin disease as one of the initial manifestations of DM. A characteristic rash preceding or accompanying muscle weakness, or a confluent, purple-red rash with swelling in surrounding tissues appears. Other rashes seen with DM include swelling at the nail beds and a scaly purple eruption over the knuckles. Muscle involvement varies from mild to severe. The muscle wall of the heart or lung tissues may also become inflamed as a consequence of DM. Some cancers have been associated with DM, a finding much more common in adults over 60 years old.

Diagnosis

A muscle **biopsy** provides a definitive diagnosis for inflammatory myopathies. Muscle biopsy is also important for the exclusion of other neuromuscular diseases. Blood levels of creatine kinase, an enzyme present in the brain and skeletal and cardiac muscles, are usually elevated in persons with muscle damage, and are useful in the diagnosis of inflammatory myopathies.

According to The Myositis Association, the main clinical features for diagnosis of inclusion body myositis (IBM) are:

• Duration of illness greater than six months

• Age of onset greater than 30 years old

• Muscle weakness that affects the arms and legs

• At least one of the following: weakness when flexing the fingers, differing degrees of weakness when flexing and extending the wrist, and weakness in the quadriceps muscle of the thigh.

In polymyositis (PM), the presence of inflammation in muscle tissue is hallmark of the disease. The diagnosis of PM is made when a person has continued elevated levels of serum creatine kinase and characteristic findings on muscle biopsy. Polymyositis is difficult to diagnose due to its ability to mimic other chronic diseases.

People with dermatomyositis (DM) often have characteristic rashes that accompany chronic weakness, making the tentative diagnosis easier for the physician and patient. Skin lesions can include red, raised areas on the surface of the joints of the arms and legs, face, or upper body.

Treatment team

A **neurologist** or rheumatologist is the primary consultant for both IBM and PM, with allied health care areas including but not limited to physical therapists and otolaryngology.

Treatment

Currently, no treatment has been shown to be effective against the different forms of IBM. Some moderate success has been obtained with the combination of corticosteroids and methotrexate or human intravenous immunoglobulins (IVIg). New therapeutic protocols are currently being tested.

In PM, however, high-dose corticosteroid therapy constitutes the first-line of treatment, and leads to improvement in more than 70% of persons with PM. Different therapeutic alternatives can be attempted with immunosuppressants, notably azathioprine, methotrexate and intravenous immunoglobulins (IVIg). The same approach is useful for DM.

Recovery and rehabilitation

In most cases of inflammatory myopathies, there is continued deterioration, in spite of any reduction of muscle inflammation that treatments may provide. Because of the slow progression, any medication regimes often continue for at least six months (possibly 12-18 months) to gain the most benefit. Physical therapy and occupational therapy help with walking, limb range of motion and positioning if the person's disability increases.

About 30% of persons with PM achieve complete recovery, with the majority of patients having a persistent deficit in movement and strength.

Clinical trials

The National Institute of Neurological Disorders and Stroke (NINDS) has sponsored a study entitled "Immune Abnormalities in Sporadic Inclusion Body Myositis." This is an investigative study intended to better define the pathogenesis of IBM. The National Institute of Arthritis and Musculoskeletal and Skin Diseases (NIAMS) is examining whether the drug infliximab (Remicade) is safe for treatment of DM and PM. Information about all current **clinical trials** can be found at the U.S government website for clinical trials: http://www.clinicaltrials.org.

Prognosis

IBM generally worsens progressively and slowly. Sometimes the condition stabilizes spontaneously or while the person is under treatment, but periods are usually transient and the inflammation reoccurs.

Before the era of corticosteroids, PM and DM were particularly severe diseases with spontaneous survival rates of less than 40%. Currently, in the absence of an underlying disease such as cancer, PM and DM in adults have a relatively favorable prognosis, with a five-year survival rate of around 90%. For children, the vascular damage of DM can be responsible for severe complications, such as perforations or hemorrhages.

Special concerns

Exercise is generally helpful to retain movement, and helps to get the most out of diseased muscles. Falls and injuries, however, can cause substantial disability for a person with an inflammatory myopathy. It is important, therefore, to maintain regular exercise within a safe capacity and avoid injury. Because weakened muscles cannot carry an excess load, keeping to an ideal weight is also helpful. A well-balanced diet is important and people with severe inflammation of the muscles may need extra protein.

Resources

BOOKS

Kilpatrick, James R., compiler. *Coping with a Myositis Disease.* Birmingham, AL: AKPE, 2000.

PERIODICALS

Mastaglia, F. L., M. J. Garllep, B. A. Phillips, and P. J. Zilko. "Inflammatory myopathies: clinical, diagnostic and therapeutic aspects." *Muscle & Nerve* (April/2003): 407–425.

OTHER

"NINDS Inclusion Body Myositis Information Page." *National Institute of Neurological Disorders and Stroke.* (February 11, 2004). <http://www.ninds.nih.gov/health_and_medical/disorders/inclusion_doc.htm>.

ORGANIZATIONS

Muscular Dystrophy Association. 3300 E. Sunrise Drive, Tucson, AZ 85718,. (800) 572-1717. mda@mdausa.org. <http://www.mdausa.org/index.html>.

Myositis Association of America. 755 Cantrell Ave., Suite C, Harrisonburg, VA 22801. (540) 433-7686; Fax: (540) 432-0206. maa@myositis.org. <http://www.myositis.org>.

Marcos do Carmo Oyama
Iuri Drumond Louro

Interferons

Definition

Interferons are a group of proteins called cytokines produced by white blood cells, fibroblasts, or T-cells as part of an immune response to a viral infection or other immune trigger. The name of the proteins comes from their ability to interfere with the production of new virus particles.

Purpose

Interferons affect the immune system in a number of ways. For example, interferon beta can enhance the activity of lymphocyte cells while simultaneously inhibiting other immune cells from becoming stimulated. Additionally, interferon beta regulates the production of interferon gamma. Interferons can also inhibit viruses from establishing an infection inside human cells. Interferon alfa displays anti-tumor activity.

The exact molecular details of how interferons act is still unclear. They may make surface-exposed antigens of tumors even more capable of stimulating the immune system, which in turn would elicit a greater response from the T-cells of the immune system. Tumor growth may also be slowed or retarded by interferon-mediated damage to the blood cells that supply the tumor with nourishment.

Description

There are three types of interferons: alfa, beta, and gamma. Alfa and beta interferons, which are grouped together as type I interferon, are produced by white blood cells and a type of connective tissue cell called a fibroblast. Gamma interferon (or type II interferon) is manufactured T-cells. Production occurs when the T-cells are activated such as during an infection.

The alfa and beta interferons share some biological activities, but also have activities that are distinct from one another. These similarities and differences reflect the common and different binding of the interferons to various targets (receptors) on the surfaces of human cells.

Alfa interferon is manufactured by Roche Products (trade name Pegasys) and Schering-Plough (Viraferon-Peg). Biogen (Avonex) and Serono (Rebif) both market an interferon-designated beta-1a. Both of the beta-1a interferons are produced in genetically engineered mammals. For example, Rebif is produced in Chinese hamster ovary cells that contain the gene coding for human interferon beta.

An interferon designated as beta-1b enhances the activity of T-cells, while simultaneously reducing the production cytokines that operate in the inflammatory

response to infection and injury. As well, this interferon retards the exposure of antigens on the surface of cells (and so lessens the development of an immune response to the antigens), and retards the appearance of white blood cells (lymphocytes) in the **central nervous system**.

The reduction of the immune response can lessen the damage to nerve cells in diseases such as **multiple sclerosis**. In this disease, the immune system is stimulated to react against the myelin sheath that surrounds the cells, a phenomenon called demyelination. Demyelination produces a malfunction in the transmission of impulses from nerve to nerve and from nerve to muscle.

Infection with the virus that causes hepatitis C is hindered by interferon via the binding to a site on human cells that is also used by the virus. Thus, the virus cannot enter and infect the host cell.

In the late 1980s, a large clinical trial conducted in the United States and Canada evaluated the influence of interferon beta-1b (Betaseron, marketed by Berlex) made in bacteria using genetic engineering technology. Specifically, the bacterium *Escherichia coli* contained a piece of genetic material (plasmid) that contains the gene coding for human beta interferon. The study was double-blind (neither the test participants or the researchers knew which person was receiving the real drug or a placebo). The two-year study demonstrated that those people receiving the interferon had fewer reappearances of the symptoms, and fewer nerves in the brain were damaged.

Betaseron was approved in 1993 by the U.S. Food and Drug Administration for use by people affected with multiple sclerosis. Avonex was approved in 1996 and Rebif in 2002.

Recommended dosage

Interferons are normally injected. They are not taken by mouth as the strong digestive enzymes of the stomach will degrade them.

For use in multiple sclerosis, interferon beta-1a is injected into the muscle (intramuscular injection), and beta-1b is injected just below the skin (subcutaneous injection). The injections are usually given every other day. The recommended dose for beta-1a and 1b is 0.03 mg and 0.25 mg, respectively. Initial doses of beta-1b should be far less (i.e., 0.0625 mg), with a gradual increase in dose over six weeks.

Precautions

Patients who have had **seizures** or who are at risk for a seizure should be closely monitored following the injection of interferon, as should those with heart disorders such as angina, congestive heart failure, or an irregular heartbeat.

It is not known if interferon can be expressed in breast milk. Concerned mothers may opt to cease breast-feeding while receiving interferon therapy.

Side effects

Interferon beta 1-a and 1-b commonly produce flu-like symptoms, including fever, chills, sweating, muscle aches, and tiredness. These side effects tend to diminish with time. Menstrual cycle changes have also been documented in a significant number of women.

Far less commonly, interferon beta 1-a and 1-b can produce suicidal feelings in someone who is already clinically depressed. Death of cells around an injection site (necrosis) can occur, as can swelling and bruising. Allergic reactions are possible. The massive and sometimes fatal allergic reaction termed anaphylaxis occurs rarely. Other side effects include liver and thyroid malfunction, and altered blood chemistry (fewer platelets and red and white blood cells).

Interactions

As of December 2003, drug interaction studies have not been conducted.

Resources

BOOKS

Lotze, M. T., R. M. Dallal, J. M. Kirkwood, and J. C. Flickinger. "Cutaneous Melanoma." In *Principles and Practice of Oncology*, edited by V. T. DeVita, S. A. Rosenberg, and S. Hellmon. Philadelphia: Lippincott, 2001.

PERIODICALS

Aguilar, R. F. "Interferons in Neurology." *Rev Invest Clin* 52, no. 6 (2000): 665–679.

Polman, C. H., and B. M. J. Uitdehaag. "Drug Treatment of Multiple Sclerosis." *BMJ* 321 (2000): 490–494.

OTHER

National Multiple Sclerosis Society. *Interferons.* National Multiple Sclerosis Society Sourcebook. December 28, 2003. (May 22, 2004). <http://www.nationalmssociety.org/%5Csourcebook-Interferons.asp>.

ORGANIZATIONS

National Multiple Sclerosis Society. 733 Third Avenue, New York, NY 10017. (800) 344-4867. <http://www.nationalmssociety.org>.

Brian Douglas Hoyle, PhD

Intestinal lipodystrophy *see* **Whipple's disease**

Intracranial cysts *see* **Arachnoid cysts**

J

Joubert syndrome

Definition

Joubert syndrome is a well-documented but rare autosomal recessive disorder. The syndrome is characterized by partial or complete absence of the cerebellar vermis (the connective tissue between the two brain hemispheres), causing irregular breathing and severe muscle weakness. Other features of the syndrome include jerky eye movements, abnormal balance and walking, and mental handicap. Additionally, there may be minor birth defects of the face, hands, and feet.

Description

Marie Joubert (whose name is given to the condition) gave a detailed description of the syndrome in 1969. She wrote about four siblings (three brothers, one sister) in one family with abnormal breathing, jerky eye movements (nystagmus), poor mental development, and **ataxia** (staggering gait and imbalance). X-ray examination showed that a particular section of the brain, called the cerebellar vermis, was absent or not fully formed. This specific brain defect was confirmed on autopsy in one of these individuals. Her initial report also described a sporadic (non-inherited) patient with similar findings, in addition to polydactyly. Another name for Joubert syndrome is Joubert-Bolthauser syndrome.

Demographics

Joubert syndrome affects both males and females, although more males (ratio of 2:1) have been reported with the condition. The reason why more males have the condition remains unknown.

Joubert syndrome is found worldwide, with reports of individuals of French Canadian, Swedish, German, Swiss, Spanish, Dutch, Italian, Indian, Belgian, Laotian, Moroccan, Algerian, Turkish, Japanese, and Portuguese origin. In all, more than 200 individuals have been described with Joubert syndrome.

Causes and symptoms

Although the underlying genetic cause remains unknown, there have been numerous instances of siblings (brothers and sisters) with Joubert syndrome. The parents were normal. A few families have also been seen where the parents were said to be closely related (i.e., may have shared the same altered gene within the family). For these reasons, Joubert syndrome is classified as an autosomal recessive disorder. Autosomal means that both males and females can have the condition. Recessive means that both parents carry a single copy of the responsible gene. Autosomal recessive disorders occur when a person inherits a particular pair of genes that do not work correctly. The chance that this would happen to children of carrier parents is 25% (one in four) for each pregnancy.

It is known that the **cerebellum** and brain stem begin to form between the sixth and twelfth week of pregnancy. The birth defects seen in Joubert syndrome must occur during this crucial period of development.

The cerebellum is the second largest part of the brain. It is located just below the cerebrum, and is partially covered by it. The cerebellum consists of two hemispheres separated by a central section called the vermis. The cerebellum is connected to the spinal cord through the brain stem.

The cerebellum (and vermis) normally works to monitor and control movement of the limbs, trunk, head, and eyes. Signals are constantly received from the eyes, ears, muscles, joints, and tendons. Using these signals, the cerebellum is able to compare what movement is actually happening in the body with what is intended to happen, then send an appropriate signal back. The effect is to either increase or decrease the function of different muscle groups, making movement both accurate and smooth.

In Joubert syndrome, the cerebellar vermis is either absent or incompletely formed. The brain stem is sometimes quite small. The absence or abnormal function of

KEY TERMS

Apnea An irregular breathing pattern characterized by abnormally long periods of the complete cessation of breathing.

Ataxia A deficiency of muscular coordination, especially when voluntary movements are attempted, such as grasping or walking.

Cerebellum A portion of the brain consisting of two cerebellar hemispheres connected by a narrow vermis. The cerebellum is involved in control of skeletal muscles and plays an important role in the coordination of voluntary muscle movement. It interrelates with other areas of the brain to facilitate a variety of movements, including maintaining proper posture and balance, walking, running, and fine motor skills, such as writing, dressing, and eating.

Iris The colored part of the eye, containing pigment and muscle cells that contract and dilate the pupil.

Nystagmus Involuntary, rhythmic movement of the eye.

Polydactyly The presence of extra fingers or toes.

Retina The light-sensitive layer of tissue in the back of the eye that receives and transmits visual signals to the brain through the optic nerve.

Vermis The central portion of the cerebellum, which divides the two hemispheres. It functions to monitor and control movement of the limbs, trunk, head, and eyes.

these brain tissues causes problems in breathing and vision, and severe delays in development.

One characteristic feature of Joubert syndrome is the pattern of irregular breathing. The individuals's breathing alternates between deep rapid breathing (almost like panting) and periods of severe apnea (loss of breathing). This is usually noticeable at birth. The rate of respiration may increase more than three times that of normal (up to 200 breaths per minute) and the apnea may last up to 90 seconds. The rapid breathing occurs most often when the infant is awake, especially when they are aroused or excited. The apnea happens when the infants are awake or asleep. Such abnormal breathing can cause sudden death or coma, and requires that these infants be under intensive care. For unknown reasons, the breathing tends to improve with age, usually within the first year of life.

Muscle movement of the eye is also affected in Joubert syndrome. It is common for the eyes to have a quick, jerky motion of the pupil, known as nystagmus. The retina (the tissue in the back of the eye that receives and transmits visual signals to the brain) may be abnormal. Some individuals (most often the males) may have a split in the tissue in the iris of the eye. Each of these problems will affect their vision, and eye surgery may not be beneficial.

The **central nervous system** problem affects the larger muscles of the body as well, such as those for the arms and legs. Many of the infants will have severe muscle weakness and delays in development. They reach normal developmental milestones, such as sitting or walking, much later than normal. For example, some may learn to sit without support around 19–20 months of age (normal is six to eight months). Most individuals are not able to take their first steps until age four or older. Their balance and coordination are also affected, which makes walking difficult. Many will have an unsteady gait, and find it difficult to climb stairs or run, even as they get older.

Cognitive (mental) delays are also a part of the syndrome, although this can be variable. Most individuals with Joubert syndrome will have fairly significant learning impairment. Some individuals will have little or no speech. Others are able to learn words, and can talk with the aid of speech therapy. They do tend to have pleasant and sociable personalities, but problems in behavior can occur. These problems most often are in temperament, hyperactivity, and aggressiveness.

Careful examination of the face, especially in infancy, shows a characteristic appearance. They tend to have a large head, and a prominent forehead. The eyebrows look high, and rounded, and the upper eyelids may be droopy (ptosis). The mouth many times remains open, and looks oval shaped in appearance. The tongue may protrude out of the mouth, and rest on the lower lip. The tongue may also quiver slightly. These are all signs of the underlying brain abnormality and muscle weakness. Occasionally, the ears look low-set on the face. As they get older, the features of the face become less noticeable.

Less common features of the syndrome include minor birth defects of the hands and feet. Some individuals with Joubert syndrome have extra fingers on each hand. The extra finger is usually on the pinky finger side (polydactyly). It may or may not include bone, and could just be a skin tag. A few of these patients will also have extra toes on their feet.

Diagnosis

The diagnosis of Joubert syndrome is made on the following features. First, there must be evidence of the cerebellar vermis either being absent or incompletely formed. This can be seen with a **CT scan** or **MRI** of the brain. Second, the physician should recognize that the in-

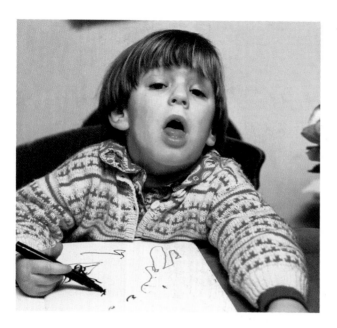

This child is diagnosed with Joubert syndrome. Common symptoms of this disorder include mental retardation, poor coordination, pendular eye movement, and abnormal breathing patterns. *(Photo Researchers, Inc.)*

fant has both muscle weakness and delays in development. In addition, there may be irregular breathing and abnormal eye movements. Having four of these five criteria is enough to make the diagnosis of Joubert syndrome. Most individuals are diagnosed by one to three years of age.

Treatment team

A pediatric **neurologist** usually sees children with Joubert syndrome. Physical, occupational, and speech and language therapists are important members of the treatment team.

Treatment

During the first year of life, many of these infants require a respiratory monitor for the irregular breathing. For the physical and mental delays, it becomes necessary to provide special assistance and anticipatory guidance. Speech, physical, and occupational therapy are needed throughout life.

Prognosis

The unusual pattern of breathing as newborns, especially the episodes of apnea, can lead to sudden death or coma. A number of individuals with Joubert syndrome have died in the first three years of life. For most individuals, the irregular breathing becomes more normal after the first year. However, many continue to have apnea, and require medical care throughout their life. Although the true life span remains unknown, there are some individuals with Joubert syndrome who are in their 30s.

Resources
ORGANIZATIONS

Joubert Syndrome Foundation Corporation. c/o Stephanie Frazer, 384 Devon Drive, Mandeville, LA 70448.

OTHER

Alliance of Genetic Support Groups. <http://www.geneticalliance.org.htm>.

Joubert Syndrome Foundation Corporation. <http://www.joubertfoundation.com>.

Kevin M. Sweet, MS, CGC
Rosalyn Carson-DeWitt, MD

K

Kennedy's disease

Definition

Kennedy's disease is a rare genetic neurodegenerative disorder that affects the motor neurons (cells that are important for normal function of the brain and spinal cord). It is a progressive disorder that leads to increasing severity of motor dysfunction and subsequent deterioration of muscle strength, muscle tone, and motor coordination. It was first described by the American physician William R. Kennedy in 1966.

Description

As Kennedy's disease is a progressive neurodegenerative disorder, affected individuals have physical, mental, and emotional impacts. Physically, the neurological degenerative process results in muscle weakness and eventual muscle wasting that can affect the patient's ability to walk or move. Kennedy's disease is also called spinal bulbar muscular atrophy, or SBMA, because both the spinal and bulbar neurons are affected.

Demographics

Kennedy's Disease is inherited through the X chromosome, and since males only have one X chromosome inherited from their carrier mother, they are usually affected while females are usually carriers. Therefore, sons of carrier mothers will be affected and all her daughters have a 50% chance of being a carrier. Although affected males often have a low sperm count or are infertile, if they are capable of reproducing, all male children will be unaffected and all female children will be unaffected carriers. In some cases, women who are carriers also exhibit clinical symptoms, although they are generally less severe. Kennedy's disease is a rare disease, with only one in 50,000 males affected and no particular pattern among various races or ethnic groups.

Causes and symptoms

Symptoms do not usually develop until between the second and fourth decades of life, although an earlier (and a later) age of onset have been documented. Symptoms initially are mild and include **tremors** while stretching hands, muscle cramps after exertion, and fasciculations (visible muscle twitches). Muscle weakness often develops in the arms and legs, beginning usually in the shoulder or midsection. It is most noticeable in the legs and the arms. Breathing, swallowing, and talking are functions that require bulbar muscles controlled by motor nerves that communicate with the brain. The effects of bulbar muscle dysfunction can be manifested by slurred speech and dysphagia (swallowing difficulties). In later stages, patients often develop aspiration pneumonia (pneumonia caused by food and fluids traveling down the bronchial tubes instead of the trachea due to poor ability to swallow).

Kennedy's disease is caused by a trinucleotide repeat expansion in the androgen receptor gene. This means that three letters in the DNA alphabet (cytosine-adenine-guanine, or CAG) that are normally repeated 10–36 times expand to produce a larger repeat size of approximately a 40–62 repeated trinucleotide sequence. This sequence is unstable and can change from one generation to the next leading to further expansions. The specific mechanism explaining how this trinucleotide repeat expansion (which leads to an increased length in the protein it encodes) causes the disease is unknown.

Diagnosis

Patients with Kennedy's disease usually receive a definitive diagnosis in a clinical molecular genetics laboratory. This requires DNA extraction from blood, followed by testing the gene that causes Kennedy's disease for a mutation. Kennedy's disease can be misdiagnosed as **spinal muscular atrophy** and Lou Gehrig's disease due to similar symptoms displayed.

Key Terms

Dysphagia   Difficulty swallowing.

Fasciculations   Fine muscle tremors.

X-linked disorder   A disorder resulting from a genetic mutation on the X chromosome. Usually, males, having only one X chromosome, are affected with X-linked disorders; females are usually carriers.

Treatment team

The treatment team caring for a patient with Kennedy's disease includes a **neurologist**, physical therapists, occupational therapists, gastroenterologists, and genetic counselors.

Treatment

Although research efforts are underway, currently there is no treatment for Kennedy's disease. Medical treatment is based on lessening the symptoms. Physical therapy is useful in reducing the side affects from the progressive muscle weakness.

Recovery and rehabilitation

In the absence of a cure, patients usually do not recover and the symptoms progress during their lifetime. Lifestyle changes may become necessary, especially late in the disease. These changes, in more severe cases, can include (but are not limited to) help eating, wheelchair access at home, and help with using the restroom and changing clothes.

Prognosis

Kennedy's disease is a neurodegenerative disorder that is slow in its progression. It is likely that individuals will become wheelchair bound during the later stages of the disease. Although individuals will have certain difficulties in motor function and may have special needs, the lifespan of affected individuals is not thought to be shortened.

Special concerns

Genetic counseling is important in this disorder since the presence of one affected offspring means that it is likely the disease gene was inherited and that there is a risk that there will be affected offspring in subsequent generations. The possibility of infertility due to low sperm count should also be discussed during the counseling, especially in cases that develop early. Also, gynecomastia (enlarged breasts) in males due to reduced virilization can also have

psychosocial consideration and need to be addressed. Erectile dysfunction and/or testicular atrophy may also affect males.

Resources

BOOKS

Cooper, D. N., M. Krawczak, and S. E. Antonarakis. "The Nature and Mechanisms of Human Gene Mutation." In *The Metabolic and Molecular Basis of Inherited Disease,* 7th ed. Edited by C. R. Scriver, A. L. Beaudet, W. S. Sly, and D. Valle. NY: McGraw-Hill, 1995.

Icon Group Publications. *The Official Parent's Sourcebook on Spinal Muscular Atrophy: A Revised and Updated Directory for the Internet Age.* San Diego: Icon Group International, 2002.

Panzarino, Connie. *Me in the Mirror.* Seal Press, 1994.

OTHER

"NINDS Kennedy's Disease Information Page." National Institute of Neurological Disorders and Stroke. (April 24, 2004). <http://www.ninds.nih.gov/health_and_medical/disorders/kennedy's.htm>.

"What Is Kennedy Disease?" Kennedy Disease Association. (April 24, 2004). <http://www.kennedysdisease.org/about.html>.

ORGANIZATIONS

National Organization of Rare Disorders. PO Box 8923, New Fairfield, CT 06812-8925. (203) 746-6518 or (800) 999-6673; Fax: (203) 746-6481. orphan@rarediseases.org. <http://www.rarediseases.org>.

Kennedy's Disease Association. PO Box 2050, Simi Valley, CA 93062-2050. (805) 577-9591. tswaite@pacbell.net. <http://www.kennedysdisease.org/about.html>.

Bryan Richard Cobb, PhD

Kinsbourne syndrome *see* **Opsoclonus myoclonus**

Klippel Feil syndrome

Definition

Klippel Feil syndrome is a rare congenital (present at birth) disorder in which there is abnormal fusion of some of the cervical (neck) vertebrae.

Description

People with Klippel Feil syndrome are often identified due to three major characteristics: a short neck, a low hairline, and restricted neck mobility due to the fused cervical vertebrae. Klippel Feil syndrome can occur as a lone defect, or in association with other abnormalities, including scoliosis (curved spine), **spina bifida** (a birth defect involving the spinal column and cord), cleft palate, and a variety of defects involving the ribs, urinary tract, kidneys, heart, muscles, brain, and skeleton. Facial defects and problems with hearing and breathing may also occur in Klippel Feil syndrome.

Klippel Feil syndrome has been organized into three basic types. In type I, all of the cervical and upper thoracic vertebrae are fused together into one block. In type II, one or two pairs of cervical vertebrae are fused together. In type III, there is lower thoracic or lumbar fusion as well as cervical fusion.

Demographics

Although not a lot of data has been collected regarding how often Klippel Feil syndrome occurs, the information available suggests that the incidence of this condition ranges from about one in 42,400 births to about three in 700 births. Boys are slightly more likely than girls to have this condition (1.5:1).

Causes and symptoms

Klippel Feil syndrome is believed to occur during very early fetal development, when the cervical vertebrae do not segment normally. The exact mechanism that causes the defect is unkown.

Although most cases of Klippel Feil syndrome occur spontaneously, there have been a few reports of Klippel Feil syndrome that showed a pattern of inheritance within a family. In some cases, maternal alcoholism and subsequent fetal alcohol syndrome seems to be associated with Klippel Feil syndrome.

Many individuals with Klippel Feil syndrome have no symptoms. Individuals who have more minimal degrees of fusion can live completely normally and partake in all activities. They may never become aware that they have any abnormality at all. Individuals with more severe degrees of fusion will be obviously impaired in terms of their neck mobility. Some individuals will suffer from torticollis or wry neck, a condition in which the neck muscles pull the neck to one side. If the spinal cord is constricted by the abnormal vertebrae, neurological symptoms (weakness, numbness, tingling) may result.

A full 30–40% of all individuals with Klippel Feil syndrome will have significant structural abnormalities of their urinary tract. These often lead to chronic kidney infections (pyelonephritis), and a high risk of kidney failure.

Diagnosis

Diagnosis is usually established through a variety of imaging techniques, such as plain x-ray films of the neck and spine, **CT scan**, or **MRI**. Other diagnostic studies

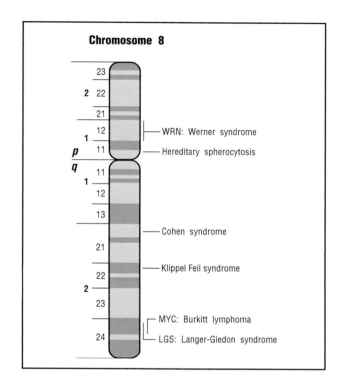

Klippel Feil syndrome, on chromosome 8. *(Gale Group.)*

should be done to uncover associated defects. For example, children diagnosed with Klippel Feil syndrome should have a thorough hearing screening performed, due to the high risk of associated hearing problems. The cardiovascular system and the kidneys and urinary tract may also require evaluation.

Treatment team

The treatment team will depend on the degree of disability brought on by the vertebral defects, and the presence of any associated problems. In more mildly affected individuals, a pediatrician and orthopedic surgeon may collaborate to achieve a diagnosis. In more severely affected individuals, a **neurologist** or neurosurgeon may need to be involved as well. Depending on what other body systems are involved, a cardiologist, nephrologist, urologist, and orofacial surgeon may be consulted. An audiologist can consult about hearing issues. A physical therapist and occupational therapist can be very helpful in helping with issues of mobility and ability to tend to activities of daily living.

Treatment

More mildly affected individuals will require no treatment. Other individuals may need surgery to improve cervical stability, correct scoliosis, and improve any constriction of the spinal cord. Depending on the degree of scoliosis, a brace may be helpful.

Physical therapy can be very helpful in order to improve strength and mobility. Occupational therapy can help more severely restricted individuals learn how to best perform activities of daily living, despite the limitations of their condition.

Prognosis

The prognosis is excellent for very mildly affected people with Klippel Feil syndrome. With careful medical attention, the prognosis can be good for more severely affected individuals as well.

Resources

BOOKS

Thompson, George H. "The Neck." In *Nelson Textbook of Pediatrics*, edited by Richard E. Behrman, et al. Philadelphia: W.B. Saunders Company, 2004.

Maertens, Paul, and Paul Richard Dyken. "Storage Diseases: Neuronal Ceroid-Lipofuscinoses, Lipidoses, Glycogenoses, and Leukodystrophies." In *Textbook of Clinical Neurology*, edited by Christopher G. Goetz. Philadelphia: W.B. Saunders Company, 2003.

Warner, William C. "Pediatric Cervical Spine" In *Campbell's Operative Orthopedics*, edited by S. Terry Canale. St. Louis: Mosby Company, 2003.

WEBSITES

National Institute of Neurological Disorders and Stroke (NINDS). *NINDS Klippel Feil Syndrome Information Page.* May 6, 2003. <http://www.ninds.nih.gov/health_and_medical/disorders/klippel_feil.htm>.

Rosalyn Carson-DeWitt, MD

Krabbe disease

Definition

Krabbe disease is an inherited enzyme deficiency that leads to the loss of myelin, the substance that wraps nerve cells and speeds cell communication. Most affected individuals start to show symptoms before six months of age and have progressive loss of mental and motor function. Death occurs at an average age of 13 months. Other less common forms exist with onset in later childhood or adulthood.

Description

Myelin insulates and protects the nerves in the central and **peripheral nervous system**. It is essential for efficient nerve cell communication (signals) and body functions such as walking, talking, coordination, and thinking. As nerves grow, myelin is constantly being built, broken down, recycled, and rebuilt. Enzymes break down, or metabolize, fats, carbohydrates, and proteins in the body including the components of myelin.

Individuals with Krabbe disease are lacking the enzyme galactosylceramidase (GALC), which metabolizes a myelin fat component called galactosylceramide and its by-product, psychosine. Without GALC, these substances are not metabolized and accumulate in large globoid cells. For this reason, Krabbe disease is also called globoid cell **leukodystrophy**. Accumulation of galactosylceramide and psychosine is toxic and leads to the loss of myelin-producing cells and myelin itself. This results in impaired nerve function and the gradual loss of developmental skills such as walking and talking.

Demographics

Approximately one in every 100,000 infants born in the United States and Europe will develop Krabbe disease. A person with no family history of the condition has a one

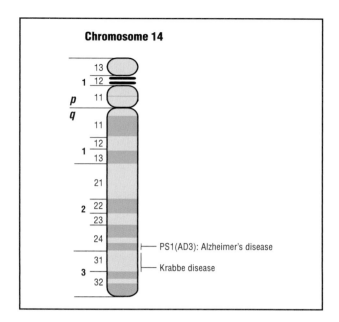

Chromosome 14

PS1(AD3): Alzheimer's disease

Krabbe disease

Krabbe disease, on chromosome 14. *(Gale Group.)*

in 150 chance of being a carrier. Krabbe disease occurs in all countries and ethnic groups but no cases have been reported in the Ashkenazi Jewish population. A Druze community in Northern Israel and two Moslem Arab villages near Jerusalem have an unusually high incidence of Krabbe disease. In these areas, about one person in every six is a carrier.

Causes and symptoms

Krabbe disease is an autosomal recessive disorder. Affected individuals have two nonfunctional copies of the GALC gene. Parents of an affected child are healthy carriers and therefore have one normal GALC gene and one nonfunctional GALC gene. When both parents are carriers, each child has a 25% chance to inherit Krabbe disease, a 50% chance to be a carrier, and a 25% chance to have two normal GALC genes. The risk is the same for males and females. Brothers and sisters of an affected child with Krabbe disease have a 66% chance of being a carrier.

The GALC gene is located on chromosome 14. Over 70 mutations (gene alterations) known to cause Krabbe disease have been identified. One specific GALC gene deletion accounts for 45% of disease-causing mutations in those with European ancestry and 35% of disease-causing mutations in those with Mexican ancestry.

Ninety percent of individuals with Krabbe disease have the infantile type. These infants usually have normal development in the first few months of life. Before six months of age, they become irritable, stiff, and rigid. They

may have trouble eating and may have **seizures**. Development regresses leading to loss of mental and muscle function. They also lose the ability to see and hear. In the end stages, these children usually cannot move, talk, or eat without a feeding tube.

Ten percent of individuals with Krabbe disease have juvenile or adult type. Children with juvenile type begin having symptoms between three and ten years of age. They gradually lose the ability to walk and think. They may also have paralysis and vision loss. Their symptoms usually progress slower than in the infantile type. Adult Krabbe disease has onset at any time after age 10. Symptoms are more general including weakness, difficulty walking, vision loss, and diminished mental abilities.

Diagnosis

There are many tests that can be performed on an individual with symptoms of Krabbe disease. The most specific test is done by measuring the level of GALC enzyme activity in blood cells or skin cells. A person with Krabbe disease has GALC activity levels that are zero to 5% of the normal amount. Individuals with later onset Krabbe disease may have more variable GALC activity levels. This testing is done in specialized laboratories that have experience with this disease.

The fluid of the brain and spinal cord (cerebrospinal fluid) can also be tested to measure the amount of protein. This fluid usually contains very little protein but the protein level is elevated in infantile Krabbe disease. Nerve-conduction velocity tests can be performed to measure the speed at which the nerve cells transmit their signals. Individuals with Krabbe disease will have slowed nerve conduction. Brain imaging studies such as computed tomography (**CT scan**) and **magnetic resonance imaging (MRI)** are used to get pictures from inside the brain. These pictures will show loss of myelin in individuals with Krabbe disease.

DNA testing for GALC mutations is not generally used to make a diagnosis in someone with symptoms but it can be performed after diagnosis. If an affected person has identifiable known mutations, other family members can be offered DNA testing to find out if they are carriers. This is helpful since the GALC enzyme test is not always accurate in identifying healthy carriers of Krabbe disease.

If an unborn baby is at risk to inherit Krabbe disease, prenatal diagnosis is available. Fetal tissue can be obtained through chorionic villus sampling (CVS) or amniocentesis. Cells obtained from either procedure can be used to measure GALC enzyme activity levels. If both parents have identified known GALC gene mutations, DNA testing can also be performed on the fetal cells to determine if the fetus inherited one, two, or no GALC gene mutations.

Key Terms

Globoid cells Large cells containing excess toxic metabolic "waste" of galactosylceramide and psychosine.

Motor function The ability to produce body movement by complex interaction of the brain, nerves, and muscles.

Mutation A permanent change in the genetic material that may alter a trait or characteristic of an individual, or manifest as disease, and can be transmitted to offspring.

Some centers offer preimplantation diagnosis if both parents have known GALC gene mutations. In-vitro fertilization (IVF) is used to create embryos in the laboratory. DNA testing is performed on one or two cells taken from the early embryo. Only embryos that did not inherit Krabbe disease are implanted into the mother's womb. This is an option for parents who want a biological child but do not wish to face the possibility of terminating an affected pregnancy.

Treatment team

The treatment team for a child with Krabbe disease should include a **neurologist**, general surgeon to place certain types of feeding tubes, and a hematologist if bone marrow or stem cell transplants are being considered. Physical and occupational therapists can help plan for daily care of the child and provide exercises to decrease muscle rigidity.

Treatment

Once a child with infantile Krabbe disease starts to show symptoms, there is little effective treatment. Supportive care can be given to keep the child as comfortable as possible and to counteract the rigid muscle tone. Medications can be given to control seizures. When a child can no longer eat normally, feeding tubes can be placed to provide nourishment.

Affected children who are diagnosed before developing symptoms (such as through prenatal diagnosis) can undergo bone marrow transplant or stem cell transplant. The goal of these procedures is to destroy the bone marrow which produces the blood and immune system cells. After the destruction of the bone marrow, cells from a healthy donor are injected. If successful, the healthy cells travel to the bone marrow and reproduce. Some children have received these transplants and had a slowing of their symptom's progression or even improvement of their symptoms.

However, these procedures are not always successful and research is being done in order to reduce complications.

Scientists are also researching **gene therapy** for Krabbe disease. This involves introducing a normal GALC gene into the cells of the affected child. The goal is for the cells to integrate the new GALC gene into its DNA and copy it, producing functional GALC enzyme. This is still in research stages and is not being performed clinically.

Prognosis

Prognosis for infantile and juvenile Krabbe disease is very poor. Individuals with infantile type usually die at an average age of 13 months. Death usually occurs within a year after the child shows symptoms and is diagnosed. Children with juvenile type may survive longer after diagnosis but death usually occurs within a few years. Adult Krabbe disease is more variable and difficult to predict but death usually occurs two to seven years after diagnosis.

Resources
BOOKS

Wenger, D. A., et al. "Krabbe Disease: Genetic Aspects and Progress Toward Therapy." *Molecular Genetics and Metabolism* 70 (2000): 1-9.

ORGANIZATIONS

Hunter's Hope Foundation. PO Box 643, Orchard Park, NY 14127. (877) 984-HOPE. Fax: (716) 667-1212. <http://www.huntershope.org>.

United Leukodystrophy Foundation. 2304 Highland Dr., Sycamore, IL 60178. (815) 895-3211 or (800) 728-5483. Fax: (815) 895-2432. <http://www. ulf.org>.

WEBSITES

Wenger, David A. "Krabbe Disease." *GeneClinics.* <http://www.geneclinics.org/profiles/krabbe/details.html>.

Amie Stanley, MS
Rosalyn Carson-DeWitt, MD

Kugelberg-Welander disease *see* **Spinal muscular atrophy**

Kuru

Definition

Kuru is the name of a progressively disabling and ultimately fatal brain infection caused by a unique protein particle called a prion.

Key Terms

Classic Creutzfeldt-Jakob disease   A rare, progressive neurological disease that is believed to be transmitted via an abnormal protein called a prion.

Fatal familial insomnia   A rare, progressive neurological disease that is believed to be transmitted via an abnormal protein called a prion.

Gerstmann-Sträussler-Scheinker syndrome   A rare, progressive neurological disease that is believed to be transmitted via an abnormal protein called a prion.

New variant Creutzfeldt-Jakob disease   A more newly identified type of Creutzfeldt-Jakob disease that

has been traced to the ingestion of beef from cows infected with bovine spongiform encephalopathy. Known in the popular press as Mad Cow Disease.

Transmissible spongiform encephalopathy   A term that refers to a group of disease, including kuru, Creutzfeldt-Jakob disease, Gerstmann-Sträussler-Scheinker syndrome, fatal familial insomnia, and new variant Creutzfeldt-Jakob disease. These diseases share a common origin as prion diseases, caused by abnormal proteins that accumulate within the brain and destroy brain tissue, leaving spongy holes.

Description

Kuru was first described in a specific tribal group in Papua, New Guinea. The word "kuru" means "to shake or tremble" in this tribal group's language. Individuals in New Guinea are believed to have acquired the infection through a cannibalistic ritual involving the blood and brains of deceased tribal members.

Because infection with kuru may occur years or decades before the advent of actual symptoms of the disease, it belongs to a group of diseases originally known as slow virus infections. Currently, slow virus infections are classed together as transmissible spongiform encephalopathies (TSE). TSEs include kuru, **Creutzfeldt-Jakob disease**, Gerstmann-Sträussler-Scheinker syndrome, and fatal familial insomnia. The TSE new variant called Creutzfeldt-Jakob disease (also known colloquially as "Mad Cow Disease") has received a great deal of public attention. The TSEs, including kuru, involve abnormal clumps of protein that accumulate throughout the brain, destroying brain tissue and leaving spongy holes.

Demographics

Kuru reached epidemic proportions among tribal members in the 1950s. Since the practice of cannibalism was halted, the disease has essentially disappeared. Some sources suggest that as few as zero to 10 cases of kuru are diagnosed each year.

Causes and symptoms

Kuru is caused by an infectious protein particle called a prion, which stands for proteinaceous infectious particle. A prion is similar to a virus, except that it lacks any nucleic acid, which prevents it from reproducing. Prions are abnormal versions of proteins that are found in the membranes of normal cells. These abnormal proteins can be

passed directly to individuals through the ingestion of prion-infected tissue or when open sores on the recipient's skin are exposed to prion-infected tissue. In addition to being transmissible (as are other infectious agents like viruses or bacteria), prions are unique because they can also be acquired through genetic inheritance.

Symptoms of kuru tend to begin in later middle age, years or decades after the prion was actually acquired. Early symptoms include lack of energy, intense **fatigue**, **headache**, weight loss, joint **pain**, difficulty walking, twitchy muscles, personality changes, mood swings, memory problems, and bizarre behavior. As the disease progresses, the individual experiences stiff muscles, involuntary movements, problems talking, hallucinations, increased confusion, blindness, and sometimes **dementia**. Death often occurs within three months to two years of the initial symptoms.

Diagnosis

Diagnosis is arrived at through characteristic abnormalities found on the electroencephalogram (EEG), a test of brain waves and electricity. Seventy-five percent of individuals with kuru will display these specific abnormalities on EEG. **MRI** studies and biopsies (tissue samples) from the brain may also show changes that are characteristic of slow virus infection.

Treatment team

Diagnosis of slow virus infection is usually made by a **neurologist**.

Treatment

There are no available treatments for kuru. It is relentlessly progressive, incurable, and fatal. Supportive care for the patient and his or her family is the only treatment.

Prognosis

Kuru is always fatal.

Resources

BOOKS

Berger, Joseph R., and Avindra Nath. "Slow virus infections." *Cecil Textbook of Medicine*, edited by Thomas E. Andreoli, et al. Philadelphia: W.B. Saunders Company, 2000.

Murray, T. Jock, and William Pryse-Phillips."Infectious diseases of the nervous system." *Noble: Textbook of Primary Care Medicine*, edited by John Noble, et al. St. Louis: W.B. Saunders Company, 2001.

PERIODICALS

Sy, Man-Sun, Pierluigi Gambetti, and Wong Boon-Seng. "Human Prion Diseases" *Medical Clinics of North America* 86 (May 2002) 551–571.

WEBSITES

National Institute of Neurological Disorders and Stroke (NINDS). *Kuru Fact Sheet.* Bethesda, MD: NINDS, 2003.

Rosalyn Carson-DeWitt, MD

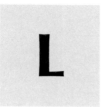

Lambert-Eaton myasthenic syndrome

Definition

Lambert-Eaton myasthenic syndrome is an autoimmune disease that causes muscle weakness and easy fatigability, particularly in the pelvic muscles and thighs.

Description

In order to understand Lambert-Eaton myasthenic syndrome, it's important to have some understanding of the basics of nerve transmission and stimulation of muscle movement. Nerve impulses in the body are electrical and chemical currents that travel down a nerve fiber. When they reach the end of that nerve fiber, they trigger the release of the neurotransmitter chemical acetylcholine. Acetycholine must cross a tiny gap called the synapse in order to stimulate the muscle to contract. The nerves leading to the synapse or synaptic junction are called the presynaptic nerves.

In the case of Lambert-Eaton myasthenic syndrome, the body's immune system accidentally treats specialized areas (called calcium channels) along the presynaptic nerve as if they were foreign. These calcium channels are vital to the presynaptic nerve's ability to release acetylcholine into the synaptic junction. The immune cells attack the calcium channels as they would attack an invader such as a virus or bacteria. When the calcium channels are damaged, the release of acetylcholine into the synapse is compromised, resulting in less acetycholine being available to stimulate the muscle.

Lambert-Eaton myasthenic syndrome has a very strong association with cancer, particularly small-cell lung cancer. The symptoms of Lambert-Eaton myasthenic syndrome often occur prior to diagnosis with lung cancer. In fact, about two-thirds of all people with Lambert-Eaton myasthenic syndrome will be diagnosed with some type of cancer, usually small-cell lung cancer, within two to three years of the onset of their initial symptoms of Lambert-Eaton myasthenic syndrome. Other types of cancer associated with Lambert-Eaton myasthenic syndrome include non-small-cell lung cancer; lymphosarcoma; malignant thymoma; and carcinoma of the breast, stomach, colon, prostate, bladder, kidney, or gallbladder.

Because of the strong connection between Lambert-Eaton myasthenic syndrome and cancer, it is sometimes considered to be a paraneoplastic syndrome (a syndrome in which substances produced by cancer cells prompt abnormalities in the body at a distance from the actual site of the malignancy). In the case of Lambert-Eaton myasthenic syndrome, it is thought that the immune system produces immune cells in response to the presence of early cancer cells. These immune cells cross-react with the calcium channels on nerve cells, resulting in the symptoms of Lambert-Eaton myasthenic syndrome.

Demographics

Lambert-Eaton myasthenic syndrome is very rare, only striking about five people per every one million annually. At any one time, there are thought to be about 400 people in the United States suffering from Lambert-Eaton myasthenic syndrome. Twice as many men than women are affected, and the average age at diagnosis is about 60 years of age. Family history of Lambert-Eaton myasthenic syndrome is a known risk factor for development of the disease, as is a personal history of smoking.

Causes and symptoms

In Lambert-Eaton myasthenic syndrome, the immune system accidentally attacks the calcium channels of the presynaptic nerve cells, preventing normal release of the neurotransmitter acetylcholine into the synaptic junction, and compromising the flow of nervous information between the presynaptic and postsynaptic nerves.

Symptoms of Lambert-Eaton myasthenic syndrome begin with weakness and some achiness and tenderness in

Key Terms

Acetylcholine A neurotransmitter that carries a signal from the nerve fiber to the muscle to direct contraction.

Autoimmune Refers to a disease in which the body's immune system is directed against parts of the body itself, causing damage.

Paraneoplastic syndrome A syndrome in which substances produced by cancer cells prompt abnormalities in the body at a distance from the actual site of the malignancy.

Plasmapheresis A procedure in which harmful cells are removed from the blood plasma.

Presynaptic Before the synapse.

Ptosis Eyelid droop.

Synapse The gap, cleft, or junction between nerve cells or between a nerve cell and the muscle fiber.

the thigh and pelvic muscles. The upper arms may also exhibit some weakness. Due to the weak thigh and upper arm muscles, the patient's walk may have a waddling appearance, and it may be difficult for the patient to lift his or her arms above the head. **Exercise** may initially improve the weakness, but the weakness may become more pronounced as exercise continues. Eyelids may droop (ptosis). Many patients notice uncomfortably dry eyes, mouth, and skin. Patients may develop difficulty chewing, swallowing, and/or speaking, as well as constipation, sudden drops in blood pressure when rising from lying down to sitting or standing, abnormalities of sweating, and erectile problems in men.

Diagnosis

Lambert-Eaton myasthenic syndrome may be diagnosed by demonstrating the presence of specific antibodies in the blood that are directed against aspects of the presynaptic nerve, such as the calcium channels. Studies of nerve conduction and muscle function will reveal a variety of abnormalities. When Lambert-Eaton myasthenic syndrome is diagnosed, a search should also be done for the presence of a previously undiagnosed cancer, especially small-cell lung cancer.

Treatment team

Patients with Lambert-Eaton myasthenic syndrome should be examined and then treated by both a **neurologist** and an appropriate cancer specialist (oncologist).

Treatment

When a cancer is identified, the first concern should be the appropriate treatment of that malignancy. Secondarily, treatment of Lambert-Eaton myasthenic syndrome may include medications to improve transmission of nerve impulses across the synaptic junction (such as pyridostigmine bromide) as well as immunosuppressant agents (such as corticosteroids, azathioprine, cyclosporine, or intravenous immungoglobulin) to decrease the immune system's ability to further damage the presynaptic nerves. A treatment called plasmapheresis may help remove damaging immune cells from the blood.

Prognosis

The prognosis of individuals with Lambert-Eaton myasthenic syndrome varies widely. In fact, the most important element of prognosis involves the prognosis associated with any existing cancer.

Special concerns

Patients who develop Lambert-Eaton myasthenic syndrome should be thoroughly screened for the presence of a previously undetected cancer. If none is found, the patient should undergo regularly scheduled surveillance to monitor for the subsequent development of a malignancy.

Resources

BOOKS

Al-Losi, Muhammad, and Alan Pestronk. "Paraneoplastic Neurologic Syndromes." *Harrison's Principles of Internal Medicine*, edited by Eugene Braunwald, et al. New York: McGraw-Hill Professional, 2001.

Gruenthal, Michael. "Lambert-Eaton Myasthenic Syndrome." *Ferri's Clinical Advisor: Instant Diagnosis and Treatment*, edited by Fred F. Ferri. St. Louis: Mosby, 2004.

Posner, Jerome B. "Nonmetastatic Effects of Cancer: The Nervous System." *Cecil Textbook of Internal Medicine*, edited by Lee Goldman, et al. Philadelphia: W.B. Saunders Company, 2000.

PERIODICALS

Bataller, L. "Paraneoplastic neurologic syndromes. " In *Neurologic Clinics* 21(1)(February 1, 2003): 221–247

WEBSITES

Lambert-Eaton Myasthenic Syndrome Fact Sheet. National Institute of Neurological Disorders and Stroke (NINDS). Bethesda, MD: NINDS, 2003.

Rosalyn Carson-DeWitt, MD

Laminectomy

Definition

Laminectomy is a surgical procedure that entails opening the spinal column to treat **nerve compression** in the spinal cord.

Purpose

Laminectomy may be performed when an abnormality causes spinal nerve root compression that causes leg or arm **pain** that limits activity. Numbness or weakness in hands, arms, legs, or feet, and problems controlling bowel movements or urination are indication for surgical consideration.

Precautions

Before surgery, patients should refrain from medications and activities as deemed appropriate by the anesthesiologist and surgeon. These precautions can include avoidance of blood thinners such as Advil or Motrin. After surgery, there can be serious complications. Patients should go to a hospital emergency department if they develop loss of bladder or bowel control (or if they cannot urinate); if they are unable to move their legs (indicates nerve or spinal cord compression); experience sudden shortness of breath (possible blood clot in the lungs causing a condition called pulmonary embolism); or if they develop pneumonia or some other heart/lung problem.

Description

Laminectomy can also be called back surgery, disc surgery, or discectomy. Laminectomy is a surgical procedure used in an attempt to treat **back pain**. The most common site for back pain is usually the lower back, or lumbar spine. A disc acts like a shock absorber for the spinal cord, which contains nerves that exit from foramina, or holes in a disc. A disc (or vertebral disc) is made up of a tough outer ring of cartilage with an inner sac containing a jellylike substance called the nucleus pulposis. When a disc herniates, the jellylike substance pushes through and causes the harder outer ring (annulus fibrosus) to compress a nerve root in the spinal cord. Herniation of a vertebral disc can cause varying degrees of pain. Approximately 25% of persons who have back pain have a herniated disc, causing a condition called **sciatica**, causing pain to be felt through the buttocks into one or both legs. The most serious compression disorder in the spinal cord is a condition called the cauda equine syndrome. The cauda equine is an area in the spinal cord where nerve roots of all spinal nerves are located. Cauda equine syndrome is a serious condition that may cause loss of all nerve function below the area of

Key Terms

Annulus fibrosus A fibrous and cartilage ring that forms the circumference of a vertebrae.

Lamina Flat plates of bone that form part of a vertebrae.

Nucleus pulposus Central core of a vertebrae.

compression, which can cause loss of bladder and bowel control. Such a condition is a surgical emergency and immediate decompression is required without delay.

Typically, conservative medical therapy is attempted for the treatment of a herniated disc. Surgery should be considered when recurrent attacks of pain cause interference with work or daily activities. The decision for surgery is indicated for chronic cases and should be made jointly between the patient and surgeon. Severe deficit can cause patients to have loss of nerve function, causing movement deficits in affected areas. Back pain is more common in men than women and more common in Caucasians than among other racial groups. Back pain results in more lost work than any other medical condition or disability. As a disorder, back pain has been documented through the ages since the first discussions date more than 3,500 years ago in ancient Egyptian writings.

Laminectomy as a procedure is not exclusive to a herniated disc. Laminectomy is used for metastatic tumor invasion of the spinal cord (which causes compression), and for narrowing of the spinal cord (a condition called spinal stenosis.)

In the United States, approximately 450 cases of herniated disc per 100,000 require surgery. Men are two times more likely to have back surgery as women and the average age for surgery is 40–45 years. More than 95% of all laminectomies are performed on the fourth and fifth lumbar vertebrae (lumbar laminectomy). Back pain is ranked second (behind the common cold) among the leading causes of missed workdays. Approximately one in five Americans, typically 45–64 years of age, will experience back pain. Each year, an estimated 13 million people will see their primary care practitioner for chronic back pain. Approximately 2.4 million Americans are chronically disabled from back pain, and another 2.4 million are temporarily disabled.

Description of surgical procedure

Typically, the patient is placed in the kneeling position to reduce abdominal weight on the spine. The surgeon makes a straight incision over the affected vertebrae (can be anywhere in the spinal cord) extending to the bony arches of the vertebrae (lamina.) The surgical goal is to completely expose the involved nerve root. To expose the nerve root(s), the surgeon removes the ligament joining the vertebrae along all or part of the lamina. The nerve root is pulled back toward the center of the spinal column, and all or part of the disc is removed. Muscle is placed to protect the nerve root(s) and the incision is closed.

Preparation

Weeks before surgery, the surgeon (a neurosurgeon or orthopedic spine surgeon) will make a general medical assessment and establish fitness for surgery. Days before the procedure, an assessment with the anesthesiologist is necessary to discuss anesthetic options during surgery: whether to use general or spinal anesthesia. A careful history should include information about all prescription and over-the-counter (OTC) medications. Anti-inflammatory agents such as aspirin or ibuprofen (Advil, Motrin) should be stopped several days before surgery. If the patient smokes, smoking should stop at least several days before surgery. Typically, imaging studies such as x rays or **magnetic resonance imaging (MRI)**, heart tracing studies (ECG), and routine blood work are performed before surgery. No food is permitted after midnight before surgery.

Anyone undergoing surgery that lasts more than two hours may be at risk of developing a blood clot, and administering heparin (an anticoagulant) may reduce the possibility of this complication. If heparin is administered to a patient receiving laminectomy, careful monitoring and blood tests are necessary to ensure that the blood is not excessively thinned, which can cause bleeding.

Aftercare

During recovery, patients will lie on a side or supine (back). There may be pain and patients will typically wear compression stockings to avoid blood-clot formation, a complication that can occur after surgery. There may be a catheter placed in the bladder to collect and measure urine output. Pain medications will be administered, and sometimes the surgeon will allow patient-controlled analgesia (PCA) with a pump that enables patients to self-deliver pain medications. Walking is encouraged hours after surgery and breathing exercises may be performed to avoid loss of air in a lung or pneumonia. It is advised to bend at the hip, not at the waist, and to avoid twisting at the shoulders or hips. The first few days after surgery may pose problems with sleeping, especially if therapeutic positions are different from normal sleeping positions. Different types of pillow positioning may be helpful (especially under the neck and knees.) To make getting out of bed easier, the patient should move the body as a unit, tighten the abdominal muscles, and roll to the side or edge of the bed and press down with arms on the bed to help raise the body while concurrently and carefully swinging legs to the floor. Typically, the surgeon will schedule an appointment with postoperative patients about one week after the procedure. At about seven days, the surgeon will remove any sutures (stitches) or staples that were placed during operation. Follow-up with the personal primary care practitioner occurs within the first month after operation.

In-home recovery

Recovery can be easier at home if patients have someone to drive for them for one or two weeks after surgery. Short, frequent walks each day may help speed recovery. Return to work is possible within one to two weeks for sedentary work, but may take more time (two to four months) if employment is strenuous with physical demands. Driving is usually not advised for one to two weeks after surgery, since postoperative medications for pain may cause drowsiness as a side effect, which can impair driving ability.

Risks

After laminectomy (postoperative), there is a risk of developing complications that can include blood clots, infection, excessive bleeding, worsening of back pain, nerve damage, or spinal fluid leak. It is possible to experience drainage at the incision site, redness at the incision area, fever (over 100.4° F), or increasing pain and numbness in arms, legs, back, or buttocks. Additionally, patients may experience inability to urinate, loss of bladder or bowel control, a severe **headache**, or redness, swelling, or pain in one extremity. If any of these signs or symptoms appears, patients are advised to immediately call the surgeon. If the sutures or staples come out, or if the bandage becomes soaked with blood, a call to the surgeon is necessary without delay.

Normal results

Some studies indicate that surgery provides better results than observation alone after one follow-up visit to the physician. However, other studies reveal that there is no statistical difference between conservative medical treatment or surgery 10 years after surgery.

Resources
BOOKS
Townsend, Courtney M. *Sabiston Textbook of Surgery,* 16th ed. New York: W. B. Saunders Co., 2001.

PERIODICALS
Petrozza, Patricia H. "Major Spine Surgery." *Anesthesiology Clinics of North America* 20, no. 2 (June 2002).

Spivak, Jeffery M. "Degenerative Lumbar Spinal Stenosis." *The Journal of Bone and Joint Surgery* 80-A:7 (July 1998).

ORGANIZATIONS

The American Back Society. 2647 International Boulevard, Suite 401, Oakland, CA 94601. (510) 536-9929; Fax: (510) 536-1812. info@americanbacksoc.org. <http://www.americanbacksoc.org>.

Laith Farid Gulli, MD
Robert Ramirez, DO

Lamotrigine

Definition

Lamotrigine is an anticonvulsant medication used in the treatment of **epilepsy**. Epilepsy is a neurological disorder in which excessive surges of electrical energy are emitted in the brain, causing **seizures**. Lamotrigine is usually reserved for difficult-to-control seizures that have not responded to other anticonvulsant medications. In psychiatry, lamotrigine is also indicated in the treatment of bipolar disorder (manic-depression).

Purpose

While lamotrigine controls seizures associated with epilepsy, there is no known cure for the disorder. Although the precise mechanism by which lamotrigine exerts its therapeutic effect is unknown, lamotrigine is thought to act at sodium channels in the neuron (nerve cell) to reduce the amount of excitatory **neurotransmitters** that the nerve cell releases. Neurotransmitters are chemicals that aid in the transfer of nerve impulses from one nerve junction to the next. With decreased levels of these neurotransmitters, the electrical activity in the brain that triggers seizures is reduced.

In the treatment of bipolar disorders, lamotrigine's effect upon neurochemicals stabilizes mood, preventing sudden, unpredictable, and severe episodes of mania and **depression**.

Description

For the treatment of epilepsy-related seizures, lamotrigine may be used alone or in combination with other anti-epileptic drugs (AEDs) or **anticonvulsants**. In the United States, lamotrigine is sold under the brand name Lamictal.

Recommended dosage

Lamotrigine is taken orally, in either tablet or chewable form. Chewable tablets may be dispersed into a liquid solution, according to the prescribing physician's instructions. Lamotrigine is prescribed by physicians in

Key Terms

Bipolar disorder A psychiatric disorder marked by alternating episodes of mania and depression. Also called bipolar illness, manic-depressive illness.

Epilepsy A disorder associated with disturbed electrical discharges in the central nervous system that cause seizures.

Neurotransmitter A chemical that is released during a nerve impulse that transmits information from one nerve cell to another.

Seizure A convulsion, or uncontrolled discharge of nerve cells that may spread to other cells throughout the brain, resulting in abnormal body movements or behaviors.

varying daily dosages, usually ranging 200–900 mg per day divided into two doses.

Beginning any course of treatment that includes lamotrigine requires a gradual dose-increasing regimen. The safety and effectiveness of lamotrigine in children under age 18 have not been proven; therefore, the drug is seldom used in children. Adults typically take an initial dose for the first two weeks that is slowly increased over time. It may take several weeks to realize the full benefits of lamotrigine, especially in those patients taking lamotrigine for the treatment of bipolar disorders.

A double dose of lamotrigine should not be taken. If a dose is missed, it should be taken as soon as possible. However, if it is within four hours of the next dose, then the missed dose should be skipped. When ending a course of treatment that includes lamotrigine, physicians typically direct patients to gradually taper down their daily dosages over a period of several weeks. Stopping the medicine suddenly may severely alter mood or cause seizures to occur, even in patients taking lamotrigine for the treatment of bipolar disorders.

Precautions

A physician should be consulted before taking lamotrigine with certain non-prescription medications. Patients should avoid alcohol and CNS depressants (medications that make one drowsy or tired, such as antihistimines, sleep medications, and some **pain** medications), while taking lamotrigine. Lamotrigine can exacerbate the side effects of alcohol and some other medications. Alcohol may also increase the risk or frequency of seizures.

Lamotrigine may not be suitable for persons with a history of liver or kidney disease, depressed renal function, mental illness, anemia, high blood pressure, angina (chest pain), or irregular heartbeats and other heart problems. Before beginning treatment with lamotrigine, patients should notify their physician if they consume a large amount of alcohol, have a history of drug use, are nursing, pregnant, or plan to become pregnant.

Lamotrigine's safety during pregnancy has not been established. Persons taking lamotrigine (and other AEDs or anticonvulsants) should be aware that many AEDs and anticonvulsants cause birth defects. Patients who become pregnant while taking any AED or anticonvulsants should contact their physician immediately.

Side effects

Lamotrigine is generally well tolerated. However, in some patients, lamotrigine may produce some of the traditionally mild side effects associated with anticonvulsants. **Headache**, nausea, and unusual tiredness and weakness are the most frequently reported side effects of anticonvulsants. Other possible side effects that do not usually require medical attention include:

- mild coordination problems
- mild dizziness
- abdominal pain
- sinus pain
- sleepiness or sleeplessness
- diarrhea or constipation
- heartburn or indigestion
- aching joints and muscles or chills
- unpleasant taste in mouth or dry mouth

Many of these side effects disappear or occur less frequently during treatment as the body adjusts to the medication. However, if any symptoms persist or become too uncomfortable, the prescribing physician should be consulted.

Other, uncommon side effects of lamotrigine can be serious and may indicate an allergic reaction. Severe and potentially life-threatening rashes have occurred during treatment with lamotrigine, occurring approximately once in every 1,000 persons who take the drug. In the unusual event that this rash develops, it normally occurs within the first eight weeks of treatment. A patient taking lamotrigine who experiences any of the following symptoms should contact a physician immediately:

- rash or bluish patches on the skin
- sores in the mouth or around the eyes
- depression or suicidal thoughts
- mood or mental changes, including excessive fear, anxiety, hostility

- general loss of motor skills
- persistent lack of appetite
- altered vision
- difficulty breathing
- chest pain or irregular heartbeat
- faintness or loss of consciousness
- persistent, severe headaches
- persistent fever or pain

Interactions

Lamotrigine may have negative interactions with some antacids, antihistamines, antidepressants, antibiotics, and monoamine oxidase inhibitors (MAOIs). Other medications such as HIV protease inhibitors (indinavir), ritonavir (Norvir), ipratropium (Atrovent), isoniazid, **phenobarbital** (Luminal, Solfoton), nefazodone, metronidazole, **acetazolamide** (Diamox), propranolol (Inderal), rifampin (Rifadin, Rimactane), and warfarin may also adversely react with lamotrigine. Oral contraceptives (birth control pills) may decrease the amount of lamotrigine absorbed by the body.

Lamotrigine may be used with other seizure prevention medications, if advised by a physician.

Resources

BOOKS

Devinsky, Orrin, M. D., *Epilepsy: Patient and Family Guide*, 2nd ed. Philadelphia: F. A. Davis Co., 2001.

Weaver, Donald F. *Epilepsy and Seizures: Everything You Need to Know.* Toronto: Firefly Books, 2001.

OTHER

"Lamotrigine." *Medline Plus.* National Library of Medicine. May 6, 2004 (June 1, 2004). <http://www.nlm.nih.gov/medlineplus/druginfo/uspdi/202786.html>.

"Lamotrigine." *Yale New Haven Health Service Drug Guide.* May 6, 2004 (June 1, 2004). <http://yalenewhaven-health.org/library/healthguide/en-us/drugguide/topic.asp?hwid=multumd03809a1>.

ORGANIZATIONS

Epilepsy Foundation. 4351 Garden City Drive, Landover, MD 20785-7223. (800) 332-1000. <http://www.epilepsy foundation.org>.

American Epilepsy Society. 342 North Main Street, West Hartford, CT 06117-2507. <http://www. aesnet.org>.

Adrienne Wilmoth Lerner

Lateral femoral cutaneous nerve entrapment *see* **Meralgia paresthetica**

Learning disorders

Definition

Learning disorders (LD) refer to a significant deficit in learning due to a person's inability to interpret what is seen and heard, or to link information from different parts of the brain.

Description

Academic deficiency is frequently associated with neurologic and psychological disorders. Severe academic problems may occur as a primary disorder of learning. Learning disorders can be classified in three major types: disorder of written expression (DWE); reading disorder (RD); and mathematics disorder (MD). The description of learning disorders corresponds to the educational legal designation of learning disabilities. Learning disabilities are legally defined by Public Law in a law called the Individuals with Disabilities Education Act, or IDEA. The IDEA defines a learning disability as a disorder in written or spoken language that results in an imperfect ability to listen, think, read, spell, write, or do mathematics. The act excludes persons who have learning impairments that are solely due to hearing problems, visual problems, motor problems, **mental retardation**, or due to environmental deprivation. The rules and related laws of IDEA stipulate that children with LD are entitled to free education and special services. A fourth category of LD has also been established for an LD that does not fulfill all the criteria (called an LD not otherwise specified.) Age of onset of LD is closely related to clinical presentation. Most cases of LD can be detected between preschool and second grade. Typically, onset of LD before first grade, often demonstrates developmental delay in learning new concepts at home, or as a delay in performance in school (delay is observed relative to other children and is observed by school officials). If the onset of LD occurs in early grade school (first or second grade), then observations typically include slow learning and difficulty completing and mastering schoolwork which often results in poor grades.

Demographics

LD occurs in approximately 5% to 10% of the population of which about 50% are classified as reading disorder. The remaining 50% of LD falls under the categories of disorder of written expression, mathematics disorder or atypical LD. LD is more common in males than females by 2:1 or 4:1 ratio. Children with LD have an increased risk for emotional behavioral problems and comorbidity (50% of the 1.6 million children with **attention-deficit hyperactivity disorder** [ADHD] have an LD). Approximately 2% to 8% of elementary school children have reading disorder (dyslexia). Speech disorder occurs in

Key Terms

Algorithms   A sequence of steps designed to calculate or determine a task.

Phoneme   A discrete unit of a language that corresponds to a similar discrete unit of speech sound.

Phonics   A system to teach reading by teaching the speech sounds associated with single letters, letter combinations, and syllables.

Rote learning   Learning by means of repitition and memorization, usually without significant understanding of the concepts involved.

approximately 10% of children younger than 8 years of age. ADHD is a comorbid condition that occurs in approximately four million school-aged children (20% of them are unable to focus their attention to required tasks in school and at home).

Causes and symptoms
Reading Disorder

The cause of reading disorder is underactivity in the left superior posterior temporal lobe (planum temporale). Research using functional and structural neuroimaging techniques, demonstrates that this underactivity is evident during reading tasks. It is believed that the planum temporale is a region that is important for phonologic processing. Genetic studies reveal that there is a higher concordance rate for RD in identical (71%) than fraternal (49%) twins. Additionally, heritability of RD may be more than 50% especially in a disorder with a focal deficit in phonologic processing (phonologic dyslexia). Some genetic investigations have identified possible genes for RD, located on chromosome six and 15. Modern research techniques have demonstrated that RD is the result of brain deficits in processing sound units and sound-symbol relationships.

Most of the persons diagnosed with reading disorder (RD) have average or higher intelligence. RD is considered synonymous with **dyslexia**, since spelling and reading are related. Persons with RD often have deficits with spelling. Affected individuals have difficulty with phonologic processing. This means that affected persons have deficits in the process of identifying and manipulating individual sounds (phonemes) within larger sound units (morphemes and words.) Symptoms usually appear before early grade school. Patients cannot translate a visual stimulus (letters) into a meaningful blend of sounds (i.e. they have deficits in phonics). Reading is slower and more mechanical even with treatment. Typically, reading takes more effort in affected patients, often requiring intense concentration, especially on the pronunciation and identification of individual words. The increased concentration required during reading can impair the person's attention ability, causing mental fatigue, attention problems (less attention available for comprehension and memory). Sometimes, but not often, children may have visualization-comprehension or memory deficits causing RD. Persons with visualization-comprehension weakness often exhibit difficulty visualizing what is being read. The cause of visualization-comprehension weakness occurs because of deficits in visual organization (nonverbal skills.) This is a vital deficit since reading comprehension is based on some visualization (nonverbal skills.) However, in the majority of affected children with RD it is the deficits in phonologic processing (processing phonemes within morphemes and words) that are responsible for difficulty with comprehension or memory.

Mathematics Disorder

The cause of mathematics disorder (MD) is thought to be due to a nonverbal weakness. MD could take various forms and therefore the causes also change. There may be deficits visualizing and visually organizing mathematical concepts and manipulations. Some patients may have short-term or working memory deficits which can interfere with processing mathematical calculations. The cause of MD can be linked to a larger atypical LD.

The symptoms of MD can vary. Patients can exhibit dyscalculia or acalculia (deficits in mathematical calculation). Dyscalculia patients may over-rely on memory and tangible aids, because they have deficits to mentally calculate arithmetic manipulations. Symptoms in some patients can include deficits in memory (short term and working memory or deficits in visual organization or mathematical concepts).

Disorder of Written Expression

The cause of the disorder of written expression in some persons may be due to deficits in visual-motor integration and motor coordination. Most causes of DWE occur because there are deficits in the brain concerning information translation from auditory-oral modality to visual-written modality. The cause of this deficit is unknown.

Patients often exhibit spelling deficits that include problems with punctuation, grammar, and development of ideas during writing. Writing samples from persons with DWE are typically brief, simple, or may be difficult to comprehend because of grammar and punctuation errors. Patients with visual-motor deficits write with so much care that they often lose track of ideas and thoughts. If motor coordination is the only cause then symptoms may be classified more appropriately as a motor skills disorder not a DWE. Typically symptoms are not apparent until the third or fourth grade, when academic exercises demand development of ideas.

Diagnosis

The diagnosis of LD can be made if there is significant discrepancy between intelligence test scores (raw ability to learn) and achievement test score (actual learning achievement). However, the diagnosis can be a complex process since there is no universal agreement concerning the magnitude of discrepancy between test scores, nor is there a consensus concerning which test scores should be analyzed to obtain a statistical analysis of discrepancy. Tests should be administered to establish that low intelligence alone is not the cause of underachievement (i.e. children with mental retardation are not diagnosed with LDs.) There are several psychological tests that separately measure intelligence (i.e. Wechsler Intelligence Scale for Children) and achievement (Kaufman Test of Educational Achievement, K-TEA).

Treatment Team

The treatment team typically includes school counselors, education specialists, specialists in learning disorders, school psychologists or clinical psychologists (with advanced clinical training in administration and interpretation of psychological tests (psychometrics). Tests for achievement and intelligence should be administered and interpreted by a clinical psychologist or a school psychologist. Only a duly licensed or certified clinical or school psychologist can administer the recommended psychological tests. A full written report of results and interpretation of results is typically prepared and submitted to concerned persons.

Treatment

Before treatment is initiated, a very comprehensive evaluation is necessary with standardized achievement and intelligence tests.

Treatment for RD-affected persons involves a plan that provides intensive tutoring to develop phonologic processing and fluent word reading with treatment objectives that emphasize comprehension. There are several treatment approaches (Gillingham-Stillman Approach, Fernald-Keller Approach or Lindamood-Bell Reading Program) that provide intensive phonic practice and phonic associations with sensory integration or mnemonic strategies to remember letter-sound blends and relationships.

Treatment for MD can vary widely since MD can have a variety of causes and presentations. The treatment program is typically highly individualized and specific to enhance and expand upon strengths to improve weaknesses and math errors. Sometimes analogies are utilized to demonstrate abstract concepts and to build upon concepts (concrete learning) until the concept becomes understood or mastered. Flash cards and practice drills can help to memorize simple mathematical operations such as multiplication tables. MD due to visual-organization deficits can be treated with visualization techniques to improve math errors.

Treatment for DWE can involve interventions that help to improve written expression caused by a deficit in the expressive task of writing. There are several treatment plans that include writing in more "natural environments" (i.e. encourages keeping a diary or making "lists"), writing notes and outlines before attempting writing prose, and talking-to-writing progression. The talking-to-writing progression approach initially involves the affected child taking the role of dictating while another person writes for the child. As the treatments progress, the roles are gradually reversed until the child is able to dictate and write without assistance. Treatment continues with dictation until the child is independently thinking and writing. Treatment interventions for atypical LDs involve objectives to expand on the child's strengths (i.e. verbal and rote learning strengths) and to provide additional experience and practice in nonverbal weakness areas. Atypical LDs are complex disorders and treatment interventions are detailed and typically include teaching social and nonverbal material with extensive practice and concrete examples; teaching the affected person in rote in a predictable fashion; and the utilization and application of known algorithms to new situations. Additionally, treatment can include practicing organizational skills at home; practicing attention to visual and auditory (verbal information); and to encourage supervised and highly structured and interactive peer experiences.

Clinical trials

There are many **clinical trials** (http://www.nlm.nih.gov) currently in progress. The studies currently sponsored by governmental agencies focus on topics that include coping, diagnosis, symptoms specific aspects of disorders, and law and public policy.

Prognosis

It is rare for persons with LD to completely improve their academic deficiencies. However, performance in the area of weakness can significantly improve with appropriate treatment interventions.

Recovery

Recovery is slow and patients are often in specialized intervention programs (MD, DWE) or are part of programs that offer specific treatments (RD).

Other Atypical LDs

There are two common patterns of working memory deficits. Nonverbal learning disability (NVLD) is a neuropsychological syndrome characterized by deficits in comprehension, motor skills, visual-perception organization, tactile perception and novel problem solving, comprehension, visual memory, concept formation, and integration/organization of information. However, NVLD patients exhibit strengths in simple verbal skills, rote learning, memory, and knowledge of facts. In addition to weakness in mathematical achievement most persons affected by NVLD also tend to have problems with written expression, reading comprehension and social skills. Persons affected with working memory deficits tend to lose track of information as they are mentally processing that information or other information. Patients with working memory deficits often have problems with mathematical manipulations (which requires working memory), and the disorder is often accompanied by ADHD. Working memory is defined as the ability to remember information while executing another cognitive task.

Resources

BOOKS

Behrman, Richard, E., et al., eds. *Nelson Textbook of Pediatrics,* 17th ed. Philadelphia: Saunders, 2004.

Goetz, Christopher G., et al, eds. *Textbook of Clinical Neurology,* 1st ed. Philadelphia: W. B. Saunders Company, 1999.

PERIODICALS

Frank, Y., and Steven G. Pavlakis. "Brain Imaging in Neurobehavioral Disorders." *Pediatric Neurology* 25, no. 4 (October 2001).

Kronenberger, William G., and David Dunn. "Learning Disorders." *Neurologic Clinics* 21, no. 4 (November 2003).

Toppelberg, Claudio O., and Theodore Shapiro. "Language Disorders: A 10-Year Research Update Review." *Journal of the American Academy of Child & Adolescent Psychiatry* 39, no.2 (February 2000).

WEBSITES

National Center for Learning Disabilities. <http://www.ld.org>.

National Institute on Deafness and Other Communication Disorders. <http://www.nidcd.nih.gov>.

ORGANIZATIONS

National Institute of Mental Health, Office of Communications. 6001 Executive Boulevard, Room

8184, MSC 9663, Bethesda, MD 20892-9663. (301) 443-4513 or 1-866-615-6464; Fax: (301) 443-4279.

Laith Farid Gulli, MD
Nicole Mallory

Lee Silverman voice treatment

Definition

Lee Silverman voice treatment (LSVT) is a technique for improving the voice volume of patients with **Parkinson's disease** (PD) and other neurological disorders.

Purpose

Most patients with PD experience a decreased voice volume and decreased intelligibility of their speech as their disease progresses. The purpose of LSVT is to reverse that decline by focusing the patient's attention on increasing voice volume through an intensive set of exercises. The treatment program was developed by two speech language pathologists, and is named after one of the first patients to undergo the program.

Precautions

The treatment program is entirely safe, as it consists only of vocal exercises.

Description

The LSVT program occurs in 16 one-hour sessions given four times per week and spaced over one month. The program includes at-home exercises the patient must complete for an additional hour (two hours on non-class days). The sessions are led by specially trained speech professionals who have been certified by the LSVT Foundation, a nonprofit organization devoted to improving speech among PD patients through the LSVT method.

During the sessions, patients are taught to "think loud," that is, to focus their conscious efforts on increasing voice volume. The intensive schedule of the workshops and frequent encouragement and reinforcement from the speech professionals provide an effective training system in which the patient learns to consistently increase voice volume. Exercises to increase breath support may also be used, although for many patients, focusing on increasing the volume is sufficient.

A consequence of the PD disease process is a decrease in the strength of vocal effort, due to the slowed movements and stiffness that characterize the disease, as well as a possible alteration in the sensory processing of sounds that is used to modulate the voice level. Despite the loss of volume, patients continue to believe their voice volume is adequate. Therefore, a key feature of LSVT is to make patients aware that their normal, pre-treatment voice level is too soft, and to help them find the correct level for normal speech. During the workshops, patients are taught methods to increase their vocal efforts by breathing more deeply and expelling air more fully and to "think shout." Patients are trained to reach the correct volume and to self-correct even when they feel they are speaking too loudly.

Another key feature of the program is building up the length and complexity of the vocalizations the patient is expected to deliver at the increased volume. Practice and feedback begin with single words to train the patient about the correct volume and the breath support required to produce that volume. Training moves on to simple and frequently used phrases so that the habit of loudness becomes associated with habitually used phrases. Sentences, reading aloud, and conversations follow.

Repetition and reinforcement are essential parts of the program. Through constant practice and reinforcement from the therapist, the patient learns to "recalibrate" the level of effort and to become accustomed to using a louder voice than beforehand. Reinforcement from family members and others in the community is also important in solidifying the gains made during the treatment program. Patients practice with tape recorders and sound-level meters to increase the degree of feedback.

Aftercare

No aftercare is involved, although the patient is instructed to continue practicing the exercises learned during the treatment program.

Risks

There are no risks to this treatment. Not all patients can sustain the prolonged and intense effort required in the program. Patients who have had cognitive decline may have difficulty complying with all of the instructions during training.

Normal results

Patients who engage in the program dramatically increase their voice volume to return to the correct levels. They learn to be understood much better and communication renormalizes.

Resources

BOOKS

Ramig, L. O., S. Countryman, A. A. Pawlas, and C. Fox. *Voice Treatment for Parkinson Disease and Other Neurologic*

Disorders. Rockville: American Speech-Language-Hearing Association, 1995.

WEBSITES

Lee Silverman Voice Treatment.
   <http://www.lsvt.org/main_site.htm> (April 19, 2004).

Richard Robinson

Leigh disease

Definition

Leigh syndrome is an early onset, progressive neurological disease that involves defects in the normal function of the mitochondria. The mitochondrion is a small organelle located in most cells and is responsible for producing energy for cells and tissues throughout the body.

Description

Leigh syndrome is caused by defective cellular respiration that supplies many tissues with energy. The disorder is severe and can be particularly difficult for family members, as infants are among the severely affected. Leigh syndrome is also known as necrotizing **encephalopathy**.

Demographics

Leigh syndrome is a very rare disease that affects different peoples relatively equally. Some studies have shown that more males are affected than females.

Causes and symptoms

In Leigh syndrome, symptoms usually develop within the first year of life; rarely, symptoms can develop during later childhood. The infant usually initially develops symptoms that include **hypotonia** (decreased muscle tone), vomiting, and **ataxia** (balance or coordination abnormalities). Overall, failure to grow and thrive is usually the primary reason parents seek medical help. Eventually, the infant experiences **seizures**, lactic acidosis (an excess of lactic acid, a normal product of carbohydrate metabolism, in the body), and respiratory and kidney impairment.

Various abnormalities of the eyes are also common in Leigh syndrome. Ophthalmoplegia (paralysis of some or all of the muscles of the eye) is a typical finding, along with optic atrophy (degeneration of the optic nerve) and pigmentary retinopathy, a disorder that eventually leads to blindness.

On the cellular level, persons with Leigh syndrome have an inability to produce ATP (an energy source for the

Key Terms

Brainstem   The portion of the brain which lies between the cerebrum and the spinal cord that controls the functions of breathing, swallowing, seeing, and hearing.

Mitochondria   A part of the cell that is responsible for energy production.

Seizure   A disorder of the nervous system due to a sudden, excessive, disorderly discharge of the brain neurons.

cell) in the mitochondria. Tissues that are not provided with adequate energy replenishment usually die. Irreversible damage can occur first in cells requiring much energy, such as the brain, leading to mental impairments and developmental delay. Many parts of the brain are affected by the lack of ATP in Leigh disease, including the basal ganglia, which helps regulate motor performance; the brainstem, which controls the functions of breathing, swallowing, seeing, and hearing; and the **cerebellum**, which coordinates balance and voluntary muscle movement.

Several genetic causes explain how persons develop Leigh disease, and several genes are involved. These genes include defects found in nuclear DNA as well as the smaller, less widely known mitochondrial DNA. Genes from both genomes contribute to the normal function of the mitochondria. Mutations in genes from the nuclear and the mitochondrial DNA have both been implicated in Leigh disease.

Diagnosis

In general, diagnosis of Leigh syndrome is often difficult due to the broad variability in clinical symptoms as well as the many different genetic explanations that cause this disease. Genetic testing for specific nuclear or mitochondrial DNA mutation is helpful in this regard.

Laboratory studies can assist in the diagnosis of Leigh syndrome. A muscle **biopsy** often determines if there are abnormalities associated with the mitochondria. Additionally, as the mitochondria are responsible for producing energy, a deficiency in a protein complex that has an important function in the mitochondria is often detected. In Leigh syndrome, this deficiency is found in one of five complexes that make up the mitochondrial respiratory system. One of these complexes, complex IV, or cytochrome c oxidase (COX), is commonly deficient. Although a COX deficiency is associated with Leigh syndrome, it can also indicate other mitochondrial abnormalities. Similarly, there are mutations found in other complexes that can cause Leigh syndrome.

Treatment team

Treatment for Leigh syndrome is aimed at easing the disease-related symptoms and involves neurologists, pediatricians, clinical geneticists, nurses, and other related caretakers. Psychological counseling and support for family members caring for a child with Leigh disease is often encouraged.

Treatment

Currently, there is no treatment that is effective in slowing the progression of Leigh disease. Thiamine or vitamin B1 is usually given. Sodium bicarbonate may also be prescribed to help manage lactic acidosis.

Recovery and rehabilitation

As there is no cure for Leigh disease and the nature of the disorder is rapidly progressive, maintaining function for as long as possible is the primary focus rather than recovery. Physical therapists often assist in exercises designed to maintain strength and range of motion. As the disease progresses, occupational therapists can provide positioning devices for comfort.

Clinical trials

As of early 2004, there are no **clinical trials** to treat or cure Leigh syndrome. However, studies are underway to better understand all mitochondrial diseases in an effort to identify treatments and, eventually, a cure.

Prognosis

Soon after the onset of symptoms, the progression of Leigh disease is unrelentingly rapid. Death usually occurs from respiratory failure within two years following the initial symptoms, and usually by age six.

Resources

BOOKS

Icon Health Publicaitons. *The Official Parent's Sourcebook on Leigh's Disease: A Revised and Updated Directory for the Internet Age.* San Diego: Icon Group International, 2002.

PERIODICALS

Schmiedel, J., S. Jackson, J. Schafer, and H. Reichmann. "Mitochondrial Cytopathies." *Neurol.* 250, no. 3 (March 2003): 267–77.

DiMauro, S., A. L. Andreu, and D. C. De Vivo. "Mitochondrial Disorders." *J Child Neurol.* 17, Suppl. 3 (December 2002): 3S35–45; 3S46–47.

OTHER

"NINDS Leigh's Disease Information Page." *National Institute of Neurological Disorders and Stroke.* February 10, 2004 (April 4, 2004). <http://www.ninds.nih.gov/health_and_medical/disorders/leighsdisease_doc.htm>.

ORGANIZATIONS

The National Leigh's Disease Foundation. P.O. Box 2222, Corinth, MS 38834. (601) 286-2551 or (800) 819-2551.

United Mitochondrial Disease Foundation. 8085 Saltsburg Road, Suite 201, Pittsburgh, PA 15239. (412) 793-8077; Fax: (412) 793-6477. info@umdf.org. <http://www.umdf.org/>.

Bryan Richard Cobb, PhD

Lennox-Gastaut syndrome

Definition

Lennox-Gastaut syndrome (LGS) is one of the most severe forms of **epilepsy** (a seizure disorder) that develops in children usually between one and eight years old. It is characterized by several types of **seizures**, developmental delay, and behavioral disturbances such as poor social skills and lack of impulse control.

Description

Lennox-Gastaut syndrome can be the result of any one of many neurological problems of childhood that begins with intractable, or hard to control, seizures. French physician Samuel Auguste A. D. Tissot (1728–1797) first described the syndrome in 1770. He reported an 11-year-old boy with frequent drop attacks, **myoclonus** (jerking movements), and progressive functional impairment. Seizure types vary among children with LGS. The tonic seizures of LGS include stiffening of the body, upward deviation of the eyes, dilation of the pupils, and altered respiratory patterns. Atonic seizures are also experienced by children with LGS and involve a brief loss of muscle tone and consciousness, which causes abrupt falls. Other seizures common in LGS include the atypical absence seizure type (staring spells) and myoclonic seizures (sudden muscle jerks).

Lennox-Gastaut syndrome frequently affects language development in children, ranging from little or no verbal ability to slowness in ideation and expression. Varying degrees of motor difficulties hinder age-appropriate activities such as walking, skipping, or using a writing instrument. Severe behavioral disorders such as hyperactivity, aggressiveness, and autistic tendencies and personality disorders are nearly always present. There is usually **men-**

tal retardation and sometimes a tendency for psychosis that eventually develops with LGS.

In young children, LGS usually begins with episodes of sudden falls. In the school-age group, behavioral disturbances may be the heralding signs, along with sudden falls. This is soon followed by frequent seizures, episodes of **status epilepticus** (a continuous seizure state that is associated with a change in the child's level of awareness), progressively deteriorating intellectual functions, and personality disturbances. By age six, most children with LGS have some degree of mental retardation.

When children grow older, the types of seizures often change. In most cases, the drop seizures subside. They are replaced by partial, complex partial, and secondarily generalized convulsions. Among teenagers, complex partial seizures are the most common form.

Demographics

In the United States, Lennox-Gastaut syndrome accounts for 1–4% of older children with epilepsy, but 10% of children with epilepsy beginning in the first five years of life. In Europe, studies demonstrated that the proportion of patients with LGS seems similar to that in the US.

No racial differences exist in the occurrence of LGS; however there are differences in respect to sex and age. Males are affected more often than females; the relative risk of occurrence of LGS is significantly higher in boys than in girls (one in 10,000 boys, and one in 50,000 girls). The average age for the onset of seizures is three years.

Causes and symptoms

Causes

Often no specific cause is identifiable, however, some of the known causes include:

- developmental malformations of the brain
- genetic brain diseases such as **tuberous sclerosis**, and inherited metabolic brain diseases
- brain injury due to problems associated with pregnancy and birth, including prematurity, asphyxia, and/or low birth weight
- severe brain infections, including encephalitis, meningitis, toxoplasmosis, and rubella

In many instances, LGS follows earlier **infantile spasms**, which are sudden spasms or body bending, either at the trunk or neck. These episodes usually begin between three and eight months of age, and may develop into the mixed seizure pattern that characterizes LGS at two to three years of age.

Key Terms

Seizure Abnormal electrical discharge of neurons in the brain, often resulting in abnormal body movements or behaviors.

Vagus nerve Tenth cranial nerve and an important part of the autonomic nervous system, influencing motor functions in the larynx, diaphragm, stomach, and heart, and sensory functions in the ears and tongue.

Symptoms

The main symptom of LGS is the occurrence of seizures. Several different seizure types occur, and a child may experience some or all of these:

- In drop attacks, the child falls suddenly to the ground. This may be because the legs suddenly fold up (atonic seizure) or stiffen (tonic seizures), or because of a violent jerk (myoclonic seizure) that throws the child to the floor.

- During atypical absences, the child appears to be vacant or to stare blankly. Sometimes these seizures are associated with blindness or nodding of the head. Often, children are able to continue their activity to some extent during the seizure. These episodes are usually very brief, but frequent. Sometimes these seizures occur so frequently that they merge into one another. Such a phenomenon can lead to what is called non-convulsive status epilepticus. During these episodes, children may appear to switch off, but can be partly responsive, drool, be unable to speak or eat properly, and be wobbly on their feet.

- Tonic seizures are often difficult to detect as they occur much more frequently at night. During these attacks, there is general stiffening of the arms or legs. This may be associated with the eyes rolling up or the head moving back. Sometimes, breathing is interrupted and the child may turn blue. If the attacks last for more than 10–20 seconds, the arms often start to tremble rapidly while remaining stiff.

Most children with LGS experience some degree of impaired intellectual functioning or mental retardation. In approximately 65% of children with LGS, intellectual disability is evident, either previous to or at the time of diagnosis. Behavioral disturbances are also usually present, including persistent attention-seeking behavior, impulsiveness, lack of regard for personal safety and fearlessness, and, in severe cases, autistic behaviors. These behavior disturbances may be the result of the condition causing LGS, effects of a particular medication, uncontrolled epilepsy, difficulty interpreting information, or even a lower level of concept understanding.

Diagnosis

LGS is diagnosed by some or all of the following symptoms, including:

• presence of a mixed seizure pattern

• some degree of developmental delay or intellectual disability

• distinct, slow, spike-and-wave pattern shown during electroencephalogram (EEG)

Magnetic resonance imaging (MRI) is an important part of the search for an underlying cause in a child with LGS. Abnormalities revealed by **MRI** associated with LGS include tuberous sclerosis, brain malformations, or evidence of previous brain injury.

Treatment team

Treatment for LGS involves a multidisciplinary team that may include a **neurologist**, a **neuropsychologist**, and a neurosurgeon. A dietitian may help with specialized diet regimens.

Treatment

The drug treatment for LGS is based on the use of anti-epileptic drugs that are effective in reducing the number of seizures. However, the improvement often only lasts for a period of months or, rarely, a year or more. **Carbamazepine**, sodium valproate, vigabatrin, **lamotrigine**, and the **benzodiazepines** (clobazam, in particular) are often prescribed.

One alternative treatment involves a ketogenic diet in which 87% of calories come from fat, 6% from carbohydrates, and 7% from protein. The diet is restrictive, difficult to follow, but has shown results in reducing seizures in some affected children. Other less conventional therapies such as intravenous immunoglobulin therapy have also been attempted.

For children with repeated drop attacks, a procedure to cut the corpus collosum (the large group of nerve fibers connecting the two halves of the brain) may be very helpful. However, this procedure involves significant surgery and is not always effective, and seizures may return after several months or years.

An implanted vagus nerve stimulator is effective in reducing seizures in many children with Lennox-Gastaut syndrome. It is a device, similar in size to a heart pacemaker, that is implanted in the chest with a lead wrapped around the vagus nerve in the neck. It is able to stimulate the vagus nerve automatically at adjustable intervals. The device may take months to show maximum benefit, and requires a surgical procedure for insertion as well as for removal. The batteries require replacement approximately every eight to ten years, which entails further surgery.

Recovery and rehabilitation

A very small percentage of children with LGS experience a spontaneous improvement in seizures, usually during adolescence. In these cases, mental function also shows some improvement. In the overwhelming majority of cases, however, emphasis is placed on maximizing quality of life rather than recovery.

Protective devices such as helmets and pads may be necessary during periods of high seizure activity, but many children and parents consider them too burdensome and restrictive for continuous daily use.

Clinical trials

Although as of early 2004 there were no ongoing **clinical trials** for LGS, the National Institutes of Health (NIH) sponsors research related to many seizure disorders. Information on the numerous current clinical trials for the study and treatment of seizure disorders can be found at the NIH Web site: <http://clinicaltrials.gov/search/term= Seizure+Disorder>.

Prognosis

The prognosis for individuals with LGS is unfavorable, but variable. Long-term studies of children with LGS found that a majority of patients continue to have typical LGS characteristics (mental retardation, treatment-resistant seizures) many years after onset. Children with an early onset of seizures, prior history of West syndrome, higher frequency of seizures, or constant slow EEG background activity have a worse prognosis than those with seizures beginning later in childhood. Tonic seizures may persist and be more difficult to control over time, while myoclonic and atypical absences become easier to control.

Special concerns

It is recognized that the frequency of seizures may be associated with the child's level of alertness. The child who is overexcited or lacks sufficient stimulation may experience more seizures. Therefore, a stable but stimulating environment may be important in reducing the number of daily seizures. This may include a strict routine of regular meals, sleep, and medication.

Providing for the safety of a child with Lennox-Gastaut syndrome is a 24-hour concern for parents. Coupled with safety concerns, children with LGS are often dependent for personal care such as toileting, management of behavioral impulses, and interpretation of attempts at communication. Often, **respite** care can provide parents with a chance to reenergize. As the child matures into adulthood, an assisted living center or group home may help provide maximum independence and social integration, along with continued medical supervision.

Resources

BOOKS

The Official Parent's Sourcebook on Lennox-Gastaut Syndrome: A Revised and Updated Directory for the Internet Age. San Diego: Icon Group International, 2002.

PERIODICALS

Frost, M., et al. "Vagus Nerve Stimulation in Children with Refractory Seizures Associated with Lennox-Gastaut Syndrome." *Epilepsia* 42 (2001): 1148–1152.

OTHER

NINDS Lennox-Gastaut Syndrome Information Page. National Institute of Neurological Disorders and Stroke. March 10, 2004 (May 23, 2004). <http://www.ninds.nih.gov/health_and_medical/disorders/lennoxgastautsyndrome_doc.htm>.

ORGANIZATIONS

Lennox-Gastaut Syndrome Group. 3872 Lyceum Avenue, Los Angeles, CA 90066. (310) 391-0335; Fax: (310) 397-2687. CandaceLGS@aol.com.

Epilepsy Foundation. 4351 Garden City Drive, Suite 500, Landover, MD 20785-7223. (301) 459-3700 or (800) EFA-1000 (332-1000); Fax: (301) 577-2684. postmaster@efa.org. <http://www.epilepsyfoundation.org/>.

NIH/NINDS Brain Resources and Information Network. PO Box 5801, Bethesda, MD 20824. (301) 496-5751 or (800) 352-9424; Fax: (301) 402-2186. <http://www.ninds.nih.gov/>.

Greiciane Gaburro Paneto
Iuri Drumond Louro, MD, PhD

Lesch-Nyhan syndrome

Definition

Lesch-Nyhan syndrome is a rare genetic disorder that affects males. Males with this syndrome develop physical handicaps, **mental retardation**, and kidney problems. It is caused by the complete absence of a particular enzyme. Self injury is a classic feature of this genetic disease.

Description

Lesch-Nyhan syndrome was first described in 1964 by Dr. Michael Lesch and Dr. William Nyhan. Males with Lesch-Nyhan syndrome develop neurological problems during infancy. Infants with Lesch-Nyhan syndrome have weak muscle tone (**hypotonia**) and are unable to develop normally. Affected males develop uncontrollable writhing movements (athetosis) and muscle stiffness (**spasticity**) over time. Lack of speech is also a common feature of Lesch-Nyhan syndrome. The most dramatic symptom of Lesch-Nyhan syndrome is the compulsive self-injury seen in 85% of affected males. This self injury involves the biting of their own lips, tongue, and finger tips, as well as head banging. This behavior leads to serious injury and scarring

Demographics

Lesch-Nyhan syndrome affects approximately one in 380,000 live births. It occurs evenly among races. Almost always, only male children are affected. Women carriers usually do not have any symptoms. Women carriers can occasionally develop inflammation of the joints (gout) as they get older.

Causes and symptoms

The syndrome is caused by a severe change (mutation) in the HPRT **gene**. Since the HPRT gene is located on the X chromosome, Lesch-Nyhan syndrome is considered an X-linked disorder and therefore only affects males.

The HPRT gene is responsible for the production of the enzyme called hypoxanthine-guanine phosphoribosyltransferase (HPRT). HPRT catalyzes a reaction that is necessary to prevent the buildup of uric acid. A severe mutation in the HPRT gene leads to an absence of HPRT enzyme activity which, in turn, leads to markedly elevated uric acid levels in the blood (hyperuricemia). This buildup of uric acid is toxic to the body and is related to the symptoms associated with the disease. Absence of the HPRT enzyme activity is also thought to alter the chemistry of certain parts of the brain, such as the basal ganglia, affecting **neurotransmitters** (chemicals used for communication between nerve cells), acids, and other chemicals. This change in the nervous system is also related to the symptoms associated with Lesch-Nyhan syndrome.

At birth, males with Lesch-Nyhan syndrome appear completely normal. Development is usually normal for the first few months. Symptoms develop between three to six months of age. Sand-like crystals of uric acid in the diapers may be one of the first symptoms of the disease. The baby may be unusually irritable. Typically, the first sign of nervous system impairment is the inability to lift their

Lesch-Nyhan syndrome

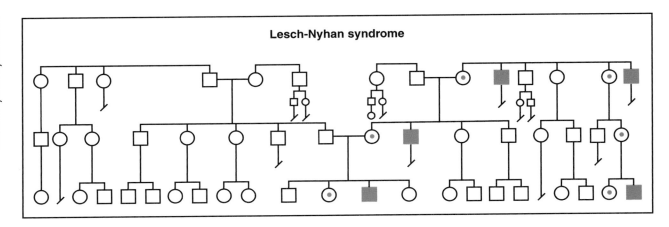

See Symbol Guide for Pedigree Charts. *(Gale Group.)*

Key Terms

Amniocentesis A procedure performed at 16-18 weeks of pregnancy in which a needle is inserted through a woman's abdomen into her uterus to draw out a small sample of the amniotic fluid from around the baby. Either the fluid itself or cells from the fluid can be used for a variety of tests to obtain information about genetic disorders and other medical conditions in the fetus.

Athetosis A condition marked by slow, writhing, involuntary muscle movements.

Basal ganglia A section of the brain responsible for smooth muscle movement.

Chorea Involuntary, rapid, jerky movements.

Chorionic villus sampling (CVS) A procedure used for prenatal diagnosis at 10–12 weeks gestation. Under ultrasound guidance a needle is inserted ei-

ther through the mother's vagina or abdominal wall and a sample of cells is collected from around the fetus. These cells are then tested for chromosome abnormalities or other genetic diseases.

Enzyme A protein that catalyzes a biochemical reaction or change without changing its own structure or function.

Mutation A permanent change in the genetic material that may alter a trait or characteristic of an individual, or manifest as disease, and can be transmitted to offspring.

Neurotransmitter Chemical in the brain that transmits information from one nerve cell to another.

Palsy Uncontrollable tremors.

Spasticity Increased muscle tone, or stiffness, which leads to uncontrolled, awkward movements.

---

head or sit up at an appropriate age. Many patients with Lesch-Nyhan will never learn to walk. By the end of the first year, writhing motions (athetosis), and spasmodic movements of the limbs and facial muscles (**chorea**) are clear evidence of defective motor development.

The compulsive self-injury associated with Lesch-Nyhan syndrome begins, on average, at three years. The self-injury begins with biting of the lips and tongue. As the disease progresses, affected individuals frequently develop finger biting and head banging. The self-injury can increase during times of stress.

Males with Lesch-Nyhan disease may also develop kidney damage due to kidney stones. Swollen and tender joints (gout) is another common problem.

Diagnosis

The diagnosis of Lesch-Nyhan syndrome is based initially on the distinctive pattern of symptoms. Measuring the amount of uric acid in a person's blood or urine can not definitively diagnose Lesch-Nyhan syndrome. It is diagnosed by measuring the activity of the HPRT enzyme through a blood test. When the activity of the enzyme is very low it is diagnostic of Lesch-Nyhan syndrome. It can also be diagnosed by DNA testing. This is also a blood test. DNA testing checks for changes (mutations) in the HPRT gene. Results from DNA testing are helpful in making the diagnosis and also if the family is interested in prenatal testing for future pregnancies.

Prenatal diagnosis is possible by DNA testing of fetal tissue drawn by **amniocentesis** or chorionic villus sampling (CVS). Fetuses should be tested if the mother is a carrier of a change (mutation) in her HPRT gene. A woman is at risk of being a carrier if she has a son with Lesch-Nyhan syndrome or someone in her family has Lesch-Nyhan syndrome. Any woman at risk of being a carrier should have DNA testing through a blood test.

Treatment team

Patients with Lesch-Nyhan syndrome should be cared for by neurologists (to monitor and treat neurological symptoms); urologists and/or nephrologists (to treat kidney stones and kidney damage); orthopedic surgeons (to treat joint problems); and psychiatrists or psychologists (to create a behavioral program).

Treatment

There are no known treatments for the neurological defects of Lesch-Nyhan. The medication Allopurinol can lower blood uric acid levels. This medication does not correct many of the symptoms. Some patients with Lesch-Nyhan syndrome have their teeth removed to prevent self-injury. Restraints are recommended to reduce self-destructive behaviors.

Prognosis

With strong supportive care, infants born with Lesch-Nyhan can live into adulthood with symptoms continuing throughout life.

At present, there are no preventive measures for Lesch-Nyhan syndrome. However, recent studies have indicated that this genetic disorder may be a good candidate for treatment with gene replacement therapy. Unfortunately, the technology necessary to implement this therapy has not yet been perfected.

Resources

BOOKS
Jinnah, H. A., and Theodore Friedmann. "Lesch-Nyhan Disease and Its Variants." *The Metabolic and Molecular Bases of Inherited Disease.* New York: McGraw-Hill, 2001.

PERIODICALS
Lesch, M., and W. L. Nyhan. "A Familial Disorder of Uric Acid Metabolism and Central Nervous System Function." *American Journal of Medicine* 36 (1964): 561–570.

Mak, B. S., et al. "New Mutations of the HPRT Gene in Lesch-Nyhan Syndrome." *Pediatric Neurology* (October 2000): 332–335.

Visser, J. E., et al. "Lesch-Nyhan Disease and the Basal Ganglia." *Brain Research Reviews* (November 1999): 450–469.

ORGANIZATIONS
Alliance of Genetic Support Groups. 4301 Connecticut Ave. NW, Suite 404, Washington, DC 20008. (202) 966-5557. Fax: (202) 966-8553. <http://www.geneticalliance.org>.

International Lesch-Nyhan Disease Association. 114 Winchester Way, Shamong, NJ 08088-9398. (215) 677-4206.

Lesch-Nyhan Syndrome Registry. New York University School of Medicine, Department of Psychiatry, 550 First Ave., New York, NY 10012. (212) 263-6458.

National Organization for Rare Disorders (NORD). PO Box 8923, New Fairfield, CT 06812-8923. (203) 746-6518 or (800) 999-6673. Fax: (203) 746-6481. <http://www.rarediseases.org>.

WEBSITES
GeneClinics <http://www.geneclinics.org/profiles/lns/details.html>.

Pediatric Database (PEDBASE) <http://www.icondata.com/health/pedbase/files/LESCH-NY.HTM>.

Holly Ann Ishmael, MS, CGC
Rosalyn Carson-DeWitt, MD

Leukodystrophy

Definition

Leukodystrophy refers to a group of rare genetic disorders affecting the central and peripheral nervous systems. They are neurodegenerative diseases characterized by abnormalities in myelin, the fatty substance that surrounds, insulates, and facilitates the function of nerve cells.

Description

Leukodystrophy derives from two Greek words; "leuko" means white, referring to the white matter (myelin) of the nervous system, and "dystrophy" means abnormal growth or development. Myelin insulates, or sheaths, nerve cells, helping them to transmit electrical nerve signals. It is a complex substance composed of a number of fat and protein molecules. Without myelin, nerve cells cease to function and eventually die. It also covers the spinal cord and the long nerve cell projections, known as axons, which innervate all of the peripheral tissues.

Key Terms

Ataxia A condition marked by impaired muscular coordination, most frequently resulting from disorders in the brain or spinal cord.

Hypotonia Having reduced or diminished muscle tone or strength.

Mitochondria Spherical or rod-shaped structures of the cell. Mitochondria contain genetic material (DNA and RNA) and are responsible for converting food to energy.

Myelin A fatty sheath surrounding nerves throughout the body that helps them conduct impulses more quickly.

Neuropathy A disease or abnormality of the peripheral nerves (the nerves outside the brain and spinal cord). Major symptoms include weakness, numbness, paralysis, or pain in the affected area.

Nystagmus An involuntary, rhythmic movement of the eyes.

Organelle A specialized structure within a cell, which is separated from the rest of the cell by a membrane composed of lipids and proteins, where chemical and metabolic functions take place.

Paraplegia Loss of voluntary movement and sensation of both lower extremities.

Peroxisome A cellular organelle containing different enzymes responsible for the breakdown of waste or other products.

Spasticity Increased mucle tone, or stiffness, which leads to uncontrolled, awkward movements.

More than 15 different types of leukodystrophy have been described, the most common of which will be discussed here. They are all caused by either an abnormality in one of the protein components of myelin, or by a defective or missing enzyme that assists in the production or normal degradation of myelin. As such, leukodystrophies are often referred to as demyelinating or dysmyelinating diseases, as well as leukoencepalopathies.

Based on the part of the nervous system that is most affected, leukodystrophies may be categorized as central (brain and spinal cord), peripheral, or combined. The neurologic symptoms vary widely, both within and between the different types. All types of leukodystrophy are genetic (present at conception), progressive, and never spontaneously resolve. None of the leukodystrophies can be cured, and effective treatments are limited.

Demographics

Most of the individual leukodystrophies are rare. The most common type is **Canavan disease**, with an incidence of about one in 8,000, followed by X-linked **adrenoleukodystrophy** (XL-ALD), which occurs in one in 40,000 male births. Some types of leukodystrophy are more common in certain ethnic groups, such as Canavan disease in Ashkenazi Jews, or globoid cell leukodystrophy (GLD) and **metachromatic leukodystrophy** (MLD) in Scandinavians.

As indicated, all types of leukodystrophy are genetic, with several patterns of inheritance represented. Genes reside on the chromosomes in the nucleus of each cell; a normal complement is 46 chromosomes arranged in 23 pairs. The first 22 pairs are the autosomes, and the last pair, designated X and Y, are the sex chromosomes. Males have one X and one Y, while females have two X chromosomes. One of each chromosome/gene pair is contributed by each parent at conception.

Autosomal recessive inheritance refers to a disorder that only occurs if both copies of a gene pair are defective. An affected individual is typically born to unaffected parents, who each silently carry one copy of the disease gene. Each time parents who both carry the same recessive gene conceive a pregnancy, there is a 25% chance they will both transmit the disease gene and have an affected child.

Autosomal dominant inheritance requires that only one copy of a gene pair be defective in order to develop the disorder. Each offspring of a parent with an autosomal dominant disorder has a 50% risk of inheriting the gene. In some conditions (e.g., **Alexander disease**), most cases are due to a new mutation of the gene in a sperm or egg (unaffected parent).

A male who inherits the gene for an X-linked recessive disorder develops the condition because he has no normal gene on a second X chromosome to compensate for it. Female carriers of an X-linked recessive disorder are usually unaffected, but not always. If they do develop signs/symptoms, they tend to have later onset and milder symptoms. A woman who carries an X-linked recessive gene faces one of four possible outcomes with each pregnancy: affected male, unaffected male, carrier female, and noncarrier female. If an affected male has children, all of his daughters will be carriers, but none of his sons will be affected.

Causes and symptoms

All of the leukodystrophies are caused by either a defective protein component of myelin, or by a malfunctioning enzyme that interacts with one of the protein or lipid constituents. In some cases, defective, deficient, or absent myelin may cause neurons in the central or **peripheral nervous system** to degenerate. In other cases the neurons remain intact, but transmission of normal signals through the nerves is affected. Brief synopses of the most common leukodystrophies are provided below.

Adrenoleukodystrophy (ALD), also called Addison disease with cerebral sclerosis, or melanodermic leukodystrophy, is inherited primarily as an X-linked recessive trait, but there is also a rare autosomal recessive form (neonatal ALD). X-linked ALD is caused by defects in the ABCD1 gene, also known as the ALDP (ALD protein) gene. A defective enzyme in the peroxisomes (organelles that assist in degrading substances, including some components of myelin) fails to break down very long chain fatty acids (VLCFA), which then accumulate to harmful levels in the nervous system and adrenal glands. About 35% of affected individuals have the childhood or adolescent cerebral form of ALD, which is the most severe. Age of onset ranges from four to ten years, with initial symptoms of behavioral changes, hyperactivity, and learning problems. The skin takes on a bronzed appearance due to adrenal gland dysfunction. Within several years, significant visual and auditory deficits develop, motor coordination worsens, and nearly all boys with the condition are in a vegetative state by their mid-teens. Adult adrenomyeloneuropathy (AMN) affects 30% of men with ALD, onset of symptoms may occur anywhere from adolescence to late adulthood, and progression of the disorder may occur over several decades. Adrenal dysfunction occurs first, and subsequent neurological impairments may include spastic paraplegia, **peripheral neuropathy**, impotence, sphincter disturbances, and hypogonadism. Approximately 10% of individuals develop an adult cerebral form, which is similar to the childhood variety, but with milder symptoms and slower progression. Another 15% have adrenal insufficiency only, and 10% of males who are positive for an ALDP gene mutation are presymptomatic at the time of testing. About 15% of carrier females develop some degree of neurologic impairment.

Alexander disease is designated as an autosomal dominant condition, but most reported cases are thought to be due to new mutations in the glial fibrillary acidic protein gene (GFAP). The average age of onset in the infantile form is six months, with death by age five. Signs/symptoms include progressive macrocephaly (large head),

psychomotor regression, **spasticity**, and **seizures**. The less common juvenile and adult forms have a slower clinical course, present with **ataxia** and spasticity, but usually have normal intellect. Affected adults may show relapsing-remitting symptoms, similar to **multiple sclerosis**. The presence of Rosenthal fibers and glial fibrillary acidic proteins (GFAP) around the nerves are classic histological signs.

Canavan disease, also referred to as spongy degeneration of the CNS, is autosomal recessive, secondary to mutations in the aspartoacylase gene (ASPA). Symptoms typically begin two to four months after birth, with death occurring by 10 years of age. Signs/symptoms include increased head circumference, deafness, optic atrophy, nystagmus, blindness, initial **hypotonia** followed by spasticity, and seizures.

Cerebrotendinous xanthomatosis (CTX) is autosomal recessive, and results from mutations in the CYP27A1 gene. Large deposits of cholesterol and one of its derivatives, cholestanol, are found throughout the body, particularly the Achilles tendons, brain, and lungs. Most individuals with CTX have been diagnosed as juveniles. Signs/symptoms include cataracts and tendon xanthomas (fatty tumors) in the early stages, with ataxia, spasticity, mild **mental retardation**, **dementia**, psychiatric symptoms, respiratory insufficiency, and myocardial infarction due to atherosclerosis developing over subsequent decades.

Globoid cell leukodystrophy (GLD), also known as **Krabbe disease** and galactocerebrosidase deficiency, is autosomal recessively inherited, and caused by defects in the glycosylceramidase (GALC) gene. The four clinical forms of GLD, based on age of onset, are infantile, late infantile, juvenile, and adult. About 90% are diagnosed with infantile GLD, with onset at several months of age, and severe neurologic deterioration progressing to death in early childhood. Signs/symptoms include deafness, blindness, irritability, episodic fever, mental deterioration, hypertonia in early stage, hypotonia later, seizures, motor deterioration, and peripheral neuropathy. The other forms of GLD vary widely in severity of symptoms and rate of progression, but those diagnosed later tend to have a better prognosis.

Leigh syndrome, also called subacute necrotizing **encephalopathy** (SNE), refers to at least eight distinct disorders inherited as autosomal recessive or X-linked recessive traits. Another six types exhibit an unusual hereditary pattern known as mitochondrial inheritance. Mitochondria are energy producing organelles that contain their own genes. With rare exceptions, all of the mitochondria in the first cell of the embryo come from the egg. Therefore, mitochondrial inheritance resembles X-linked recessive inheritance in that the disease can only be transmitted by women, with the difference, though, that both male and female children are equally affected. Symptoms of Leigh syndrome usually develop in infancy or early childhood (classic form), but later onset with milder symptoms may also occur. Age of onset and symptom severity can be quite variable in families with mitochondrial inheritance. Signs/symptoms include failure to thrive, optic atrophy, nystagmus, pigmentary retinopathy, abnormal respiratory patterns, respiratory failure, hypotonia, psychomotor retardation, ataxia, **dystonia**, spasticity, brainstem lesions, and mental retardation.

Leukoencephalopathy with Vanishing White Matter (LVWM) includes childhood ataxia with **central nervous system** hypomyelinization (CACH), Cree leukoencephalopathy (CLE), and ovarioleukodystrophy. All forms show autosomal recessive inheritance, and are caused by mutations in the EIF2B class of genes. Individuals with LVWM are typically diagnosed in childhood, but later diagnoses have been described. Symptoms mainly include ataxia, spasticity, and seizures. Optic atrophy may also be present, along with mild intellectual decline. Neurologic symptoms are progressive, and episodes of dramatic deterioration may follow infection or minor head trauma. Average age of onset of CLE is six months, followed by a rapid progression and death by two years of age. Symptoms include hypotonia, seizures, spasticity, vomiting, and diarrhea. Ovarioleukodystrophy presents with neurologic symptoms similar to those of LVWM, with the added finding in women of ovarian dysgenesis.

Metachromatic leukodystrophy (MLD), also called sulfatide lipidosis and arylsulfatase A (ARSA) deficiency, is inherited as an autosomal recessive trait, due to mutations in the arylsulfatase A (ARSA) gene. The late infantile form has onset at six to 24 months, and the primary early symptoms are speech difficulties, gait disturbance, behavioral problems, and intellectual decline. The disease progresses rapidly; seizures, blindness, and severe muscle contractions may occur, and most children are bedridden by early childhood. Juvenile and adult forms of MLD typically first present with psychological symptoms and decreasing intellectual performance. Disease progression is similar to the late infantile form, but may occur over several years to several decades.

Pelizaeus-Merzbacher disease (PMD), which includes spastic paraplegia 2 (SPG2), is X-linked recessive, and caused by mutations in the PLP1 gene. Signs/symptoms in the classical form (type 1) develop in infancy and progress slowly, with death occurring in late adolescence or early adulthood. The connatal form (type 2) also develops in infancy, but progresses more rapidly. Initial, stereotypical symptoms involve rotary movements of the head and eyes, which may later disappear. Other symptoms include hypotonia, choreoathetosis (slow or jerky involuntary movements), spasticity, cerebellar ataxia, dementia, and parkinsonian symptoms. Spastic paraplegia is the primary, initial symptom in SPG2. Depending on the type of gene mutation in the family, occasional carrier females may develop some neurologic symptoms.

Refsum disease, also called hereditary motor and sensory neuropathy (HMSN) IV, shows autosomal recessive inheritance, and is caused by mutations in the PAHX/PHYH or PEX7 genes. Individuals with Refsum disease are unable to metabolize phytanic acid, which then accumulates in tissues to harmful levels. Onset of symptoms occurs anywhere from childhood to late adulthood, but most individuals are diagnosed by age 20. Signs/symptoms include retinitis pigmentosa (vision loss), polyneuropathy, ataxia, **anosmia** (no sense of smell), nerve deafness, and ichthyosis (scaly skin).

Zellweger syndrome (ZS), also known as cerebrohepatorenal (CHR) syndrome, is autosomal recessively inherited, and caused by mutations in seven different genes affecting peroxisome function. They are especially numerous in the brain, liver, and kidneys. A set of distinctive facial/physical signs, anomalies, and neurologic symptoms are present at birth. The primary neurologic symptoms are failure to thrive (poor weight gain and lack of development of normal motor skills), mental retardation, hypotonia, and seizures. Most babies with ZS do not survive past 12 months.

Diagnosis

A wide variety of tests and procedures to diagnose leukodystrophy are available. The methods employed depend upon a clinician's suspected diagnosis, and this is based on physical and neurological findings, along with the presence or absence of a positive family history. Testing falls into several categories:

- Imaging studies, such as specialized **magnetic resonance imaging (MRI)**, to visualize any abnormalities of the white matter of the brain

- Histological (microscopic) studies on small samples of neural tissue to look for abnormal myelin and/or nerve cell structure

- Testing of peripheral nerve function using a procedure such as nerve conduction velocity (NCV), which measures how quickly electrical signals pass through nerves

- Biochemical studies to look for excess/diminished components or breakdown products of myelin, or defective/absent myelin-related enzymes

- Genetic testing to screen for mutations in one or more genes associated with the suspected leukodystrophy

Different types of leukodystrophy may mimic each other, as well as other neurodegenerative diseases (e.g., multiple sclerosis), so multiple tests could be attempted before a diagnosis is reached. A few individuals with a neurodegenerative disorder may never receive a diagnosis. A board-certified geneticist is most likely to make the correct diagnosis, using the fewest tests in the least amount of time.

Carrier testing, as well as prenatal diagnosis, depends upon the availability of an established biochemical or genetic marker. The availability and accuracy of these tests are constantly changing for all genetic disorders, and the interpretation of results may be complicated. For rare disorders such as the leukodystrophies, it is especially critical to seek a consultation with a genetics counselor or geneticist to obtain the most complete and current information available.

Treatment team

A **neurologist** manages the basic care of an individual with a neurodegenerative disorder. Given their special training and greater familiarity with these rare diseases, a geneticist would likely be consulted to make or confirm the diagnosis. The geneticist and/or genetics counselor also provides support for the family, along with the most current information on the natural history and inheritance of the disorder, options for diagnostic and prenatal testing, availability of specialized reproductive procedures, and referrals to other specialists and support groups. A diagnosis of leukodystrophy might also require involvement of neonatal intensive care unit (NICU) staff, a developmental pediatrician, occupational and physical therapists, and health professionals associated with institutional or specialized home care.

Treatment

In the majority of cases, there is no effective treatment for an individual diagnosed with a leukodystrophy. However, several of the conditions do respond to specific treatments.

Bone marrow transplantation has been shown to be successful in treating XL-ALD (and MLD), but only in very specific situations. The use of "Lorenzo's oil," a food product consisting of oleic acid, to treat XL-ALD has not been shown in multiple studies to provide any consistent benefit. Adrenal insufficiency in ALD can be successfully managed with the use of glucocorticosteroids.

Effective treatment of Refsum disease is possible with a diet low in phytanic acid. Improvements in ataxia, neuropathy and ichthyosis are seen, but the diet cannot restore any vision or hearing loss that has occurred.

The use of chenodeoxycholic acid and cholic acid (CDCA), in combination with a cholesterol lowering drug, for the treatment of CTX has been successful in stopping the progression of the disease.

In general, all that can be offered to most individuals with a leukodystrophy is supportive care and therapy to address their neurologic symptoms.

Clinical trials

As of 2004, a primary focus for research on the treatment of leukodystrophies is on the use of stem cells from umbilical cord blood for transplantation, known as allogeneic hematopoietic stem cell transplantation. The cells are easily obtained, and are less likely than bone marrow to elicit immune system reactions in the patient. There has been some success in treating GLD, and there is hope that both XL-ALD and MLD will respond favorably as well. Both the United Leukodystrophy Foundation (ULF) and the National Institute of Neurological Disorders and Stroke (NINDS) (see below) are excellent sources of information for research being conducted on the various forms of leukodystrophy.

Prognosis

The prognosis for leukodystrophy depends on the specific diagnosis. In general, a younger age of symptom onset implies a worse prognosis. With few effective treatments, and the progressive nature of hereditary, myelin-related disorders, the overall prognosis for individuals with leukodystrophy is poor.

Resources

BOOKS

Bradley, Walter G, et al, eds. *Neurology in Clinical Practice.* 3rd ed. Boston: Butterworth-Heinemann, 2000.

Victor, Maurice and Allan H. Ropper. *Adams' and Victor's Principles of Neurology.* 7th ed. New York: The McGraw-Hill Companies, Inc., 2001.

Wiederholt, Wigbert C. *Neurology for Non-Neurologists.* 4th ed. Philadelphia: W.B. Saunders Company, 2000.

PERIODICALS

Kristjansdottir, R., et al. "Cerebrospinal Fluid Markers in Children with Cerebral White Matter Abnormalities." *Neuropediatrics.* 32 (August 2001): 176-182.

Moroni, I., et al. "Cerebral White Matter Involvement in Children with Mitochondrial Encephalopathies." *Neuropediatrics.* 33 (April 2002): 79-85.

Moser, H.W., et al. "X-Linked Adrenoleukodystrophy: Overview and Prognosis as a Function of Age and Brain Magnetic Resonance Imaging Abnormality. A Study Involving 372 Patients." *Neuropediatrics.* 31 (October 2000): 227-239.

Schiffmann, Raphael and Marjo S. van der Knaap. "The latest on leukodystrophies." *Current Opinions in Neurology*. 17 (April 2004): 187-192.

ORGANIZATIONS

Association for Neuro-Metabolic Disorders. 5223 Brookfield Lane, Sylvania, OH 43560-1809. 419-885-1497.

Kennedy Krieger Institute. 707 North Broadway, Baltimore, MD 21205. 888-554-2080. <http://www.kennedykrieger.org>.

MLD Foundation. 21345 Miles Drive, West Linn, OR 97068-2878. 800-617-8387; Fax: 503-212-0159. <http://www.MLDfoundation.org>.

National Tay-Sachs and Allied Diseases Association, Inc. 2001 Beacon Street, Boston, MA 02135. 800-906-8723. <http://www.NTSAD.org>.

NIH/NINDS Brain Resources and Information Network. PO Box 5801, Bethesda, MD 20824. 800-352-9424. <http://www.ninds.nih.gov/>.

United Leukodystrophy Foundation. 2304 Highland Drive, Sycamore, IL 60178. 800-728-5483. <http://www.ulf.org/>.

Scott J. Polzin, MS, CGC

Levetiracetam

Definition

Levetiracetam is an anti-epileptic drug (AED). It is often used in combination with other medications in the treatment of **epilepsy**, a neurological dysfunction in which excessive surges of electrical energy are emitted in the brain.

Purpose

While levetiracetam controls the partial **seizures** (focal seizures) associated with epilepsy, there is no known cure for the disorder. In partial epileptic seizures, neural disturbances are limited to a specific region of the brain and the affected person usually remains conscious throughout the seizure. Although the precise mechanisms by which it works are unknown, levetiracetam is thought to exert its therapeutic effect by decreasing the abnormal activity and excitement within the area brain that may trigger partial seizures.

Research indicates that levetiracetam may also be effective in treating neurogenic **pain**.

Description

In the United States, levetiracetam is sold under the brand name Keppra. A newer generation medication, levetiracetam lacks many of the usual side effects commonly

---

Key Terms

Epilepsy A disorder associated with disturbed electrical discharges in the central nervous system that cause seizures.

Neurogenic pain Pain originating in the nerves or nervous tissue.

Partial seizure An episode of abnormal activity in a localized (specific) part of the brain that causes changes in attention, movement, or behavior.

---

assiocated with other AEDs. Levetiracetam has fewer negative interactions with other AEDs or anti-convulsants, and may be used in combination with other AEDs in the treatment of epilepsy.

Recommended dosage

Levetiracetam is taken by mouth in tablet form. It is available in 250 mg, 500 mg, and 750 mg tablets. Levetiracetam is prescribed by physicians in varying total daily dosages, usually from 1000 mg to 3000 mg. Patients typically take divided doses (equal to one half of the total daily dose) twice daily.

Like many other AEDs, beginning a course of treatment which includes levetiracetam requires a gradual dose-increasing regimen. Adults and teenagers 16 years or older typically take 1000 mg a day for the first two weeks. Daily dosages of levetiracetam may then be increased by as much as 1000 mg every two weeks until reaching the maximum therapeutic dose (usually not more than 3000 mg). It may take several weeks to realize the full benefits of levetiracetam.

It is important not to take a double dose of levetiracetam. If a dose is missed, it should be taken as soon as possible. However, if it is almost time for the next dose, then the missed dose should be skipped.

When ending treatment of AEDs, including levetiracetam, physicians typically direct patients to gradually reduce their daily dosages over a period of several weeks. Stopping the medicine suddenly may cause seizures to return or occur more frequently.

Precautions

A physician should be consulted before taking levetiracetam with certain non-perscription medications. Patients should avoid alcohol and CNS depressants (medications that make one drowsy or tired, such as antihistimines, sleep medications, and some pain medications) while taking levetiracetam. It can exacerbate the side effects of alcohol and other medications.

Levetiracetam may not be suitable for persons with a history of kidney disease, depressed renal function, or mental illness.

Before beginning treatment with levetiracetam, patients should notify their physician if they consume a large amount of alcohol, have a history of drug use, are pregnant, or plan to become pregnant. Levetiracetam's safety during pregnancy has not been established. Patients taking levetiracetam with other AEDs or anti-convulsants should be aware that many AEDs and anti-convulsants have been shown to cause birth defects in animals. Patients who become pregnant while taking any AED or anti-convulsants should contact their physician immediately.

Side effects

Research indicates that levetiracetam is generally well tolerated and lacks many of the traditional side effects associated with AEDs. However, levetiracetam may case a variety of usually mild side effects in some patients. Cough, **dizziness**, and muscle weakness are the most frequently reported side effects of levetiracetam. Other possible side effects that do not usually require medical attention include:

- dryness or soreness of throat
- fever
- hoarseness or voice changes
- sleepiness or unusual drowsiness
- tender, swollen glands in neck
- numbness, prickling, "pins and needles," or tingling feelings
- loss of appetite or weight loss

Many of these side effects disappear or occur less frequently during treatment as the body adjusts to the medication. However, if any symptoms persist or become too uncomfortable, consult the prescribing physician.

Other, uncommon side effects of levetiracetam can indicate a potentially serious condition. A patient taking levetiracetam who experiencs any of the following symptoms should immediately contact their physician:

- clumsiness or unsteadiness
- depression, paranoia, or other significant mood changes
- double vision
- problems with memory
- lower back or side pain
- painful or difficult urination
- shortness of breath, wheezing, or troubled breathing.

Interactions

Levetiracetam is often used with other other seizure prevention medications, as prescribed by a physician. Unlike many other AEDs and anti-convulsants, levetiracetam does not decrease the effectiveness of oral contraceptives (birth control pills).

Resources

BOOKS

Weaver, Donald F. *Epilepsy and Seizures: Everything You Need to Know.* Firefly Books, 2001.

PERIODICALS

Hadjikoutis, S., et. al. "Weight loss associated with levetiracetam." *British Medical Journal* 327, no. 7420 (October 18, 2003): 905.

Shorvon, S. D., and K. van Rijckevorsel. "A new antiepileptic drug: levetiracetam, a pyrrolidone recently licensed as an antiepileptic drug." *Journal of Neurology, Neurosurgery and Psychiatry* 72, no. 4 (April 2002): 426.

OTHER

"Levetiracetam (Systemic)." *Medline Plus.* National Library of Medicine. (April 20, 2004). <http://www.nlm.nih.gov/medlineplus/druginfo/uspdi/500101.html>

ORGANIZATIONS

Epilepsy Foundation. 4351 Garden City Drive, Landover, MD 20785-7223, USA. (800) 332-1000. <http://www.epilepsyfoundation.org>.

American Epilepsy Society. 342 North Main Street, West Hartford, CT 06117-2507, USA. <http://www.aesnet.org>.

Adrienne Wilmoth Lerner

Levodopa *see* **Antiparkinson drugs**

Lewy body dementia

Definition

Lewy body **dementia** (LBD) is a neurodegenerative disorder that can occur in persons older than 65 years of age, which typically causes symptoms of cognitive (thinking) impairment and abnormal behavioral changes.

Description

The condition was first described by Frederick Lewy in 1941 when he described Lewy bodies, which are abnormal inclusions in the cytoplasm (components of a cell outside the nucleus) of cells found in patients who had

Parkinson's disease (PD). There is some controversy concerning the relationship between Lewy body dementia and Parkinson's disease. When cognitive impairment and behavioral disturbance are early and prominent symptoms, then LBD is the likely diagnosis. When motor symptoms are the predominant and early symptoms, then Parkinson's disease is likely to be the diagnosis. Typically, on autopsy examination of the brain, both PD and LBD would probably demonstrate Lewy bodies. Autopsy examination is the only method to available for a definitive diagnosis.

The signs and symptoms of LBD stem from a multifactorial cause of disrupted bidirectional (two-way) information flow in neurons, especially those located in the frontal lobe; that is, there are abnormalities in the chemicals that regulate and pass on message signals between neurons in the brain. Alterations in neurotransmitter chemicals can also impair nerve cell circuitry, causing abnormalities in bidirectional information flow.

Most patients with LBD also have brain evidence of Alzheimer's disease pathology. Additionally, most patients with LBD possess amyloid plaques in their cerebral cortex. Lewy bodies can also occur in a genetically transmitted form of Alzheimer's disease, Pick's disease, and Down syndrome.

Demographics

Dementia (used as a general term) has been an increasingly common disorder that is especially more frequent in the elderly. Dementia affects 7% of the general population older than 65 years and that incidence increases with age to 30% of those age 80 years and older. Autopsy results in the United States estimate that LBD accounts for 10–20% of dementia cases. Approximately 40% of patients with Alzheimer's disease also have LBD. Data from autopsy results in Europe and Japan reveal similar frequencies as reported in studies from the United States. No data is available concerning age, gender, or potential risk factors.

Causes and symptoms

The formation of Lewy bodies is thought to occur because of an abnormal increase in the production of a normally occurring protein in nerve cells called alpha-synuclein. Called upregulation, this overproduction can cause substances to accumulate or multiply in increased numbers. Other theories propose that alpha-synuclein may become insoluble (unable to mix in a watery environment), which could make the molecule more prone to accumulate abnormally in the brain.

Symptoms can include cognitive impairment, neurological signs, sleep disorder, and autonomic failure. Cognitive impairment is the presenting feature of LBD in most cases. Patients have recurrent episodes of confusion that progressively worsen. The fluctuation in cognitive ability is often associated with shifting degrees of attention and alertness. Cognitive impairment and fluctuations of thinking may vary over minutes, hours, or days.

Psychological manifestations

Psychological manifestations of LBD predominantly include:

- delusions, false beliefs, or wrong judgments held to be true despite incontrovertible evidence to the contrary
- visual hallucinations, strong subjective perception of an imaginary event or object
- apathy, an indifference or absence of interest in the environment
- anxiety, apprehension, or dread that causes symptoms of rapid heart rate, restlessness, tension, and shortness of breath

Neurological symptoms in patients affected with LBD include extrapyramidal features early in the disease. The extrapyramidal symptoms in LBD can be differentiated from other dementias such as Parkinson's disease. Patients affected with LBD tend to show axial involvement with greater postural instability and facial impassivity, and less tremor. Disorders of sleep in patients with LBD typically can include impairment of rapid-eye-movement (REM) sleep; REM sleep behavior disorder causes vivid and frightening dreams. Patients may also exhibit loss of muscle tone or cataplexy, hypersomnolence (an increased inclination to sleep), hallucinations, and **narcolepsy**. Patients with LBD also have deficits in the autonomic nervous system, part of which regulates specific body functions such as blood pressure and bladder control. Autonomic abnormalities can cause **orthostatic hypotension** and urinary incontinence.

Diagnosis

Clinically, patients have features of fluctuating cognitive impairment such as from alert to confused state, recurrent visual **hallucination**, **depression**, and REM sleep disorder. Patients may have impairment of memory retrieval and they often do poorly on tests that measure visuospatial skills such as copying figures or drawing a clock. Patients may have mild gait (walking) impairment. An accurate diagnosis can include identification of target symptoms, including cognitive impairment, psychological disorders (hallucinations, depression, sleep disorder, and behavioral disturbances), extrapyramidal motor features or **autonomic dysfunction** (orthostatic hypotension), or urinary incontinence. Standard blood tests are ordered and additional tests are typically required, including thyroid studies, vitamin B-12 levels, and, if appropriate, tests for **Lyme disease**, syphilis, or HIV since these infections can affect the brain. Currently, there are no specific tests used

Key Terms

Alzheimer's disease A neurodegenerative disorder that causes nerve-cell death and symptoms that typically include loss of thinking and language ability, and memory impairment.

Autonomic failure Refers to failure in the autonomic nervous system, which comprises two divisions called the parasympathetic nervous system, which slows heart rate, increases intestinal and gland activity, and relaxes sphincter muscles; and the sympathetic nervous system, which accelerates heart rate, raises blood pressure, and constricts blood vessels.

Cataplexy A sudden loss of muscle tone.

Dementia A progressive loss of intellectual functions without impairment of consciousness or perception. The condition is often associated with brain disease and persons exhibit symptoms such as disorientation and impaired memory, judgment, and intellect.

Down syndrome A genetic disorder, also called trisomy 21, characterized by mental retardation, heart defects, slanting eyes, short fingers, broad short skull, and broad hands.

Hallucinations False perceptions that can occur without a true sensory stimulus.

Narcolepsy A genetically determined disorder characterized by recurrent episodes of daytime sleep, disrupted nighttime sleep, cataplexy, hallucinations, and sleep paralysis.

Orthostatic hypotension A fall in blood pressure due to a change in body position, usually from the sitting position to an erect or standing position.

Parkinson's disease A neurodegenerative disorder that results in changes to neurons in the brain stem, causing affected persons to have symptoms that include a resting tremor, speech impairments, movement disorders, shuffling walk, stooped posture, and dementia.

Pick's disease A neurological degenerative disorder that causes deterioration of social skills and personality, and causes impairment of memory, language, and intellect.

Urinary incontinence Unable to control urinary excretion.

to diagnose LBD. A **magnetic resonance imaging (MRI)** scan is indicated to distinguish LBD from another disorder called vascular dementia, which can present with similar clinical signs and symptoms. It is important to exclude diseases or drugs that can cause **delirium**.

Treatment team

The treatment team can be broad, including general practitioners, geriatric psychotherapists, emergency services, or movement disorder specialists. Additionally, the team can include family members, primary care practitioners, caregivers, and neurologists. Special consultations from a **neurologist** with special expertise in dementias may be appropriate for caregiver education.

Treatment

The management of LBD can be approached in four stages: accurate diagnosis, identification of target symptoms, nonpharmacological treatment, and pharmacological treatment. Nonpharmacological interventions include management of environment and other necessities associated with LBD patient care. Caregiving skills should be specifically tailored to the patient. Pharmacological treatment can include several different medications, most notably a class of drugs called **cholinesterase inhibitors**.

These medications tend to increase a brain neurochemical called acetylcholine, which is an excitatory brain chemical that is decreased in persons with LBD. With a typical dose of a cholinesterase inhibitor (Donepezil or Aricept), the symptoms of visual hallucinations, apathy, anxiety, sleep disorder, and cognitive impairments can be improved. Generally, medications can be utilized to slow the rate of cognitive decline, treat agitation and hallucinations, treat depression, and improve cognition and/or alertness.

Recovery and rehabilitation

Generally, there are no dietary restrictions for persons affected with LBD, except for those who have swallowing impairment. Physical therapy and an **exercise** program can be useful to maintain mobility. There are potential problems for patients who drive a motor vehicle, and family members and caregivers should be advised.

Clinical trials

Currently, the National Institute of Neurological Disorders and Stroke (NINDS) supports research concerning diagnosis, prevention, and treatment. Research efforts studying the biological consequences of Lewy body formation and mechanisms of disease progression are funded by NINDS.

Prognosis

LBD is a slowly progressive chronic disorder. However, the rate of progression may be faster than in Alzheimer's disease. The disease is fatal from complications of poor nutrition, swallowing difficulties, and immobility.

Special concerns

Primary caregivers and family members require information concerning management of symptoms such as hallucinations, agitation, and cognitive changes. Children of patients with LBD may require genetic counseling. Family members should be aware that LBD affects job performance and medical leave of absence or early retirement may be advisable. Driving may become problematic and should be addressed with the medical treatment team, patient, and family.

Resources

BOOKS

Goetz, Christopher G., et al, eds. *Textbook of Clinical Neurology*, 1st ed. Philadelphia: W. B. Saunders Company, 1999.

Goldman, Lee, et al. *Cecil's Textbook of Medicine*, 21st ed. Philadelphia: W. B. Saunders Company, 2000.

PERIODICALS

McKeith, Ian. "Dementia with Lewy bodies." *The Lancet Neurology* 3, no. 1 (January 2004).

WEBSITES

Crystal, Howard A. *eMedicine—Dementia with Lewy Bodies.* November 11, 2003 (May 23, 2004). <http://www.emedicine.com/neuro/topic91.htm>.

Lewy Body Dementia. <http://www.alzheimer.ca> (May 23, 2004).

National Organization for Rare Disorders (NORD). <http://www.rarediseases.org> (May 23, 2004).

ORGANIZATIONS

National Institute on Aging, National Institutes of Health. Building 31, Room 5C27, Bethesda, MD 20892-2292. (301) 496-1752. <http://nih.gov/nia>.

Laith Farid Gulli, MD
Robert Ramirez, DO
Nicole Mallory, MS, PA-C

Lidocaine patch

Definition

Lidocaine belongs to a class of local and topical anesthetic medications. As lidocaine causes a temporary numbness or loss of sensation when injected in the tissues, it is used as a local anesthetic and in the treatment of **pain**.

When given intravenously, lidocaine is also an antiarrythmic agent, capable of correcting some ventricular arrythmias of the heart. The lidocaine patch is a topical treatment that is especially helpful in the treatment of pain associated with postherpetic neuralgia, a condition that can occur after infection with the herpes varicella zoster (**shingles**) virus. Additionally, the lidocaine patch is sometimes used in the treatment of some chronic forms of nerve pain such as the pain associated with fibromyalgia.

Purpose

The lidocaine patch relieves pain and discomfort by blocking signals sent to nerve endings in the skin. Almost 20% of the one million Americans who develop shingles yearly experience long-term pain after the infection has resolved. People over age 60 are especially prone to postherpetic neuralgia.

Description

The lidocaine patch is composed of an adhesive material containing 5% lidocaine that is applied to a polyester felt backing. When it is applied to the skin, lidocaine is released into the epidermal and dermal layers of the skin, reducing pain at the site of the dysfunctional nerves damaged by the prior herpes zoster infection. The lidocaine patch provides pain reduction without numbness of the affected skin.

In the United States, the lidocaine patch is sold under the name of Lidoderm.

Recommended dosage

The lidocaine patch is available in varying doses. Patches are applied directly to healthy, non-broken skin close to the source of pain or discomfort. Patients may typically apply up to three patches at one time. However, patches should not be worn longer than 12 hours in a 24-hour period. Patches can be cut into smaller pieces before removing the release liner and applying to the skin. Clothing may be worn over the applied patch.

If a dose is missed, it should be taken as soon as possible. However, if it is almost time for the next dose, then the missed dose should be skipped. More patches than are instructed by the prescribing physician should never be applied.

Precautions

Lidocaine may not be suitable for persons who have had a past reaction to any local anesthetic. Patients should discuss past adverse reactions to anesthetics with their physician before using the lidocaine patch. The lidocaine patch may also not be suitable for persons with a history of severe liver disease. Additionally, the lidocaine patch should be used with caution in persons receiving antiar-ryhthmic drugs.

Hand-washing is important after handling or applying the lidocaine patch. Contact with eyes should be avoided. The zipper pouch containing the lidocaine patches should be completely closed after opening, as the patches will lose potency if allowed to dry. Patches can be cut with scissors to the size and shape necessary to fit facial areas, but care should be used not to allow the material in the lidocaine patch to enter the eye. The lidocaine patch should never be chewed or ingested, or used to relieve pain inside the mouth.

Side effects

As only minute amounts of lidocaine enter the bloodstream from the patch, side effects are few. Most patients tolerate normal use of the lidocaine patch well, but some patients may experience usually mild side effects. Localized tingling may occur. If a rash or burning sensation occurs after application, the patch should be removed and not reapplied until the irritation subsides. If any symptom becomes uncomfortable, patients should consult the prescribing physician.

Some patients may be allergic to topical lidocaine and the lidocaine patch. Medical treatment should be sought immediately if any of the following symptoms occur:

- cough
- difficulty breathing or swelling of the tongue
- dizziness, **fainting**, or loss of consciousness
- hives or swelling of the face
- trouble breathing

Other less common side effects of the lidocaine patch may be serious, potentially indicating that too much medication is being absorbed into the body. A patient should seek medical treatment if experiencing:

- excessive, all-over numbness

- blurred or double vision
- ringing or buzzing in the ears
- uncontrollable nervousness, shaking
- slow heartbeat

Interactions

As the lidocaine patch is topical treatment and only minute amounts of the drug are absorbed into the bloodstream, interactions with other drugs are few. The lidocaine patch may have rare negative interactions with digoxin (Lanoxin) or any medications for irregular heartbeats. Some antibiotics, antidepressants, and monoamine oxidase inhibitors (MAOIs) may adversely react with the lidocaine patch or lessen its effectiveness.

Resources

PERIODICALS

Alper, B. S., and P. R. Lewis. "Treatment of Postherpetic Neuralgia: A Systemic Review of the Literature." *Journal Fam. Pract.* (2002): 51: 121–8.

Argoff, C. E. "New Analgesics for Neuropathic Pain: The Lidocaine Patch." *Clin. Journal Pain* (2000): 16: S62–66.

Watson, C. P. "A New Treatment for Postherpetic Neuralgia." *New England Journal Med.* (2000): 343: 1563–65.

OTHER

"Lidocaine Patch Effective in Relieving Nerve Pain After Shingles." *The Doctors' Guide.* June 4, 1999. May 13, 2004 (June 1, 2004). <http://www.pslgroup.com/dg/102db6.htm>.

"Lidocaine Transdermal." *Medline Plus.* National Library of Medicine. <http://www.nlm.nih.gov/medlineplus/druginfo/medmaster/a603026.html>.

Adrienne Wilmoth Lerner

Lissencephaly

Definition

Lissencephaly is a neurological disorder of early brain development that leads to the gross appearance of a smooth brain. The malformed brain lacks the characteristic convolutions of the normal cerebral cortex and is abnormally thick. Lissencephaly is part of a spectrum of brain malformations, which are referred to as the agyria-pachygyria-band spectrum and are caused by abnormalities in neuronal migration, a critical process in brain development. These disorders range from complete absence of folds (agyria) to milder forms such as subcortical band heterotopia or double cortex syndrome, a neurological disorder where the malformed brain has two distinct

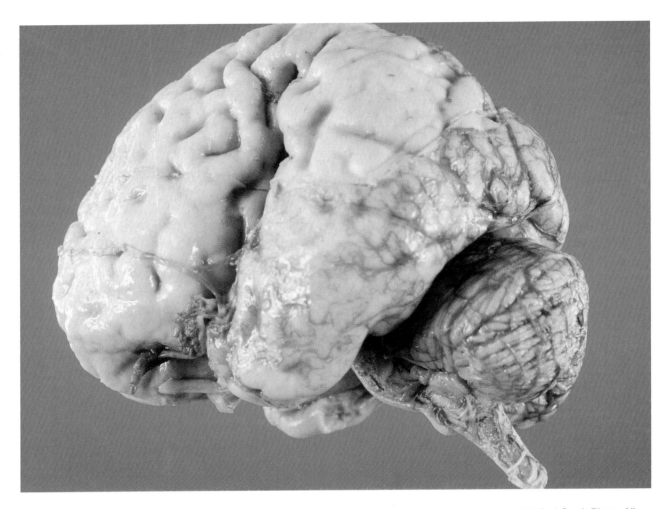

The disconnected hemispheres of a brain affected with agenesis of the corpus callosum. *(Custom Medical Stock Photo. All Rights Reserved.)*

layers of cerebral cortex. In pachygyria, there are localized areas of abnormally large folds and, in general, it is less severe than agyria. Scientific research on mice and humans has revealed several important genes responsible for causing lissencephaly.

Description

Lissencephaly was first described by Owen in 1868 and means "smooth brain," which describes the gross appearance of the brain. Microscopically, the brain appears abnormally thick and disorganized. The layering of the cerebral cortex is grossly abnormal, with four layers instead of the normal six layers.

Lissencephaly can be divided into two main subtypes. Type I, also known as classical lissencephaly, is distinguished by the smooth surface of the cerebral cortex and an abnormal four-layered cortex. Classical lissencephaly can be associated with abnormalities of the rest of the brain, including malformation of the corpus callosum or

cerebellum. Lissencephaly can also be associated with other developmental abnormalities such as facial deformities in a syndrome known as the Miller-Dieker syndrome. Type II, or "cobblestone" lissencephaly, is characterized by a bumpy appearance of the abnormal surface of the brain. The cortex in Type II lissencephaly is completely abnormal and there are no distinguishable layers. This subtype tends to be associated with genetic syndromes affecting muscles, as in the Walker-Warburg syndrome. Different genes and distinct processes are thought to be responsible for causing the two types of lissencephaly.

Demographics

Type I lissencephaly is more common and comprises 43% of lissencephaly syndromes in some studies. Type II lissencephaly accounted for 14% of lissencephalies. The remainder in these studies were comprised of various disorders such as pachygyria.

Key Terms

Cerebral cortex The layer of gray matter that makes up the surface of cerebral hemispheres of the brain. It is responsible for controlling sensation, movement, and higher cognitive functions.

Causes and symptoms

Lissencephaly is due to a defect in neuronal migration, a sequence of events in early brain development in which nerve cells travel to their final destinations to populate and form the six layers of the cerebral cortex. This process occurs between 12 and 16 weeks gestation. When the brain first forms, neurons are generated in a region of the brain known as the ventricular zone. From there, they travel by crawling outward along other cells, known as radial glia, to reach the cortical surface. The traveling neurons need instructions on when to start, continue, and stop moving, and these processes are controlled by a complicated molecular machinery.

Several genes have been implicated in causing lissencephaly, and their roles in neuronal migration are currently being characterized. The first gene causing lissencephaly, LIS1, was identified in patients with Miller-Dieker syndrome, a genetic syndrome caused by deletions of chromosome 17 that is a combination of lissencephaly and other facial deformities. So far, five genes have been identified that cause type I lissencephaly in humans. Among them, LIS1, DCX, and RELN have been implicated as important at various steps during neuronal migration. DCX, a gene on the X-chromosome, is responsible for the double cortex syndrome, a milder subtype of lissencephaly, which has the unusual appearance of a brain with two layers of cerebral cortex, one normal and one abnormally situated in the white matter. This abnormal layer, called a band heterotopia, represents the neurons that have started and failed to migrate completely to their destination. For type II lissencephaly, only one gene, fukutin, has been identified. Presumably, the disorder in type II lissencephaly is an abnormal overmigration of neurons, which causes nerve cells to accumulate beyond the cortical surface, leading to the cobblestone appearance. Other nongenetic causes of lissencephaly include cytomegalovirus infection.

Babies with lissencephaly may appear normal at birth, but then progress to severe developmental delay, **seizures**, and failure to thrive at several months of age. There may be abnormally small head size, known as **microcephaly**. Seizures are usually difficult to treat and start out in the first few months of life. Patients may also develop **cerebral palsy** and decreased muscle tone. Patients with milder forms such as double cortex syndrome may not develop symptoms until later in early childhood. They may have only mild developmental delay and seizures without microcephaly.

Diagnosis

Diagnosis is usually made by neuroimaging. A computer tomography (**CT**) or **magnetic resonance imaging (MRI)** scan shows a smooth brain with the lack of characteristic folds. MRI may delineate the band of abnormal nerve cells in the double cortex syndrome. MRI may also show abnormalities in other areas of the brain in certain forms of lissencephaly. Genetic testing can be performed in patients with lissencephaly to identify abnormalities in the LIS1 or DCX gene.

Treatment team

Management of lissencephaly usually involves a pediatrician, pediatric **neurologist**, and physical therapists. A geneticist may be involved to provide counseling and advice about family planning. Depending on the age of onset of symptoms, an adult neurologist may be involved in treating symptoms of seizures. A case manager may be involved in coordinating the different care needs of the patient and families.

Treatment

Currently, there is no cure for lissencephaly. Treatment of individuals with lissencephaly depends on the manifesting symptoms. Patients may need anticonvulsant drug therapy for treatment of seizures. Muscle relaxants may be used for symptoms of increased tone.

Recovery and rehabilitation

Due to the congenital nature of lissencephaly, patients show little recovery from their symptoms. Physical therapists may help treat symptoms of weakness or increased tone associated with lissencephaly.

Clinical trials

A clinical trial is currently ongoing and is funded by the National Institutes of Health to identify genes responsible for **neuronal migration disorders** such as lissencephaly and **schizencephaly**.

Prognosis

There is no known cure for lissencephaly. Most individuals will die at an early age due to failure to thrive or infections such as pneumonia. Patients with milder forms such as double cortex syndrome may have mild retardation and seizures only. The response to treatment varies from individual to individual.

Special concerns

Due to developmental disability, children with lissencephaly who survive beyond the age of two may benefit from special education programs. Various state and federal programs are available to help individuals and their families with meeting these needs.

Resources

BOOKS

Menkes, John H., MD, and Harvey Sarnat, MD, eds. *Childhood Neurology*, 6th edition. Philadelphia: Lippincott Williams & Wilkins, 2000.

"Congenital Anomalies of the Nervous System." *Nelson Textbook of Pediatrics*, 17th edition, edited by Richard E. Behrman, MD, Robert M. Kliegman, MD, and Hal B. Jenson, MD. Philadelphia: Saunders, 2004.

PERIODICALS

Gleeson, J. G. "Neuronal Migration Disorders." *Mental Retardation and Developmental Disabilities Research Reviews* 7 (2001): 167–171.

Guerrini, R., and R. Carrozzo. "Epilepsy and Genetic Malformations of the Cerebral Cortex." *American Journal of Medical Genetics* 106 (2001): 160–173.

Kato, M., and W. B. Dobyns. "Lissencephaly and the Molecular Basis of Neuronal Migration." *Human Molecular Genetics* 12 (2003): R89–R96.

Ross, M. E., and C. A. Walsh. "Human Brain Malformations and Their Lessons for Neuronal Migration." *Annual Review of Neuroscience* 24 (2001): 1041–1070.

WEBSITES

National Institutes of Neurological Disorders and Stroke (NINDS). *Cephalic Disorders Information Page.* (February 19, 2004.) <http://www.ninds.nih.gov/health_and_medical/pubs/cephalic_disorders.htm>.

ORGANIZATIONS

Lissencephaly Network. 10408 Bitterroot Court, Ft. Wayne, IN 46804. (260) 432-4310. LissencephalyOne@aol.com. <http://www.lissencephaly.org>.

March of Dimes Birth Defects Foundation. 1275 Mamaroneck Avenue, White Plains, NY 10605. (914) 428-7100 or (888) MODIMES; Fax: (914) 428-8203. askus@marchofdimes.com. <http://www.marchofdimes.com>.

National Information Center for Children and Youth with Disabilities. P.O. Box 1492, Washington, DC 20013-1492. (202) 884-8200 or (800) 695-0285; Fax: (202) 884-8441. nichcy@aed.org. <http://www.nichcy.org>.

National Institute of Child Health and Human Development (NICHD). Bldg. 31, Rm. 2A32, Bethesda, MD 20892-2425. (301) 496-5133 or (800) 370-2943. NICHDClearinghouse@mail.nih.gov. <http://www.nichd.nih.gov>.

Walsh Lab Web Site. 4 Blackfan Circle, Boston, MA 02115. (617) 667-0813; Fax: (617) 667-0815. cwalsh@bidmc.harvard.edu. <http://walshlab.bidmc.harvard.edu/>.

Peter T. Lin, MD

Locked-in syndrome

Definition

Locked-in syndrome is a condition in which an individual is fully conscious, but all the voluntary muscles of the body are completely paralyzed, with the exception of the muscles controlling eye movement.

Description

Locked-in syndrome is a catastrophic condition that prevents an individual from voluntarily moving any muscles of the body, other than those that control eye movement. As a result, the individual cannot move or speak, although some communication is possible through blinking or eye movements. Despite the devastating loss of function, an individual with locked-in syndrome is completely conscious and aware, able to think and reason normally. Luckily, locked-in syndrome is exceedingly rare.

About 40–70% of people suffering from locked-in syndrome die within a short time of suffering the causative injury.

Causes and symptoms

Locked-in syndrome can occur after severe, catastrophic brain injuries due to massive **stroke**, traumatic head injury, or ruptured aneurysm. Diseases that destroy the myelin sheath around nerves and the toxic effects of medication overdose can also cause locked-in syndrome. The most common cause involves any condition that affects an area of the brain called the ventral pons; all of the nerve tracts responsible for voluntary movement pass through the ventral pons. Areas of the brain responsible for cognition and consciousness are above the level of the ventral pons, and are therefore preserved.

Symptoms include complete inability to control any voluntary muscles in the body, other than those for eye movements and blinking. Reasoning, thinking, consciousness, and awareness are preserved. Normal sleep and wake cycles persist throughout the locked-in state.

Diagnosis

Diagnosis is evident in a conscious individual with no muscle functioning, save for the ability to respond to questions by blinking a certain number of times per the interviewer's directions. Further diagnostic tests will be required to determine the underlying cause of the condition; **CT** or **MRI** scans can reveal the presence of an aneurysm or stroke.

Treatment team

Patients with locked-in syndrome are cared for by critical care specialists, neurologists, and physiatrists. A variety of therapists may also work with such patients, including physical therapists, occupational therapists, speech and language therapists, and psychotherapists.

Treatment

There is no cure for locked-in syndrome. Treatment is supportive.

Recovery and rehabilitation

One of the most important goals of rehabilitation involves finding assistive devices that can help with communication. A technique of stimulating muscle groups with electrodes (called functional neuromuscular stimulation) sometimes can help restore some small degree of functioning; however, even being able to move one finger can greatly improve an individual's ability to communicate or operate assistive devices that could improve that person's level of functioning.

Prognosis

Locked-in syndrome has a very poor prognosis, although some individuals have lived as long as 18 years with the condition.

Special concerns

Ethical dilemmas regarding the treatment and wishes of patients with locked-in syndrome are complicated.

Resources
BOOKS
Hammerstad, John P. "Strength and Reflexes." In *Textbook of Clinical Neurology*, edited by Christopher G. Goetz. Philadelphia: W. B. Saunders Company, 2003.

Simon, Roger P. "Coma and Arousals of Disorder." In *Cecil Textbook of Internal Medicine*, edited by Lee Goldman, et al. Philadelphia: W. B. Saunders Company, 2000.

PERIODICALS
Hayashi, H. "ALS patients on TPPV: totally locked-in state, neurologic findings and ethical implications." *Neurology* 61, no. 1 (July 2003): 135–137.

Rosalyn Carson-DeWitt, MD

Lou Gehrig disease *see* **Amyotrophic lateral sclerosis**

Lumbar radiculopathy *see* **Radiculopathy**

Lupus

Definition

Lupus, also known as lupus erythematosus, is an autoimmune inflammatory disorder that occurs mostly in women.

Description

Lupus produces widely varying symptoms, although joint **pain** is reported by most patients and skin lesions are common. Lupus can cause short periods of symptoms alternating with healthy periods, or can progress into a life-threatening disorder affecting the heart, kidneys, and other organs.

Why the disease is termed lupus is unknown, but it has been known as a distinct disorder and called lupus by European physicians since at least the tenth century A.D. The term erythematosus was first attached to the disease in the 1850s, and it refers to the patchy congestion of skin capillaries with blood (erythema) that often accompanies the disease.

Demographics

Between one million and 1.5 million Americans have some form of lupus. The incidence among women is 10–15 times greater than among men, and it is two to three times more common among African Americans, Hispanics, Asians, and Native Americans than among whites. Lupus most often appears for the first time in women between the ages of 15 and 44. Twenty thousand people die of lupus-related causes in the United States annually.

Causes and symptoms

Lupus is an autoimmune disorder, a disease in which the body's immune system turns against the body itself. In a healthy person, the immune system defends against invading organisms but does not, in general, attack the body's own tissues. The cause of lupus is unknown. However, it is known that lupus has a genetic component, which means a predisposition to lupus can be inherited. Approximately 10% of lupus patients have one or more direct relatives with lupus. (Note that this means that 90% of lupus patients have no such relatives; however, it shows a

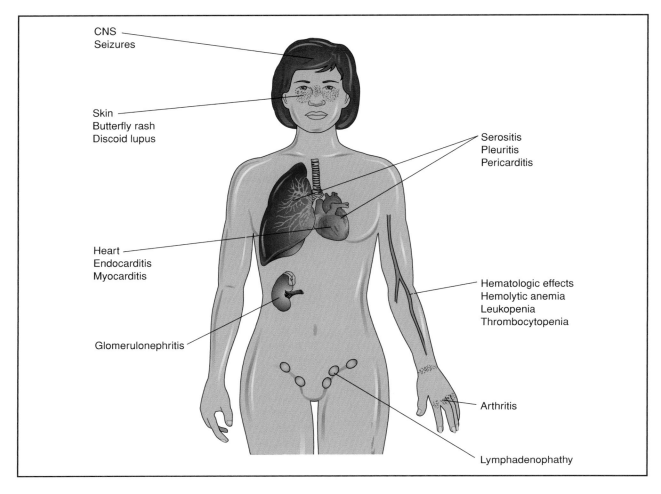

CNS
Seizures

Skin
Butterfly rash
Discoid lupus

Serositis
Pleuritis
Pericarditis

Heart
Endocarditis
Myocarditis

Hematologic effects
Hemolytic anemia
Leukopenia
Thrombocytopenia

Glomerulonephritis

Arthritis

Lymphadenophathy

Systemic lupus erythematosus (SLE) is an autoimmune disease in which the individual's immune system attacks, injures, and destroys the body's own organs and tissues. Nearly every system of the body can be affected by SLE, as depicted in the illustration above. *(Illustration by Electronic Illustrators Group.)*

Key Terms

Autoimmune disorder   A disorder characterized by abnormal functioning of the immune system that causes the body to produce antibodies against its own tissues.

Cutaneous   Relating to the skin.

Erythema   Redness of the skin due to congestion of the capillaries, usually due to injury, infection, or inflammation.

genetic connection because 10% is a much higher figure for familial lupus than can be attributed to chance alone.) Lupus has been definitely linked to genes on chromosome 1 and less certainly to genes on chromosomes 4 and 6.

Given genetic susceptibility, the disease may either develop spontaneously or be triggered by some environmental factor. Environmental factors known to trigger lupus include infections (e.g., Epstein-Barr virus, which infects 99% of children with lupus, but only 70% of healthy children), antibiotics, ultraviolet light (the rays in sunlight or sunlamp-light that causes sunburn), stress, smoking, certain medications, and hormones (especially estrogen, the female sex hormone).

Lupus manifests as a continuum or spectrum of disorders. However, it is common to divide lupus cases into four categories or groups:

• Systemic lupus erythematosus. This is the most serious form of lupus and affects about 70% of all persons with lupus. It is termed systemic because, in this variety of lupus, the body's immune system attacks one or more essential body systems. Targets may include the brain, kidneys, heart, pancreas, or other organs.

• Discoid or cutaneous lupus erythematosus. This variety of lupus is less severe, in that it attacks the skin only. However, it can be disfiguring, often attacking the skin of the face. The term discoid is derived from the round (disc-shaped) lesions that appear on the skin. About 10–15% of lupus patients have cutaneous lupus.

• Drug-induced or drug-related lupus erythematosus. This term refers to lupus that develops after a patient has taken a medication. Medications that can trigger drug-induced lupus include procainamide or hydralazine. Many of the substances that can potentially trigger lupus fall into the class of aromatic amines, or hydrazines. For example, the aromatic amine paraphenylenediamine is present in certain hair dyes and has been associated with lupus or lupus-like syndrome. Tartrazine (a food coloring, FD&C yellow No. 5), which is present in thousands of foods and medications, has also been associated with lupus. Cocaine abuse can induce lupus and several other connective-tissue diseases, as can exposure to certain metals (e.g., mercury). Between 10,000 and 15,000 people are diagnosed with drug-induced lupus annually in the United States.

• Mixed connective tissue disease. Approximately 10% of patients with lupus also have symptoms of one or more additional connective-tissue diseases.

The symptoms of lupus are quite varied. In discoid lupus, red patches (erythema) appear symmetrically on the cheeks, possibly extending to the face, neck, scalp, and other parts of the body. No organ other than the skin is affected (or the disease is classified as systemic, rather than discoid). Systemic lupus may begin suddenly, signaled by fever, or develop slowly over months or years. Chronic **fatigue** is a common symptom. Symptoms related to impairment of any organ may occur. The lupus disease process in a given organ is named after that organ; for example, inflammation of the kidneys is termed lupus nephritis, and inflammation of the brain is termed lupus cerebritis. Kidney involvement may be fatal. Over 50% of all systemic lupus patients in the United States presently have some degree of lupus cerebritis; 25–75% have neuropsychiatric symptoms at some time in their illness. Symptoms of lupus cerebritis may include headaches, **seizures**, **stroke**, psychosis, **dementia**, **peripheral neuropathy**, cerebellar **ataxia** (failure of muscular coordination, usually on one side of the body), **chorea** (jerky, involuntary movements), and others. Duration of **central nervous system** involvement may be transient (as with a migraine **headache**) or long lasting (as with dementia). Stroke incidence is 3–20% in systemic lupus patients, and is highest in the first five years of the disease. Peripheral neuropathy (**carpal tunnel syndrome**, for example) occurs in more than 20% of systemic lupus patients and cranial nerve palsies occur in 10–15%.

Exposure to the ultraviolet rays in sunlight can trigger lupus or, in a person who already has the disease, cause it to flare up. Worsening flare-ups of the disease can be life threatening because they can include inflammation and failure of the kidneys. Also, declining memory and mental sharpness with long-term lupus is common.

Diagnosis

Lupus is notoriously difficult to diagnose. Many cases are not diagnosed until the patient has suffered irreversible kidney damage; for patients who do not have organ-threatening disease, diagnosis takes an average of two years of searching among physicians and conditions. The telltale erythematous skin lumps or rashes that give lupus erythematosus the latter half of its name eventually appear in 90% of systemic lupus patients and all discoid lupus patients, but may not appear early enough in the course of the disease to guarantee timely diagnosis. Additionally, no single lab test can confirm lupus, although certain antibody tests can help to distinguish lupus from other diseases.

Diagnosis of systemic lupus is based on a list of 11 criteria listed by the American College of Rheumatology. If four or more of the 11 criteria are met, a patient is deemed to have systemic lupus. The criteria include discoid or macular rash (often in a classic facial butterfly pattern across the nose and cheeks), photosensitivity, ulcers in the mouth, kidney dysfunction, and the presence of various blood factors such as anti-DNA antibody or anti-nuclear antibody (antibody that targets cell nuclei).

Approximately 15% of diagnoses of lupus may be misdiagnoses of other disorders, including fibromyalgia, seronegative spondyloarthropathies such as ankylosing spondylitis or Reiter's syndrome, autoimmune thyroiditis, and **multiple sclerosis**.

Although diagnosis of lupus cerebritis is particularly difficult, even if a patient has lupus, this does not necessarily mean that the neurological symptoms are due to lupus. Imaging studies cannot necessarily distinguish lupus cerebritis, although **magnetic resonance imaging (MRI)** studies are considered helpful. **Positron emission tomography (PET)** imaging has a high sensitivity to changes in the brain resulting from lupus cerebritis.

Treatment team

As with other neurological diseases in which the spectrum of symptoms varies widely, the treatment team must be designed for each individual case of lupus. A dermatologist will be involved if skin lesions are present; a **neurologist**, if cognitive loss is a possibility; a nephrologist will monitor kidney function; and a rheumatologist is often involved because of the frequency of joint pain. Other specialists will be needed depending on what organ systems are affected.

Treatment

There is no known cure for lupus. However, there are numerous interventions designed to lessen the severity of the disease. These interventions can be classed as pharmacologic (drug-based) or nonpharmacologic.

Pharmacologic interventions (drug therapies)

Five categories of medication are used to treat systemic lupus patients: sunscreens and steroid lotions, nonsteroidal anti-inflammatory drugs (NSAIDs, e.g., acetaminophen or ibuprofen), corticosteroids (e.g., prednisone to suppress the autoimmune response and control inflammation), anti-malarial drugs, and cytotoxic agents (i.e., chemotherapy drugs that are used for cancer, such as methotrexate, azathioprine, and cyclophosphamide).

Cytotoxic agents are used in order to decrease steroid dosage. Anticoagulants (blood thinners) may also be prescribed. For patients with non-organ-threatening disease, the antimalarial drug hydroxychloroquine is often prescribed; prednisone is often prescribed in cases of organ-threatening disease. New lupus drugs are under investigation; with recent increases in knowledge about the genetic and molecular basis of autoimmune disorders, including lupus, pharmacological treatment breakthroughs are possible at any time.

Nonpharmacologic (non-drug) interventions

All persons with lupus should guard against exposure to the sun and use protective clothing, sunscreen, and common sense when going outdoors. Adequate **exercise** can protect against fatigue, obesity, osteoporosis (weakening of the bones), and hyperlipidemia (excessive fats in the blood plasma). In some cases, dietary restrictions may be helpful, including especially the avoidance of food allergens and foods that may trigger lupus symptoms (such as alfalfa seeds). Vitamins, minerals, and dietary fatty acids have been shown to moderate lupus symptoms in some cases. On the other hand, some dietary supplements such as melatonin and Echinacea can worsen symptoms of some autoimmune diseases.

For lupus cerebritis, therapy choices include all the above options for alleviating the disorder throughout the rest of the body. Drug therapy can also include psychotropic medications such as antipsychotics, antidepressants, and **benzodiazepines** to stabilize mood, if this is affected. Unfortunately, long-term use of corticosteroids, one of the mainstays of pharmacological lupus treatment, may itself cause psychiatric symptoms. Experimental investigation of pheresis of cerebrospinal fluid for treatment of lupus cerebritis (cerebrospinal fluid is withdrawn from, filtered, and returned to the patient) was begun in the early 1990s.

Clinical trials

As of mid-2004, approximately 25 lupus-related **clinical trials** were in progress, including investigations of monoclonal antibody therapy, the genetics of lupus, quality-of-life improvement, ultraviolet light therapy, stem-cell transplantation therapy, the mechanisms of kidney and brain damage, and many other aspects of lupus. Updated information on these trials can be found at the National Institutes of Health clinical trials website at <http://www.clinicaltrials.gov> for up-to-date information.

Prognosis

Prognosis for the individual patient depends on the severity of the disease process. Lupus can be fully compatible with a normal lifespan, or can result in fatal organ failure, depending upon the progression of the disorder in each individual.

Before corticosteroids became available, half of all patients with systemic lupus died within two years. Today, half of systemic lupus patients with organ-threatening complications survive for 20 years or longer. However, most systemic lupus patients eventually die from infections or from heart disease complicated by long-term use of corticosteroids.

There is some evidence that lupus may spontaneously resolve in part or whole, or resolve in response to treatment, in some lupus patients who have had the disease long term (i.e., 10 years or more).

Special concerns

Psychological counseling may be helpful, given that a diagnosis of lupus is life altering, and stress and frustration can enhance symptoms while searching for a diagnosis. Genetic counseling may be appropriate, as children of women with lupus have a 10% chance of developing lupus if female and 2% if male, while 20% of offspring overall will develop an autoimmune disorder of some type.

Resources

BOOKS

Phillips, Robert H., et al. *Coping with Lupus: A Practical Guide to Alleviating the Challenges of Systemic Lupus Erythematosus*, 3rd ed. New York: Avery Penguin Putnam, 2001.

Wallace, Daniel J. *The Lupus Book: A Guide for Patients and Their Families*. New York: Oxford Press, 2000.

PERIODICALS

Marshall, Eliot. "Lupus: Mysterious Disease Holds Its Secrets Tight." *Science* (April 26, 2002).

Nickens, Candice. "Treating Systemic Lupus Erythmatosus." *Minority Health Today* (July 1, 2000).

Rushing, Jill D. "Managing Organ-threatening Systemic Lupus Erythematosus." *MedSurg Nursing* (December 1, 2003).

"Systemic Lupus Erythematosus: Guidelines for Control." *Consultant* (February 1, 2000).

OTHER

"NINDS Neurological Sequelae Of Lupus Information Page." *National Institute of Neurological Disorders and Stroke.* April 24, 2004 (June 1, 2004). <http://www.ninds.nih.gov/health_and_medical/disorders/lupus_doc.htm>.

ORGANIZATIONS

Lupus Foundation of America. 2000 L Street, N.W., Suite 710, Washington, DC 20036. (202) 349-1155; Fax: (202) 349-1156. <http://www.lupus.org/>.

Larry Gilman

Lyme disease

Definition

Lyme disease, which is also known as Lyme borreliosis, is an infection transmitted by the bite of deer ticks carrying the spirochete (spiral-shaped bacterium) *Borrelia burgdorferi*. The disease was named for Lyme, Connecticut, the town where it was first diagnosed in 1975 after a puzzling outbreak of juvenile arthritis. The organism that causes the disease was identified in 1982 and named for its discoverer, Willy Burgdorfer.

Description

Lyme disease is classified as a zoonosis, which means that it is a disease of animals that can be transmitted to humans under natural conditions; it cannot be transmitted person-to-person. *B. burgdorferi* is carried by infected deer ticks (more precisely known as black-legged ticks) and passed to humans or household pets when they are bitten by the ticks. In the United States, the white-footed mouse is the usual host of immature (nymphal and larval) ticks, while deer are the most common hosts of the adult ticks. In Europe, sheep are the usual hosts of adult infected ticks. Adult black-legged ticks are hard to detect because of their small size; an adult male tick, for example, is about 0.039 in (1 mm) long. An adult female is slightly larger, about 0.051 in (1.3 mm) long.

Ticks feed on their hosts by piercing the skin and slowly sucking blood through the broken tissue. The spirochete enters the host as the tick fills itself with blood. After the spirochete has been introduced into the person's skin, it may be destroyed by the body's defense mechanisms. If it is not eliminated, it may either remain in the skin or spread throughout the body through the lymphatic system or the bloodstream. *B. burgdorferi* can spread to the heart, joints, or **central nervous system** once it has gained access to the person's circulation. Studies show that *B.*

burgdorferi can penetrate the central nervous system relatively early in the course of the infection without causing any neurologic symptoms. It can also remain in the person's skin for years without causing symptoms.

Lyme disease is a systemic illness, which means that it affects all parts of the body. The most commonly affected areas and organs, however, are the skin, nervous system, heart, joints, and eye. The symptoms of Lyme disease typically emerge in three stages.

It is possible for a person to contract Lyme disease more than once; having the disease does not lead to immunity.

Demographics

The risk of getting Lyme disease depends more on geographical location and the amount of time spent outdoors in tick-infested areas than on age, sex, or race per se, although about 25% of cases in the United States are reported in children younger than 14. Cases of Lyme disease have been reported in 49 of the 50 states; however, 92% of the 17,730 cases reported to the Centers for Disease Control and Prevention (CDC) in 2000 were from only nine states (Connecticut, Rhode Island, New York, Pennsylvania, Delaware, New Jersey, Maryland, Massachusetts, and Wisconsin). The disease is also found in Scandinavia, continental Europe, the countries of the former Soviet Union, Japan, and China; in addition, it is possible that it has spread to Australia.

Lyme disease is seasonal in occurrence. In the United States, humans are most likely to be infected from May through August, when the ticks are most active and people are spending more time outdoors.

The number of cases reported in the United States continues to increase each year; the CDC attributes this increase to the growing size of the deer herd and the geographical spread of infected ticks rather than to improved diagnosis. In addition, some epidemiologists believe that the actual incidence of Lyme disease in the United States may be five to ten times greater than that reported by the CDC. The reasons for this difference include the narrowness of the CDC's case definition as well as frequent misdiagnoses of the disease.

Causes and symptoms

Lyme disease itself is caused by a bacterium known as *Borrelia burgdorferi*, which enters the skin through the bite of an infected tick belonging to the genus *Ixodes*. In Europe, the disease is caused by related species known as *B. afzinii* and *B. garinii*.

Currently, scientists do not completely understand exactly how *B. burgdorferi* produces the variety of symptoms that characterize Lyme disease. Some symptoms are

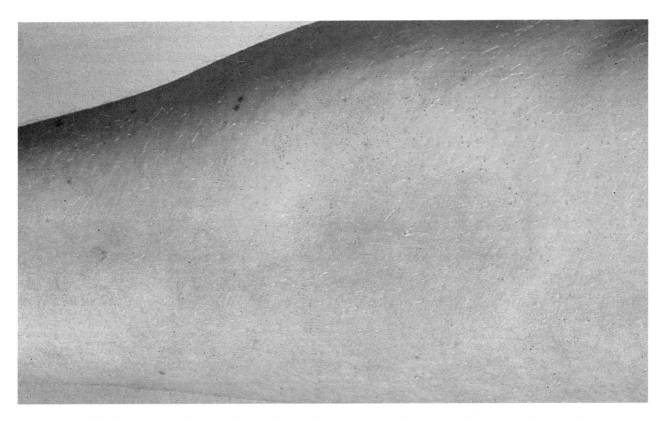

Lyme disease. The image shows the side of a leg at the calf with an insect bite enclosed by a distinctive, slightly raised red ring. The rash is called erythema chronicum migrans. *(© 1993 Science Photo Library. Custom Medical Stock Photo. Reproduced by permission.)*

directly caused by the spirochete, but others may result from the body's immune response to the organism.

The symptoms of Lyme disease are typically divided into three stages: early localized, early disseminated, and late. Neurologic complications are most common in disseminated and late-stage Lyme disease.

EARLY LOCALIZED DISEASE Early symptoms of Lyme disease include low-grade fever and erythema migrans, or EM, a red spot or patch on the skin that is found in about 75% of patients with Lyme disease. The initial spot is usually found on the arms, legs, armpits, or trunk within 3–32 days after the tick bite. Erythema migrans often has a ring-like or "bull's-eye" appearance, with the bite itself in the center of the affected area, surrounded by a ring of reddened and inflamed skin. The ring grows outward around the central lesion, sometimes growing as large as 27 in (70 cm) in diameter. Secondary EM lesions appear in about 20% of patients. The rash does not usually itch or burn, and typically fades in a few weeks even if untreated.

Other symptoms of early-stage Lyme disease include flu-like muscular aches and pains, **headache**, a stiff neck, and **fatigue**. Nausea and vomiting or sore throat occur in some patients, but are less common symptoms.

EARLY DISSEMINATED DISEASE Early disseminated Lyme disease is characterized by ongoing fatigue; arthritis-like pains in the joints; a headache that comes and goes; inflammation of the tendons and their protective sheaths (synovitis); and red or itchy eyes (conjunctivitis). It is common for the aches and pains in muscles and joints to move from one part of the person's body to another. About 8% of people with Lyme disease develop cardiac complications, which may include heart block and inflammation of the walls of the heart (myocarditis).

Neurologic symptoms in early disseminated Lyme disease affect about 15% of people, usually within a few weeks to months after the onset of EM. The following may be the first symptoms in people who did not develop EM, however:

• **Bell's palsy**. This refers to weakness or paralysis of the facial muscles caused by inflammation or swelling of the seventh cranial nerve. People with facial palsy caused by Lyme disease may be affected on both sides of the face.

Key Terms

Babesiosis A disease caused by protozoa of the genus *Babesia* characterized by a malaria-like fever, anemia, vomiting, muscle pain, and enlargement of the spleen. Babesiosis, like Lyme disease, is carried by a tick.

Bell's palsy Facial paralysis or weakness with a sudden onset, caused by swelling or inflammation of the seventh cranial nerve, which controls the facial muscles. Disseminated Lyme disease sometimes causes Bell's palsy.

Cerebrospinal fluid A clear fluid found around the brain and spinal cord and in the ventricles of the brain.

Disseminated Scattered or distributed throughout the body. Lyme disease that has progressed beyond the stage of localized EM is said to be disseminated.

Erythema migrans (EM) A red skin rash that is one of the first signs of Lyme disease in about 75% of patients.

Lyme borreliosis Another name for Lyme disease.

Prophylactic Treatment given to protect against or ward off disease. Many doctors give antibiotics to patients who have been bitten by ticks as a prophylactic measure against Lyme disease.

Radiculoneuropathy Disease of the nerve roots and nerves.

Spirochete A bacterium shaped like a loosely coiled spiral. The organism that causes Lyme disease is a spirochete.

Vector An animal carrier that transfers an infectious organism from one host to another. The vector that transmits Lyme disease from wildlife to humans is the deer tick or black-legged tick.

Zoonosis (plural, zoonoses) Any disease of animals that can be transmitted to humans under natural conditions. Lyme disease and babesiosis are examples of zoonoses.

This symptom may be important in diagnosis, as Bell's palsy caused by other disorders typically affects only one side of the face.

- Radiculoneuropathy. This is the medical term for disease affecting nerves and nerve roots. In Lyme disease, neuropathy often takes the form of abnormal sensations (paresthesias) in the hands or feet.

- Meningoencephalitis. This refers to inflammation of the brain tissue and the protective membranes that cover it (the **meninges**). This complication of Lyme disease often causes sleep disturbances, memory problems, difficulty concentrating, mood swings, headache, **ataxia** (loss of muscular coordination), paresis (mild paralysis), and disturbances in the person's deep tendon reflexes. To test these reflexes, or involuntary responses of certain muscles to a stimulus, the physician gently taps with a small hammer below the person's kneecap, behind the elbow, over the Achilles tendon at the back of the heel, and over the biceps and triceps muscles in the upper arm. The deep tendon reflexes are often weakened or asymmetrical in people with meningoencephalitis related to Lyme disease.

LATE DISEASE The most common symptom of late disseminated Lyme disease is swelling and **pain** in a few large weight-bearing joints, most often the knee. The affected joints are typically much more swollen than painful, but the arthritis may be accompanied by low-grade fever

and fatigue. Lyme-related arthritis develops within weeks to months after the initial eruption of erythema migrans. About 10% of people diagnosed with Lyme disease develop chronic arthritis of the knee.

A late-stage complication of Lyme disease that affects the skin is acrodermatitis chronica atrophicans, a disorder in which the skin on the person's lower legs or hands becomes inflamed and paper-thin. This disorder is seen more frequently in Europe than in the United States.

People with late-stage Lyme disease may develop a neurologic disorder characterized by personality changes and problems with thinking or memory that persist in spite of antibiotic treatment. This syndrome has been called persistent Lyme disease, or PLD. One study of 33 patients diagnosed with PLD found that the most common symptoms were headache (36.4% of patients); memory problems (27.3%); insomnia (33.3%); problems with gait and coordination (36.4%); and impaired deep tendon reflexes (9%). Children with PLD have difficulty getting along with classmates in school as well as making academic progress, and are at increased risk of developing long-term psychiatric disturbances.

Diagnosis

Early diagnosis and prompt treatment are critical to preventing the neurologic complications of Lyme disease.

Patient history and symptoms

The diagnosis of Lyme disease is complicated by the fact that about 25% of patients do not develop the characteristic rash. It is important for the doctor to determine the likelihood of Lyme disease by taking a careful history of exposure to ticks, as only about 25% of patients recall being bitten. In addition to the history, the doctor will examine the patient for the following symptoms:

• Erythema migrans. When present, EM has a characteristic "bull's-eye" pattern. In addition, the bite location is often significant; tick bites are more frequently found in such body folds as the armpits or on areas on the trunk near elastic bands in bra straps or underwear.

• Fever. The fever that accompanies early Lyme disease is usually low; a high fever indicates either concurrent infection with babesiosis or a different diagnosis altogether.

• Absence of digestive or respiratory symptoms.

• Presence of fatigue, headache, and muscle or joint pains.

Laboratory tests

Blood testing is not considered necessary if the patient has EM, a history of exposure to ticks, and other indications of a high likelihood of Lyme disease. Moreover, it is difficult to culture *B. burgdorferi* from human tissues and body fluids. Timing is another important factor in interpreting blood tests for Lyme disease; patients in the early stages of the disease may continue to test negative for several weeks after being infected. Blood testing is, however, recommended for patients with Bell's palsy or myocarditis. The CDC advises doctors to perform a two-step blood test: a screening ELISA test, followed by a Western blot test for confirmation.

Polymerase chain reaction (PCR) testing may not be available in all hospitals, but can be used to detect the DNA of *B. burgdorferi* in fluid drawn from the joints of untreated patients with late-stage symptoms.

Imaging studies

Imaging studies are rarely used to diagnose Lyme disease with the exception of late-stage arthritis. X rays of patients with Lyme-related arthritis usually show considerable swelling of soft tissue; erosion of bone or cartilage also appears in a small minority of these patients.

Treatment team

Patients are usually treated initially by an emergency physician (if they have gone to an emergency room to have the tick removed) or by a primary care physician (PCP).

The PCP may consult a **neurologist**, dermatologist, or infectious disease specialist to confirm the diagnosis or advise about medications, particularly in cases of chronic or late-stage disease.

Treatment

Initial treatment

Immediate removal of an attached tick is the first step in treatment for people who know they have been bitten. Because black-legged ticks are slow feeders, it takes about 36 hours for *B. burgdorferi* to make its way into the body; infection is unlikely if the tick is removed within 24 hours of attachment. People who find ticks on themselves should *not* use a hot match, petroleum jelly, nail polish, or similar items to remove the tick. They should use fine-tipped tweezers, grasp the tick as close to the skin as possible, and pull the tick away from the skin with a steady motion. The area should then be cleansed with an antiseptic.

If the person has been bitten in an area with a high percentage of infected ticks, the doctor will usually prescribe a prophylactic (disease-preventing) course of antibiotics. The usual dosage is 10 days of oral amoxicillin, doxycycline, or cefuroxime, although a study published in 2001 reported that a single 200-mg dose of doxycycline is also effective.

Aspirin or NSAIDs may be given to relieve fever, aching muscles, and other flu-like symptoms of early Lyme disease.

Treatment of disseminated disease and neurologic complications

Patients who have developed heart block as a complication of disseminated Lyme disease may require a temporary pacemaker. Those with swollen knee joints may need to have excess fluid removed by aspiration, a procedure in which the doctor withdraws the fluid through a fine needle.

Patients with Bell's palsy may be given oral antibiotics for 21–30 days. Patients who have neurologic symptoms together with Lyme-related arthritis are usually treated with intravenous ceftriaxone.

Recovery and rehabilitation

Most patients with neurologic complications of Lyme disease recover completely following treatment with antibiotics. Those who do not respond are usually given an additional course of antibiotics. As of 2003, however, treatment recommendations for central nervous system (CNS) complications of Lyme disease are still evolving, and there is ongoing disagreement among specialists regarding the effectiveness of various treatments for PLD.

Clinical trials

As of October 2003, the National Institute of Neurological Disorders and Stroke (NINDS) is recruiting patients for a 24-week treatment study of persistent Lyme disease (PLD). The investigators will be using brain imaging (**MRI** and **PET** scans) to study the effects of intravenous antibiotic treatment on the neurologic symptoms of PLD. Two other trials are recruiting patients with Lyme disease in order to study the immune system's response to the disorder and to evaluate various treatment regimens.

Prognosis

Patients who are treated early with antibiotics and take their medications on schedule should recover completely from Lyme disease. Most long-term effects of the infection result from misdiagnosis or delayed treatment. Co-infection with such other tick-borne diseases as babesiosis and ehrlichiosis may lead to treatment failures or more severe symptoms. The few fatalities reported with Lyme disease occurred in patients who had also contracted babesiosis.

Neurologic symptoms of early disseminated Lyme disease may last for several months but usually resolve completely. Late neurologic complications of Lyme disease, however, may not respond to antibiotic therapy, particularly if diagnosis and treatment were delayed.

Special concerns

A vaccine for Lyme disease known as LYMErix was available from 1998 to 2002, when it was removed from the United States market. The decision was influenced by reports that LYMErix may be responsible for neurologic complications in vaccinated patients. Researchers from Cornell-New York Hospital presented a paper at the annual meeting of the American Neurological Association in October 2002 that identified nine patients with neuropathies linked to vaccination with LYMErix. In April 2003, the National Institute of Allergy and Infectious Diseases (NIAID) awarded a federal grant to researchers at Yale University School of Medicine to develop a new vaccine against Lyme disease.

Resources

BOOKS

"Bacterial Diseases Caused by Spirochetes: Lyme Disease (Lyme Borreliosis)." Section 13, Chapter 157 in *The Merck Manual of Diagnosis and Therapy*, edited by Mark H. Beers, MD, and Robert Berkow, MD. Whitehouse Station, NJ: Merck Research Laboratories, 2002.

PERIODICALS

Adams, H. B., G. A. Blasko, and L. A. DiDomenico. "An Unusual Case of Bilaterally Symmetrical Neuropathic Osteoarthropathy of the Midfoot as a Result of Lyme Disease-Induced Peripheral Neuropathy: A Case Report." *Foot and Ankle International* 23 (February 2002): 155–157.

Coyle, P. K. "Lyme Disease." *Current Neurology and Neuroscience Reports* 2 (November 2002): 479–487.

Edlow, Jonathan A., MD. "Tick-Borne Diseases, Lyme." *eMedicine*, 13 December, 2002 (February 20, 2004). <http://www.emedicine.com/emerg/topic588.htm>.

Gustaw, K., K. Beltowska, and M. M. Studzinska. "Neurological and Psychological Symptoms after the Severe Acute Neuroborreliosis." *Annals of Agricultural and Environmental Medicine* 8 (2001): 91–94.

Tager, F. A., B. A. Fallon, J. Keilp, et al. "A Controlled Study of Cognitive Deficits in Children with Chronic Lyme Disease." *Journal of Neuropsychiatry and Clinical Neurosciences* 13 (Fall 2001): 500–507.

OTHER

National Institute of Neurological Disorders and Stroke (NINDS) Fact Sheet. *Bell's Palsy.* Bethesda, MD: NINDS, 2003.

NINDS Information Page. *Neurological Complications of Lyme Disease.* Bethesda, MD: NINDS, 2003.

WEBSITES

Centers for Disease Control and Prevention, Division of Vector-Borne Infectious Diseases. *CDC Lyme Disease Home Page.* (February 20, 2004.) <http://www.cdc.gov/ncidod/dvbid/lyme/>.

ORGANIZATIONS

Centers for Disease Control and Prevention (CDC). 1600 Clifton Road, NE, Atlanta, GA 30333. (800) 311-3435. inquiry@cdc.gov. <http://www.cdc.gov>.

Lyme Disease Foundation. One Financial Plaza, Hartford, CT 06103. (860) 525-2000 or (860) 525-TICK or (800) 886-LYME. lymefnd@aol.com. <http://www.lyme.org>.

National Institute of Allergy and Infectious Diseases (NIAID). 31 Center Drive, Room 7A50 MSC 2520, Bethesda, MD 20892. (301) 496-5717. <http://www.niaid.nih.gov>.

NIH Neurological Institute. P. O. Box 5801, Bethesda, MD 20824. (301) 496-5751 or (800) 352-9424. <http://www.ninds.nih.gov>.

Rebecca J. Frey, PhD

For Reference

Not to be taken from this room

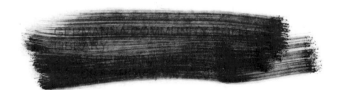